GERIATRIC PALLIATIVE CARE

GERIATRIC PALLIATIVE CARE

A Practical Guide for Clinicians

EDITED BY:

EMILY CHAI, MD
Associate Professor, Geriatrics and Palliative Medicine
Icahn School of Medicine at Mount Sinai
New York, New York

DIANE MEIER, MD, FACP
Professor, Geriatrics and Palliative Medicine
Icahn School of Medicine at Mount Sinai
New York, New York

JANE MORRIS, MS, RN, ACHPN
Clinical Coordinator, Palliative Care
New York Hospital
Queens, New York

SUZANNE GOLDHIRSCH, MA, MsED
Program Coordinator, Geriatrics and Palliative Medicine
Icahn School of Medicine at Mount Sinai
New York, New York

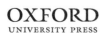
OXFORD
UNIVERSITY PRESS

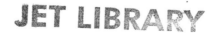

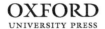

Oxford University Press is a department of the University of Oxford.
It furthers the University's objective of excellence in research, scholarship,
and education by publishing worldwide.

Oxford   New York
Auckland   Cape Town   Dar es Salaam   Hong Kong   Karachi
Kuala Lumpur   Madrid   Melbourne   Mexico City   Nairobi
New Delhi   Shanghai   Taipei   Toronto

With offices in
Argentina   Austria   Brazil   Chile   Czech Republic   France   Greece
Guatemala   Hungary   Italy   Japan   Poland   Portugal   Singapore
South Korea   Switzerland   Thailand   Turkey   Ukraine   Vietnam

Oxford is a registered trademark of Oxford University Press
in the UK and certain other countries.

Published in the United States of America by
Oxford University Press
198 Madison Avenue, New York, NY 10016

Library of Congress Cataloging-in-Publication Data
Geriatric palliative care : a practical guide for clinicians / edited by Emily Chai ... [et al.].
p. ; cm.
Includes bibliographical references and index.
ISBN 978-0-19-538931-9 (alk. paper) — ISBN 978-0-19-987489-7 (alk. paper)
I. Chai, Emily.
[DNLM: 1. Palliative Care.   2. Aged.   3. Hospice Care.   4. Patient Care Team. WB 310]
616.02'9—dc23
2012046220

9 8 7 6 5 4 3 2 1
Printed in the United States of America
on acid-free paper

This book is dedicated to the late Dr. Robert Butler, pioneer in the field of Geriatrics, founding Chair of our Department, and early advocate of palliative care.

Emily Chai
Diane Meier
Jane Morris
Suzanne Goldhirsch

CONTENTS

SECTION V: *Diseases and Syndromes*

SECTION VI: *The Interdisciplinary Team*

PREFACE

This clinical guide to geriatric palliative care is being published at a time of robust national debate over how to improve the US health care delivery system, especially for older patients with multiple chronic and serious conditions. The complexity of this patient population, and the fact that they are typically going to live for years with these chronic conditions, poses a challenge for our health care providers. Training in geriatric and palliative medicine is going to be critically important if these patients—and their family members—are to receive high-quality care that meets their needs and helps them avoid unnecessary trips back and forth to the emergency room and hospital. The demand for expertise in the complex needs of the frail, functionally and cognitively impaired, and those with one or more serious illnesses far outstrips the capacity of the e trained workforce-hence the reason for this practical guide for all clinicians who serve this patient population. In this volume, we aim to integrate the core principles and practices of these two related and complementary specialties in a clear, user-friendly format to assist physicians, nurses, social workers and other disciplines who want to offer comprehensive person-centered care for older persons and their families.

What does person-centered geriatric palliative care look like? What are the hallmarks which distinguish it from other clinical approaches? Perhaps the defining characteristic is that person-centered care matches treatment to informed patient and family priorities, their goals and preferences.

Other key geriatric palliative care themes that clinicians will find woven through the pages of this volume include a commitment to expert communication skills allowing clinicians to understand what is most important to our patients and their families in the context of the medical realities, and then developing a care plan that honors these priorities; evidence-based practice; recognition of the necessity of the interdisciplinary team approach for quality of care for complex populations; support for integrated co-management from both disease-specific specialists (such as cardiologists) and clinicians with a "whole-person" quality of life focus (such as primary care providers); and attention to the meticulous management of pain and other distressing physical and psychological symptoms that steal the will to live and stand in the way of an acceptable quality of life.

Patients and families will benefit when we deliver this care, and so will we, because our satisfaction lies in the genuine human connection with the patients we are privileged to serve.

"The reward is to be found in that personal bond which forms the greatest satisfaction of the practice of medicine. One of the essential qualities of the clinician is interest in humanity, for the secret of the care of the patient is caring for the patient."

Francis Peabody, Harvard University 1921 (cite Peabody F. The care of the patient. JAMA 88: 877–882, 1927)

CONTRIBUTORS

Robert Aiken, MD

Department of Neuroscience
Division of Neurological Oncology
Rush University Medical Center
Chicago, IL

Melissa D. Aldridge, PhD, MBA

Brookdale Department of Geriatrics and
    Palliative Medicine
Icahn School of Medicine at Mount Sinai
New York, NY

Shahla Baharlou, MD

Brookdale Department of Geriatrics and
    Palliative Medicine
Icahn School of Medicine at Mount Sinai
New York, NY

Ana Blohm, MD

Division of General Internal Medicine
Mount Sinai Hospital
New York, NY

Patricia A. Bloom, MD

Brookdale Department of Geriatrics and
    Palliative Medicine
Icahn School of Medicine at Mount Sinai
New York, NY

Sara M. Bradley, MD

Brookdale Department of Geriatrics and
    Palliative Medicine
Icahn School of Medicine at Mount Sinai
New York, NY

Tracy Breen, MD

Long Island Jewish Medical Center
New Hyde Park, NY

Mark E. Burnett, MD

Department of Dermatology
Icahn School of Medicine at Mount Sinai
New York, NY

Gina Caliendo, BS, Pharm.D, BCPS

Department of Pharmacy
Icahn School of Medicine at Mount Sinai
New York, NY

Eileen H. Callahan, MD

Brookdale Department of Geriatrics and
    Palliative Medicine
Icahn School of Medicine at Mount Sinai
New York, NY

Kathryn E. Callahan, MD

Department of Internal Medicine
Section on Gerontology and Geriatric Medicine
Wake Forest School of Medicine
Winston Salem, North Carolina

Patrick Chae, MD

Department of Medicine
Division of Pulmonary, Critical Care, and Sleep
    Medicine
Icahn School of Medicine at Mount Sinai
New York, NY

Christine Chang, MD

Brookdale Department of Geriatrics and
    Palliative Medicine
Icahn School of Medicine at Mount Sinai
New York, NY

Peter K. Chang, MD

Department of Medicine
Division of Gastroenterology
Icahn School of Medicine at Mount Sinai
New York, NY

Sita Chokhavatia, MD

Department of Medicine
Division of Gastroenterology
Icahn School of Medicine at Mount Sinai
New York, NY

Audrey Chun

Brookdale Department of Geriatrics and
    Palliative Medicine
Icahn School of Medicine at Mount Sinai
New York, NY

Candace Coggins, RN-C, ACHPN, APRN-BC

Allergy and Immunology of Hilton Head
Hilton Head, NC

Susan E. Cohen, MD

New York University School of Medicine
Palliative Care Program
Bellevue Hospital Center
New York, NY

Jessica Cook-Mack, MD

Visiting Doctors Program
Brookdale Department of Geriatrics and
    Palliative Medicine
Icahn School of Medicine at Mount Sinai
New York, NY

Bruce Darrow, MD, PhD

Department of Medicine
Division of Cardiology
Icahn School of Medicine at Mount Sinai
New York, NY

Linda V. DeCherrie, MD

Brookdale Department of Geriatrics and
    Palliative Medicine
Icahn School of Medicine at Mount Sinai
New York, NY

Yasmin deLeon-Kraus, MS, ANP-C

Martha Stewart Center for Living
Mount Sinai Hospital
New York, NY

Anca Dinescu, MD

Department of Internal Medicine
George Washington University
Washington, DC

Leslie Dubin Kerr, MD

Departments of Medicine and Geriatrics
Icahn School of Medicine at Mount Sinai
New York, NY

Jennifer Egert, PhD

Department of Family and Social Medicine
Montefiore Medical Center
Bronx, NY

J.D. Elder, MA, LMT

Hertzberg Palliative Care Institute
Brookdale Department of Geriatrics and
    Palliative Medicine
Icahn School of Medicine at Mount Sinai
New York, NY

Helen Fernandez, MD

Brookdale Department of Geriatrics and
    Palliative Medicine
Icahn School of Medicine at Mount Sinai
New York, NY

Beverly A. Forsyth, MD

Department of Medicine
Department of Medical Education
Icahn School of Medicine at Mount Sinai
New York, NY

Amy Frieman, MD

Jersey Shore University Hospital
Neptune, NJ

Rebecca B. Fuller, MS, APRN- BC, ACHPN

The George Washington University School of
    Nursing
Washington, DC

**Marianne P. Wientzen Gelber, MSN,
GNP, ACHPN**

Hertzberg Palliative Care Institute
Brookdale Department of Geriatrics and
    Palliative Medicine
Icahn School of Medicine at Mount Sinai
New York, NY

Gabrielle Goldberg, MD

Hertzberg Palliative Care Institute
Brookdale Department of Geriatric and Palliative
    Medicine
Icahn School of Medicine at Mount Sinai
New York, NY

Leanne Goldberg, MS, SLP-CCC

Department of Rehabilitation Medicine
Icahn School of Medicine at Mount Sinai
New York, NY

Nathan Goldstein, MD

Hertzberg Palliative Care Institute
Brookdale Department of Geriatrics and
    Palliative Medicine
Icahn School of Medicine at Mount Sinai
New York, NY

Carl Grey, MD

Department of Medicine
West Virginia University Health Sciences Center
Morgantown, West Virginia

Cameron R. Hernandez, MD

Visiting Doctors Program
Brookdale Department of Geriatrics and
    Palliative Medicine
Icahn School of Medicine at Mount Sinai
New York, NY

Jay R. Horton, PhD, ACHPN, FNP-BC, MPH

Hertzberg Palliative Care Institute
Brookdale Department of Geriatrics and
    Palliative Medicine
Icahn School of Medicine at Mount Sinai
New York, NY

Sharon Houlihan, LMT

Swedish Institute
New York, NY

William W. Hung, MD, MPH

James J. Peters VA Medical Center
Icahn School of Medicine at Mount Sinai
New York, NY

Shirish Huprikar, MD

Department of Medicine
Icahn School of Medicine at Mount Sinai
New York, NY

Serge Khaitov, MD

Department of Surgery
Division of Colorectal Surgery
Icahn School of Medicine at Mount Sinai
New York, NY

Amit Khanna, MD, MPH

Department of Colorectal Surgery
Temple University School of Medicine
Philadelphia, PA

Jane Knowles, MPH, LCSW

Department of Social Work
Mount Sinai Hospital
New York, NY

Beatriz Korc-Grodzicki, MD, PhD

Department of Medicine
Geriatrics Service
Memorial Sloan-Kettering Cancer Center
New York, NY

Stephen Krieger, MD

Department of Neurology
Icahn School of Medicine at Mount Sinai
New York, NY

Jacob Levitt, MD, FAAD

Department of Dermatology
Icahn School of Medicine at Mount Sinai
New York, NY

Betty Lim, MD

Brookdale Hertzberg Palliative Care Institute
Department of Geriatrics and
    Palliative Medicine
Icahn School of Medicine at Mount Sinai
New York, NY

Hannah I. Lipman, MD, MS

Department of Medicine
Divisions of Geriatrics and Cardiology
Montefiore Medical Center
Bronx, NY

Evgenia Litrivis, MD

Hertzberg Palliative Care Institute
Brookdale Department of Geriatrics and
    Palliative Medicine
Icahn School of Medicine at Mount Sinai
New York, NY

Anna Loengard, MD

St. Francis Healthcare System of Hawaii
Honolulu, HI

Adriana Malone, MD

Department of Medicine
Division of Hematology and Medical
    Oncology
Icahn School of Medicine at Mount Sinai
New York, NY

Arlene Manso Witt, MA, LCAT, MT-BC

NHS Human Services
Philadelphia, Pennsylvania

Susan McHugh-Salera, NP

Lawrence Hospital Center
Bronxville, NY

Devandra Mehta, MD, PhD

Department of Medicine
Division of Cardiology
Icahn School of Medicine at Mount Sinai
New York, NY

Rabbi Edith M. Meyerson, DMin, BCC

Hertzberg Palliative Care Institute
Brookdale Department of Geriatrics and
    Palliative Medicine
Icahn School of Medicine at Mount Sinai
New York, NY

Denise Mohess, MBBS

Center for Geriatric Medicine
Providence Hospital
Washington DC
George Washington University School of
    Medicine
Washington, DC

Sonni Mun, MD

Director, Inpatient Hospice Unit
Bellevue Medical Center
New York, NY

Florida Olivieri, MD

Brookdale Department of Geriatrics and
    Palliative Medicine
Icahn School of Medicine at Mount Sinai
New York, NY

Lynn B. O'Neill, MD

Department of Medicine
Division of Geriatrics
Duke University School of Medicine
Durham, North Carolina

Arik Olson, MD

Visiting Nurse Service of New York
New York, NY

Cynthia X. Pan, MD

Division of Geriatrics and Palliative Care
    Medicine
New York Hospital Queens
Flushing, New York

Stacie T. Pinderhughes, MD

Palliative Medicine Program
Banner Good Samaritan Medical Center
Phoenix, Arizona

Debra Ann Pollack, MD

Director, Sleep Medicine
Center for Comprehensive Care
Shelton, CT

Dennis M. Popeo, MD

Department of Psychiatry
Bellevue Hospital Center
New York University School of Medicine
New York, NY

Meenakshi Mehrotra Rana, MD

Department of Medicine
Division of Infectious Diseases
Icahn School of Medicine at Mount Sinai
New York, NY

Lisa Rho, MD

Department of Medicine
Division of Pulmonary, Critical Care and
    Sleep Medicine
Icahn School of Medicine at Mount Sinai
New York, NY

Nisha Rughwani, MD

Brookdale Department of Geriatrics and
    Palliative Medicine
Icahn School of Medicine at Mount Sinai
New York, NY

Skandan Shanmugan, MD

Division of Colon and Rectal Surgery
Perelman School of Medicine
University of Pennsylvania
Philadelphia, PA

Joanna Sheinfeld, MD

Departments of Medicine
Brookdale Department of Geriatrics and
    Palliative Medicine
Icahn School of Medicine at Mount Sinai
New York, NY

Parag Sheth, MD

Department of Rehabilitation Medicine
Icahn School of Medicine at Mount Sinai
New York, NY

Jennifer Shin, MD

Department of Medicine
Division of Hematology and Oncology
Massachusetts General Hospital
Boston, MA

David Skovran, BSN, ANP-BC

Visiting Doctor's Program
Mount Sinai Hospital
New York, NY

Cardinale B. Smith, MD, MSCR

Department of Medicine
Hematology and Medical Oncology
Brookdale Department of Geriatrics and
    Palliative Medicine
Icahn School of Medicine at Mount Sinai
New York, NY

Earl L. Smith, MD, PhD

Department of Medicine
Icahn School of Medicine at Mount Sinai
Elmhurst Hospital Center
Elmhurst, NY

Lorie N. Smith, MD

Department of Palliative Care
Massachusetts General Hospital
Boston, MA

Rainier Soriano, MD

Brookdale Department of Geriatrics and
    Palliative Medicine
Department of Medical Education
Icahn School of Medicine at Mount Sinai
New York, NY

Theresa Soriano, MD, MPH

Department of Medicine
Brookdale Department of Geriatrics and
    Palliative Medicine
Icahn School of Medicine at Mount Sinai
New York, NY

Harry Spiera, MD

Division of Rheumatology
Department of Medicine
Icahn School of Medicine at Mount Sinai
New York, NY

Ruth Spinner, MD

Brookdale Department of Geriatrics and
    Palliative Medicine
Icahn School of Medicine at Mount Sinai
New York, NY

Carol Stangby, LCSW

Visiting Nurse Service of New York Hospice
New York, NY

Susan Sturgess, MS

Hospice Care Network
Woodbury, NY

Mahesh Swaminathan, MD

Department of Medicine
Division of Infectious Disease
Icahn School of Medicine at Mount Sinai
New York, NY

Mark A. Swidler, MD

Department of Medicine
Division of Nephrology Brookdale
Brookdale Department of Geriatrics and
    Palliative Medicine
Icahn School of Medicine at Mount Sinai
New York, NY

Winona Tse, MD

Department of Neurology
Icahn School of Medicine at Mount Sinai
New York, NY

Sarina Van der Zee, MD

Pacific Heart Institute
Santa Monica, CA

Michal Sarah Wall, MD
Internal Medicine Physician
West Palm Beach, FLA

Daniel E. Wollman MD, PhD
Medical Director, Palliative Care
St. Vincent's Medical Center
Bridgeport, CT

Herrick H. Wun, MD
Department of Surgery
Weill Cornell Medical College
New York Downtown Hospital
New York, NY

Svetlana Zhovtis, MD
New York University Langone Medical Center
New York, NY

SECTION I

Overview

1

Geriatric Palliative Care

INTRODUCTION

The median age at death in the United States is 78.5 years, associated with a steady and linear decline in age-adjusted death rates since 1940. While in 1900 life expectancy at birth was less than 50 years, a girl born in 2012 may expect to live to age 81 and a boy to age 76. Life expectancy is currently projected to increase to 86 years for women and 79 years for men.[1,2]

The result of these changes in demographics has been an enormous growth in the number and increased longevity of elderly Americans, so that by the year 2030, 20% of the U.S. population will be over age 65, as compared to fewer than 5% in the early 1900's.

HOW WE DIE

- While death a century ago typically followed an acute infectious illness, today the leading causes of death are chronic diseases such as heart disease, cancer, and stroke. Advances in treatment of atherosclerotic vascular disease and cancer have turned these previously rapidly fatal diseases into chronic illnesses that people often live with for many years before death.
- The location of death in the US has also shifted. Deaths that occurred at home in the early part of the 20th century now occur primarily in institutions (39% in hospitals and 24% in nursing homes). The reasons for this shift in location of care prior to death are complex but are related to financial incentives[3] and to the care burdens of chronic illness and functional dependency that typically accompany life-threatening disease in the elderly. The older the patient, the higher the likelihood of death in a nursing home or hospital, with an estimated 58% of persons over 85 spending at least some time in a nursing home in the last year of life.[4]

THE EXPERIENCE OF SERIOUS ILLNESS FOR OLDER ADULTS

- In the United States, the overwhelming majority of people who suffer from serious illness are elderly. They typically die of chronic diseases, over long periods of time, with multiple coexisting problems, progressive dependency on others, and heavy care needs met mostly by family members. They spend the majority of their final years at home but, in most parts of the country, most die in hospitals or nursing homes, surrounded by medical technology and a phalanx of specialist physicians who believe there is nothing else that they can offer.
- In institutional settings, deaths become protracted and negotiated processes, with health care providers and family members making difficult, often wrenching, decisions about the use or discontinuation of life-prolonging technologies, such as feeding tubes, ventilators, and intravenous fluids.
- Although illness occurs far more commonly in the elderly than in any other age group, most research on the experience has been done in younger populations, and relatively little is known about the experience of serious illness and death in the oldest old, those over age 75. There are data, however, suggesting that the last years of life for elderly persons are often characterized by significant physical distress that is neither identified nor properly treated. For example, studies have shown consistently high levels of untreated or undertreated pain in the elderly. In one study of elderly cancer patients in nursing homes, 26% of patients with daily pain received no analgesics, and 16% received only acetaminophen, a percentage that rose with increasing age and minority status.[5] Other

studies, comparing pain management in cognitively intact versus demented elderly with acute hip fracture, found high rates of undertreatment of pain in both groups, a phenomenon that worsened with increasing age and cognitive impairment.[6,7]

IMPACT OF SERIOUS ILLNESS ON PATIENTS AND FAMILIES

- Aside from pain and other sources of physical distress, the key characteristic that distinguishes serious illness in the elderly from that experienced by younger groups is the nearly universal occurrence of long periods of functional dependency and need for family caregivers in the last months to years of life. Unlike in younger adults, for whom one disease is often the sole cause of death, death in older adults typically results from one or more major acute illnesses superimposed on multiple comorbidities (e.g., diabetes, hypertension, osteoarthritis, gait disturbances), age-related changes in organ physiology (e.g., decreased glomerular filtration rate), and progressive functional decline.
- A survey by the National Alliance for Caregiving and AARP found that 21% of people over 18 in the United States were caregivers, representing 44.4 million people.[8] The annual cost to U.S. businesses of productivity losses associated with intense caregiving by full-time employees is estimated to be over $17 billion.[9] Most family caregiving is provided by women (spouses, adult daughters, and daughters-in-law), placing significant strains on the physical, emotional, and socioeconomic status of the caregivers.[10] More than 87% of caregivers say they need more help with transportation (62%), homemaking (55%), nursing (28%), and personal care (26%) for the patient. Caregiving in itself is a risk factor for death, major depression, and associated comorbidities.[11]
- Those patients who are ill and dependent and have no family caregivers, or those whose caregivers can no longer provide or afford needed services, are placed in nursing homes, where 20% of the over age 85 population resides.[12,13]

(See Chapter 4: Special Issues in Caregiving, and Chapter 23: Caregiving.)

GERIATRIC PALLIATIVE CARE

- Geriatrics is the medical specialty that focuses the diagnosis and treatment of diseases and problems specific to older adults. Recognizing the complex interaction of medical, social, economic, and mental health issues that may impact their patients, geriatricians proactively emphasize disease prevention and improvement in function, not just treatment of acute illness or injury.
- Palliative care provides specialized medical care for people with serious illness. It focuses on providing patients with relief from the symptoms, pain, and stress of a serious illness, whatever the diagnosis may be. The goal is to improve quality of life for both the patient and the family. Palliative care is provided by a team of doctors, nurses, and other specialists who work with a patient's other doctors to provide an extra layer of support. It is appropriate at any age and at any stage of a serious illness, and can be provided together with curative treatment.
- Geriatric palliative care integrates these two related and complementary specialties to provide sophisticated and comprehensive management for older patients entering the later stage of their lives, and their families. The core principles and practices of geriatric palliative care, which are outlined in this volume, will aid physicians, nurses, social workers, and other disciplines as they accompany patients and their families through one of the most important and most challenging stages of late life. (See Chapter 2: Principles of Geriatric Palliative Care.)

WHEN IS GERIATRIC PALLIATIVE CARE APPROPRIATE FOR OLDER ADULTS?

- The palliative approach to patient care differs not in kind but in emphasis for the geriatric patient. As with younger patients, meticulous attention is given to symptom distress and the management of side effects. Repeated discussions are held about the changing goals of medical care as the disease progresses, and support for family caregivers is a priority. The differences are related to the lengthy duration of most geriatric chronic illnesses, the high prevalence of long-term functional and cognitive impairment in this patient population, and the stressful burden of the associated long-term caregiver role.

- Indications for geriatric palliative care include:

    1. **Geriatric syndromes:** Markers for initiation of palliative care in the elderly are most appropriately centered on the identification and amelioration of functional and cognitive impairment, development of frailty, dependency on family caregivers, and burden of symptom distress, rather than identification of a specific and advanced terminal illness or signs of poor prognosis or imminent death, as is typical in advanced cancer and in traditional hospice settings (Box 1.1).

    2. **Presence of symptom distress:** Whether or not it is secondary to a discrete terminal illness, symptom distress should prompt a comprehensive assessment and plan of treatment (Box 1.1). When the time remaining is short (measured in months or years, not in decades), the quality of each of those days becomes proportionately more important, and

the priority accorded to the goal of improving quality of life should increase accordingly.

    3. **Stage of disease:** While palliative care will prioritize different goals depending upon the needs and aims of each individual patient and family, the stage of a chronic illness helps determine the range and intensity of appropriate palliative care interventions (Table 1.1). (See Chapter 7: Prognostication.)

        - In the early stages of a 10-year-long dementing illness, for example, appropriate palliative interventions might include early attention to advance care planning; discussion about the preferred goals of care during later stages of illness and appointment of a health care proxy; financial planning; attention to other important tasks that need to be completed while cognition allows; disease-modifying therapies; and education, support, and counsel for family caregivers. (See Chapter 67: Dementia.)

        - In the middle stages of dementia, when progressive functional dependency, behavioral and physical symptoms, and increasing family burden and distress become prominent, palliative care should focus on meticulous assessment

---

BOX 1.1   MARKERS FOR INITIATION OF PALLIATIVE CARE IN GERIATRICS

Disease-independent markers	Frailty
	Functional dependency
	Cognitive impairment
	Symptom distress
	Family support needs
Disease-specific markers	Symptomatic congestive heart failure
	Chronic lung disease
	Dementia
	Stroke
	Cancer
	Recurrent infection
	Degenerative joint disease causing functional impairment and chronic pain

TABLE 1.1: STAGING OF GERIATRIC PALLIATIVE CARE DURING THE COURSE OF A CHRONIC ILLNESS

	Early	Middle	Late
Goals of care	Discuss diagnosis, prognosis, what to expect	Review understanding of diagnoses/prognosis	Communicate Assess understanding of diagnosis, disease course, prognosis
	Discuss and offer disease-modifying therapies if appropriate	Review efficacy and benefit/ burden of disease-modifying treatment	Review appropriateness of disease-modifying treatments
	Discuss patient-centered goals, hopes, and expectations from medical treatment	Reassess goals of care and expectations; prepare patient/family for shift in goals	Review goals of care and recommend appropriate shifts in the context of advanced disease
			Explicitly plan for a peaceful death
		Encourage completion of important tasks, relationships, financial affairs	Encourage completion of important tasks, relationships, financial affairs
Advance care planning	Advance care planning Appoint health care proxy	Review current preferences for care, concordance of treatment with wishes, and understanding of proxy role	Review for accuracy For patient without decisional capacity, ensure alignment of treatment decisions with patient's previously stated wishes
Financial planning	Advise financial planning and consultation about estate planning, long-term care options and insurance	Reassess adequacy of financial planning for medical, home care, prescription, long-term care and family support needs	Review financial resources and needs Inform patient and family of financial options for home care and long-term care (hospice, Medicaid) if resources are inadequate for patient/family needs
		Consider hospice referral	Explicitly recommend hospice and review advantages to patient and family
Symptom management	Formal symptom assessment using validated instruments	Formal symptom assessment using validated instruments	Formal symptom assessment using validated instruments
	Treat identified symptoms Manage side effects Reassess and adjust medications if necessary	Treat identified symptoms Manage side effects Reassess, and adjust medications if necessary	Treat identified symptoms, Manage side effects Reassess and adjust medications if necessary
Functional dependency and rehabilitation	Formal assessment of functional impairments and ADL and IADL needs	Review functional impairments and benefit-burden of interventions aimed at improved functional capacity	Utilize interventions to promote comfort, sense of control, ease of care for family
	Seek rehab evaluation, and home safety assessment Issues include: conditioning exercises, support for I/ADLs, reducing fall risk, option for gait assist devices		Reassess equipment needs, safe transfers, and positioning for purposes of comfort

(continued)

TABLE 1.1: (CONTINUED)

	Early	Middle	Late
Comorbid disease management	Manage comorbid illness Review drug interactions Seek close coordination with other specialists	Review benefit/burden of comorbid disease management in terms of impact on quality and length of life	Evaluate comorbid disease management in terms of contribution to quality of life discontinue treatments no longer of benefit
Family support	Inform patient and family about support groups; Ask about practical support needs (transportation, prescription drug coverage, respite care, personal care) Listen	Encourage support/ counseling for family caregivers Screen family caregivers for practical resource needs, stress, depression, adequacy of medical care Identify respite and practical support resources Recommend help from family/friends Introduce possibility of hospice and review its benefits	Encourage out of town family to visit; Refer to disease-specific support groups and counseling programs and bereavement support groups for family caregivers, Routinely inquire about caregiver health, well-being, practical needs; Offer respite care alternatives After death, send bereavement card, and call after 1–2 weeks Screen for high-risk bereavement Maintain occasional contact after patient's death
Spiritual care	Assess need for spiritual counseling and support	Inquire about spiritual support and current engagement with religious community; Refer as appropriate	Ask if referral to clergy or other spiritual support resources would be helpful for patient or family, especially in last days of life

and treatment of symptom distress, practical and psychosocial support for families, and explicit planning for expected long-term care needs. (See Chapter 33: Behavioral Disorders in Dementia, and Chapter 4: Special Issues in Caregiving.)

- In the advanced stages of dementia, the primary goals are: the patient's physical and emotional comfort; helping families decide about the benefits and burdens of life-sustaining treatments such as tube feeding; helping families decide when and if placement in a nursing home is necessary and appropriate; attention to the family's anticipatory grief and bereavement associated with advanced stage illness; planning for a peaceful and controlled death; and

appropriate support and counseling during the bereavement process. (See Chapter 27: Artificial Nutrition and Hydration, Chapter 15: Dying at Home, and Chapter 20: Bereavement.)

THE SIMULTANEOUS PALLIATIVE AND LIFE-PROLONGING CARE MODEL

- For the vast majority of older patients living with chronic illness, both life-prolonging and palliative treatments are necessary and appropriate. The artificial distinction and forced choice between hospice and "curative" care that is required by the Medicare Hospice Benefit only results in inappropriate, burdensome, and costly life-prolonging treatments long after the time that they are beneficial to the patient.

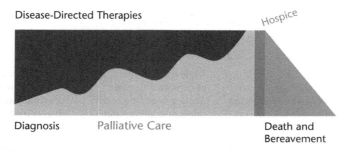

FIGURE 1.1: Model of palliative and disease-directed therapies.

It also frequently causes a great deal of preventable suffering during all stages of a serious illness. (See Chapter 5: Financing Palliative Care and Hospice, and Chapter 13: Health Insurance.)

• The model of care that makes more sense for older adults with serious illness is a simultaneous model of palliative care delivered at the same time as disease-directed and life-prolonging treatments, with the ratio and nature of these treatments varying in response to patient needs and preferences. (See Chapter 12: The Hospice Model of Palliative Care.) This integrated and simultaneous model of palliative and disease-directed therapies is illustrated in Figure 1.1.

• Late in the course of any serious illness, when the burden of continued life-prolonging treatments outweighs their benefit, the goals of care may shift to a predominant and eventually exclusive focus on ensuring comfort for the patient, and practical and emotional support for family caregivers. A patient who has been receiving excellent palliative care along with life-prolonging measures will make the transition to hospice far more easily because the change in type of care will be a gradual change in emphasis over time rather than an abrupt shift in kind of care, and the transition will be driven by the patient's needs, and not by the rigid and inflexible demands of the payment system.

TAKE-HOME POINTS

• For older adults, serious illness is frequently characterized by a high prevalence of untreated pain and other symptoms due to chronic conditions, associated with progressive functional dependency,

unpredictable disease course, and extensive family caregiver needs.

• Geriatric palliative care integrates two related and complementary specialties to provide sophisticated and comprehensive interdisciplinary management for older patients entering the later stage of their lives and for their families. The focus on disease prevention and maximizing function and quality of life provides patients with relief from the symptoms, pain and stress of a serious illness, whatever the diagnosis may be.

• For the vast majority of older patients living with chronic illness, both life-prolonging and palliative treatments are necessary and appropriate. The rigid distinction between hospice and "curative" care results in inappropriate, burdensome, and costly life-prolonging treatments long after the time that they are beneficial to the patient, causing a great deal of preventable suffering during all stages of a serious illness.

• The model of palliative care that makes more sense is a simultaneous model of palliative care delivered at the same time as disease-modifying and life-prolonging treatments, with the ratio and nature of these treatments varying in response to patient needs and preferences.

REFERENCES

1. National Vital Statistics Report, Vol. 60, No. 3, December 29, 2011. http://www.cdc.gov/nchs/data/nvsr/nvsr60/nvsr60_03.pdf. Accessed August 31, 2012.
2. Field MJ, Cassel CK, ed, Committee on Care at the End of Life, Institute of Medicine. *Approaching Death: Improving Care at the End of Life.* Washington DC: National Academy Press, 1997.

3. Meier DE, Morrison RS. Autonomy reconsidered. *N Engl J Med*. 2002;*346*:1087–1089.

4. National Center for Health Statistics. *National mortality followback survey: 1986 Summary, United States*. Hyattsville, Maryland: Vital and Health Statistics, series 20, 1992.

5. Bernabei R, Gambassi G, Lapane K, et al. Management of pain in elderly patients with cancer. *JAMA* 1998;*279*:1877–1882.

6. Feldt KS, Ryden MB, Miles S. Treatment of pain in cognitively impaired compared with cognitively intact older patients with hip-fracture. *J Am Geriatr Soc* 1998;*46*:1079–1085.

7. Morrison RS, Siu AL. A comparison of pain and its treatment in advanced dementia and cognitively intact patients with hip fracture. *J Pain Symptom Manage* 2000;*19*:240–248.

8. Caregiving in the U.S. A report from the National Alliance for Caregiving and AARP. April 2004. http://www.caregiving.org/data/04finalreport.pdf. Accessed September 1, 2012.

9. The MetLife Caregiving Cost Study: Productivity Losses to U.S. Businesses. MetLife Mature Market Institute & National Alliance for Caregiving, July 2004.

10. Emanuel EJ, Fairclough DL, Slutsman J, Alpert H, Baldwin D, Emanuel L. Assistance from family members, friends, paid caregivers, and volunteers in the care of terminally ill patients. *N Engl J Med* 1999;*341*:956–963.

11. Schulz R, Beach S. Caregiving as a risk factor for mortality: the Caregiver Health Effects Study. *JAMA* 1999;*282*:2215–2219.

12. Ferrell BA, Ferrell BR, Rivera LSO. Pain in cognitively impaired nursing home patients. *J Pain Symptom Manage* 1995;*10*:591–598.

13. Ferrell B. Overview of Aging and Pain. In: Ferrell B, ed. *Pain in the Elderly*. Seattle: IASP, 1996.

2

Principles of Geriatric Palliative Care

INTRODUCTION

The United States is undergoing a longevity revolution. Average life expectancy in 1959 was 69.9 years[1] vs. 77.7 years in 2009.[2] Those who are 65 and over constitute an increasingly large number and proportion of the U.S. population. In 1994, this age group accounted for 13% of the population, and it is predicted that in 2030, 20% of the U.S. population will be over age 65. According to a recently released report from the National Institute on Aging, the number of nonagenarians was 1.9 million in 2010, and that number is expected to quadruple by 2050.[3]

Geriatric patients are very different from younger patients because of physiological changes associated with aging, atypical presentation of disease, dependence on a range of health care providers, and a continuum of care settings. Caring for these elderly patients is a complex endeavor involving medical, social, and psychological issues, and is best achieved by the interdisciplinary and patient-centered approach of geriatric palliative care.

PATHOPHYSIOLOGY OF AGING

Pathophysiologic changes experienced during aging impose special challenges in caring for older adults. The rates of aging vary not only with tissue types and also among individuals Table 2.1 describes common age-related changes by organ system, and selected clinical implications of these changes.

PRINCIPLES OF GERIATRIC PALLIATIVE CARE[4,5,6]

- Geriatrics is the branch of medicine that deals with the diagnosis and treatment of diseases and problems specific to the aged. Geriatricians are trained to focus on disease prevention and improvement in function of older people in a proactive manner, not just treatment of illnesses and diseases as they occur.

- Palliative care is an approach that improves the quality of life of patients and their families as they face the problems associated with serious illness. The goal is to prevent and relieve suffering by means of early identification, assessment, and treatment of pain and other symptoms, including physical, psychosocial, and spiritual domains. Palliative care is offered throughout continuum of illness and strives to facilitate patient autonomy, access to information, and choice.

- Geriatric palliative care combines these two specialties and is based on the following shared core principles:
  1. Clarifying and documenting individual and family preferences and goals of care
  2. Providing care that is patient/family-centered and evidence-based
  3. Employing an interdisciplinary team approach
  4. Careful attention to medication management
  5. Using interpersonal and communications skills that result in effective information exchange with patients, their families, and other health professionals
  6. Coordination of care, especially as patients transition across settings of care and stages of illness
  7. Respecting the importance of family caregivers, and recognizing and addressing their needs
  8. Offering treatment plans that are developed with consideration of cost effectiveness, economic burden, and insurance reimbursement issues
  9. Maximizing quality of life and functionality
  10. Providing psychosocial, spiritual, and bereavement support to patients and caregivers

TABLE 2.1: COMMON AGE-RELATED CHANGES BY ORGAN SYSTEM

Organ System	Age-Related Changes/Consequences	Clinical Implications/Disease Outcomes
Central nervous system	Reduced quantity of axons, dendrites, synapses, and neurons Decreased cerebral blood flow Altered neurotransmitters	Aging does not affect all domains of cognition equally Affected functions may include: speed of information processing, divided attention, learning/recall of new information, verbal fluency, reaction time
Cardiovascular	Ventricular and atrial hypertrophy Sclerosis of aortic and mitral valves Large arteries become less compliant Decreased maximal oxygen consumption, 7.5%–10% per decade of adult's life	Heart failure Aortic stenosis Hypertension Stroke Syncope
Pulmonary	Decreased thoracic muscle strength and chest wall compliance Reduced maximum vital capacity and forced expiratory volume Increased residual volume and lung compliance	Decreased pulmonary reserve Decreased exercise tolerance
Renal	Decreased renal function due to structural and functional changes	Renal insufficiency worsened by concomitant comorbidities such as diabetes mellitus, hypertension, heart failure, and nephrotoxic medication exposure
Urinary	Decreased bladder wall elasticity and tone	Increased risk of urinary retention or incontinence, especially associated with comorbidities such as BPH and uterine prolapse
Musculoskeletal	Decreased muscle mass Bone loss exceeds replacement after age 35	Muscle weakness and sarcopenia Frailty Falls Osteoporosis Hip fracture
Digestive	Reduced liver size and blood flow Reduced pancreatic enzyme reserves and insulin secretion Decreased colonic contractions Loss of tensile strength of colonic wall muscle	Impaired clearance of drugs Increased insulin resistance
Skin	Reduced melanocytes Reduced vitamin D production Impaired wound healing	Skin cancers Osteomalicia Persistent wounds, weak scars
Vision	Presbyopia may begin in the 40s and continues to worsen until around age 60 Lenses become harder and less flexible, and circular muscles may also get weaker	Decreased visual acuity Vision loss and blindness Increased susceptibility to glare, poor night vision, and more difficulty in detecting moving objects
Auditory	Presbycusis (sensorineural hearing impairment in the elderly) is most likely multifactorial	Bilateral high-frequency hearing loss associated with difficulty in speech discrimination and central auditory processing of information

11. Delivery of ethical care that is aligned with patient and family preferences and that always balances the benefits and burden of therapeutic interventions

CARING FOR THE WHOLE PATIENT

As a result of age-related changes described in Table 2.1, clinicians caring for the geriatric patient population must treat the whole person in the context of the patient's family and community, and not just the illness or syndrome. It is essential to be vigilant in regard to multiple contributing factors that can have a cumulative and deleterious impact on a geriatric patient in the domains of care shown in Table 2.2.

IMPORTANCE OF ASSESSMENT

A cornerstone of comprehensive geriatric palliative care is multidimensional assessment. Early identification of physical, cognitive, or psychosocial problems enables clinicians to plan timely and appropriate interventions to maintain or improve

TABLE 2.2: DOMAINS OF CARE

Domain	Conditions	Impact on Patient
Medical	Diseases and disorders in elderly patients, as well as geriatric syndromes, are usually multifactorial, involve multiple organ systems, and encompass physical, social, and psychosocial elements Typical disorders have atypical presentations	Chronic illness(es) Comorbidities, with polypharmacy Geriatric syndromes Depression risk Sensory losses (hearing, vision)
Functional	Multisystem comorbidities Osteoarthritis affects gait and use of hands, causes chronic pain, creates a fall risk, and limits functional independence in activities such as dressing, driving, shopping, housekeeping, etc.	Consideration of alternative care settings Need for special equipment and assistive devices Safety risks must be evaluated (indoor and outdoor) Dependence on others for activities of daily living
Social	Multiple comorbidities can lead to serious impact on overall quality of life Causes for social withdrawal include medications, disorders of bladder or bowel, gait dysfunction, hearing and visual impairment Social interactions also affected by isolation, death of spouse and friends, limited access to transportation, move to alternate care setting, forced migration to live with adult children or other relatives	Social isolation Unacceptable quality of life Accumulated losses Depression risk Functional decline Loss of family and community support Family caregiver burden
Economic	Fixed income/pensions after retirement are often not sufficient Investment reverses can lead to difficulty managing finances Increased cost of health care Reduced ability to afford to stay at home with home care, but with increased debility, causing ever-increasing need for care/assistance May need long-term care Elders are at increased risk for financial fraud and scams	Difficulty managing cost of personal long-term care, health insurance and medications Inability to identify and afford foods with adequate nutrition Limited funds to visit friends/family or to seek entertainment can lead to depression risk Stress of having to choose between rent, medicines, and food

functional status, address debilitating symptoms such as pain or depression, prevent complications, reduce risks associated with chronic disease states, and avoid unnecessary hospitalization for the older patient.

GERIATRIC PALLIATIVE CARE ASSESSMENT "TOOLBOX"

While there are many assessment tools that can be utilized to obtain important clinical data, clinicians who treat older adults should be familiar with at least one in each domain that requires evaluation. Table 2.3 below lists the key assessment areas and recommended instruments to gather clinical data in each domain.

Other assessments that should be pursued, but that do not have validated instruments, include:

- Medication review: Conduct a "brown bag review" of medications by asking patients to bring all medications and supplements to their next appointment. This review helps you to advise patients to take medications

TABLE 2.3: COMPREHENSIVE GERIATRIC ASSESSMENT[10]

Domain	Instruments
Delirium	Confusion Assessment Method (CAM)
Dementia	Mini Mental Status Exam Three-item recall Clock draw Animal Naming Test FAST SCALE (moderate to severe dementia)
Depression	Screening: Ask two questions: "During the last month, have you often been bothered by feeling down, depressed or hopeless?" "During the last month, have you often been bothered by having little interest of pleasure in doing things?" Assessment: Geriatric Depression Scale (Short form) Cornell Scale for Depression in Dementia (CSDD) Patient Health Questionnaire (PHQ-9)
Physical function	Assess for ADLs Assess for IADLs Palliative Care Performance Scale Karnofsky Performance Scale PPS (Palliative Performance Scale)
Falls	"Get up and Go" test: Patient is asked to get up from a chair without armrest and walk several steps, turn, and then return to his or her seat; patient with difficulty needs further evaluation Functional Reach Test: As reach decreases, the chance of falling increases John Hopkins Hospital Falls Assessment Tool
Vision and hearing	Hearing Handicap Inventory for the Elderly (HHIE-S) Snellen chart, visual field testing, intraocular eye pressure
Skin	Braden scores Chailey score (for patients in wheelchair)
Nutrition	Weight chart Nestle Mini Nutritional Assessment
Psychosocial issues	FICA Spiritual History Tool Needs at the End-of-life Screening Tool (NEST) Norbeck Social Support Questionnaire
Caregiver Stress	Famcare Zarit Burden Interview Modified Caregiver Strain Index (CSI)

correctly and identify/avoid medication errors and drug interactions. (See Chapter 3: Medication Management.)

- Advance care plans: See Chapter 8: Advance Care Planning.
- Safety concerns: See Chapter 24: Assistive Technology.
- Driving history.
- Sleep patterns.

EXPLORING PREFERENCES AND GOALS FOR CARE

- Once assessment data and relevant clinical information are gathered, the clinician should initiate a dialogue with the patient and family (or health care surrogate decision makers) about identifying appropriate care options and matching treatment plans to patient- and family-determined goals for care. (See Chapter 9: Communication Skills.)
- Clarifying preferences and achievable goals of care is a key requirement of care planning. Identifying and documenting care preferences can help avoid tests, treatments, or procedures that might be clinically appropriate but may not be consistent with the patient's overall health care goals.

DEVELOPING THE CARE PLAN

- Patients and their families should be offered the opportunity to work collaboratively with their medical providers to formulate appropriate and feasible care plans that best meet the needs and goals of the patient. (See Chapter 9: Communication Skills.)
- Using an interdisciplinary approach, a plan of care is developed that is tailored to patient's needs, goals, and preferences. An appropriate care plan will also take into account any psychosocial, spiritual, and economic considerations, as well as strategies to mitigate caregiver burden and stress.

RE-EVALUATING THE PLAN

- The trajectory of illness in older adults typically starts with diagnosis, intervention, and establishment of prognosis; often leads to the need for chronic and comorbid disease management; and eventually approaches the end of life. A care plan should thus be reevaluated on a regular basis, and especially in light of certain sentinel events or changes in clinical status that may cause goals of care to evolve (Figure 2.1).
- A review of the care plan should always include a benefit/burden analysis that takes into consideration the patient's current or past expression of achievable goals for care, estimated disease prognosis in the context of comorbidities, expectations for quality of life, and the resources available to the patient and family.

TAKE-HOME POINTS

- Geriatric patients differ from younger patients due to physiological changes, atypical presentation, multiple involved health care providers, and a continuum of care settings.
- Caring for older patients is a complex endeavor involving medical, social, and psychological issues, and is best achieved by the interdisciplinary and patient-centered approach.
- Geriatricians focus on disease prevention and improvement in function, not just treatment of illnesses and diseases as they occur.
- Palliative care is an approach that improves the quality of life of patients and their families facing the problems associated with serious illness.
- A cornerstone of comprehensive geriatric palliative care is multidimensional assessment. Early identification of physical, cognitive, or psychosocial problems enables clinicians to plan timely and appropriate interventions.
- Clarifying preferences and achievable goals of care is a key requirement of care planning.
- Medical providers should work collaboratively with patients and their families to develop an appropriate care plan that is tailored to patient's needs, goals, and preferences.
- Care planning should also take into account any psychosocial, spiritual, and economic considerations, as well as strategies to mitigate caregiver burden and stress.

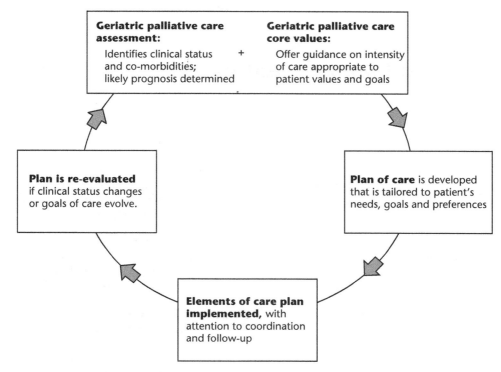

Geriatric palliative care assessment:
Identifies clinical status and co-morbidities; likely prognosis determined   +

Geriatric palliative care core values:
Offer guidance on intensity of care appropriate to patient values and goals

Plan is re-evaluated if clinical status changes or goals of care evolve.

Plan of care is developed that is tailored to patient's needs, goals and preferences

Elements of care plan implemented, with attention to coordination and follow-up

FIGURE 2.1: Geriatric palliative care planning.

REFERENCES

1. Congressional Research Service (CRS) compilation from National Center for Health Statistics (NCHS). United States Life Tables, 2002, *National Vital Statistics Reports*, vol. *53*, no. 6, Nov. 10, 2004. For 2003, NCHS, Deaths: Final Data for 2003, *National Vital Statistics Reports*, vol. 54, no. 13, Apr. 19, 2006.

2. U.S. Census Bureau. The 2010 Statistical Abstract | Page Last Modified: December 17, 2009.

3. He W, Muenchrath MN. U.S. Census Bureau, ACS 17; 90+ in the United States: 2006-2008. U.S. Government Printing Office, Washington DC, 2011.

4. The Principles of Geriatric Care. *The American Geriatrics Society.* July 2011. http://www.americangeriatrics.org/files/documents/Adv_Resources/PayReform_fact3.pdf. Accessed March 20, 2012.

5. Kapo J, Morrison LJ, Liao S. Palliative care for the older adult. *Journal of Palliative Medicine.* 2007;*10*(1):185–209.

6. Morrison RS, Meier DE. Palliative care. *N Engl J Med.* 2004;*350*:2582–2590.

7. Rosen SL, Rueben D. Geriatric assessment tools. *Mount Sinai Journal of Medicine.* 2011;*78*:489–497.

3

Medication Management in Older Adults

INTRODUCTION

Pharmacotherapy of the elderly is a complex topic due to age-related physiologic changes, multiple comorbidities, multiple medications, and multiple providers (prescribers and pharmacies). In addition, cognitive impairment, functional difficulties, and caregiver issues play a key role in errors and compliance. To prescribe appropriately, clinicians must consider not only the pharmacological properties of the drugs but also clinical, epidemiological, social, cultural, and economic factors.

PHARMACOTHERAPY OF OLDER ADULTS

Most older adults have several chronic conditions, and they stand to benefit the most from best practice guidelines. They also are at a greater risk of toxicity given diminished physiologic reserve and our increasingly complex pharmacopoeia. Providers must minimize side effects and avoid potentially harmful drug interactions. Age-related physiologic changes in organ function affect drug handling (pharmacokinetics) and response (pharmacodynamics).

Pharmacokinetics

- Pharmacokinetics describes the process of drug handling by the tissue, organ, or body. The four traditional components of pharmacokinetics are absorption, distribution, metabolism, and excretion.[1,2]
- Absorption, a passive process that takes place mostly in the small intestine, shows the least changes with aging.
- Distribution refers to the locations in the body that a drug penetrates, and the time required for the drug to reach such locations. It is expressed as the volume of distribution (Vd) and it is altered by age-associated changes in body composition.
- Metabolism is most commonly carried out by the liver through type I (cytochrome

p450 oxidation/reduction) and type II (conjugation/acetylation) reactions.
- Excretion refers to the drug's final route of exit from the body. For most drugs it involves elimination by the kidney.
- A summary of the pharmacokinetic changes during aging, their clinical and therapeutic implications, and clinical recommendation is presented in Table 3.1.

Pharmacodynamics

- Pharmacodynamics describes how drugs exert their effect at the site of action, the time course, and the intensity of pharmacological effect.
- Pharmacodynamics of specific drugs are determined not only by the concentration of the drug at the receptor but also by drug-receptor interactions (variation in receptor number, receptor affinity, second messenger response, and cellular response), variations in physiological or homeostatic mechanisms, and changes in functional reserves.
- Pharmacodynamics have been more difficult to define than pharmacokinetic changes because the effect of many drugs is magnified in the elderly by reduced drug clearance, resulting in increased serum concentration. However, there are well documented age-related changes in pharmacodynamics with significant clinical consequences (Table 3.2).

ADVERSE DRUG REACTIONS

- **Adverse drug reactions** (ADRs) are undesirable or noxious effects that occur at standard drug treatment doses. They are very common in the geriatric population.[3] They account for approximately 10% of emergency department visits and 10% to 17% of hospital admissions.

TABLE 3.1: AGE-RELATED CHANGES IN PHARMACOKINETICS

Component	Age-Related Changes	Clinical Consequences	Clinical Recommendations
Absorption	Little change in absorptive capacity of small bowel Changes in gastric motility and bowel transit time Changes in blood flow to the gut	None described	When prescribing, be aware of other medications that may impact absorption and patient comorbid conditions
Distribution	Decrease in lean body mass and total body water Increase in body fat Decrease in serum binding proteins	Decreased volume of distribution of water-soluble drugs with higher blood levels Increased volume of distribution of fat-soluble drugs with increased half-life Decreased binding of acidic drugs to albumin with elevation of free drug level even if the total concentration of the drug is decreased Increased binding of basic drugs; clinical consequence unclear	Drug doses should be started lower and increased more slowly to account for these changes Check levels of free drug when the assay is available
Metabolism[1]	Reduced liver mass and reduced hepatic blood flow Reduced enzyme activity of the cytochrome p450 system	Reduced rate of drug metabolism Increased variability in drug bioavailability	Different drugs metabolized through the same pathway may cause drug-drug interactions Always check whether a newly prescribed drug inhibits/induces the cytochrome p450 enzymes[1]
Elimination	Reduced renal blood flow and renal mass mostly in the cortical area; sclerotic changes of the glomeruli and infiltration of chronic inflammatory cells, and fibrosis in the stroma	Loss of glomerular filtration capacity Decrease in concentrating and diluting ability Decreased elimination Increased half-life	Serum creatinine is NOT an accurate reflection of creatinine clearance in elderly patients Always calculate creatinine clearance[2]

[1] There are multiple resources (PDR, online sites, textbooks, pharmacists, etc.) where interactions can be checked. A useful website for health care professionals is www.drug-interactions.com, which provides up-to-date information about CYP substrates, inhibitors, and inducers.
[2] Glomerular filtration rate (GFR) × serum creatinine clearance (SCr) = Urine creatinine concentration (UCr) × Urine volume (V)

- The majority of the ADRs experienced by older adults are considered to be predictable. ADRs include amplified drug effects, side effects, interactions with other drugs, and interactions with nutrients or diseases. The most common ADRs include electrolyte, renal, gastrointestinal tract, hemorrhagic, and endocrine abnormalities.
- Most common drug categories implicated in ADRs in the elderly include cardiovascular drugs, antibiotics, diuretics, anticoagulants, hypoglycemics, steroids, opioids, anticholinergics, benzodiazepines,

TABLE 3.2: AGE-RELATED CHANGES IN PHARMACODYNAMICS

Age-Related Changes	Clinical Consequences	Clinical Recommendations
Reduced sensitivity of arterial pressure receptors with decreased in baroreceptor reflex response	Postural hypotension Post-prandial hypotension	Check orthostatic changes in blood pressure before and after starting a new antihypertensive
Decreased responsiveness of B-adrenergic receptors	Limits heart rate and contractile response to stress	Start beta-blockers at low doses and increase gradually
Decreased sensitivity of respiratory centers to hypoxia and hypercapnia	Delayed and/or diminished ventilatory response	Check oxygen saturation as part of the patient's vital signs
Loss of neuronal substance, decreased synaptic activity, impaired glucose metabolism in the brain, and more ready penetration of drugs in the CNS	Higher susceptibility and exaggerated response to drugs that interact with the peripheral and central nervous system	Avoid medications with significant CNS side effects

and nonsteroidal anti-inflammatory drugs (NSAIDs).

- Adverse drug reactions can mimic or precipitate geriatric syndromes and in many cases produce additional unnecessary prescriptions. Drug-induced cognitive impairment is among the most common causes of reversible dementia; falls can be precipitated by a wide variety of drugs; the anticholinergic effect of many drugs can result in dry mouth, constipation, urinary retention, blurred vision, and confusion.
- If the physician does not consider medications as responsible for the patient's symptoms, additional drug therapy may be prescribed to treat the adverse effect of another drug, causing what is called a "prescribing cascade." Any symptom in an older patient may be a drug side effect until proven otherwise.
- Multiple clinical and treatment-related factors increase the frequency of ADRs in older adults.
  - Clinical factors:
    Reduction of stimuli-induced adaptation capacity
    Inappropriate homeostatic response
    Frailty
    Multiple comorbidities
    Cognitive/visual/hearing impairment
  - Treatment-related factors:
    Number of drugs prescribed/ polypharmacy
    Pharmacokinetic interactions
    Patient adherence
    Fragmented care

PATIENT ERROR

- ADRs may result from patient errors.[4] The patient errors leading to adverse events most often occur in administration of the drug, modification of the medication regimen, and failure to follow clinical advice about medication use. Health care providers have an opportunity at every visit to review medication issues.
- The most common reasons for errors are the complexity of the medication regimen (administration pattern, frequent changes, as-needed drugs based on patient monitoring, medication handling that disrupts a patient's lifestyle) and the presence of dementia, confusion, and sensory problems.

DRUG-DRUG INTERACTION

- Drug-drug interaction (DDI) is a pharmacological or clinical response to the administration of a drug combination that differs from that anticipated from the known effects of each of the agents given alone. DDIs can occur at any level of pharmacokinetics since one drug may affect the absorption, distribution, metabolism, and/or excretion of another drug.
- The most common pharmacokinetic interactions involve the inhibition of the cytochrome P450 metabolism. Risk factors include multiple medications, multiple prescribing clinicians, and multiple pharmacies.

- The risk of drug-drug interaction increases with the number of medications used, occurring in 13% of patients taking two medications and 82% of patients taking more than six medications.

ADR AND DDI PREVENTION STRATEGIES

Medication Review

- A "brown bag checkup" is the single best thing that physicians can do to avoid medication mistakes and cut down unnecessary medications. To assist in the medication review, patients should bring all their medications in a bag to each office visit.
- Throw away expired medications. Provide the patient with a pill box and a large-font typed medication list with clear directions and indications in plain English, and in translation if necessary.
- For cognitively impaired patients, it is important to review the medications with the person responsible for administering them. When indicated for patient safety, a referral to home care should be considered for further assessment and management of medication.

Prevention Guidelines

1. For the treatment of the primary disease, choose the drug that is recognized as being most efficient and safe. Also remember that medications are not always the only way to treat a patient.
2. Be familiar with a source of drug interaction information.
3. Screen for drug-drug interactions when adding a new drug to the regimen.
4. Evaluate renal function and adapt the treatment dosing and schedule accordingly.
5. Recognize that a clinical sign or symptom could be an ADR. Do not add a medication to combat the side effect of another one unless it is absolutely necessary.
6. Use the least possible number of medications. Eliminate those that have no benefit. Try not to start two drugs at the same time.
7. Drugs that have the simplest administration schedule are preferred.
8. Recognize that self-medication and nonadherence are common and can induce ADRs.
9. Eliminate PRN (i.e. take-as-needed) medications that have not been used for the last month.
10. Print a legible and plain English medication list for your patient.
11. Evaluate cognitive function.
12. Use an interdisciplinary approach. Involve the family, caregiver, nurse, and pharmacist. Look for caregivers able to take responsibility for drug administration.

POTENTIALLY INAPPROPRIATE MEDICATION (PIM)

- Potentially inappropriate medications (PIMs) are medications that pose more risk than benefit to the patient, either because they are ineffective, because they pose unnecessary risks, or because there are safer alternatives available.
- A consensus guideline known as the "Beers criteria," first published in 1991 and last updated in 2003, provides a list of drugs that a panel of experts thought to be particularly problematic for older patients.[5, 6]
- Forty-eight individual medications or classes of medications to avoid in older adults and their potential concerns are listed. Examples include indomethacin (causes the most CNS side effects of all NSAIDs), muscle relaxants (anticholinergic side effects), digoxin (at doses >0.125 mg daily may cause toxic effects due to decreased renal clearance), diphenhydramine (may cause confusion or sedation).
- Beers criteria also include diseases or conditions, and medications to be avoided in older adults with these conditions, such as gastric/duodenal ulcers—avoid NSAIDs and Aspirin>325 mg daily; constipation—avoid calcium channel blockers, anticholinergics; blood clotting disorders—avoid aspirin, NSAIDs, clopidogrel; Parkinson's disease—avoid conventional antipsychotics.
- The Beers criteria are widely used. They are vitally important to managed-care organizations, pharmacy benefit plans,

and both acute and long-term care institutions. However, clinicians should be aware that the Beers criteria system has multiple deficiencies that are being addressed in the literature, e.g., rarely prescribed drugs are included; presentation criteria lack structure; frequently written inappropriate prescriptions are omitted; and inappropriate underutilization of drugs is not addressed.

OVER-THE-COUNTER AND HERBAL MEDICATIONS

- Americans of all ages have increasingly turned to herbal medicines. However, older adults are the biggest consumers not only of prescription drugs but also of over-the-counter (OTC) medications and dietary supplements.[7]
- The use of OTC agents and herbal preparations adds to the challenge of prescribing appropriate medications for older patients. It presents a further risk for ADRs and herb-drug interactions.
- Many health providers do not ask about herbals and OTC medications, and many older patients do not disclose their use to their physicians. In fact most patients do not recognize that herbals are pharmaceutical agents that may cause serious adverse effects.
- Older persons may be more vulnerable to drug interactions and toxicities of herbal medicines due to polypharmacy and age-related changes in pharmacokinetics. However, there is little information about the pharmacokinetics of the herbal agents, and the level of risk is not well known.
- Over-the-counter and herbal medicine use should be assessed frequently, and patients should be educated about potential side effects and interactions.

TAKE-HOME POINTS

- There are significant age-associated changes in drug pharmacokinetics and pharmacodynamics, so remember to "Start Low and Go Slow."
- Different drugs metabolized through the same pathway may cause drug-drug interactions. Therefore, always check whether a newly prescribed drug inhibits/induces the cytochrome P450 enzymes.
- Serum creatinine is not a good representation of kidney function in the elderly, so always calculate creatinine clearance [Glomerular filtration rate (GFR) × serum creatinine clearance (SCr) = Urine creatinine concentration (UCr) × Urine volume (V)].
- Know your patients' medications. Ask frequently about prescription medications, OTC supplements, and herbal preparations.
- Communicate with caregivers and other health care providers to increase adherence and decrease medication errors.
- Explicitly weigh benefits and burdens of all medications in the context of the patient's life expectancy, functional and cognitive status, and achievable goals of care.

REFERENCES

1. Cusak BJ. Pharmacokinetics in older persons. *Am J Geriatr Pharmacotherapy.* 2004;2:274–302.
2. Avorn J, Gurwitz JH. Principles of Pharmacology. In: Cassel CK, Leipzig R, Cohen HJ, Larson ED, Meier DE, eds. *Geriatric Medicine An Evidence-Based Approach.* New York, NY: Springer-Verlag; 2003; 55–70.
3. Kohn LT, Corrigan JM, Donaldson MS, eds. *To Err Is Human: Building a Safer Health System.* Washington, DC: National Academies Press; 2000.
4. Field TS, Mazon KM, Brusacher B, Debellis KR, Gurwitz JA. Adverse drug events resulting from patient errors in older adults. *J Am Geriatr Soc.* 2007;55:271–276.
5. Beers MH. Explicit criteria for determining potentially inappropriate medication use by the elderly. An update. *Arch Intern Med.* 1997;157:1531–1536.
6. Fick DM, Cooper JW, Wade WE, Waller JL, Maclean JP, Beers MH. Updating the Beers criteria for potentially inappropriate medication use in older adults: results of a US consensus panel of experts. *Arch Intern Med.* 2003;163:2716–2724.
7. Qato DM, Alexander GC, Conti RM, Johnson M, Schumm P, Lindau ST. Use of prescription and over-the-counter medications and dietary supplements among older adults in the United States. *JAMA.* 2008;300(24):2867–2878.

4

Special Issues in Caregiving

"There are only four kinds of people in this world—those that have been caregivers, those who currently are caregivers, those who will be caregivers, and those who will need caregivers."

ROSALYNN CARTER

INTRODUCTION

From the beginning, the medical specialties of geriatrics and palliative care have understood the critical role of the patient's social network in facilitating encounters with the complex modern health care system and its vast array of choices, constraints, benefits, and burdens. This chapter will focus on several key changes in our evolving understanding of the role of the caregiver that are very relevant to the patient and family-centered approach of the primary clinician and other care providers.

WHO ARE THE CAREGIVERS?

- The term "caregiver" refers to family members, friends, or others in the patient's social, religious, or neighborhood networks who provide help to an older adult who is no longer able to perform the tasks of everyday life independently.
- Assistance is frequently offered voluntarily and without compensation, though usually with a profound combination of love and obligation.
- The patient may have a network of these "informal" caregivers who assume various responsibilities at different times over the course of care, with one person assuming a lead role as the primary caregiver.
- The term "formal caregiver" is often used to describe a paid care provider who may have specific training and supervision.

CAREGIVING DEMOGRAPHICS

- 15% of caregivers for older adults are age 65 or older.[1]
- Old age accounted for 12% of care recipients in 2009, followed by Alzheimer's disease (10%), mental/emotional illness (7%), cancer (7%), heart disease (5%), and stroke (5%). Diabetes, currently receiving increased attention from health providers and public health experts, accounts for 6%.[1]
- Caregivers provide an average of 4.6 years of care. Persons with Alzheimer's and other dementias require 1–4 years more care than that provided to persons with other conditions.[2]
- Long-distance caregivers, those who live an hour or more from the care recipient, account for 15% of caregiving.
- The cost to businesses of productivity losses associated with intense caregiving by full-time employees is estimated to be over $17 billion annually. The total for caregiving at all levels of intensity is estimated at over $33 billion. This includes losses from absenteeism, interruptions in the workday, employee replacement, and shifts from full-time to part-time to accommodate caregiving responsibilities.[3]

IMPLICATIONS FOR THE FUTURE[2]

- Dramatic growth in the population over 85 years old will create extended periods of functional dependence and the need for assistance with Instrumental Activities of Daily Living (IADL) and Activities of Daily Living (ADL).
- For all conditions and illnesses, the duration and intensity of caregiving is related to higher rates of emotional, physical, and financial stress. Alzheimer's caregivers face the greatest risk of profound emotional and physical stress, as well as decline in their own health status.[4]
- Decrease in U.S. birthrates over the past 50 years points to a smaller pool of available

family caregivers. Many experts consider the approaching surge in the national caregiving burden to be a public health issue meriting attention from health policy makers.

- The current economic situation has led to decreased flexibility in how families fund eldercare, based on the following factors:
  - Americans generally have a low rate of savings from which to fund the care needs of old age.
  - Lower home values mean less available equity for the care recipient to draw upon.
  - Caregivers, particularly those who are older, may have added anxiety about time off from work to provide care, despite the Family Medical Leave Act and corporate efforts to provide employee assistance programs.
  - Reductions in state and local budgets may reduce the availability of services that offer respite and relief to caregivers.
  - Medicare is examining hospital readmission rates, making it essential to enlist the patient and family in discussions of realistic options that will ensure the patient's smooth discharge and transition to the appropriate level of care.

NEW ROLES FOR CARE RECIPIENTS AND CAREGIVERS

- For patients, the recognition that they need help can be painful and may be met with sadness or with expressions of hurt, anger, or denial. The patient with dementia may lack the cognitive or emotional capacity to recognize the problems, or to appreciate and accept the care required.[4]
- Becoming a "caregiver" can be a gradual process or it may happen suddenly, as an adult child, sibling, or spouse comes to the realization that changes in the patient's function must be addressed. Acceptance of the new role of caregiver frequently occurs when hospital staff engage the family in discussions to ensure a safe discharge. In this context, the interdisciplinary team may find that long-standing friction between patient and caregiver, or the need to coordinate multiple caregivers, can complicate discharge planning. (See Chapter 10: Managing Conflict.)

- Ideally, family members will communicate well with each other and react creatively to the process of shifting roles and responsibilities, with expressions of compassion, respect and support for the patient and for each other. Family meetings can help outline the needs of the patient as perceived by the various involved individuals. Participants can then divide the caregiving tasks according to their abilities, time constraints, and financial resources. Most importantly, a pattern of communication must be established that will enable the caregivers to respond effectively to the patient's changing needs and to prepare for the more complicated challenges to come.
- A helpful resource to begin this communication process is the Family Caregiver Alliance's Fact Sheet entitled "Holding a Family Meeting" (available online at www.caregiver.org).
- In situations where there is conflict over caregiving needs and roles, family members and friends will often withdraw until the patient experiences a health crisis. An office visit to the primary care physician or a trip to the hospital emergency room then provides the clinical team with an opportunity to begin a constructive process with the family to organize care for the patient.
- Numerous healthcare agencies and organizations provide guidance for caregivers on their websites. Resource materials for families are also available in most public libraries. (See the reference section below; also see Chapter 28: Caregivers.)

LONG-DISTANCE CAREGIVING[5,6]

- About 15% of caregivers (approximately 7 million people) live more than one hour from the care recipient. Of these, 23% are the sole caregiver. Workforce mobility and retirement relocation are common reasons that families live apart.
- These long-distance caregivers and their care recipients have a special set of needs. Some unique challenges encountered by the long-distance care relationship include the following:
  - Being at a distance requires the caregiver to thoughtfully interpret reports from the care recipient or other members of the

care network about how the caregiving plan is working. Additional expenses related to travel and transportation may be incurred.

- A sudden change in the care recipient's health status may require an unplanned visit or even an immediate revisit.
- The care recipient may have less time to adapt to a new care plan, given the long-distance caregiver's time constraints for a visit.
- Distance may make the caregiver feel inadequate, ineffective, or guilty for not being more available.
- In an emergency, the caregiver may need to quickly assemble data, including health provider information, advance directives, neighbors' addresses and phone numbers, financial papers, copies of important documents such as birth certificate, Medicare and other insurance cards, and signed permissions to represent the patient to various entities such as banks, Social Security Administration, etc. Resources are available online, including forms to help organize all necessary information. (See Family Caring Alliance and AARP web sites).
- Strategies to help the caregiver become organized as efficiently and as soon as possible include:
  - Be sure that all important parties, such as key neighbors and health providers, have the caregiver's contact information.
  - The family meeting, held early in the course of an illness when the care recipient can participate, is critical to assemble information, establish tasks and schedules, and open lines of communication to prepare for an uncertain future.
  - The local agency on aging, county senior services office, or entities such as the local chapter of AARP, Alzheimer's Association, and community nursing agencies can provide information about local resources.
  - Those who are financially able may find the services of a geriatric care manager to be helpful. The care manager is typically a nurse or social worker who is familiar with local sources, knowledgeable about geriatrics, and able to function as the long-distance caregiver's eyes and ears between visits.

- For the clinician, the long-distance caregiver may require a special attention to communication strategies. For example, expediting lab work, consultant appointments, and changing medications or dosages during a caregiver's visit to the area may ensure better implementation of the plan of care. Between visits, the long-distance caregiver can participate via speaker phone during the care recipient's visit with the physician.

THE HEALTH PROVIDER'S RELATIONSHIP WITH THE CAREGIVER

- The education and training of health professionals, particularly outside of geriatrics and palliative care, has largely focused on providing care to one person-- the patient. The evolving demographics of aging and caregiving, with the young-old caring for the old-old, will prompt the clinician to also develop a relationship with the family caregiver.
- While the primacy of the patient-centered relationship will remain intact, the clinician is likely to find that, over time, the health and well-being of the caregiver is his or her concern as well. Specific clinical aspects of this relationship will be found in the chapter on Caregivers. Health care professionals are also developing ethical and practice guidelines to address caregiver issues and concerns.[7]
- Discussion of advance directives before a health crisis arises, and while the patient is able participate, is essential. The health provider should discuss the patient's preferences for early inclusion of the caregiver, with the goal of establishing the caregiver as a recognized partner on the care team.

CHANGES IN THE CAREGIVING ROLE OVER TIME

- As family members devote more hours, attention, and expenses to caregiving, the incidence of caregiver depression, stress, and physical illness rises. Current research on caregiving identifies levels of physical and emotional intensity as factors which add to the burden of caregiving. Advancing dementia is particularly associated with a decrease in caregiver well-being.

- Unfamiliar care needs present a special challenge to both the caregiver and the care recipient. Special tasks that may be new, overwhelming, and complicated for the caregiver, and potentially upsetting to the care recipient include:
  - Making an occupied bed
  - Lifting, turning, and repositioning
  - Giving a bed bath
  - Transfer techniques
  - Toileting and incontinence care
  - Hygiene
  - Feeding
- These skills and techniques should be acquired by family caregivers for the safety and well-being of both the patient and themselves. Some caregivers have the intuition or natural ability to do what is needed; others will acquire essential skills through trial and error. Health providers, however, should be attentive to potential learning needs for the many caregivers who may face increased burden and earlier burnout due to ignorance of the most ergonomic or sensible approach to providing care.
- Increasingly, community-based programs and agencies are recognizing the need for these skills and are providing caregivers with training. Educational sessions focus on techniques that can support the patient, promote confidence, and build skills, potentially reducing the need for paid home help or increased hours of home help, premature nursing home placement, and excessive office, outpatient or emergency room visit.
- Caregiver training is also available in person or online through caregiver organizations or disease-related associations. Some are free of charge, and others request a donation or fee. See the Family Caregiver Alliance web site (www.caregiver.org) and the Alzheimer's Association (www.alz.org).

EMERGING CAREGIVING ISSUES[8]

- Many clinicians are noting that some "blended" families, particularly in the context of late-life second marriage, may experience difficulty establishing caregiving priorities. For example, adult children of a caregiver in a second marriage may express concerns or even anger about the demands

that caregiving for an elderly spouse places on their biological parent.
- Families of couples who were older at the time of remarriage may not have developed a set of expectations about caregiving in their parents' later life. When a crisis occurs, roles are unclear, and expectations may cause tensions.
- Family meetings to bring all parties together for discussion are critically important. Research is also underway that promises to offer guidance to clinicians on this topic.

TAKE-HOME POINTS

- For frail or seriously ill older adults, the viability of the caregiving plan depends on the effectiveness of a caregiving network that may include spouse, children, friends, neighbors, and others. There is usually a primary caregiver who will serve as the contact point for the health care team.
- Care tasks may be new to the caregiver(s), who will benefit from instruction and support from the clinical team.
- Caregiving for the patient with Alzheimer's or other dementias is associated with longer duration of care and greater decline in caregiver health status than other health conditions.
- The clinical team faces special challenges when the primary caregiver lives at a distance. Good communication strategies will help ensure a timely response by the caregiver to changes in the patient's functional status and well-being.
- Many on-line resources offer support and information for caregivers. Special assistance will be helpful for the non-English speaking caregivers, or those who are not familiar with computers.

REFERENCES

1. Caregiving in the U.S. 2009 National Alliance for Caregiving in collaboration with AARP, November 2009.
2. Talley RC, Crews JE. Framing the public health of caregiving. *Am J Public Health*. Feb 2007;*97*(2): 224–228.
3. The MetLife Caregiving Cost Study: Productivity Losses to U.S. Businesses. MetLife Mature Market Institute & National Alliance for Caregiving, July 2004.
4. 2012 Alzheimer's Disease Facts and Figures. Alzheimer's Association. *Alzheimer's & Dementia*. Mar 2012;*8*(2):131–168.

5. Handbook for Long-Distance Caregivers. Family Caregiver Alliance, 2003.
6. Miles Away: the MetLife Study of Long Distance Caregiving. MetLife Mature Market Institute & National Alliance for Caregiving, July 2004.
7. Mitnick S, Leffler, C, and Hood VL, for the American College of Physicians Ethics, Professionalism and Human Rights Committee. Family caregivers, patients and physicians: ethical guidance to optimize relationships. *J Gen Intern Med.* 2010: doi: 10.1007/s11606-009-1206-3.
8. Sherman CW, Boss P. Spousal dementia caregiving in the context of late-life remarriage. *Dementia.* May 2007;6(2):245–270. doi:10.1177/1471301207080367.

5

Financing Hospice and Palliative Care

INTRODUCTION

Older adults are an increasingly vulnerable population due to a high prevalence of chronic illness that is often combined with fixed and limited financial resources. The U.S. population aged 65 and older will exceed 70 million by 2030, roughly twice the number in 2000. The number of nonagenarians reached 1.9 million in 2010, and that number is expected to quadruple by 2050.[1]

The incidence of chronic conditions and disability rates increases with age, placing older adults at greater risk of incurring high medical costs than younger adults.[1] It has been estimated that 65% of Medicare patients with two or more chronic conditions account for 95% of Medicare expenditures.[2]

ACCESS TO PALLIAITVE CARE

- Despite the increased spending on health care services for our older adults with chronic and comorbid illnesses, there is evidence that they receive less than optimal care. In fact, these vulnerable patients and their families often endure untreated pain and other distressing symptoms, unmet psychosocial and home care needs, high caregiver burden, and low patient and family satisfaction.[3]
- Given this convergence of an aging population, costly chronic illness, and less than optimal care, there is growing realization among health care professionals that our society must put policies in place that assure widespread access to palliative care so that older patients with serious illnesses and their families can get the care they need and deserve.
- Unfortunately, existing financing and reimbursement mechanisms have erected barriers to timely access to hospice care, and they also effectively limit the delivery of palliative care at appropriate points in the continuum of a serious illness.

- The goals of this chapter are to (1) describe the key elements of palliative and hospice care; (2) explain the current U.S. reimbursement methods for these two models of care; (3) outline the shortcomings of these financing mechanisms; and (4) describe the challenge of finding policy solutions that will allow increased and more timely access to palliative care at appropriate points in the care continuum for patients with serious illness.

PALLIATIVE CARE AND HOSPICE

- Palliative care is specialized medical care for people facing serious and chronic illness. It focuses on relief from symptoms, pain, and stress, whatever the diagnosis. The goal is to improve quality of life for both patient and family. Palliative care is provided by a team that includes physicians, nurses, and other specialists who work together with a patient's own doctor to provide an extra layer of support. It is appropriate at any age and any stage in a serious illness and can be provided along with curative treatment.
- The differences between palliative care and hospice relate primarily to the timing and eligibility criteria, the care setting, and financing of care services (Table 5.1).
- Palliative care is available to patients who continue to benefit from life-prolonging treatments. It is not dependent on prognosis. This independence from prognosis is especially important for individuals with chronic, debilitating diseases such as heart failure, stroke, or dementia[4] because prognostication is particularly difficult for these diseases. (See Chapter 7: Prognostication.)
- To be eligible for the Medicare Hospice Benefit, however, an individual must be certified by two physicians as "terminal"

TABLE 5.1: COMPARING PALLIATIVE CARE AND HOSPICE

	Palliative Care	Hospice
Timing	Upon diagnosis with serious illness	Terminal prognosis
Eligibility	Based on patient need	Based on prognosis
Setting	Primarily hospital-based	Primarily home care
Reimbursement	Fee for service; Medicare for physician and nurse only	Medicare Hospice Benefit; Medicaid; private insurance

(defined as a prognosis of six months or less); and the patient must also agree to give up Medicare coverage for life-prolonging therapies. (See Chapter 12: The Hospice Model of Palliative Care.)

- While both palliative care and hospice can be offered in any setting, palliative care in the United States is primarily hospital-based, and hospice care is usually provided in the patient's home.
- Palliative care in hospice and outside of hospice is paid for by two entirely difference reimbursement systems. (See Chapter 13: Insurance.)

CURRENT FINANCING MECHANISMS

Palliative Care Reimbursement

- Private insurance fee-for-service reimbursement for palliative care outside of hospice is currently limited in both amount and scope. Reimbursement categories and rates are typically not sufficient for the level and intensity of care that is required by patients and families.
- Existing Medicare reimbursement policy for palliative care covers only the services of the physician and nurse practitioner. Reimbursement for the balance of care provided by the comprehensive interdisciplinary team (e.g., social worker, chaplain, and other disciplines) is excluded.
- As a result of these payment barriers, gaps in financing for palliative care programs must currently be filled by institutional support and/or philanthropy.

Hospice Reimbursement

- Hospice is covered by the Medicare Hospice Benefit (MHB), which is fairly comprehensive and reimburses the hospice on a per-diem basis for the care provided to

patients and families. (See Chapter 13: Health Insurance.) Significant growth in the number and size of hospice agencies during the past decade[5] indicates that providing hospice care within the context of existing reimbursement guidelines is a profitable endeavor.

- The MHB eligibility criteria include limited life expectancy of six months or less and the patient's agreement to discontinue any curative treatment of the terminal condition that prompted the decision to receive hospice care.

NEGATIVE IMPACT OF THE MHB ELIGIBILITY CRITERIA

- The MHB is acknowledged by most experts to be a comprehensive benefit that facilitates compassionate interdisciplinary care (provided primarily in the place the patient calls home) for a targeted population of patients with limited life expectancy, in a manner that is consistent with the core mission of hospice's founders.
- The criteria of limited life expectancy[6] and waiver of Medicare reimbursement for the curative treatment of the terminal condition that prompted election of hospice care[7] are also considered by many to be necessary and appropriate to define the target hospice population.
- The drawback of the Medicare Hospice Benefit as currently structured, however, is that these eligibility criteria limit timely access to hospice for a growing number of very seriously ill patients in two very significant ways:
  1. **Prognostic uncertainty**: Although there has been significant growth in the number and variety of diagnoses of individuals receiving hospice care,[8] the difficulty in certifying that a patient

has six months or less to live remains a significant barrier to hospice referral,[9-12] particularly for individuals with non-cancer diagnoses.

2. **Choosing curative vs. palliative therapies**: The line between curative and palliative treatments has become more difficult to define because a number of recently developed curative treatments also simultaneously provide symptom relief. Because of this increasingly blurred boundary between disease-directed treatment and palliative care, most hospice referrals are delayed, usually occurring only within one month of death. The result of this trend to late referral is that patients and families do not benefit from comprehensive end-of-life hospice care, and what they often do experience is basically crisis management health care at the end of life.

A BETTER MODEL OF CARE

- As described above, the current payment systems for palliative care inside and out of hospice do not align with the optimal continuum of care for patients with serious illness. There is inadequate reimbursement for the initial palliative care consultation and for services that should begin at the time of diagnosis. This limited coverage for palliative care continues until there is documentation of a terminal prognosis. At that point, if a choice is made to forego life-prolonging care, an abrupt shift to hospice care takes place, and subsequent costs are covered by the Medicare Hospice Benefit.
- Alternatively, an ideal model of care would be that illustrated in Figure 5.1. At the time of diagnosis of a serious or life-threatening

illness, a patient would receive a palliative care consultation. The patient and family would then decide with their health care providers which disease-directed therapies to pursue, while simultaneously receiving an increasing proportion of palliative care that is discussed and reevaluated when and if the disease progresses. When life-prolonging care is no longer effective or desired, the patient could transition to hospice care, with the family receiving bereavement care following the patient's death.

SEARCHING FOR SOLUTIONS

- Experts in the field of palliative care agree that changes in how and when palliative care and hospice are paid for would improve the care that can be offered to seriously ill patients and their families. There exists considerable uncertainty among policy experts, however, over how the financing of palliative and hospice care should be restructured to achieve this important goal. Potential solutions that currently frame the debate include:

1. **Expanding patient eligibility for the Medicare Hospice Benefit**: Eligibility for enrollment in the Medicare Hospice Benefit could shift from a prognosis-based to a needs-based criterion, with no restriction on the ability to receive reimbursement for curative treatments while also receiving hospice care. The potential economic implications of this option are widely debated.[13]

2. **Hospice concurrent care pilot programs**: There are a number of ongoing concurrent care pilots in which patients are able to receive simultaneous

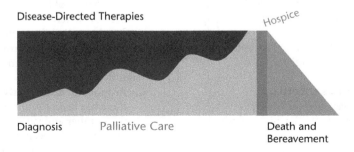

FIGURE 5.1: Model of palliative and disease-directed therapies.

hospice and life-prolonging care. Data regarding patient and family outcomes and system-level cost saving must still be evaluated.

- Any policy "fix" must provide adequate reimbursement for a patient's evolving interdisciplinary health care needs at each point along the care continuum, from initial diagnosis through a possibly extended period of chronic and debilitating illness, followed by inevitable but not always predictable disease progression, and eventually leading to the time when life-prolonging therapies are no longer desired or effective, and a transition to hospice care is appropriate.
- Careful study of the proposed options and evaluation of the potential impact of any proposed changes in the payment system will be needed to meet the challenge of finding the best solution not only for patients, families, health care providers, and organizations, but also for the American taxpayers who will subsidize the costs.

TAKE-HOME POINTS

- Palliative care is appropriate at any point in a serious illness. It is provided at the same time as curative and life-prolonging treatment. Palliative care does not require enrollment or benefit choice; there are no prognostic criteria, or choosing between treatment approaches.
- Hospice provides palliative care for those in the last weeks/months of life under the Federal Medicare Hospice Benefit. The patient must be certified as terminally ill with six months or less to live and must agree to give up Medicare coverage for curative or life-prolonging therapies.
- The current payment system for palliative care inside and out of hospice does not match the optimal continuum of care for patients with serious illness. One of the most pressing issues facing the field is how to improve the financing mechanisms for palliative care, thus improving access to the best possible care for patients with serious and chronic illnesses and their families.

REFERENCES

1. He W, Muenchrath MN. U.S. Census Bureau, American Community Survey Reports, *ACS-17, 90+ in the United States: 2006–2008*, U.S. Government Printing Office, Washington, DC, 2011.
2. Wolfe JL, Starfield B, Anderson G. Prevalence, expenditures, and complications of multiple chronic conditions in the elderly. *Arch Intern Med.* Nov 11, 2002;*162*(20):2269–2276.
3. Morrison RS, Meier DE. Palliative care. *N Engl J Med.* 2004;*350*(25):2582–2590.
4. Zerzan J, Stearns S, Hanson L. Access to palliative care and hospice in nursing homes. *JAMA.* Nov 15, 2000;*284*(19):2489–2494.
5. Carlson MD, Gallo WT, Bradley EH. Ownership status and patterns of care in hospice: Results from the National Home and Hospice Care Survey. *Med Care.* 2004;*42*:432–438.
6. U.S. Government Printing Office. Code of Federal Regulations 42CFR418.22, Certification of Terminal Illness 2002.
7. U.S. Government Printing Office. Code of Federal Regulations 42CFR418.24, Election of Hospice Care 2002.
8. Connor SR. Development of hospice and palliative care in the United States. *OMEGA.* 2007;*56*(1):89–99.
9. Brickner L, Scannell K, Marquet S, Ackerson L. Barriers to hospice care and referrals: survey of physicians' knowledge, attitudes, and perceptions in a health maintenance organization. *J Palliat Med.* Jun 2004;*7*(3):411–418.
10. Simpson DA. Prognostic criteria for hospice eligibility. *JAMA.* May 17, 2000;*283*(19):2527.
11. Fox E, Landrum-McNiff K, Zhong Z, Dawson NV, Wu AW, Lynn J. Evaluation of prognostic criteria for determining hospice eligibility in patients with advanced lung, heart, or liver disease. SUPPORT Investigators. Study to Understand Prognoses and Preferences for Outcomes and Risks of Treatments. *JAMA.* Nov 3, 1999;*282*(17):1638–1645.
12. Christakis N. *Death Foretold: Prophecy and Prognosis in Medical Care.* Chicago: University of Chicago Press; 1999.
13. Carlson MD, Morrison RS, Bradley EH. Improving access to hospice care: informing the debate. *J Palliat Med.* Apr 2008;*11*(3):438–443.

6

Ethical Decision-Making

INTRODUCTION

Ethics is the branch of philosophy concerned with standards of right and wrong that prescribe human behavior. These standards are usually framed in terms of rights, obligations, benefits to society, fairness, or specific virtues. The standards used to determine the appropriateness and desirability of human actions, behaviors, and practices are based on accepted ethical principles.

ETHICAL PRINCIPLES

- One of the basic questions that ethicists have debated throughout history is the source and validity of these ethical principles. Are they merely subjective recommendations that differ across societies and according to circumstances? Or are they universal values that do not vary across cultures, circumstances, or history?
- Whatever their position on how moral principles are derived, ethicists agree that two central questions inform all ethical theories:[1]
  1. What is the good for which we should strive, and what is the evil we would like to or must avoid?
  2. What is the proper or desired course of action, and what is the inappropriate or forbidden course of action?

MODERN MEDICAL ETHICS

- Ancient codes of ethics governing the practice of medicine were written by small groups of people, usually physicians. The Oath of Hippocrates is considered to be the first code to describe the proper relationship between the physician and patient.[1] In the mid-19th century, medical organizations began to formulate ethical standards for their members. The first formal code of professional medical ethics, outlining the rights of patients and care providers, was published by the American Medical Association (AMA) in 1847.

- Modern medical ethics began to develop as a separate and distinct field of inquiry, discussion, and debate in the 1950s, when fundamental ethical principles were applied to clinical practice situations and to the implementation of medical research. Since that time, the field of medical ethics has expanded dramatically. Ethics courses are now taught in all health care training programs. Research in medical ethics has grown exponentially, and health care journals now devote considerable space to discussion of ethical topics. The adoption of the term "biomedical" ethics indicates a broadening of the field to include ethical inquiry relating to all branches of knowledge about life and health.
- Several factors have contributed to the increased importance of medical ethics:[2]
  1. Technological and scientific advances in all fields of medicine, and the exponential growth of medical research with human subjects, have produced new ethical dilemmas and exacerbated old ones.
  2. The physician monopoly on decision-making has waned with the philosophical shift from paternalism to autonomy in the physician-patient relationship.
  3. Many additional groups are now deeply involved stakeholders in the health care environment, including various medical disciplines and health professionals, students and trainees, administrators, research scientists, and patient advocacy organizations. Each of these groups has its own cultural and professional value system, and the result is an increased intensity of ethical debate on a variety of health care topics.
  4. The public's involvement in the health care system, through the print media, Internet, social networking, courts, and legislatures, has redefined the parameters

of the relationship between society and the health care provider.

CLINICAL ETHICS

- Clinical ethics is the category of medical ethics that addresses the identification, analysis, and resolution of ethical questions arising during the course of delivering health care to patients and their families.[3] Four fundamental principles have been widely adopted as the basis for making ethical decisions in medicine:[4,5]
  1. Autonomy is the principle of self-governance or self-determination.
  2. Beneficence is the duty to do good and provide benefit.
  3. Nonmaleficence is the obligation to act in a manner that does not inflict harm on others.
  4. Justice refers to the duty to treat patients fairly, free of any bias and based on medical need.

ETHICAL DILEMMAS

- The question of what is in the patient's best interest can be complicated or even contentious, and a single, unanimously agreed-upon course of action often cannot be determined. The resulting stalemate is frequently based on an ethical dilemma. An ethical dilemma is a difficult problem that does not appear to have a satisfactory solution, or a situation involving a choice between equally unsatisfactory alternatives.
- There are two primary reasons that ethical dilemmas arise:[4]
  1. A "prima facie" or universally accepted principle is ethically binding unless there is conflict with another moral principle. In the event of divergence, a choice has to be made between the two competing principles.
  2. Because of the variations in time and place, as well as cultural, religious, and personal values, ethical principles may be applied or prioritized differently by different people, even when they are considering the same set of facts.

COMMON ETHICAL DILEMMAS IN GERIATRIC PALLIATIVE CARE[5,6]

- While all physicians encounter ethical dilemmas in their clinical practice, many unique factors can generate complex ethical questions in the field of geriatric palliative care. The treatments offered to older adults who face chronic illnesses are often expensive or risky, may have uncertain outcomes and burdensome side effects, or may not offer meaningful disease modification. When life-prolonging interventions cannot achieve cure, but do significantly reduce the patient's quality of life, discussions also arise about changing the focus of care from curative treatment to palliative care. Conditions that profoundly impair communication and cognitive function also pose questions of informed consent and surrogate decision-making for seriously ill older patients. Additional areas of ethical dilemma in geriatric palliative care include:
  - Maintaining patient confidentiality
  - Responding to requests for interventions that may not be effective, advisable, or safe
  - Honoring patient and family preferences for care
  - Withholding or withdrawing treatment in order to deliver medical care concordant with achievable patient and family goals
  - Unresolved family tensions and conflict over decision-making and establishing goals of care
  - Caring for patients who do have decisional capacity, but who make seemingly ill-advised or unsafe decisions about treatment, discharge planning options, or a preferred setting for their care

ETHICAL DECISION-MAKING

- Medical ethicists agree that health care professionals have a moral and legal obligation to act for the patient's good. A key role of the health care team is therefore to try to avoid situations where ethical dilemmas can negatively impact patient care. Clear, effective communication between providers and patients and families is the key to avoiding potential scenarios where ethical principles could result in conflict. Carefully exploring and respecting ethnic, cultural, and religious values is essential in these discussions.

- Resolving ethical dilemmas when they do arise is an important skill for the palliative care clinician to master. Even with clear communication, situations involving ethically based conflict and disagreement can develop between a patient and family members, or a between the patient and the health care team, or one or more clinicians involved in the patient's care. (See Chapter 10: Managing Conflict.)
- Ideally, the ethical questions can be identified and resolved without too much difficulty. The relative merits of alternative actions should be considered and weighed by the patient, family, and health care team in structured and facilitated discussions. A choice will then be made based on the relevant ethical principles and consideration of the context in which the decision is being made. (See Chapter 9: Communication Skills.)
- Navigating an ethically complicated decision-making scenario can be a challenge to even the most experienced clinicians. Multiple clinical facts must be analyzed, patient and family goals and preferences must be considered, and the concerns of involved colleagues and interdisciplinary team members must be acknowledged.

THE FOUR TOPICS APPROACH

The "Four Topics" framework provides a systematic approach for successfully resolving an ethically complicated clinical question.[7,8] This method offers a protocol for sorting through and analyzing the facts of a clinical scenario (medical indications, patient preferences, quality of life considerations, and contextual features), and then connecting these circumstances to the relevant underlying ethical principle(s) (i.e. autonomy, beneficence, nonmaleficence, and justice). The four topics and the specific questions to be considered for each topic are as follows:

1. **Gathering the Clinical Information**
   - What is the patient's medical problem? History? Diagnosis? Prognosis?
   - Is the problem acute? Chronic? Critical? Emergent? Reversible?
   - What are the goals of the treatment and care?
   - What are the probabilities of successful outcome?

- What are the plans in case of therapeutic failure or if the goals of treatment are not achieved?
   - In sum, will medical and nursing care benefit the patient and will harm be avoided?

2. **Identifying Patient and Family Preferences**
   - What has the patient expressed about preferences for treatment?
   - Has the patient been informed of benefits and risks, understood this information, and given consent?
   - Does the patient have decisional capacity? What is evidence of incapacity?
   - Has the patient expressed prior preferences (e.g., advance directives)?
   - How does the patient want to include family or friends in the decision-making process?
   - If the patient lacks decisional capacity, who is the appropriate surrogate? Is the surrogate using appropriate standards?
   - Is the patient unwilling or unable to cooperate with medical treatment? If so, why?
   - Are there family issues that might influence treatment decisions?
   - In sum, is the patient's right to choose being respected to the extent possible in ethics and law?

3. **Evaluating Quality-of-Life Issues**
   - What are the prospects, with or without treatment, for the patient to return to a level of functional health he or she would deem acceptable?
   - What biases might prejudice provider evaluations of the patient's quality of life (e.g., whose definition of quality of life is being used as the basis for discussion used)?
   - What physical, mental, and social deficits is the patient likely to experience if treatment succeeds?
   - Is the patient's present or future condition such that, if it continues, he or she might judge life undesirable?
   - Is there any plan and rationale to forgo treatment?
   - What are the plans for comfort and palliative care?

4. **Considering Contextual Factors**
   - Are there provider (physician, nurse, etc.) issues that might influence treatment decisions?

- Are there financial and economic factors?
- Are there religious or cultural factors?
- Is there any justification for breaching confidentiality?
- Are there resource allocation problems?
- What are the legal implications of treatment decisions?
- Is clinical research or teaching involved?
- Is there any provider or institutional conflict of interest?

After using the Four Topics method to collect and analyze all the relevant information, the clinician should attempt to distill the identified ethical dilemma into one or two key questions that can be used to address the ethical issues, arrive at a decision that is agreeable to all parties, and then create a plan of care based on the resolution. (See Chapter 78: End-Stage Renal Disease for a clinical case illustration of decision-making using the Four Topics method.)

MANAGING UNRESOLVED ETHICAL CONFLICT

When health care providers cannot agree with or support a patient/family decision that appears unreasonable, unsafe, illegal, or futile, a situation of moral distress is created.

Options to resolve such an impasse include:

- Continue to pursue reasonable efforts at rational discussion and persuasion.
- Request an ethics consultation. Evidence for the effectiveness of consultation with a hospital ethics committee has not been clearly established; however, there may be value in the process when two or more ethical principles are in conflict. Many hospitals have ethics committees that are staffed by professionals with training in bioethics who come from a range of health care disciplines. While the recommendations of these committees are rarely legally binding, an ethics consultation may be an effective forum that facilitates conflict resolution.
- If all other options to resolve the conflict are unsuccessful, the provider-patient relationship can be dissolved and arrangements made for an orderly transfer of patient care to a provider who can meet the patient/family needs.

TAKE-HOME POINTS

- Ethics is the branch of philosophy concerned with standards of right and wrong that govern human behavior. These standards are usually framed in terms of rights, obligations, benefits to society, fairness, or specific virtues.
- Clinical ethics is concerned with the identification, analysis, and resolution of ethical questions that arise during the course of delivering health care to patients and their families. Four fundamental principles have been widely adopted as the basis for making ethical decisions in medicine: autonomy, beneficence, nonmaleficence, and justice.
- Many factors combine to generate ethical dilemmas in the field of geriatric palliative care, including questions of informed consent and surrogate decision-making, modifying the focus of care from curative treatment to palliative care, responding to requests for interventions that may not be effective, honoring patient and family preferences for care, and unresolved family tensions and conflict over decision-making and establishing goals of care.
- An ethically complicated decision-making scenario can be challenging, even to experienced clinicians. The "Four Topics" framework provides a systematic approach for successfully resolving ethically complicated clinical questions.
- When the health care providers cannot support a patient/family decision that may appear unreasonable, unsafe, illegal or futile, the options to resolve such an impasse include continuing efforts at rational discussion and persuasion, requesting an ethics consultation, or dissolving the provider-patient relationship and arranging for an orderly transfer of patient care to a provider who can meet the patient/family needs.

RESOURCES

Current professional codes of ethics for selected health care disciplines may be reviewed on the following Internet sites:

National Association of Social Workers
http://www.socialworkers.org/pubs/code/code.asp

American Pharmacists Association
http://www.pharmacist.com/code-ethics

American Nursing Association
http://ana.nursingworld.org/
MainMenuCategories/EthicsStandards

American Medical Association
http://www.ama-assn.org/ama/pub/
category/2512.html

REFERENCES

1. Steinberg A. Secular ethics. *Encyclopedia of Jewish Medical Ethics*. 2003; Vol *II*:389–404. Feldheim Publishers (English edition).
2. Steinbereg A. The foundation and the development of modern medical ethics. *Journal of Assisted Reproduction and Genetics*. 1995; *12*(8):473–476.
3. Jonsen AR, Siegler M, Winslade WJ. *Clinical Ethics*. 5th ed. New York, NY: McGraw-Hill; 1998.
4. Beauchamp TL, Childress JF. *Principles of Biomedical Ethics*. 4th ed. New York, NY: Oxford University Press; 1994.
5. Gillon R. Medical ethics: four principles plus attention to scope. *BMJ*. 1994;*309*:184–88.
6. Mueller PS, Hook CC, Fleming KC. Ethical issues in geriatrics: a guide for clinicians. *Mayo Clin Proc*. 2004;*79*:554–562.
7. Bottrell MM, Cassel CK, Felzenberg ER. Ethical and policy issues in end-of-life care in Geriatric Medicine; an evidence based approach. Cassel CK (ed). Springer-Verlag New York, Inc; 4th ed. 2003.
8. Schumann JH, Alfandre D. Clinical ethical decision making: the four topics approach. *Semin Med Pract*, 2008;*11*:36–42.

7

Prognostication

INTRODUCTION

Prognostication can be defined as "a prediction of future medical outcomes of a treatment or a disease course based on medical knowledge."[1] Prognosticating involves two essential skills:[2]

- Foreseeing, or formulating the prediction
- Foretelling, or communicating the prediction

The incidence of chronic end-organ disease is increasing as a consequence of the aging of the population and the advances in life-sustaining technologies. An understanding of nonmalignant disease trajectories, end-stage indicators, and treatment needs at each stage of disease is vital to providing comprehensive and medically appropriate care for seriously ill patients.

WHY IS MEDICAL PROGNOSTICATION IMPORTANT?

- Patients and families often base decisions about treatment and advance care planning on their perception of prognoses, e.g., decisions regarding code status.
- Prognosis guides health care providers in the development of appropriate treatment plans for their patients, e.g., recommendation of health maintenance screening, or continuing disease-modifying care options.
- Establishing a prognosis can enable access to comprehensive services, e.g., home hospice.
- Prognostic information provides patients and families with information about the future, allowing them the opportunity to set their own goals and individualized priorities, e.g., plan for future care, advise friends and other family members about expected course of a serious illness, get financial affairs in order, say goodbye, etc.

PATIENTS AND FAMILIES WANT TO KNOW THE PROGNOSIS

- The majority of patients and family members want to be informed about prognostic information, regardless of whether it is good or bad.[2,3]
- In a multicenter, prospective, longitudinal cohort study, conversations about prognosis were associated with improved quality of life for patients near the end of life. Lack of such discussions was associated with aggressive hospital care in the last weeks of life, increased rates of major depression and post-traumatic stress disorder among bereaved caregivers, and diminished patient quality of life.[4]

FORMULATING A PROGNOSIS

- Clinicians also formulate a prognosis through knowledge of disease trajectories, identification of end-stage indicators, and assessment of symptom and care needs of older adults at each stage of chronic disease progression (Table 7.2).
- Table 7.1 describes hospice prognostic criteria and also identifies validated prognostic models for some common end-organ diseases.

COMMUNICATING PROGNOSIS

- Honoring patient goals of care and matching treatment preferences with medical care are core principals of geriatric and palliative medicine that are essential for the provision of high quality medical care.
- Prognostic information is the framework required for informed decision-making regarding medical treatment options and advance care planning. Patients and their family members often base their treatment decisions on their understanding of the prognosis. These perceptions of prognosis are in turn often guided by

TABLE 7.1: PROGNOSTIC MODELS FOR SELECTED END-ORGAN DISEASES

Diagnosis	Hospice Criteria for Determining Diagnoses of 6 Months or Less[5]	Other Helpful Prognostic Models
Congestive Heart Failure	*Primary Factors*: NYHA Class IV, and patient care medically optimized *Secondary Factors*: Decreased ejection fraction, symptoms in the setting of an underlying arrhythmia, prior cardiac arrest, comorbid HIV disease, stroke of cardiac origin, syncope of unknown etiology	**Seattle Heart Failure Model**: a validated prediction model that estimates survival for out-patients with heart failure [6] Incorporates basic demographic and clinical information to provide short- and long-term survival predictions Easily accessible at http://depts.washington.edu/shfm Provides survival estimates and illustrates differences in prognosis with and/or without the addition of medical and/or surgical interventions **Note**: Does not take comorbidities into account when formulating survival predictions; was validated in an ambulatory population and may not be generalizable to hospitalized patients
COPD	*Primary Factors*: Dyspnea at rest, increasing hospital utilization for respiratory distress or pulmonary related infections, hypoxemia at rest on supplemental oxygen (oxygen saturation of $\leq 88\%$) OR hypercapnia (pCO2 50 mmHg) *Secondary Factors:* unintentional weight loss, resting tachycardia in patients with advanced COPD, right-sided heart failure as a sequelae of advanced pulmonary disease, or FEV1 < 30% of predicted for normal patients	**Bode Index**: a validated grading scale that predicts mortality in patients with COPD[7] Based on the degree of airflow obstruction, body mass index, exercise capacity, and functional dyspnea Greater predictive capability than FEV_1 alone for formulating mortality risk assessments Was recently updated in an effort to improve its calibration[8] Index available at: http://www.eperc.mcw.edu[9] See also Fast Facts #141: Prognosis in End-Stage COPD
Liver Failure	Advance grade cirrhosis and not eligible for liver transplantation Coagulopathy as evidenced by Prothrombin time > 5 sec over control, or INR > 1.5 Serum albumin < 2.5 g/dL At least one of the following complications: ascites despite treatment, spontaneous bacterial peritonitis, hepatorenal syndrome, hepatic encephalopathy, recurrent variceal bleed	**Model for end stage liver disease (MELD):** a prognostic scoring system that has been validated in patients with ESLD[10] Due to its precision in assessing mortality estimates, MELD plays a large role in determining liver transplant distribution Calculation of the MELD score is based upon three easily obtainable laboratory variables: bilirubin, INR, and creatinine Well validated for predicting short- and long-term survival Online MELD calculator available at: http://www.mdcalc.com[11]
Dementia	FAST (Functional Assessment Staging) $\geq$ Stage 7–C: dependent in walking, dressing and bathing, urinary and fecal incontinence, incapable of speaking greater than 6 intelligible words/day Severe dementia-related complications in the past 6 months: aspiration pneumonia, septicemia, multiple stage 3–4 decubiti, fever despite recent antibiotic course Decreased caloric and fluid intake in the setting of a feeding tube; serum albumin < 2.5 gm/dl or weight loss > 10% in the past 6 months	**The Mortality Risk Index**: a model that estimates short-term mortality rates for nursing home residents who have advanced grade dementia[12] Total scale based on 12 risk factors easily obtainable from the Minimum Data Set (MDS) Validated in a cohort of >11,000 nursing home residents with advanced grade dementia who were recently admitted MRI has greater 6-month predictive value than the FAST 7-C

(continued)

TABLE 7.1: (CONTINUED)

Diagnosis	Hospice Criteria for Determining Diagnoses of 6 Months or Less[5]	Other Helpful Prognostic Models
Kidney Disease	*Primary factors:* Chronic renal insufficiency and forgoing dialysis or opting for the withdrawal of dialysis Creatinine clearance < 10 cc/min and creatinine >8.0 mg/dL Symptoms associated with advanced renal failure: uremia, treatment refractory fluid overload or hyperkalemia, uremic pericarditis, hepatorenal syndrome *Secondary factors:* advanced age, cachexia or low serum albumin, coagulopathies	**The Modified Charlson Comorbidity Index**: a prognostic scoring system based on age and comorbidities[13] Can be used to predict prognoses in individuals who are receiving dialysis Patients are characterized into one of four groups based on their index score. Patients with a score of ≥ 8 have a predicted 1-year mortality rate of approximately 50% Index available at: http://www.eperc.mcw.edu[14] See also Fast Facts 191: Prognostication in Patients Receiving Dialysis

patients' impressions of their physicians' recommendations for or against treatment.[4]

- Once a prognosis is developed, the clinician should then begin a dialogue with patients and/or their appointed health care decision-makers about appropriate care options based on the trajectory of illness (Table 7.2). Examples of statements that communicate prognosis to a patient or a family member include:
  - "From my clinical experience, and given your advanced stage of disease, it is likely that you will live several months to possibly a year."
  - "Given your father's functional status and likely disease course, his time is limited and is best measured in weeks to months..."
- If an overly optimistic picture of underlying prognosis is given or implied, patients and family members naturally assume that their physician's treatment recommendations will be effective, even when physicians and care teams may be aware that a proposed treatment plan will provide minimum benefit given the expected course of the underlying disease.
- Realistic prognostic information offers patients and their families the opportunity to work collaboratively with their medical teams to formulate appropriate and feasible care plans that best meet the needs and goals of the patient.
- Before realistic prognostic information is conveyed, however, clinicians should

ask patients and or family members what information they want to know and who should receive the information.

FUNCTIONAL STATUS AND PROGNOSIS

- Performance or functional status is a factor that reliably correlates with prognosis, especially in cancer.[17] In the oncological literature, the Karnofsky Performance Scale, the ECOG (Eastern Cooperative Oncology Group), and the Palliative Performance Scale (PPS) have all been found to predict survival and serve as a basis for determining patients' eligibility for oncological treatments.
- In the geriatric literature, functional status as determined by one's ability to perform activities of daily living and/or instrumental activities of daily living has been shown to correlate directly with future functional decline and transition to a nursing facility as well as to mortality.[18,19,20]
- Multiple studies have illustrated that functional deconditioning during acute illnesses is a strong predictor of mortality.[21,22] Functional status should therefore be evaluated routinely and weighed as an important factor in a clinician's overall assessment of an older adult's underlying prognosis.

TAKE-HOME POINTS

- Prognostication is vital to providing comprehensive and medically appropriate care for seriously ill patients.

TABLE 7.2: COMMUNICATING PROGNOSIS BASED THE TRAJECTORY OF ILLNESS

Prognosis	Suggested Next Steps for the Health Care Provider[15]
Years	Begin discussion of patient's overall goals of care, values, beliefs, and preferences in the context of the patient's diagnosis, expected prognosis, and expected illness trajectory
	Encourage completion of advance directives—particularly the assignment of a health care proxy
	Consider recommending that the patient meet with a lawyer who specializes in elder law to assist with financial and/or insurance matters
	Become familiar with other individuals and groups who form the patient's social network and who are or can be providers of care over the course of the patient's illness
Months	Review patient's understanding of prognosis and overall expected course of illness
	Review advance directives and ensure that medical goals are up to date
	Assess family caregiver burden and family's need for information about what to expect
	Discuss the option of hospice care. The EPERC fast fact guide on discussing hospice provides a helpful template for clinicians. The patient's goals of care and understanding of illness are woven into an introduction of the benefits of hospice support services.[16] http://www.eperc.mcw.edu
Weeks	Reassess goals of care
	Discuss hospice if not previously referred
	Assess family caregiver burden and family's need for information about what to expect
	Provide ongoing pain and symptom assessment and communications regarding disease progression
	Reevaluate the benefit-to-burden ratio of treatment plan
Days	Discuss the expected signs and symptoms of the dying process
	If hospice is not involved, ensure that family has 24/7 access to care provider
	Assess family caregiver burden and family's need for information about what to expect
	Encourage visits from family members and friends
	Provide psychosocial and bereavement support
	Prepare family for the time of death: what to do, whom to contact
	Screen for complicated grief among family and friends

- Prognosis is formulated through knowledge of disease trajectories, identification of end-stage indicators, and assessment of symptom and care needs of the patient and family at each stage of chronic disease progression.
- The majority of patients and family members want to know prognostic information, regardless of whether it is good or bad.
- Prognostic information is the framework required for informed decision-making regarding medical treatment options and advance care planning.

REFERENCES

1. Li JMW, Feinbloom D. Evidence-Based Prognostication for Medscape Internal Medicine. Based on the Society of Hospital Medicine Annual Meeting Presentation quoted by Sinclair, C., 2007.

2. Christakis N. *Death Foretold: Prophecy and Prognosis in Medical Care*. University of Chicago Press: Chicago; 1999.

3. Steinhauser KE, Christakis NA, Clipp EC, et al. Factors considered important at the end of life by patients, family, physicians, and other care providers. *JAMA*. 2000;*284*:2476–2482.

4. Wright A, Zhang MS, Ray A, et al. Associations between end-of-life discussions, patient mental health, medical care near death, and caregiver bereavement adjustment. *JAMA*. 2008;*300*: 1665–1673.

5. Storey P, Knight CF, Schonwetter RS. *Summary of the National Hospice & Palliative Care Organization's Guidelines for Determining Prognosis of 6 Months or Less: Pocket Guide to Hospice/Palliative Medicine*, American Academy of Hospice and Palliative Medicine, 2003. Glenview, IL.

6. Levy WC. The Seattle Heart Failure Model: prediction of survival in heart failure. *Circulation*. 2006;*113*(11):1424–1433.

7. Celli BR, Cote CG, Marin JM, et al. The body-mass index, airflow obstruction, dyspnea, and exercise capacity index in chronic obstructive pulmonary disease. *N Engl J Med.* 2004;4(350):1005–1012.

8. Puhan MA, Garcia-Aymerich J, Riet G, et al. Expansion of the prognostic assessment of patients with chronic obstructive pulmonary disease: the updated BODE index and the ADO index. *The Lancet.* 2009;373:9691.

9. Childers JW, Arnold R, Curtis JR. Fast Facts #141: Prognosis in End-Stage COPD; April, 2009. End-of-Life Physician Education Resource Center. http://www.eperc.mcw.edu.

10. Kamouth P. A model to predict survival in patients with end stage liver disease. *Hepatology.* 2001;33(2):464–470.

11. http://www.mdcalc.com

12. Mitchell SL et al. Estimating prognosis for nursing home residents with advanced dementia. *JAMA.* 2004;291:2734–2740.

13. Beddhu S, Bruns FJ, Saul M, Seddon P, Zeidel ML. A simple co-morbidity scale predicts clinical outcomes and costs in dialysis patients. *Am J Med.* 2000;108:609–613.

14. Hudson M, Weisbord S, Arnold R. Fast Facts# 191: Prognostication in Patients Receiving Dialysis; May 2009. End-of-Life Physician Education Resource Center. http://www.eperc.mcw.edu.

15. Morrison RS, Meier DE. Palliative care. *N Engl J Med.* 2004;25(350):2582–2590.

16. von Gunten CF, Ferris F, Weissman DE. Fast Facts and Concepts #38: Discussing Hospice; April, 2001. End-of-Life Physician Education Resource Center. http://www.eperc.mcw.edu.

17. Glare P, Christakis N. Predicting survival in patients with advanced disease. Section 2.4. In: Doyle D, Hanks G, Cherney N, Calman K, eds. *Oxford Textbook of Palliative Medicine.* 3rd ed. Oxford University Press; 2005:29–42. New York.

18. Walter LC, Brand RJ, Counsell SR, et al. Development and validation of a prognostic index for 1-Year mortality in older adults after hospitalization. *JAMA.* 2001;285(23):2987–2994.

19. Reuben DB, Rubenstein LV, Hirsch SH, Hays RD. Value of functional status as a predictor of mortality: Results of a Prospective Study. *Am J Med.* 1992;93:663–669.

20. Gaugler JE, Duval S, Anderson KA, Kane RL. Predicting nursing home admission in the U.S: a meta-Analysis. *BMC Geriatrics.* 2007;7:13.

21. Baztán JJ, Gálvez CP, Socorro A. Recovery of functional impairment after acute illness and mortality: One-year follow-up study. *Gerontology.* 2009;55:269–274.

22. Sleiman I, Rozzini R, Barbisoni P, Morandi A, Ricci A, Giordano A, Trabucchi M. Functional trajectories during hospitalization: A prognostic sign for elderly patients. *J Gerontol A Biol Sci Med Sci.* 2009;64(6):659–663.

8

Advance Care Planning

INTRODUCTION

Advance care planning (ACP) allows individuals to specify how they want to be treated should serious illness or injury leave them without the capacity to make decisions or communicate.[1] Advance care planning should not be viewed as a single event in an individual's life. Rather, it is a process that should take place over time and should then be revisited frequently, especially if there are changes in health status or goals of care.

A PLANNING FRAMEWORK

Research data shows that when the appropriate process is followed, care plans can be created and made available to providers that are specific enough to assist with clinical decision-making, even as the patient moves to different care settings.[2] While the trajectory of advance care planning should be tailored to the specific needs of patients and families, the following steps provide a helpful framework:

1. Exploration of values, priorities, preferences, what gives meaning to one's life, and discussions about what constitutes an acceptable quality of life.
2. Identification of personal goals of care in the event of a severe illness, and discussions of different treatment options in the context of these goals. Specific personal preferences typically explored during advance care planning may include these topics:[3]
   - Future hospitalizations
   - Hospice/home care preferences
   - Resuscitation
   - Goals and expectations for comfort and symptom management
   - Spiritual support options
   - Life-sustaining treatments at the end of life, e.g., ventilator support, artificial hydration, and nutrition
3. Naming a trusted person as proxy or surrogate decision-maker to help medical providers apply overarching care goals to specific clinical situations in the event that the patient loses decisional capacity.
4. Translating the individual's expressed care preferences into an advance directive document (e.g., Health Care Proxy or Living Will).
5. Health care providers are made aware of existence of ACP documents; written plans are stored and retrievable.
6. Advance care plans are updated and should become more specific in the event of a change in health status or modification of goals for care.

EXPLORING PREFERENCES AND ESTABLISHING GOALS FOR CARE

- Advance care planning can be discussed in the outpatient setting, where the main focus should be on identifying "big picture" goals and preferences in the context of a hypothetical life-limiting illness, or in the hospital setting, when the patient may be facing a serious and potentially life-threatening illness.
- In the outpatient setting, appointing a health care proxy may be just the first step of a broader dialogue with the patient about preferences and goals for care. The advance care planning process should then proceed incrementally, with multiple conversations over a period of weeks or months. Discussing specific interventions may not be worthwhile at this time because future decisions will vary according to the clinical context. For example, short-term artificial nutrition and hydration or mechanical ventilation during a hospital admission may be acceptable during recovery from surgery, but as long-term

interventions after discharge, they may not be consistent with patient goals for care.

- When a patient is in the hospital, the clinician may have to approach the advance care planning discussion with a narrower focus. In the event of serious illness, for example, discussions offer a framework for exploring patient's current life goals and preferences, and how these might evolve in the event of changing clinical realities. Determining the patient's personal preferences for comfort, symptom management, and code status should be a priority.

- Planning for both in- and out-patient settings will employ the same ACP tools and documents (such as a health care proxy, living will, etc.). The language recommended for both types of advanced planning discussions will be similar (Table 8.1).

DOCUMENTING PREFERENCES FOR CARE

An Advance Directive (AD) is a statement that describes a patient's preferences for medical treatment and care if he/she is unable to express these wishes and preferences due to a serious illness or injury.

- Advance directives are essential to the delivery of quality health care. Regulatory bodies such as the Joint Commission now require hospitals to:
  - Ask individuals at the time of admission if they have an advance directive
  - Provide every patient with a written summary of the patient's health care decision-making rights and the institution's policies with respect to ADs
  - Provide education to staff and the community about ADs

- Advance care planning and documentation helps to:
  - Identify, respect, and implement patients' wishes about their care, especially as they approach the end of life
  - Improve care from the patients' and families' points of view[4]
  - Reduce the incidence of stress, anxiety, and depression in surviving family members[5]

- Giving expression to care preferences can be informal, for example, a verbal expression of preferences to a family member, friend, or physician. It is preferable, however, to create formal advance directive documents that are signed in presence of a witness or notary. Advance directives generally fall into two broad categories, as shown in Table 8.2:

1. Designation of a proxy decision maker; that is, drawing up a durable power of attorney for health care, or appointing a health care proxy (HCP).
2. Instructional directives: i.e., creating a living will (LW) or completing the Five Wishes document.

IMPORTANT ADVANCE CARE PLANNING ISSUES

1. **Living will versus appointing health care agent:** The scenarios described in a living will often do not correspond with the clinical events and circumstances that may arise during the course of a serious illness or at the end of life. A health care agent or proxy can analyze, interpret, and respond to the actual facts and variables when a health care decision has to be made. Hence, appointment of an agent is both more important and more useful than completion of a LW.

2. **Communicating preferences:** Designating a health care agent does not constitute adequate advance care planning. The agent must also be informed about and familiar with the patient's wishes for care. Several initiatives to promote the use of ADs have employed trained facilitators to help ensure a comprehensive dialogue between patients and their health care agents and family members.[6]

3. **Barriers to advance care planning:** Helping patients discuss, select, and document health care preferences in advance is an important part of the clinician's professional responsibility. Obstacles that can interfere with this planning process include:
   - Patients and families may be reluctant to address difficult or frightening health care issues.
   - Comprehensive advance care planning involves conversations between physician and patient or proxy that can be time-consuming and may also be non-reimbursable.
   - Providers may also lack the expert communication skills required for

TABLE 8.1: HELPFUL LANGUAGE FOR ADVANCE CARE PLANNING DISCUSSIONS

	Outpatient Setting	Inpatient Setting
Starting the conversation	*"I would like to talk to you about another aspect of your care—advance care planning. These conversations are part of my routine with all my patients."* *"ACP will help your doctors and your family understand how to focus your medical care in case you lose the ability to make these decisions."*	*"I would like to talk with you about how we should plan for your care from now on."* *"Knowing the time is short, I would like to discuss your goals regarding your care."*
Assessing patient goals	*"Have you had any previous experience with making decisions about medical care during a serious illness? Please tell me about that experience."* *"You might have heard public discussion or debate in the media about keeping very sick people alive by artificial means. Have you thought about this issue?"* *"If you were weeks away from death, how would you like to spend your last days?"* [Examples of potential goals in the event of a life-limiting illness: Cure Prolong life See a family milestone Taking a family trip]	*"Can you help me understand what is most important to you at this time?"* [Examples of potential goals in the event of a diagnosis of life-threatening illness: Symptom management Comfort Staying in control Receiving care at home] *"Can you tell me about your greatest hopes and fears?"* *"Are there any important goals or tasks left undone?"* *"How do you picture your death?"*
Translating goals into a care plan	*"You have told me that if you are not able to recover sufficiently to recognize and interact with your family, you would not want to be fed artificially. If am understanding your preference correctly, I will document them in the chart."*	*"Given what you have told me about your wish to die peacefully and naturally, if you agree, I will document that and I will write an order in the chart that when you die, no attempt will be made to restore your heartbeat. Is this acceptable to you?"*
Identifying the preferred surrogate decision-maker	*"Who do you count on for support?"* *"Is there someone that you trust to be involved in making medical decisions on your behalf, if you are not able to do so? For example, family member, a friend, and religious or spiritual adviser?"*	*"Who should make medical decisions for you in case you are not able to do so?"* *"I understand that your daughter is the person you trust most to make medical decisions in case you are not able to do so. If you agree, I will fill out an HCP and ask you to sign the form."*
Documenting the advance care planning discussion	Complete appropriate forms, i.e., health care proxy, living will Document all previous discussions leading to the ACP in the patient's chart	Complete appropriate forms (i.e., health care proxy) and Physician Orders for Life-Sustaining Treatment (POLST) Issue the appropriate orders (i.e., DNR) Communicate with family and caregivers Communicate with other members of the patient's care team Document all previous discussions supporting the ADs in the patient's chart

TABLE 8.2: ADVANCE DIRECTIVE DOCUMENTATION

Advance Directive	Definition	Characteristics	Advantages	Limitations
Health Care Proxy (HCP) Durable Power of Attorney for Health Care	A document in which an individual with decisional capacity appoints another trusted person to make medical decisions regarding treatment and care in the event of future loss of decisional capacity	The designated HCP has the same legal right to request or refuse treatment that the person would have if still capable of making health care decisions. The HCP is a person trusted to make medical decisions on a patient's behalf, e.g., family member, close friend, attorney The HCP cannot be a health professional involved in the patient's care because of potential for ethical conflict	Permits application of patient values to the particular clinical situation Can be changed by a patient with decisional capacity	HCP may distort or misinterpret patient wishes in a specific clinical situation Not portable across states HCP may not be available when needed Requires MD cooperation to translate goals and preferences into actual treatment plans
Living Will (LW)	A written document created to inform health care providers and caregivers of an individual's preferences about the course of treatment and care that is to be followed in the event he or she loses decisional capacity	In most cases, living wills express preferences concerning various medical treatments, e.g., artificial hydration and nutrition. More detailed living wills may include an individual's wishes for analgesia (pain relief), antibiotics, hydration, feeding, and the use of ventilators or cardiopulmonary resuscitation. A LW is limited to medical decisions only.	Completed ahead of time Represents "patient's voice" Can be changed by a patient with decisional capacity	Impossible to anticipate in advance every clinical situation that should be addressed Decisions are made based on interpretation of a document, rather than discussion of treatment options with a person acting on behalf of patient Not portable across states Document may not be available Requires MD translation into actual medical orders
The Five Wishes	Document that combines aspects of health care proxy and a living will; also addresses matters of comfort and spirituality at the end of life	Document first developed in Florida, with funding from the Robert Wood Johnson Foundation, then adopted by 40 states Requires two witnesses; some states require notarization of the signature of the patient and/or witnesses	Communicates wishes for medical care, but also addresses spiritual, emotional, and existential issues	Does not meet the legal requirements in some states, e.g., California, Connecticut, Delaware, Georgia, New York, North Dakota, South Carolina, Vermont, Wisconsin, Michigan, and District of Columbia In these states, the Five Wishes can be used as an attachment to the state's required forms. Portability Availability

discussions of prognosis, disease trajectory over time, and possibly limited options for care.

4. **Availability across care settings:** Completed advance care directives are of little value if the health provider is not aware that a directive exists, or if the directive is not made available when a patient is admitted to the hospital. Most importantly, the directive must be translated by health care providers into documented medical orders consistent with the patient's preferences and goals for care.

5. **Portability:** Many states have different requirements about medical decision-making. Because some states may not honor directives from another state, it is important to execute ADs that comply with law of the state where patient resides.

ALIGNING MEDICAL ORDERS WITH ADVANCE DIRECTIVES

- When death would not be unexpected, it is essential to convert patient preferences into specific medical orders that are documented and that will be honored across different care settings.
- The POLST paradigm (Physician Orders for Life-Sustaining Treatment) is a coordinated system for eliciting, documenting, and communicating the life-sustaining treatment wishes of seriously ill patients (Table 8.3).

TAKE-HOME POINTS

- Advance care planning is a process that ideally should take place over time and should then be revisited frequently when changes in health status or goals of care may occur.
- Advance directives become applicable only if a patient loses the capacity to express his/her preferences regarding medical treatment and care. If the patient recovers decisional capacity, advance directives are no longer in force.
- The preferences addressed in advance directives usually concern the appointment of a health care agent and identifying goals for treatment near the end of life, when patients often lose decisional capacity due to serious illness.

TABLE 8.3: POLST PARADIGM

Document	Definition	Characteristics	Advantages	Limitations
Physician Orders for Life-Sustaining Treatments (POLST) Paradigm[7,8]	"POLST Paradigm" describes a set of medical orders, developed on a state-or community-wide basis, having different program names, forms, and policies in different locales. Printed on distinctive, brightly colored paper meant to be easily identifiable to all health care providers, and portable across care settings	These documents contain actionable medical orders that provide explicit instructions about medical interventions at the end of life. Directions are given regarding CPR, artificial nutrition and hydration, and other life-sustaining treatments. Endorsing states include New York, California, Pennsylvania, Washington, West Virginia, and Wisconsin. Each has a state-specific form.	Provides explicit instructions to be used directly as medical orders State-wide, uniform physician order designed to be transported with patient from one residential or medical setting to another Honored by emergency responders in the community Can be modified or revoked based on new information or changes in patient's preferences or prognosis	Only for patients with prognosis of less than 1 year Must be completed and signed by a state-licensed physician or nurse practitioner Portability Availability

- Ensuring that the patient designates a health care agent does not constitute adequate advance care planning. The decision-maker must be fully informed and familiar with the patient's wishes for care.
- In the outpatient setting, advance care planning may consist of multiple conversations over a period of weeks or months. During a hospital admission, however, the clinician may have to approach the advance care planning discussion with a narrower focus, i.e., exploring the patient's goals and preferences in the context of serious illness.
- To ensure that care is aligned with a patient's goals and preferences, advance care directives must be translated by health care providers into documented medical orders that will be available across all care settings.

REFERENCES

1. Field MJ, Cassel CK (eds). *Approaching Death: Improving Care at the End of Life*. Washington, DC: National Academies Press; 1997:198.
2. Hammes BJ, Rooney BL, Gundrum JD. A comparative, retrospective, observational study of the prevalence, availability, and specificity of advance care plans in a county that implemented an advance care planning microsystem. *JAGS*. 2010;58:1249–1255.
3. Caring Connections. http://www.caringinfo.org/i4a/pages/index.cfm?pageid=3277. Accessed January 29, 2012.
4. Kass-Bartelmes BL, Hughes R, Rutherford MK. *Advance care planning: preferences for care at the end of life*. Rockville (MD): Agency for Healthcare Research and Quality; 2003. Research in Action Issue #12 AHRQ Pub No. 03-0018.
5. Detering KM, Hancock AD, Reade MC, Silvester W. The impact of advance care planning on end of life care in elderly patients: randomized controlled trial. *BMJ*. Mar 23, 2010;340:c1345.
6. Schwartz CE, Wheeler HB, Hammes B, et al. Early intervention in planning end-of-life care with ambulatory geriatric patients. *Arch Intern Med*. 2012;162:1611–1618.
7. Citko J, Moss AH, Carley M, Toll S. The National POLST Paradigm initiative. *Journal of Palliative Medicine*. 2011;14(2):241–242.
8. Physician Orders for Life-Sustaining Treatment (POLST) Paradigm. http://www.ohsu.edu/polst/, Accessed February 6, 2012.

9

Communication Skills

INTRODUCTION

Geriatric palliative care clinicians have multiple daily encounters requiring communication about very complex issues. Mastering key communication skills will help all health care providers to improve patient care by:

- Building trust between provider and patient and family
- Determining information needs of patient and family
- Eliciting patient and family care requirements
- Obtaining properly informed consent
- Enhancing collaborative process of establishing goals of care
- Facilitating realistic decision-making
- Navigating difficult conversations
- Effectively interacting with colleagues including referring physicians, other consultants, and other members of the interdisciplinary team

CONSEQUENCES OF POOR COMMUNICATION

The risks of ineffective communication are grave. Small misunderstandings can lead to bigger problems if not appropriately corrected. Consequences of poor communication include:

- Lack of trust between provider and patient and family
- Misconceptions or misunderstandings by patient and family about diagnosis, treatment, and prognosis
- Decisions regarding goals of care that are based on incorrect information or misperceptions
- Medical errors
- Litigation

CHALLENGING CONVERSATIONS

- Geriatrics and palliative care clinicians must frequently conduct conversations about challenging topics with patients, families and other health care providers.

Some examples of complex discussions include:
- Advance care planning
- Breaking bad news
- Discussing goals of care
- Facilitating a family meeting
- Discussing discontinuation of treatments
- Discussing a transition from efforts to achieve a cure to an approach focused on comfort, quality of life, and possibly discussing hospice referral
- For providers, these conversations are difficult because they often involve highly emotional content in a situation where the underlying problem—the patient's disease—cannot be solved. Additional factors that contribute to clinicians' difficulties with communication include:[1]
  - Inadequate skills due to lack of training
  - Fear of causing emotional distress
  - Not knowing how to handle an emotional outburst
  - Concerns about containing one's own emotions
  - Fear of being blamed by patients and families for failure
  - Overidentification with certain patients
  - Having to confront one's own fears of death
- This juxtaposition of stressors may challenge the identity of clinicians as healers. It may be helpful, therefore, when navigating difficult conversations, to expand the definition of "healing." Healing can come in many forms. Conversations themselves can be healing.

CONVERSATIONS ARE DIFFICULT FOR PATIENTS AND FAMILIES

- For patients and families, these conversations are also very emotional and can be overwhelming, whether due to the charged content or to the presence of many "white coats" in the room.

- It is important for providers to recognize when patients and/or families have reached their saturation point, i.e., the point beyond which they are unable to process any additional information. This saturation point may be cognitive (they are overwhelmed with medical facts) or emotional (they are overcome by stressful emotions). In both cases, a skilled clinician will recognize that the limit has been reached, will allow silence and time for cognitive and/or emotional processing, and will accept that the conversation may have to be continued at a later date.

TOOLS TO HELP NAVIGATE DIFFICULT CONVERSATIONS

Many people think that communication is an innate skill. You're either good at it or you're not. Fortunately, this is not true. In fact, there are skills that can be taught, practiced, and incorporated into a health care provider's personal communication "toolbox." Four communication strategies that can be used to improve communication with patients, families, and colleagues in challenging situations are described below.

1. Breaking Bad News

- Clinicians are frequently faced with the task of delivering bad news. It is important to remember that bad news should be broadly defined. News that clinicians might consider unremarkable may be perceived as "bad" by some patients. Of course certain information always constitutes bad news: a diagnosis of dementia, a cancer recurrence, or a prognosis of months to live. However, a new diagnosis of insulin-dependent diabetes may also be a life-changing event for a patient. Therefore, conversations should be approached carefully and with sensitivity in any encounter when there is new and important information to be conveyed to the patient.
- SPIKES is a six-step protocol developed by Robert Buckman and Walter Baile to help clinicians communicate bad news to patients[2] (Table 9.1).

TABLE 9.1: SPIKES FOR COMMUNICATING BAD NEWS

Step	Things to Consider	Suggested Language
Setup	Who should be present? Create a conducive environment (private, adequate seating, quiet) Allow adequate time	*"We will be discussing some important information regarding your health today. Are there others who you would like to be present?"*
Perception	Establish what the patient knows already Get a sense of the big picture for this patient (i.e., any declines in functional status, ADLs or IADLs)	*"Tell me what you understand about your illness."* *"It sounds like this illness has really had a profound effect on your life. When were you last able to go out and do the grocery shopping?"* (or other ADL/IADL as appropriate)
Invitation	Ask the patient's permission to proceed with providing additional information	*"Would it be all right if I shared some additional information with you now?"*
Knowledge	Warning shot Give information in small bits Avoid jargon Pause frequently Check for understanding	*"Unfortunately, the news is not what we'd hoped."* *"I've just given you a lot of information. Let me stop and see if you have any questions."*
Emotion	Be prepared for a wide range of emotions Don't underestimate the importance of silence and presence Continue to respond to emotion until the patient has calmed down enough to proceed with more cognitive information	*"Would it be alright if we move forward to talk about our next steps?"* If the answer is anything other than "Yes," then you must continue to respond to the emotion.
Summarize	Allow for questions Have the patient summarize Plan for next steps	*"We've talked about a lot of things. What questions do you have?"* *"Who will you call when you leave here?"* *"How will you explain all of this to them?"*

TABLE 9.2: A 7-STEP APPROACH TO DISCUSSING GOALS OF CARE

Step	Things to Consider	Suggested Language
Setup	Who would the patient like to be present? Create a conducive environment (private, adequate seating, quiet) Allow enough time	*"A lot has been going on recently in regards to your illness. I'd like an opportunity to meet with you to discuss how things are going and how we should best proceed together. Is there anyone else who you'd like to be present for this meeting?"*
Perception	Establish what the patient knows already Pay close attention to the emotional cues that the family is displaying while talking Get a sense of the big picture for this patient (i.e., any declines in functional status, ADLs or IADLs)	*"Since so much has been happening with your health, it would be helpful for me to hear your understanding of what's going on so that I can make sure we're on the same page."* *"It sounds like this illness has really had a profound effect on your life. When were you last able to go out and do the grocery shopping?"* (or other ADL/IADL as appropriate)
Invitation	Ask permission to proceed with providing additional information	*"Thank you for sharing with me your understanding of what's going on. You've done an amazing job of wrapping your head around what I'm sure was a lot of overwhelming information. Can I share with you a few additional things that I think are also important?"*
Knowledge	Give information in small bits Avoid jargon Pause frequently Check for understanding If the knowledge you hope to impart is related to prognosis, follow the same Perception-Invitation-Knowledge framework	*"Some people find that it's helpful to have information about what to expect going forward, both in terms of the time course of their illness as well as what to expect physically and emotionally."* **Perception:** *"Have you discussed this with any of your other doctors? What have you understood from those conversations?"* **Invitation:** *"Would it be helpful if I shared my thoughts with you? If so, what would be helpful to you? Some people prefer more specific information while others prefer less specific information but rather reassurance that they will be well cared for no matter what. What type of person are you?"* **Knowledge:** *"Given your illness as we've discussed, your life will now likely be measured in months rather than years."*
Explore	Elicit the patient's values, goals, fears, and concerns by asking open-ended questions If there are multiple people in the room, make sure that everyone present is able to air his or her concerns	*"What things are most important to you now?"* *At this point, people often hope for many different things. What are you hoping for? What else?"* *"You have been through a tremendous amount. What helps you cope?"* *"What's the hardest part?"* *"What are your biggest worries right now?*
Emotion	Pay attention to displays of emotion from the patient and others in the room throughout the conversation Often, different people in the room can display differing emotions or other feelings through nonverbal cues	*"I noticed, Mrs. Burns [the patient's wife], that you shook your head when I mentioned using morphine to treat your husband's pain. Can you tell me more about what you're thinking?"*

(continued)

TABLE 9.2: (CONTINUED)

Step	Things to Consider	Suggested Language
Strategize	Make a treatment recommendation based upon the patient's values If your recommendation is for hospice care, follow the same **Perception-Invitation-Knowledge** framework Allow time and space for the patient to accept or reject this recommendation; negotiation may be required	*"Based on all that we've discussed, including the fact that you hope to remain at home for as long as possible with a good quality of life, I recommend that we provide you with the best care at home to help you achieve this. Hospice is a service that can help you and your wife to achieve your goals."* **Perception:** *"What is your understanding of hospice?"* **Invitation:** *"Would it be helpful if I shared with you more information about hospice?"* **Knowledge:** Clarify misconceptions (e.g., explain that hospice is not just for people with a few days to live; it's not always a place like a hospital that you actually go to, but instead is care primarily provided at home) Provide information about who is included in the hospice interdisciplinary team
Summarize	Allow for questions Outline next steps Be specific including by when you will complete a given task, or by whom a task will be done (if another member of the team will be involved)	

2. Discussing Goals of Care

Geriatricians and palliative care physicians are frequently asked to address goals of care with patients and families. (See Chapter 8: Advanced Care Planning). Table 9.2 outlines a seven-step approach for discussing goals of care with patients.

3. Facilitating a Family Meeting

Most patients do not make decisions in isolation. Families are frequently included in the planning and decision-making process. For patients without capacity, the family will often be called upon to make the decisions on behalf of the patient.

Family meetings are a key forum for difficult decision-making. The 10-step approach to facilitating a family meeting described in Table 9.3 is built on the SPIKES protocol outlined in Table 9.1, but also incorporates additional steps that are specific to conducting a family meeting.

4. Responding to Emotion

- Responding to emotion is one of the most difficult aspects of communicating with patients and families. A common pitfall for clinicians is the tendency to stay in the cognitive realm for the entire encounter. But simply presenting factual information, asking if there are any questions, and then listing a series of "next steps" is not an adequate or effective communication strategy.
- If the emotion in the room is ignored, it is likely that the main concerns of the patient and/or family members will remain unresolved. What seemed to the clinician to be a quick, straightforward meeting where everything was clarified may have left the patient and family with the same unresolved questions and untapped emotions that they brought into the meeting.
- To avoid this common tendency to present just the facts, the first step is to observe the emotion in the room. Noticing and naming the emotion is the prelude to being able to acknowledge the emotion using a

TABLE 9.3: A 10-STEP APPROACH TO FACILITATING A FAMILY MEETING

Step	Things to Consider	Suggested Language
Setup	All family members who want to be present should be Is there an advance directive and/or designated health care proxy or health care power of attorney? Pre-meeting with other providers will allow a consistent message Identify a facilitator Private venue, quiet setting Minimize interruptions Adequate seating	
Introduction	All clinicians should introduce themselves and their role. All family members should state their relationship and caregiving responsibilities. Outline the purpose of the meeting Negotiate an agenda Write down family's additional questions, acknowledge their importance, and let them know that you'll come back to them	*"The purpose of this meeting is to ensure that everyone has a clear understanding of what's going on with your brother medically, and specifically what we are doing for him."* *"We also want to hear from all of you about him as a person so that we can help facilitate decisions that are consistent with his values and goals."* *"Are there other things that you want to make sure we cover?"*
Perception	Establish what the family already knows about the patient's illness Pay close attention to the emotional cues that the family is displaying while talking	*"I've carefully reviewed your brother's chart and spoken with his other doctors, but it would be helpful for me to hear what you understand about your brother's illness."*
Invitation	Ask permission to proceed with providing additional information	*"Would it be all right if I shared some additional information with you now?"*
Knowledge	Clarify, correct, or explore what the family has shared Focus on the "big picture"	*"All of the information you've shared is exactly right. Unfortunately, all of these problems combine to create an overall burden of disease from which your brother is unlikely to recover."*
Elicit concerns	Ask explicitly for questions and concerns Keep asking until there are no more questions Make sure that everyone present has a voice and is able to air his or her concerns	*"I recognize that that was a lot of information. What questions do you have?"* *"What are your concerns?"* *"What else?"*
Explore	Explore the patient's values Ask if the patient had ever discussed what he might want in this type of situation Gain additional information about the patient's former functional status and quality of life Based on values, try to elicit what would be an acceptable quality of life for the patient	*"Tell me about your brother. What type of person is he?"* *"Did he ever talk about what he might want were he ever in this situation?"* *"Tell me how your brother was doing prior to this illness."* *"It seems like from everything you've told me, your brother has always been fiercely independent. Given that, I'm wondering what he would say if he was able to be part of this conversation right now."*
Emotion	Pay attention to displays of emotion from all family members throughout the meeting Often, different family members can display different or conflicting emotions.	

(continued)

TABLE 9.3: (CONTINUED)

Step	Things to Consider	Suggested Language
Strategize	Make a treatment recommendation based upon the patient's values and goals Allow for questions and negotiation	*"Based on all that you've shared with me about your brother, I would recommend that…"*
Summarize	Allow for questions Outline next steps	

Note. Adapted from Back A, Arnold R, Tulsky J. *Mastering Communication with Seriously Ill Patients: Balancing Honesty with Empathy and Hope.* New York: Cambridge University Press, 2009, pp. 85–88.

nonverbal response (e.g., touch, silence, shifting position, or eye contact), a verbal response, or a combination of both.[3]

- NURSE is a communication tool for responding to emotion that provides a menu of five types of verbal empathic responses (Table 9.4).[4] NURSE responses are not meant to be used in sequence. The most appropriate empathic response is the one that should be employed, depending upon the emotion to be acknowledged.
- While utilizing nonverbal and verbal responses to emotion, it is important to focus on being present with the patient or family and their emotion, but not trying to fix the emotion. Simple presence and a few choice words from the NURSE framework are the keys to helping the patient or family to feel acknowledged and validated.
- By responding to the emotion, the clinician addresses critical issues that must be attended to before moving forward with the next steps of strategizing and summarizing.

IMPROVING COMMUNICATION SKILLS

- As described in an article published in the Harvard Business Review in 2007 entitled "The Making of an Expert," one answer to improving communication skills is deliberate practice.[5]

Key elements of deliberate practice to improve existing communication skills and to extend their effectiveness include:

1. **Practice must be out of one's comfort zone.** Easy communication encounters—those within one's comfort zone—can lead to communication by rote and reliance on intuition. Communication encounters that are not so comfortable, and that challenge existing skills, are required for deliberate practice.
2. **Deliberate practice should ideally occur in a simulated setting.** Utilizing simulated patients or family members allows one to make mistakes in a low-risk environment. It also affords time to reflect upon skills and word choices and to experiment with different skills in a protected, low-risk environment.

TABLE 9.4: NURSE

Name the emotion	*"It sounds like you're really angry."* *"I'm wondering if you're worried about what will happen next."*
Understand	*"I can only imagine how frustrating it must be to be in your situation."*
Respect	*To a family:* *"You're doing such a good job of advocating for your mom."* *"I can tell how much love there is in your family just by seeing how you talk about your mom and by the fact that you're all here."*
Support	*"I know this is difficult, and I will be here with you through this."*
Explore	*"Tell me more about how this illness is affecting you."* *"Help me to understand what is the hardest part for you."*

3. **Performance should be continually analyzed** using the following questions:
What worked?
Where did I go wrong?
How can I improve?
4. **Find a communication coach**. The coach's role is to provide supervision for deliberate practice and to offer constructive feedback. Ideally the coach should be someone who has more advanced communication skills.

OTHER STRATEGIES

Busy clinicians may find it impossible to follow these steps to improve the communication skills. As alternatives to applying this method, the following strategies may be helpful:

1. Attend a continuing medical education course dedicated to improving communication skills (e.g., a yearly course is sponsored each June by the American Academy on Communication in Healthcare, www.aachonline.org).
2. Recruit a colleague who is also interested in improving his or her communication skills and agree to serve as peer coaches for one another.
3. After enough deliberate practice, one may be able to adopt an inner coach perspective by consistently reflecting on communication skills and planning adjustments that could be made to help encounters go more smoothly.

TAKE-HOME POINTS

- While many health care providers believe that they possess good communication skills, they are often unable to name the skills that they use in order to communicate effectively.
- Mastering specific skills and recommended strategies will allow a clinician to progressively improve his or her communication capability over time.
- One technique for improving communication skills is deliberate practice.

REFERENCES

1. Fallowfield L. *Communication with the patient and family in palliative medicine.* Oxford Textbook of Palliative Medicine. Oxford University Press. New York; 2009: 335.
2. Baile WF, Buckman R, et al. SPIKES—a six-step protocol for delivering bad news: application to the patient with cancer. *Oncologist.* 2000;5(4): 302–311.
3. Back A, Arnold R, Tulsky J. *Mastering Communication with Seriously Ill Patients: Balancing Honesty with Empathy and Hope.* New York, NY: Cambridge University Press; 2009:26–27.
4. Fischer G, Tulsky J, Arnold R. Communicating a poor prognosis. In: R. Portenoy and E. Bruera, eds. *Topics in Palliative Care.* New York: Oxford University Press; 2000.
5. Ericsson KA, Prietula MJ, Cokely ET. The Making of an Expert. Harvard Business Review. July–August 2007:115–121.

10

Managing Conflict

INTRODUCTION

Conflict is a universal life experience that is encountered every day in our professional or personal lives. There is considerable literature on how to identify and negotiate conflict, regardless of the setting in which it arises.[1,2] This chapter will focus on applying helpful general guidelines to conflicts arising in the clinical practice of geriatric palliative care.

In the health care setting, conflict has been defined as "a dispute, disagreement, or difference of opinion related to the management of a patient involving more than one individual and requiring some decision or action."[3]

STAKEHOLDER VERSUS MEDIATOR

- While clinicians may be asked to act as strictly neutral mediators in a situation of conflict (e.g., as ethics consultants), more commonly they will also have an opinion about the given conflict. When they have a point of view on the issue, providers become stakeholders rather than mediators.
- A health care provider is a primary stakeholder when he or she is directly involved in the conflict (Table 10.1). For instance, the provider can disagree with a patient, a family member, or another provider on goals of care or management issues.
- If the provider is not directly involved in the conflict, he or she may be a secondary stakeholder. For example, a provider may recommend a colonoscopy to determine the

source of a patient's lower gastrointestinal bleed. The patient does not wish to have the procedure, but the patient's son is strongly in favor of it. In this conflict, the patient and his son are the primary stakeholders and the health care provider is a secondary stakeholder.
- Other situations in which the provider may be a secondary stakeholder include conflict between multiple family members and conflict between two or more other providers.

COMMON CAUSES OF CONFLICT

Common causes of conflict encountered by geriatric palliative care providers can arise in the context of the following situations or issues (see also Table 10.2):

- Establishing goals of care:
  - Duration/intensity of disease-modifying treatment
  - Duration/intensity of life-sustaining treatment
  - Provision of artificial nutrition and hydration
- Perception or allegation of medical error
- Disclosure of medical details and/or prognosis to patient

Issues involving perceived medical error and requests for nondisclosure are common and important sources of conflict. While specific ways to address these issues are beyond the scope of this

---

TABLE 10.1: THE PROVIDER AS STAKEHOLDER IN SITUATION OF CONFLICT

Provider as Primary Stakeholder	Provider as Secondary Stakeholder
Provider/Patient conflict	Patient/Family conflict
Provider/Family conflict	Family/Family (within family) conflict
Provider/Provider conflict	Provider/Provider conflict (between two or more other providers)

TABLE 10.2: ISSUES THAT CAN RESULT IN CONFLICT

Issue/Situation	Type of Conflict	Examples
Goals of care	Provider/Patient	Patient wishes to continue with disease-modifying treatment that the provider feels is futile.
		Patient refuses treatment or testing that the provider feels is necessary; often this situation leads to the provider questioning the patient's capacity (although it should not be assumed that the patient lacks capacity simply because he or she asserts authority to refuse a recommended treatment or test).
	Provider/Family	Surrogate decision-makers wish to take steps different than what is stated in the advance directive.
		Provider and surrogate decision-maker disagree about whether life-sustaining treatment would be beneficial or might increase patient suffering in the absence of advantages.
	Family/Family	Family members disagree about what the patient without capacity would have wanted in a given situation (when no advance directive is available).
		A patient lacks capacity, and family members have differing interpretations of an advance directive.
	Provider/Provider	Two providers disagree about the most appropriate treatment plan.
		Treating physicians disagree about whether or not an advance directive applies to the current situation.
Medical error	Provider/Patient or Family	Patient or family member believes that a medical error caused undue harm to the patient; provider believes that there is another explanation for the outcome in question.
Disclosure	Provider/Family	A family member feels that nondisclosure would be in the best interest of the patient, and the provider feels that he or she must respect the patient's autonomy by asking what the patient wants to know.

chapter, some of the suggestions found below will be applicable.

MANAGING CONFLICT

Stone et al.[1] developed a step-wise approach to dealing with difficult conversations that was adapted and translated into a medical context by Back, Arnold, and Tulsky.[4,5] The steps of this approach as well as pitfalls that providers may encounter when attempting to manage conflict are described here, and also summarized in Table 10.3.

Step 1: Notice the Conflict

Many conflicts are not addressed, at least initially, because they are not noticed. Noticing conflict requires self-reflection. The clinician must consciously recognize his or her own feelings of annoyance or frustration, or the

sensation of mentally "checking out" of the conversation. Recognizing conflict also requires paying close attention to the emotions and nonverbal clues being exhibited by others. Emotions such as anger, frustration, or even despair may signal conflict. Subtle body language such as a rolling of the eyes or a relaxed posture indicative of loss of interest in the conversation may also herald conflict.[5] All of these cues suggest that conflict may be simmering just under the surface.

Pitfall: Ignoring the Conflict

Clinicians may find many reasons to avoid dealing with conflict or to deny that it exists. These include trying to preserve the relationship with the patient or the family, avoiding discussions that will take too much time, or lack of confidence in the ability to negotiate effectively.[4] Beware of this pitfall

TABLE 10.3: SUMMARY OF A STEP-WISE APPROACH TO DEALING WITH CONFLICT

Step Number	Description	Pitfall
Step 1	Notice the conflict	Ignoring the conflict
Step 2	Prepare for the conversation Take a deep breath Examine the 3 stories How will success be defined?	Believing there is only *one* truth Assuming the intentions of the other person Placing blame Having a fixed agenda
Step 3	Find an unbiased starting point Acknowledge the importance of the issue Invite each perspective	Beginning to share one's own perspective before hearing everyone else's point of view
Step 4	Listen, acknowledge, and empathize Actively listen for the 3 stories Respond to emotion (*See NURSE tool in Chapter 9: Communication*)	Preparing counterarguments
Step 5	Reframe the conflict as a shared interest	
Step 6	Describe the potential options	Providing too many options (limit the options to no more than 3)
Step 7	Summarize and strategize	Failure to recognize that not all negotiations end in conflict resolution

because conflict, if ignored, will likely become an even bigger problem later.

Step 2: Prepare for the Conversation

Providers should take to time to clear the mind, identify and examine personal thoughts and feelings, and mentally prepare for the interaction that will follow. If something or someone has just provoked the conflict, it is very helpful to pause and calm down before attempting a discussion or negotiation. Anger interferes with the ability to listen to others. Two preparation strategies include

- **Examine the "Three Stories"**: Stone et al. suggest that at its heart, each conflict has three stories:[1]
  1. *The "What Happened?" Story*: At the heart of every conflict is the question of what happened: who's right, who meant what, and who's to blame.
  2. *The "Feelings" Story*: There are emotions attached to conflict situations. It's important to recognize and acknowledge one's own feelings before beginning negotiations. Also consider how the other person may be feeling.

  3. *The "Identity" Story*: Providers should reflect on how the conflict may threaten their personal or professional identity. Likewise, they should think about how the conflict may threaten the personal identity of the other person.

- **Determine how success will be defined**: Setting up the wrong definition of success when negotiating a conflict can result in an "us versus them" mentality. Resolving conflict should never be about who will "win." It is more productive to explore what the shared interests of the parties might be. In this approach, success can be predefined as: (1) identifying the shared interests, (2) creating a working relationship, and (3) collaborating to seek solutions that focus on the shared interests.[4]

Pitfall: Having a Fixed Agenda

Having a fixed agenda (e.g., a DNR must be in place after this conversation) leads to a mindset of rigidity rather than one of negotiation. While it's important to have a framework of how to approach the conversation and a predetermined definition of success, these should be broadly conceived to allow flexibility for negotiation.

Step 3: Find an Unbiased Starting Point

Often the best way to accomplish Step 3 is by asking a neutral, open-ended question. Try to gain
a better understanding of each party's perception of the situation. This can be accomplished
by acknowledging the importance of the issue at
hand and then asking each party to describe his
or her perspective. An example of language that
could be used in Step 3:

> "I recognize that providing the best care for
> your mother is of utmost importance to you, as
> it is to me. So that I can have a better under-
> standing of your perspective, maybe you could
> start by sharing with me your hopes for your
> mother at this point in her illness."

Pitfall: Dominating the Discussion

The provider should refrain from expressing personal opinions and perspectives before hearing
everyone else's point of view. Also, if there are
multiple perspectives represented, be sure to allow
time for all to be shared.

Step 4: Listen, Acknowledge, and Empathize

After asking an open-ended question, the provider should pause and listen to the other person's response. In particular, it is important
to actively listen for how the other party con-
ceptualizes the three stories described in Step
2 (what happened, feelings, and identity).[5]
Acknowledge that the other person has been
heard and understood by restating their thoughts
and concerns in a reflective way. This will also
involve responding empathically to any emotion that is expressed as they tell the story. (See
Chapter 9: Communication Skills.)

Pitfall: Preparing Counterarguments

Thinking about what to say next in response
and preparing counterarguments interferes with
listening fully to the perspective of others in the
conversation. The provider's full attention should
be on them and what they're saying.

Step 5: Reframe the Conflict as a Shared Interest

Once the other person's goals and concerns are
understood, the conflict can be identified. The art
of negotiation, and indeed mediation, lies in finding common ground in relation to the conflict. In
medicine the shared interest can often be stated as
focusing on offering the "best treatments," given
the situation at hand.[5]

Step 6: Describe the Potential Options

In a discussion of intensity of treatment, for
example, this step will involve outlining in a nonjudgmental way all potential treatment options,
including the most aggressive, least aggressive, and
the middle road. Often, the "middle road" can be
defined as a time-limited trial, a very important
concept when negotiating next steps for treatment.
By including a time-limited trial of treatment with
more aggressive measures, you both acknowledge
the patient's or family's need to provide the "best"
care, while also agreeing that this may be a situation in which the "best" care does not necessarily
mean the most aggressive. In this way, time-limited
trials can be "win-win" solutions when negotiating
conflict regarding goals of care.

Pitfall: Too Many Options

While there may be limitless options depending
on all of the various combinations of treatments
that could be continued, withheld, or withdrawn,
it is helpful to restrict the treatment options to
no more than three. More than three options will
quickly overwhelm any patient or family member
in the setting of conflict.

Step 7: Summarize and Strategize

As recommended in the SPIKES protocol for
communicating bad news (See Chapter 9:
Communication Skills), it is imperative to end
the conversation with a summary which includes
agreed-upon next steps.

Pitfall: Failure to recognize that not all negotiations end in conflict resolution

NEXT STEPS

Remember that in a conflict resolution situation,
success can be defined as:
- Identifying shared interests

- Creating a working relationship
- Collaborating to seek solutions that focus on the shared interests
- By following the above stepwise approach to addressing conflict, shared interests can be identified and a working relationship created. However, a solution which is acceptable to all parties may not be reached every time. In these situations, the next steps may include involving an impartial third party such as an ethics consultant or a patient representative who mediates disputes within the hospital.[5]
- Even in the most difficult conversations, agreeing on next steps is key to maintaining a working relationship with the other party.

TAKE-HOME POINTS

- Managing conflict can be one of the most difficult and challenging tasks faced by geriatricians and palliative medicine clinicians.
- Having a framework for how to approach these situations is invaluable for their management.

- Making time for self-reflection (Steps 1 and 2) prior to engaging with the other stakeholders will allow clinicians to approach the negotiation in a nonjudgmental way and offers the best opportunity for success.

REFERENCES

1. Stone D, Patton B, Heen S. *Difficult Conversations: How to Discuss What Matters Most*. New York: Viking; 1999.
2. Fisher R, Ury W, Patton B. *Getting to Yes: Negotiating Agreement Without Giving In*. 2nd Ed. New York: Penguin; 1991.
3. Studdert DM, Burns JP, Mello MM, Puopolo AL, Truog RD, Brennan TA. Nature of conflict in the care of pediatric intensive care patients with prolonged stay. *Pediatrics*. 2003;*112*:553–558.
4. Back AL, Arnold RM. Dealing with conflict in caring for the seriously ill: "It was just out of the question." *JAMA*. 2005;*293*(11):1374–1381.
5. Back AL, Arnold RM, Tulsky J. *Mastering Communication with Seriously Ill Patients: Balancing Honesty with Empathy and Hope*. New York, NY: Cambridge University Press, 2009, pp. 95–98.

11

Care Transitions

INTRODUCTION

Care transition is defined as a set of actions designed to ensure the coordination and continuity of health care as patients transfer between different locations or different levels of care within the same location.[1] These care settings commonly include hospitals, subacute rehabilitation facilities, long-term care facilities, the patient's home, and emergency departments.

WHY ARE CARE TRANSITIONS IMPORTANT?

In 1999 the Institute of Medicine (IOM) published a report on medical errors entitled *To Err is Human: Building a Safer Health System*.[2] The report documented an alarming rate of medical errors in U.S. hospitals, resulting in a rate of 45,000 to 98,000 preventable deaths every year. This report had a dramatic impact on the way health care organizations approached the problem of medical errors and injury. It also galvanized a national movement to develop a "culture of medical safety" in health care facilities with the goal of improving the reliability and safety of care for patients.

Since *To Err is Human* was published, a central concept of the report—that bad systems and not bad people lead to most errors—has become a mantra in the U.S. health care system.[3] Care transitions are critical points in a patient's care when preventable "systems" errors may occur. Older patients and those with acute or chronic care needs are especially vulnerable during these transitions, when the important elements of the care plan developed by one set of clinicians may not be clearly communicated to the clinicians in the next care setting.

CONSEQUENCES OF POOR CARE TRANSITIONS

- Lack of coordination, information gaps, inadequate follow-up, and inconsistent patient monitoring during care transitions can subsequently increase a patient's length of stay, impose unnecessary stress on patients and families, cause readmission to the hospital, or result in a patient's death.[4]
- Frail older patients with complex health care issues are at higher risk for adverse medical events in general, and at even higher risk during transitions across care settings.[5]
- Contributing to the risk for older patients is the fact that they receive care from many providers. Patents with chronic conditions, a number expected to reach 125 million in the United States by 2020, may see up to 16 physicians in one year.[6] They also typically move within and between care settings more frequently than younger patients.[1]
- Medication errors are a particular concern when older patients transfer from one care setting to another. The number of medications typically prescribed for older patients, their uncertainty about which medications they should be taking, and the lack of coordination between clinicians across settings pose a serious threat of dangerous polypharmacy. (See Chapter 3: Medication Management in Older Adults.)

BARRIERS TO EFFECTIVE CARE TRANSITIONS[7]

There are multiple ways that care systems and processes can break down, resulting in poorly executed transitions. These include:

- Poor communication
- Incomplete transfer of information
- Inadequate education of patients and their caregivers
- Limited access to essential services
- Lack of a single person to ensure continuity of care
- Language and health literacy issues
- Cultural considerations

ELEMENTS OF SUCCESSFUL CARE TRANSITIONS

Standards and guidelines promulgated by the American Geriatrics Society, the National Transitions of Care Coalition (NTOCC), as well as a consensus statement from a broad group of national medical professional societies have identified key elements that must be in place to facilitate successful care transitions:[8,9,10]

1. Establish specific points of accountability for sending and receiving care, especially for hospitals, skilled nursing facilities, primary care physicians, and specialists, including:
   - Common plan of care
   - A description of patient's goals, preferences, and advance directives
   - A current list of problems, physical and cognitive functional status, medications, and allergies
   - Contact information for caregivers and primary care physician
2. Patient and family members should know what to expect at the next care setting.
3. Caregivers should be encouraged to offer candid assessment of whether proposed plan is feasible.
4. Medications should be reconciled before transfer.
5. A plan should be in place for forwarding test results and arranging follow-up appointments, if they are necessary.
6. Patient and family should be made aware of specific signs and symptoms that indicate a condition has worsened, and should be given the name and phone number of whom to contact.
7. Receiving physician must evaluate a patient who has been transitioned in a timely manner to identify possible areas of concern and to assure that the care plan is implemented.
8. Additional infrastructure, performance, and educational standards include:
   - Implement electronic medical records (include standardized medication reconciliation elements).
   - Develop performance measures to encourage better transitions of care.
   - Require that health care professionals who treat patients with acute and chronic illness receive training in transitional care as a core competency.

COMMUNICATION IS A KEY FACTOR IN TRANSITIONS

- The IOM report implicated failure of communication as a key factor in the high rate of medical errors. Specific examples of communication lapses that put patients at risk included transfer of information that was insufficient, faulty exchanges of existing information, frequently ambiguous and unclear information, and lack of timely and effective exchange of pertinent information. As the report pointed out, "Especially when patients see multiple providers in different settings, none of whom has access to complete information, it becomes easier for things to go wrong."[8]
- Several initiatives have been proposed and implemented to increase the safety of older patients during transitions. A recent literature review analyzed 10 years of interventions (2000 to 2010) to improve patient safety during transitional care of the elderly, with a specific focus on discharge interventions.[11] The authors identified a range of interventions that aimed to contribute to safe transitional care by improving communication at all levels. Although the review did not conclude that one approach was more valid than another, the features of successful interventions included:
  - Interventions that commence at an early stage and are maintained throughout the hospital stay and the post-discharge period
  - A key health care worker acting as a discharge coordinator
  - Patient participation and education
  - Involving family caregivers
  - Using a multidisciplinary approach
  - Teaching transitional care
  - Pharmacy interventions, especially medication reconciliation
  - Standardized medication reports
  - Comprehensive programs with multi-interventional components

SPECIFIC TRANSITION STRATEGIES

Hand-Off Communication

To help ensure that every clinician who cares for a patient gets an accurate picture of the patient's status, the Joint Commission requires that every health care facility devise a standardized, consistent "hand-off" communication protocol to be used whenever patients are transitioned into, out of, and within the facility.[12]

- A widely adopted tool used to ensure effective hand-offs from one health care provider to another is the **Situation-Background-Assessment-Recommendation (SBAR)** technique:[13]

  *S*ituation: What is currently happening? Include vital signs, advance directives, symptom status, and your concerns.

  *B*ackground: What circumstances led to the patient's current condition? Include objective data.

  *A*ssessment: What do you think the patient's current problem is?

  *R*ecommendations: What does the person who is receiving the patient need to do next to address the problem?

- Utilizing the SBAR format has been shown to reduce hospital errors and improve safety outcomes during transitions within an institution by enhancing provider-provider communication and relations.

TABLE 11.1: CHECKLIST: TRANSITION FROM SAR FACILITY TO HOME

Physical Needs
Check activities of daily living and instrumental activities of daily living (ADLs and IADLs)
Assess the caregiver's willingness and ability to help with ADLs and IADLs
Establish home environment safety and ongoing skilled nursing or physical therapy need: refer to home health care agency, a home visit doctor, community social services
Assess need for home attendant services, making sure services are in place before the patient is discharged

Social Needs
Discuss with patient/caregiver plan of action once the patient is at home and what is to be expected, and how to access help regarding questions, concerns, or in an emergency
Assess caregiver's burden/stress prior to patient's discharge. When appropriate, give information for support groups

Financial Needs
Reassess health insurance (e.g., Is Medicaid active? Are the medications covered by the patient's insurance program especially with Medicare part D? Is there long-term care insurance or VA eligibility?)
In younger elderly patients, assess the impact of illness on the patients' ability to work and provide for themselves, and refer to appropriate community agency for unemployment insurance benefits
When possible, give options on how to maximize benefits for the patient's medical, social, and financial problems

Psychological Needs
Attempt to assess patient's/caregiver's expectations once back in the home
Look for adjustment disorder in the face of new diseases, new medications, possible decreased functional status, increased dependency on caregiver, etc.
Evaluate the patient's mental status to establish a new baseline
Identify community services, e.g., support groups or even psychiatric consultation

Spiritual/Religious Needs
Assess the patient's possible new view on meaning of life in the face of a new illness
Assess how the patient's beliefs may help or hinder progress with an illness; and encourage patient and caregiver to utilize religious resources

Medical Needs
Give prescriptions for all medications (new and old)
Assess the patient's/caregiver's understanding of the medications, including side effects
Assess the patient's cognitive status and the need of the caregiver to be present during discussions about medical changes and/or problems
Reassess the goals of care and the advance directives. Give the patient the required documentation, e.g., DNR, health care proxy form
Review the patient's understanding of their disease and their symptoms
Review follow-up appointments and home care plan with agency name and number
Communicate with primary care doctor using the SBAR format
Give a copy of the discharge summary to the patient/caregiver

Safety Checklists

- Safety checklists, or "medical checklists," are written guides that walk the practitioner through the key steps in any complex procedure. The concept of a medical checklist is increasingly being utilized to improve health care processes and patient safety outcomes.[14] Checklists for different types of care transitions (e.g., emergency department to hospital care, acute care to long-term care) can help clinicians minimize care transition mistakes.
- Table 11.1 offers a sample checklist to guide the transition of a seriously or chronically ill older adult from a subacute rehabilitation (SAR) facility to home. The move out of a subacute rehabilitation facility and back to home is one of the most challenging transitions for the clinicians, the patient, and the caregivers. Multiple factors need to be assessed before the patient can be safely discharged.
- The domains of this checklist include the physical, social, financial, psychological, spiritual/religious, and medical needs. The checklist items should be assessed by a care team coordinator and should include provider input for medical and physical issues; social worker input for social, financial, and psychological concerns; and a chaplain, if available, for spiritual/religious needs.

TAKE-HOME POINTS

- Care transitions are critical points in a patient's care when dangerous mistakes may occur. Older patients with acute or chronic care needs are especially vulnerable during these care transitions from one setting to another or within an institution.
- Poor transitions can increase a patient's length of stay, impose unnecessary stress on patients and families, cause readmission to the hospital, or result in a patient's death.
- Frail older patients with complex health care issues are especially at risk for adverse medical events caused by poor transitions across care settings.
- Features of successful interventions to improve care transitions include provider education and training, systems initiatives (e.g., transfer nurse, discharge protocols, discharge planning, medication reconciliation, standardized discharge letter, electronic tools), and patient- and family-oriented approaches (patient awareness and empowerment, discharge support).
- Using standardized communication procedures and medical checklists are two specific strategies to minimize "hand-off" gaps and reduce the potential for errors during care transitions of seriously or chronically ill older adults.

REFERENCES

1. Coleman EA, Boult CE. American Geriatrics Society Health Care Systems Committee. Improving the quality of transitional care for persons with complex care needs. *JAGS*. 2003;*51*(4): 556–557.
2. Forster AJ, Murff HJ, Peterson JF, et al. The incidence and severity of adverse events affecting patients after discharge from the hospital. *Ann Intern Med*. 2003;*138*:161–167.
3. Naylor M, Keating SA. Transitional care: moving patients from one care setting to another. *Am J Nurs*. 2008;*108*(9):58–63.
4. Bodenheimer T. Coordinating care—a perilous journey through the health system. *N Engl J Med*. 2008;*358*(10):1064–1071.
5. Naylor MD. Nursing intervention research and quality of care. *Nursing Research*. 2003;*52*(6): 380–385.
6. Coleman EA. Falling through the cracks: challenges and opportunities for improving transitional care for persons with continuous complex care needs. *JAGS*. 2003;*51*:549–555.
7. Kohn LT, Corrigan JM, Donaldson MS (eds), and the Committee on Quality of Health Care in America. *To err is human: building a safer health care system*. Washington DC: Institute of Medicine, National Academy of Sciences, National Academy Press; 2000.
8. Leape LL, Berwick DM. Five years after "To Err is Human": what have we learned? *JAMA*. 2005;*293*(19):2384–2390.
9. National Transitions of Care Coalition. Improving transitions of care: findings and considerations of the "Vision of the National Transitions of Care Coalition." September 2010. http://www.ntocc.org/Portals/0/PDF/Resources/NTOCCIssueBriefs.pdf. Accessed August 13, 2012.
10. Snow V, Beck D, Budnitz T, et al. Transitions of care consensus policy statement. American College of Physicians-Society of General Internal Medicine-Society of Hospital Medicine-American Geriatrics Society-American College of Emergency Physicians-Society of Academic Emergency Medicine. *J Gen Intern Med*. 2009;*24*(8):971–976.

11. Laugaland K, Aase K, Barach P. Interventions to improve patient safety in transitional care—a review of the evidence. *Work.* 2012;*41*:2915–2924.

12. Agency for Healthcare Research and Quality. *Patient Safety Network, Handoffs and Signouts.* http://www.psnet.ahrq.gov/primer.aspx?primerID=9. Accessed August 10, 2012.

13. Leonard M, Graham S, Bonacum D. The human factor: the critical importance of effective teamwork and communication in providing safe care. *Qual Saf Health Care* 2004;*13*(Suppl 1): i85–i90.

14. Halasyamani L, Kripalani S, Coleman E, et al. Transition of care for hospitalized elderly patients—development of a discharge checklist for hospitalists. *Journal of Hospital Medicine.* 2006;*1*(6):354–360.

12

The Hospice Model of Palliative Care

WHAT IS HOSPICE?[1]

- Hospice provides comprehensive interdisciplinary team-based palliative care, usually in the patient's home, for terminally ill patients who have an identified prognosis of six months or less to live, and who agree to forego life-prolonging therapies or interventions.
- Hospice programs typically include comprehensive interdisciplinary services that address physical, psychological, social, and spiritual suffering at the end of life.
- Hospice is appropriate when patients and their families make the decision to focus on maximizing comfort and quality of life, when life-prolonging treatments are no longer beneficial or when the burden of treatment outweighs the benefit, or when patients are entering their last weeks or months of life.
- Hospice also supports the family caregivers throughout the illness and provides bereavement follow-up services to family members after the patient's death.

PAYING FOR HOSPICE[2]

- Approximately 80% of people who use hospice care are over the age of 65 and are thus entitled to the services offered by the Medicare Hospice Benefit. Initiated in 1983, the MHB is covered under Medicare Part A (hospital insurance).
- Medicare beneficiaries who choose hospice care receive a full range of medical and support services for their life-limiting illness. (See Chapter 13: Health Insurance.)
- Most private health plans and Medicaid in most states also cover hospice services.

WHAT SERVICES DOES HOSPICE PROVIDE?

The Medicare Hospice Benefit (MHB) defines a set of core services that hospice providers are required to make available to each person they serve. The MHB covers the following services and pays nearly all of the costs:

Physician services
Nursing care
Medical equipment (e.g., wheelchairs or walkers)
Medical supplies (e.g., bandages and catheters)
Medications for symptom control and pain relief
Short-term care in the hospital, including respite and inpatient for pain and symptom management
Home health aide and homemaker services
Physical and occupational therapy
Speech therapy
Social work services
Dietary counseling
Grief support for patient and family

The MHB does not cover:

Treatment where the goal is curative
Medications not directly related to the hospice diagnosis
Care from another provider that is not part of the hospice team, unless the hospice team arranged for such care
Nursing home room and board
Patient/family may also have to pay part of the cost for outpatient drugs and inpatient respite care

WHO IS ELIGIBLE TO RECEIVE HOSPICE CARE?

To be eligible for Medicare hospice benefits, the following criteria must be met:

- Patient must be eligible for Medicare Part A (Hospital Insurance).
- Primary care physician and hospice medical director must certify the diagnosis of a

life-limiting illness and that death may be expected in six months or less if the illness follows a normal course.

- Patient must agree to choose hospice care instead of routine Medicare-covered benefits for the qualifying illness. (Note: Medicare will continue to pay for covered benefits for any health needs that are not related to the life-limiting illness.)
- Care must be provided by a Medicare-approved hospice program. (More than 90% of hospices in the United States are certified by Medicare.)

WHERE IS HOSPICE CARE PROVIDED?

- **At Home:** More than 70% of hospice services are provided in the place the patient calls home, where primary caregivers (family, friends, or private-hire caretakers) are trained to recognize and help manage distressing symptoms.
- **Long-Term Care Facility:** In nursing homes and other facilities, hospice providers give recommendations to the nursing staff on symptom management and also communicate with the family.
- **Inpatient Hospice:** Inpatient hospice units can either be freestanding inpatient facilities, or be located within a dedicated area in a hospital. Inpatient hospice offers:
  - Hospital-level medical treatments (such as intravenous medications requiring frequent titrations)
  - Short-term assistance for acute symptom management during an episode of symptom exacerbation, or at the very end of life when patients have a prognosis of days to weeks to live

MISCONCEPTIONS ABOUT HOSPICE

Erroneous beliefs and negative attitudes about hospice are widely held by patients, families, and many health care professionals. These misconceptions, contrasted with the actual realities include:[3, 4]

1. *People die sooner if they enroll in hospice.*
   - **Reality:** The goal of hospice is to improve the quality of a patient's life to allow time with family and friends and to assure conditions that facilitate a natural, comfortable death. Hospice does not hasten death. Studies suggest that hospice actually improves survival for some patients by an average of 30 days, while also relieving caregiver distress and the reducing the risk of complicated bereavement.[3]

2. *Hospice means "giving up" and abandoning hope.*
   - **Reality:** Discontinuing uncomfortable and painful curative treatments that are fruitless allows hospice patients to receive pain and symptom management as well as other supportive care services from an interdisciplinary team of experienced, compassionate caregivers. Most terminally ill patients experience less anxiety by refocusing hope on realistic goals for the time remaining for them to spend with friends and family.

3. *A hospice patient cannot decide to resume curative treatment.*
   - **Reality:** If patients' conditions improve, or if they change their minds about hospice care, they can be discharged from hospice and return to curative treatment. A hospice patient may also enter the hospital for certain types of treatment if the goal is to improve quality of life.

4. *Medicare coverage is forfeited when a patient chooses hospice.*
   - **Reality:** A patient who elects hospice retains full Medicare coverage for health care needs not related to the hospice diagnosis. Patients must continue to pay the applicable deductible and coinsurance amounts under their Medicare plan.

5. *If hospice patients live longer than six months, they can no longer receive hospice services.*
   - **Reality:** Hospice can be provided as long as a person is identified by a physician as having a six-month life expectancy. This does not mean, however, that hospice services are abruptly stopped after six months. The hospice team, along with the physician, can recertify the patient for additional 60- to 90-day periods of hospice.

6. *Hospice is only for people who have terminal cancer.*
   - **Reality:** At the beginning of the hospice movement in the United States, 90% of hospice patients had a primary diagnosis of cancer. By 2005, however,

the percent of hospice admission of patients with a cancer diagnosis dropped below 50%.

BARRIERS TO USE OF HOSPICE

1. Restrictions on "Curative" or Life-Prolonging Treatment

Restrictions on "curative" or life-prolonging treatment constitute one of the primary barriers to timely referral to hospice, especially now that the distinction between curative and palliative treatments has become less clear. Indeed, a number of recently developed "curative" treatments also provide symptom relief for patients who would otherwise benefit from hospice services.

2. Requirement of Six-Month Prognosis

To be eligible for the MHB, a patient must have a formal prognosis of six months or less to live if the disease runs its normal cause. Patients and families understandably find it difficult to acquiesce to this "public" declaration of the probability of approaching death, and thus it is not easy for a physician to document the prognosis as required.

3. Prognostic Uncertainty

The MHB prognosis requirement is more suitable for the relatively predictable downward trajectory of late-stage cancers or AIDS, but it makes referral difficult for patients living with the unpredictable, multi-year course of other common causes of death in the elderly, such as congestive heart failure, chronic lung disease, stroke, and dementing illnesses.[5]

PALLIATIVE CARE AND HOSPICE[1,4]

- Palliative care principles and practices are applicable across the full range of diagnoses, settings, stages of illness, and prognoses. Hospice is a palliative care delivery model restricted to persons willing to give up insurance coverage for life-prolonging care, and for whom two physicians are willing to certify a prognosis of six months or less. The goal is to provide compassionate, patient-centered clinical care focused on achieving the best possible quality of life for patients and their family caregivers.
- Palliative care models employ an interdisciplinary team composed of physicians, nurses, social workers, chaplains, and other health professionals to control pain and other distressing symptoms, facilitate informed decision-making, mobilize practical assistance for patients and caregivers, and identify resources in the community to ensure safe and supportive care environment. While palliative care is expanding to community settings, in the United States it is currently primarily hospital-based. Hospice is usually delivered in the place the patient calls home.
- The key point of divergence is that palliative care offered outside of hospice is available independently of prognosis and can be accessed simultaneously with life-prolonging and disease-directed therapies (Figure 12.1). The Medicare Hospice Benefit is restricted to patients with a prognosis of six months or less and who agree to forego curative treatment.
- This prognosis-based distinction between who can receive palliative care and who is eligible for hospice exists only in the United

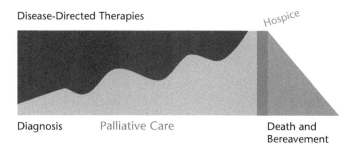

FIGURE 12.1: Model of palliative and disease-directed therapies.

States. The growing need for palliative care that is independent of prognosis has in fact driven the rapid growth of hospital-based palliative care teams in the U.S. over the last several years.

TAKE-HOME POINTS

- Hospice provides interdisciplinary team-based palliative care, usually in the patient's home, for terminally ill patients with six months or less to live, and who agree to forego life-prolonging therapies.
- Hospice care for older adults in the United States is paid for primarily through the Medicare Hospice Benefit (MHB) of Medicare Part A. Eighty percent of people who use hospice care are over the age of 65, and are thus entitled to use the MHB.
- More than 70% of hospice services are provided in the place the patient calls home, but hospice care is also available in long term care facilities and inpatient hospice units.
- Erroneous beliefs and negative attitudes about hospice, widely held by patients, families, and health care professionals, pose barriers to increased use of hospice in the United States. Other barriers to timely referral include the six-month prognosis requirement and the restriction on curative therapies.
- While the Medicare Hospice Benefit limits hospice care to those with a prognosis of six months or less and who agree to forego curative treatment, palliative care outside of hospice is offered independently of prognosis and simultaneously with life-prolonging and disease-directed therapies.
- The growing need for palliative care that is independent of prognosis has driven the rapid growth of hospital-based palliative care teams in this country over the last several years.

REFERENCES

1. Meier DE. Increased access to palliative care and hospice services: opportunities to improve value in health care. *The Millbank Quarterly.* 2011;89(3):343–380.
2. National Hospice and Palliative Care Organization Caring Connections. www.caringinfo.org. Accessed August 13, 2012.
3. Connor SR, Pyenson B, Fitch K, Spence C, Iwaskai K. Comparing hospice and non-hospice patient survival among patients who die within a three-year window. *Journal of Pain and Symptom Management.* 2007;33:238–246.
4. Connor SR. Development of hospice and palliative care in the United States. *OMEGA* 2007; 56(1):89–99.
5. Field MJ, Cassel CK. (Eds) *Approaching death: Improving care at the end of life.* Institute of Medicine, ed. Washington DC: National Academies Press; 1997.

13

Health Insurance

INTRODUCTION

Health insurance for older adults is an ever-changing landscape marked by cycles of program growth and budgetary cutbacks, as well as innovations designed to meet the needs of America's growing elderly population.

In 2009, 7.4 million adults aged 65 and over were covered by Medicare, with 22% of them choosing to enroll in private health plans that contracted with Medicare.[1] An additional 5 million older adults also received coverage from Medicaid services.[2]

HEALTH INSURANCE AND THE OLDER ADULT

For clinicians caring for older adults with significant health problems, it is important to have a general understanding of the patient's and caregivers' finances, and what services can be covered by Medicare, Medicaid, or their private insurance. Exploring these questions ahead of time, before an acute need arises, is preferable. When illness progression triggers the need for more services, or if a transfer to a setting with a more appropriate level of care becomes necessary, insurance considerations will determine what options will be available.

This chapter will help to explain how the costs of health care services for older Americans are typically shared by a combination of public and private health care insurance plans, after deductible and out-of-pocket expenses are paid by the patient and family.

For more information on the Medicare/Medicaid program addressed here, call 1-800-MEDICARE, visit www.medicare.gov, or consult "Medicare and You," the official U.S. government Medicare handbook.[3] Helpful information for caregivers is also available at www.medicare.gov/caregivers.

MEDICARE

Medicare, a federal program essentially for older adults, is the largest single-payer of health services in the United States. Currently, to qualify for Medicare benefits, one has to be a U.S. citizen or permanent resident age 65 and over, or if under 65, have a disability or end-stage renal disease.

Medicare is divided into several parts, each covering a different range of services:

Part A: Hospital Insurance
Part B: Medical Insurance
Part C: Medicare Advantage Plans
Part D: Prescription Drug Coverage

Medicare Part A (Hospital Insurance) and Part B (Medical Insurance)

Table 13.1 below lists the services covered, premiums, and other information for Medicare Parts A and B (together referred to as "Original Medicare") in 2012.[3]

Services not covered by Medicare Part A and B include:

Long-term care (i.e., custodial care)
Routine dental care
Dentures
Cosmetic surgery
Acupuncture
Hearing aids or exams for fitting hearing aids

Medicare Home Care Benefit

- Home health care services are covered by Medicare Part A or Part B. Medicare Part A covers the first 100 days of home health care after a hospital stay; Part B covers subsequent days. Home services covered under Medicare Part B do not require hospital stay for coverage.
- To qualify for services, a homebound beneficiary with a doctor's order must have a medically necessary, part-time or intermittent need for skilled nursing care and/or require physical therapy or speech therapy.
- Coverage includes skilled nursing or home health services up to seven days a week, no more than eight hours a day, for a total

TABLE 13.1: MEDICARE, PARTS A AND B ("ORIGINAL MEDICARE")

	Medicare Part A	Medicare Part B
Types of services	Hospital insurance	Medical insurance (optional)
Premium	No premium if pt. worked for 10 years for Medicare-covered employment If fewer than 10 years covered work, may need to pay premium	Monthly premium (income dependent) There are plans to help pay for premiums and payments for low-income individuals (Medicare savings programs)
Covered services	Inpatient hospital care Skilled nursing facility (SNF) care (not custodial or long-term care) Home health care Hospice care Inpatient care in a religious nonmedical health care institution	Physician visits Outpatient hospital care Durable medical equipment OT/PT services Some home health care
Deductibles and Copayments	For specific information on Medicare Part A and B monthly premiums, deductibles and copayments, and covered services, visit www.medicare.gov; call 1-800-MEDICARE; or consult "Medicare and You," the official U.S. government Medicare handbook.[3]	

of 28 hours a week. A Medicare-certified home health agency must provide the care. (Note: Availability of coverage for home care services is dependent on many factors. For more information, call 1-800-MEDICARE, visit www.medicare.gov; or consult "Medicare and You," the official U.S. government Medicare handbook.[3])

- Skilled nursing care includes wound care, tube feedings, catheter changes, assessment of patient's condition, injections. Home health aide services include bathing, toileting, and dressing. Other items covered include skilled physical, occupational, and nutrition therapy services; medical social services; outpatient mental health care; certain medical supplies; and durable medical equipment. (Copays and deductibles may apply for some services, supplies, or equipment.)
- Medicare home care benefit does not cover 24-hour care at home, prescription drugs, meals delivered to the home, homemaker, or custodial care services.

Medicare Hospice Benefit
- Medicare beneficiaries with a terminal condition can elect to switch from Medicare coverage to the Medicare Hospice Benefit (MHB). Hospice provides supportive and comfort care to those patients who have a prognosis of six months or less

and their families. Hospice care offers comprehensive services that address physical, psychological, social, and spiritual suffering at the end of life.
- The cost of hospice care is covered under Medicare Part A. The cost of health care for conditions not related to the terminal illness is covered under the original Medicare plan. A beneficiary can opt out of the hospice benefit and resume Medicare coverage at any time.
- Hospice care is delivered by a Medicare-certified agency. The patient's physician must certify eligibility, but the hospice physician, not the primary care doctor, is responsible for recertification of the patient's continued hospice stay.
- Services covered by the Medicare Hospice Benefit include skilled nursing services, skilled therapy services, home health aide and homemaker services, durable medical equipment, social services, prescription drugs for hospice-related diagnoses, pastoral care, respite care, and nutrition counseling. Hospice physician services are also covered. (See Chapter 12: The Hospice Model of Palliative Care.)

Medicare Part C (Medicare Advantage Plans)
- Medicare Advantage plans are health plan options approved by Medicare but administered by private companies. They

are optional plans that, if selected, replace Medicare Part A and Part B and usually have lower out-of-pocket costs to the participant.

- These plans cover all of the services of Medicare Part A and Part B, and some may have additional drug coverage. They often have a network of physicians and hospitals, may have different copays for in-network or out-of-network visits, and may require referrals for coverage of specialist services.
- There are different types of managed care plan options, including Preferred Provider Organization (PPO), Health Maintenance Organization (HMO), and Private Fee-for-Service (PFFS) plans.
- With Medicare Advantage Plans, a supplemental Medigap policy is unnecessary. (See explanation of Medigap plans below.)
- Medicare Advantage Plans are not required to provide any hospice benefits. Those patients who are eligible and elect hospice care may receive the benefit outside of the Medicare Advantage Plan under Original Medicare.
- For more information about Medicare Advantage plans, visit www.medicare.gov for details, or consult "Medicare and You," the official U.S. government Medicare handbook.[3]

Medicare Part D (Medicare Prescription Drug Coverage)

- Medicare Part D plans are additional insurance plans offered by private insurance companies to provide prescription drug coverage. When electing a plan, it is important for the beneficiary to carefully consider coverage, convenience, and costs, because different companies have different formularies of medications.
- Out-of-pocket costs for the Medicare Part D plans include monthly premiums, a yearly deductible, and copays.
- Most Medicare drug plans have a "coverage gap" (also called the "donut hole"). This is a temporary limit on what the plan will cover for drugs, over and above a certain amount per beneficiary. Once the coverage gap is entered, the beneficiary gets a 50% discount on covered brand-name drugs and pays 86% of the cost of generic drugs until the end of the coverage gap.

- If there are additional costs beyond the coverage gap, part D plans have "catastrophic coverage," which pays for the majority of the rest of drug costs, with a small coinsurance amount or copay for covered drugs for the rest of the policy year.
- For more information about Medicare Part D, what is covered, and the coverage gap, visit www.medicare.gov for details or consult "Medicare and You," the official U.S. government Medicare handbook.[3]

MEDIGAP PLANS

(Medicare Supplement Insurance)

- Medigap plans are additional insurance plans offered by private insurance companies to fill the gaps of Original Medicare. These plans help to cover coinsurance, copay, deductibles, and certain other costs. They are standardized plans (identified in most states as A thru N) that are offered by different insurance companies.
- If an individual has Original Medicare and buys a Medigap policy, Medicare will pay its share of the Medicare-approved amount for covered health care costs. The Medigap policy pays its share.
- Although the Medigap plans are standardized, different insurance companies may charge different premiums for the same coverage. It is important to compare plans from more than one carrier.
- For more information about the types of Medigap plans and what they cover, visit www.medicare.gov for details or consult "Medicare and You," the official U.S. government Medicare handbook.[3]

OTHER INSURANCE OPTIONS

- Older adults may have additional health insurance from their employers if they have not retired, or their retiree benefits may include a health insurance plan. The insurance that pays first is called the "primary payer," and the other one is the "secondary payer." For retirees, and those currently employed under group plans with less than 20 employees, Medicare is the primary payer. If the current coverage is from an employer with more than 20 employees, the group health plan pays first.

- Veteran Health Benefits and the Indian Health Service (IHS) provide coverage to older adults meeting certain criteria. These benefits may help to decrease costs for pharmacy, physician visits, and other services. For example, medication costs through the U.S. Department of Veterans Affairs (VA) may be lower than what is offered in Medicare prescription drug benefit or Medicare Advantage Plans. Most clinicians know little about the services offered by the VA and the IHS which can be very generous and enormously helpful to qualified beneficiaries. Encourage eligible patients, their families, and social workers to explore possible benefits.
- Program of All-inclusive Care for the Elderly (PACE) is a program administered by both Medicare and Medicaid but is available only in certain areas. It is a benefit for frail older adults who meet their state's criteria for nursing home care but who continue to stay at home. PACE generally provides care in an adult day care setting by a team of doctors, nurses, and other health professionals, who provide a comprehensive health care plan. PACE receives a monthly fixed payment from Medicare and Medicaid. Those who are enrolled in PACE may also pay a monthly premium.

MEDICAID

- Medicaid is a joint federal and state program that helps pay medical costs for individuals with limited income, and who meet other eligibility requirements. It can cover many long-term care services such as home attendant and housekeeper services, home health aide services, and nursing home care, even in the absence of a skilled nursing need.
- Some people qualify for both Medicare and Medicaid and are described as "dual eligible." For dual eligible patients, Medicare will cover prescription drugs, but Medicaid will cover some drugs and other care services that Medicare doesn't provide. Most Medicaid programs include hospice benefits.
- Financial eligibility guidelines for Medicaid vary from state to state and program to program, depending on income,

assets, and the need for long-term care. Higher-income individuals may still qualify for Medicaid because certain income may not be counted, or in some states may be "spent down" by depleting savings and certain other assets on medical expenses or by transferring funds if possible. Some families choose to consult with an attorney specializing in Medicaid eligibility.

- For more detailed information on specific Medicaid eligibility criteria, visit www.medicare.gov/contact, or call 1-800-MEDICARE to get the number of a specific state Medical Assistance (MEDICAID) office.

PLANNING FOR LONG-TERM CARE

Historical Background

- The approach to financing and provision of supportive social services in the United States evolved very differently compared to the ways medical care is subsidized for older citizens. These key differences in organization and financing become clear when the need arises for long-term care. Long-term supportive care services, such as custodial nursing home and personal care, were considered as "social services" rather than "medical care" by the designers of early health insurance plans. Today, most private health insurance plans still will not pay for custodial long-term care services.
- This social vs. medical dichotomy was also adopted by Medicare, which does not provide long-term care benefits. There are some exceptions, such as long-term care for rehabilitation, e.g., care after a stroke or a hip replacement. But these rehab benefits are time-limited.

Current Financing Options for Long-Term Care

- As more Americans are living longer, there has been a corresponding increase in utilization of long-term care by older adults. Medicaid is currently the only major source of public funding for older people with functional limitations who are in need of long-term care. (See program description of Medicaid above.) Generally, eligibility criteria include both functional limitation and financial criteria. Ironically, because of better coverage for supportive services under Medicaid, a low-income older adult is likely to be eligible for a wider array of appropriate services than is a middle-income person.

- In addition to qualifying for Medicaid, other current options for providing long-term care include relying on family support and care giving, using personal savings, or accessing veterans' benefits. Many retiring adults may also consider purchasing long-term care insurance, specifically to cover future long-term care needs such as nursing home care, assisted living, or home care services.
- These long-term care insurance plans can be purchased for lower premiums when adults are in their 50s or 60s. Health status changes over time, however, so there should be a periodic review to make sure that the policy in place is sufficient for current and future health care needs.
- Long-term care insurance plans are not well regulated. It is therefore important to examine terms in detail, compare different plans carefully and seek advice before purchase.

Researching Long-Term Care Insurance

In discussions about the long-term care insurance options with patients and their caregivers, clinicians should urge careful research and consideration of the following aspects of a plan before any purchase is made[4]:

- **Long-term viability of insurance carrier**: Those who purchase long-term care insurance usually begin enrollment well ahead of when the benefits are needed. It is therefore essential to consider the long-term viability of the insurance company.
- **Details of coverage**: Terms of coverage vary widely from company to company and from plan to plan. To select the right plan, it is important to understand exactly what is covered. Some plans may cover only nursing home costs, while others may cover home care or assisted living costs. Most plans do not cover all the costs that may be incurred, but rather allow a certain fixed cost with capitation.
- **Inflation protection**: It is important to consider inflation protection in the plan because in 10 or 20 years, when one may

need the benefit, the daily costs for long-term care may have increased substantially.

- **Maximum benefit**: Plans also include a maximum lifetime benefit, i.e., the maximum duration of time that benefits can be claimed.
- **Eligibility for benefits**: Plans have criteria stating when benefits will become available. For most plans, it is the impairment of functional ability to carry out activities of daily living; for some plans, eligibility certification from any health provider is acceptable, but some others require certification by providers designated by the insurance company. Some plans may also include a hospital stay requirement, which may be an unfavorable eligibility criterion for the insured.
- **Out-of-pocket payments**: Some plans may have a period of time when one is eligible for benefits but must pay out-of-pocket before benefit begins. These "elimination periods" are similar to a deductible expense in other types of health insurance plans.

TAKE-HOME POINTS

- Health insurance for older adults is an ever-changing landscape of public programs and private plans designed to help America's growing elderly population pay for the cost of their health care.
- Health care providers should understand the insurance options in order to help guarantee that their older patients have access to the medications, health care procedures, and supportive services that they require.
- Medicare, a federal insurance program essentially for older adults, is the largest single payer of health services in the United States. Medicare is divided into four parts, each covering a different range of services: hospital insurance, medical insurance, Medicare Advantage Plans, and prescription drug coverage.
- For older adults who meet the eligibility criteria, Medicaid will cover long-term care services such as home attendant and housekeeper services, home health aide services, and nursing home care in the absence of a skilled nursing need.
- Many retiring adults may consider purchasing long-term care insurance specifically to cover future long-term care needs. Long-term care

insurance plans are not well regulated, so patients and families should be advised to examine the terms of a plan in detail, compare different plans carefully, and seek expert advice before purchase.

REFERENCES

1. Annual Report of the Board of Trustees of the Federal Hospital Insurance and Federal Supplementary Medical Insurance Trust Funds, 2009.
2. Truffer CJ, Klemm JD, et al. Actuarial report on the Financial Outlook for Medicaid. Centers for Medicare and Medicaid Services, United States Department of Health and Human Services, 2008.
3. Medicare & You. US Dept of Health and Human Services: Centers for Medicare and Medicaid Services. CMS Product #10050-38. August 2011.
4. National Clearing House for Long-term Care. http://www.longtermcare.gov/LTC/Main_Site/Index.aspx.

SECTION II

Special Issues in Geriatric Palliative Care

14

Palliative Care Emergencies

INTRODUCTION

The literature on emergencies in palliative medicine focuses on a number of serious medical events including superior vena cava syndrome, cardiac tamponade, hypercalcemia, hemorrhage, and seizures.

Sudden worsening of pain or other physical symptoms, acute confusion, and the urgent need for reassurance in the face of life-threatening illness and loss of independence may also be considered emergencies and are covered in other sections of this handbook. (See Chapter 29: Pain Management, Chapter 35: Terminal Delirium, and Chapter 15: Dying at Home.)

For family caregivers, preparing for an anticipated death is often perceived as an emergency as well. It is important for clinicians who are caring for a dying patient to prepare the family for what to expect by discussing issues such as normal signs and symptoms of the dying process, making funeral arrangements, pronouncement of death, and obtaining death certificates. (See Chapter 15: Dying at Home.)

SUPERIOR VENA CAVA (SVC) SYNDROME

Definition

SVC syndrome is a complex of signs and symptoms associated with compression of the SVC. SVC syndrome causes distressing symptoms that are difficult to treat.

Etiology

- SVC syndrome may occur from tumor or lymph nodes compressing the vessel wall, intraluminal thrombosis, as well as through direct infiltration of the vessel by tumor.
- About 75% of cases of SVC syndrome are caused by primary bronchial carcinomas, with the remaining cases resulting from lymphomas and other infiltrating tumors.

- It is rarely due to nonmalignant conditions such as aortic aneurysm or goiter.

Prevalence

About 3% of patients with bronchial carcinoma and 8% of those with lymphoma will develop SVC syndrome.

Diagnosis

- History: shortness of breath often described as the sensation of drowning, facial swelling, chest pain, cough, hoarseness of voice, dysphagia, headache made worse by stooping.
- Physical exam: tachypnea, periorbital edema, injected conjunctiva, facial, upper chest, and arm edema, neck and upper chest vein distension, enlarged neck circumference ("Stokes collar"), Horner's syndrome (the classic triad of one-sided miosis, ptosis, and anhidrosis), cyanosis.

Treatment Options

Management of dyspnea by pharmacologic means with opiates and possibly benzodiazepines should be initiated immediately while more specific treatment of SVC syndrome is arranged. Options include:

1. **Interventional**: Stenting of the SVC by an interventionalist offers prompt and lasting improvement of symptoms in the majority of patients, does not interfere with tissue diagnosis, and is rapidly becoming standard of care.[1] A low incidence of risks has been described including infection, pulmonary embolus, stent migration, hematoma at the insertion site, bleeding, stent failure due to reocclusion, and rarely perforation or rupture of the SVC. Anticoagulation is usually required at least for the short term after stent placement, although there is debate about long-term anticoagulation after SVC stenting.

2. **Radiotherapy (XRT):** SVC syndrome typically responds well to local radiotherapy, with one study reporting that 70% of patients with SVC syndrome due to non-small cell lung cancer responded to XRT symptomatically for a mean duration of 3 months.[2] Because XRT can make histologic diagnosis of a yet-undiagnosed malignancy difficult, this treatment is usually avoided when tissue diagnosis is still desired.

3. **Pharmacologic:** If radiotherapy is contraindicated or delayed, corticosteroids may be considered for SVC syndrome. Usual doses of dexamathasone for SVC syndrome are 16 mg per day for 5 days. If no benefit is obtained, dexamethasone should be stopped after 5 days. For patients who do show benefit, dexamethasone dose should be gradually tapered.

4. **Chemotherapy:** For patients with non-radiosensitive tumor, palliative chemotherapy may be considered for SVC syndrome.

HYPERCALCEMIA OF MALIGNANCY

Definition

Hypercalcemia can occur as an early symptom of a yet undiagnosed cancer, or as the terminal event for a patient during an expected death. Hypercalcemia of malignancy usually occurs in patients with bone metastases, though 20% of cases occur in patients with no known bone metastases via paraneoplastic syndrome.

Etiology

- Various cytokines are implicated in the pathogenesis of hypercalcemia. These include IL-1 and tumor necrosis factor (TNF), 1,25 dihydroxyvitamin D in Hodgkin's lymphoma, and the production of either ectopic PTH or PTH-related peptide in a number of malignancies.
- Cancers likely to cause hypercalcemia include multiple myeloma, lung, breast, and renal cell cancer. Less common causes include lymphoma and cancers of the prostate, thyroid, ovary, colon, and head and neck.

Prevalence

Although the majority of hypercalcemia cases are related to the overproduction of PTH or PTH-like peptide (hyperparathyroidism), hypercalcemia is also quite common in malignancy, occurring in approximately 20–30% of patients with cancer.[3]

Diagnosis

- History: Significant findings include anorexia, nausea, vomiting, constipation, lethargy, excessive thirst, confusion, and muscle weakness, all of which are also common symptoms in patients with terminal illness.
- Tests: Two important issues to keep in mind when testing for hypercalcemia:
  1. Because much of total serum calcium is bound to albumin, serum calcium must be corrected for serum albumin level.
  2. Serum calcium is usually reported in units of mg/dL in the US, although some labs use other units of measurement. Be sure to check the units when making decisions about hypercalcemia.
- In general, the plasma calcium concentration falls by 0.8 mg/dL (0.2 mmol/L) for every 1.0 g/dL (10 g/L) fall in the plasma albumin concentration. The measured plasma calcium concentration can be corrected for the presence of hypoalbuminemia from the following equation: Corrected $[Ca]$ = Measured total $[Ca]$ + $(0.8 \times (4.5 - [alb]))$.
- Corrected calcium under 12 mg/dL is considered mild hypercalcemia; values of 12–14 mg/dL are considered moderate hypercalcemia, while values above 14 mg/dL are considered severe hypercalcemia.
- Free ionized calcium testing is becoming routine.
- EKG changes common in hypercalcemia include bradycardia, PR interval prolonged, QT interval reduced, wide T waves, and widened QRS complexes.

Treatment Options

- Hypercalcemia causes an array of distressing symptoms and mental status changes that usually respond to treatment.
- Treatment should begin with aggressive IV hydration with a minimum of 2 liters of normal saline. While treatment with a loop diuretic such as furosemide has long been

advocated, a recent review questions the evidence for this treatment.[4]

- Salmon calcitonin (4–8 international units/kg) administered intramuscularly or subcutaneously every 6–12 hours is relatively nontoxic and works rapidly, lowering the serum calcium concentration by a maximum of 1 to 2 mg/dL beginning within 4–6 hours. However, because of a decrease in response due to exposure, the effectiveness of calcitonin is short-lived. (Note: Nasal application of calcitonin has not been shown to be effective for treatment of hypercalcemia.)

- Treatment with bisphosphonates, particularly IV infusion of pamidronate and zoledronic acid has been effective for hypercalcemia of malignancy. There is also some evidence that bisphosphonates can be used as an adjuvant for the treatment of the pain associated with bone metastases.[5]

- Intravenous bisphosphonates should be given only after adequate fluid resuscitation. The doses of pamidronate usually given are 60 mg for mild hypercalcemia and 90 mg for moderate or severe hypercalcemia as an infusion over 2–4 hours.

- Be aware that intravenous bisphosphonates may worsen underlying kidney disease, and the median duration of normocalcemia after pamidronate infusion is only 3 weeks. For patients whose life expectancy is longer than a month, maintenance of normocalcemia will require periodic bisphosphonate therapy or treatment of the underlying disease.

- Repeat infusions of IV bisphosphonates have been associated with osteonecrosis of the jaw. There is some evidence that this complication is more likely with the more potent zoledronic acid than pamidronate.[6] This finding can help guide treatment decisions.

Prevention

Hypercalcemia can be prevented in patients at risk by keeping them well hydrated, avoiding diuretics, and avoiding excessive vitamin D supplements.

CARDIAC TAMPONADE

Definition

Cardiac tamponade occurs when the pressure from a pericardial effusion approaches intracardiac pressures, leading to impaired filling of the ventricles and decreased cardiac output. When this condition occurs acutely after trauma (or cardiac catheterization), it is considered a true emergency with immediate invasive treatment required in order to prevent death.

Etiology

Cancer can cause large pericardial effusions to accumulate subacutely until a critical threshold of pressure (often patient-specific) is reached. The most common tumors implicated in cardiac tamponade include cancers of the lung or breast, as well as leukemia and lymphoma.

Prevalence

The prevalence of cardiac tamponade among patients with terminal malignancy has been estimated at 0.2% based on an autopsy series performed at the Mayo Clinic from 1942 to 1958.[7]

Diagnosis

- History: Chest pain, shortness of breath, cough, orthopnea, weakness, and dizziness
- Exam: "Becks triad" of muffled heart sounds, distended neck veins, and hypotension has been described. Friction rub, tachycardia, and "pulsus paradoxicus" (decreased blood pressure during inspiration) also are commonly seen.
- Tests:
  - EKG: low voltage or electrical alternans (beat-to-beat shift in the QRS axis associated with mechanical movement of the heart within a large effusion)
  - Chest x-ray: check for new or worsening cardiomegaly
  - Echocardiogram: diastolic collapse of cardiac chambers can be diagnostic

Treatment Options

- Pharmacologic: For many patients with cancer and subacute tamponade, symptoms can be managed with corticosteroids, nonsteroidal anti-inflammatory agents, and opiates.
- Surgical: A variety of treatment options should be considered in the context of the patient's wishes, overall prognosis, functional status, and perceived quality of life. These options include:
  - Catheter pericardiocentesis with echocardiographic guidance

- Balloon pericardiotomy
- Surgical creation of a pericardial window

It is beyond the scope of this handbook to discuss surgical indications and risks in detail, although it should be mentioned that pericardial fluid often recurs after pericardiocentesis and that a pericardial window (if appropriate) is often the more definitive treatment.

MASSIVE HEMORRHAGE

Definition
Exsanguination, or massive hemorrhage, has been defined as a loss of greater than 150 ml of blood per minute or a loss of whole blood volume within 24 hours.

Etiology
This occurs when tumor invades into an artery and can unfortunately be a frightening final cause of death.

Prevalence
Massive hemorrhage has been estimated to affect less than 2% of patients in the palliative care setting.

Treatment Options
- Massive hemorrhage can be particularly distressing for caregivers who often do not know how to respond. There may also be concerns about the infectious risk due to handling of blood.
- For patients at risk of developing massive hemorrhage (especially those with an invasive tumor near a large artery), an early discussion involving both the patient and the caregiver specifically addressing these concerns should take place to determine the best and most appropriate care setting for the patient.
- If home is selected as the care setting, families should be advised to buy dark sheets along with a kit containing gloves and dark-colored towels for compression and absorption of blood. Families should be reassured that patient will not be in pain and that unconsciousness will follow quickly. Compression with dark towels will prevent the sight of large amounts of blood.

SEIZURES

Definition
The International League Against Epilepsy (ILAE) defines an epileptic seizure as a transient occurrence of signs and/or symptoms due to abnormal excessive or synchronous neuronal activity in the brain.

Etiology
Seizures are commonly reported at the end of life and can be attributed both to disease-related electrolyte abnormalities (such as hyponatremia) and to CNS disease such as brain metastases.

Prevalence
Seizures requiring treatment have been described to occur in about 1% of patients receiving inpatient palliative care.[8]

Diagnosis
It should be cautioned that opioid-induced myoclonus is often misinterpreted as seizure activity by caregivers and clinicians. The distinction is important, as treatment may differ. (For management of opioid-induced myoclonus, please see Chapter 29: Pain Management.) Terminal delirium can also be misinterpreted as seizure.

Treatment Options
- Seizures cause discomfort for the patient and are distressing for caregivers. The management of seizures at the end of life should therefore focus on symptom control. In the setting of advanced illness, workup with brain imaging or EEG is often not necessary, and there is less concern about long-term side effects of seizure medication.
  - Diazepam is often a medication of choice because of its availability in rectal formulations and its stability for storage at room temperature.
  - Lorazepam (Ativan) is also widely used in home hospice because of ease of administration by family caregivers.

OTHER EMERGENCIES
For management of other conditions that may be geriatric palliative care emergencies, please see:
- Pain crises (Chapter 29: Pain Management)
- Delirium (Chapter 34: Delirium, and Chapter 35: Terminal Delirium)
- GI obstruction (Chapter 44: Bowel Obstruction)
- Urinary retention (Chapter 54: Urinary Retention)
- Anxiety, panic attack (Chapter 65: Anxiety)
- Spinal cord compression (Chapter 71: Malignant Spinal Cord Compression)

TAKE-HOME POINTS

- Because older patients and patients with serious illness are often frail with a limited lifespan, they receive less benefit and often suffer a greater burden of side effects and distress from aggressive and invasive treatments for medical emergencies.
- When managing a medical emergency for a geriatric palliative care patient, clinicians should use prudent judgment and consider not just what can be done, but rather what should be done, in the context of the goal of achieving a peaceful and dignified death in accordance with the patient's wishes, goals of care, and overall prognosis.
- Preparing for an anticipated death can also be perceived as an emergency for caregivers. It is thus important for clinicians to prepare caregivers of dying patients in a reassuring and supportive manner, and by discussing what to expect and how to respond.

REFERENCES

1. Courtheoux P, Alkofer B, Al Refai M, et al. Stent placement in superior vena cava syndrome. *Ann Thorac Surg.* 2003;75:158.

2. Rowell NP, Gleeson FV. Steroids, radiotherapy, chemotherapy and stents for superior vena caval obstruction in carcinoma of the bronchus: a systematic review. *Clin Oncol* (R Coll Radiol). 2002;14:338.

3. Stewart, AF. Clinical practice. Hypercalcemia associated with cancer. *N Engl J Med.* 2005;352:373.

4. LeGrand SB, Leskuski D, Zama I. Narrative review: furosemide for hypercalcemia: an unproven yet common practice. *Ann Intern Med.* 2008;149:259.

5. Mancini I, Dumon JC, Body JJ. Efficacy and safety of ibandronate in the treatment of opioids-resistant bone pain associated with metastatic bone disease: a pilot study. *J Clin Oncol.* 2004;22:3587.

6. Dimopoulos MA, Kastritis E, Anagnostopoulos A, et al. Osteonecrosis of the jaw in patients with multiple myeloma treated with bisphosphonates: evidence of increased risk after treatment with zoledronic acid. *Haematologica.* 2006;91:968.

7. Thurber D, Edwards J, Achor R. Secondary malignant tumors of the pericardium. *Circulation.* 1962;26:228–241.

8. Stirling LC, Kurowska A, Tookman A. The use of phenobarbitone in the management of agitation and seizures at the end of life. *J Pain Symptom Manag.* 1999;17:363–368.

15

Dying at Home

INTRODUCTION

Although 70–80% of people indicate a preference to die at home, only about 20% of people actually do. Most Americans die in health care facilities such as hospitals or nursing homes.[1,2] With better understanding of palliative care and hospice services, health care providers will be empowered to assist patients and their families to fulfill their wish to spend the last days to weeks of life in a familiar environment they call "home."

HOME AS THE PLACE OF DEATH

Before offering home as a continuing care option at the end of life, clinicians should evaluate the patient's clinical condition, determine the availability of an able and willing caregiver, and identify services and resources adequate to meet the patient's care needs.[3] This assessment should include the following three areas:

1. **Patient and family preference**: Some patients and/or their caregivers may hold personal or cultural (e.g., ethnic, religious) beliefs in which death at home is not preferred, or may even be perceived as a negative occurrence.

2. **Complex symptom management**: Symptoms at the end of life can generally be managed at home, but some conditions, therapies, or treatments may be more complex or too distressing for the patient or caregiver. For example:
   - Active bleeding, requiring skilled care and continuous monitoring, even if goals of care are for comfort
   - Complex pain syndrome, requiring continuous intravenous infusion with frequent titration of opiates
   - Uncontrollable agitation requiring palliative sedation
   - Extensive wound care
   - Medical emergencies that may not be adequately managed in the home (see below; also see Chapter 14: Palliative Care Emergencies)

3. **Caregiver availability**: For patients to be safely cared for at home, there needs to be a designated primary caregiver who is willing and able to assume this role, even when paid caregivers are also employed.
   - Caregivers must be prepared and comfortable with the care they are expected to give, and also be supportive of agreed-upon goals of care.
   - Most insurance benefits, including home hospice, do not provide 24-hour home health aide services. Primary caregivers are therefore central members of the care team.
   - Full-time caregiving is essential because the patient's care needs will typically increase as the end of life approaches, and this may require round-the-clock monitoring for symptom management, administration of medications, and personal care such as turning and transferring from bed to commode or chair.

PLANNING FOR CARE AT HOME

- Once it has been determined that the patient can be cared for safely at home, a meticulous process of assessment, planning, and coordination will ensure that the medical, practical (services, equipment, transportation), emotional, spiritual, and educational needs of the patient and caregivers will be met.
- Medicare data reveals that 20% of patients are rehospitalized within 30 days of discharge, and that half of the readmissions occur before the patient has seen his or her outpatient provider.[4] Without a comprehensive plan at home, the readmission rate is likely even higher for this at-risk population.

The Care Team

- Several components of care must be in place for care at home near the end of life. The care team should consist of:
  1. Family caregiver(s) who are available on a 24-hour/7-day-a-week basis
  2. Primary medical provider (PMP):
     - May be primary care physician or hospice or palliative care clinician
     - Acts as coordinator for all services and disciplines caring for patient
     - Ideally can make home visits
  3. Interdisciplinary team of providers with expertise in palliative care
- Home hospice is the only program that provides around-the-clock telephone support and nursing visits whenever indicated, with an option for inpatient care when clinically necessary. (See Chapter 12: The Hospice Model of Palliative Care, and Chapter 13: Insurance.)
- When available, community-based palliative care can often serve as a bridge to home hospice under the following circumstances:
  1. Patient/family may not be emotionally ready to accept hospice.
  2. Patient is receiving palliative treatments (e.g., XRT, chemotherapy) not covered under the Medicare Hospice Benefit.
  3. Patient resides in a nursing home and cannot access his or her hospice benefit.

Emergency Access to Care

- Emergency availability and access to clinical staff on a 24-hour basis is essential. Clear instructions should be given about whom to call after hours for questions and concerns, or in the event of patient's death. Hospice should be the first call if the patient is enrolled in home hospice.
- If there is a nonhospital DNR in place, it is important to reconfirm it every 90 days so that it will be current in the event that 911 is called.

MEDICATIONS

- When a patient is in the hospital, the clinician may have to approach the advance care planning discussion with a narrower focus. In the event of serious illness, for example, discussions offer a framework for exploring patient's current life goals and preferences, and how these might evolve with changing clinical realities. Determining the patient's personal preferences for comfort, symptom management, and code status should be a priority.
- There should be timely and adequate access to appropriate medications for symptom management in the home. (See Chapter 19: Last Hours of Living.) For patients enrolled in home hospice, medications related to a terminal diagnosis are covered under hospice benefit and are delivered to the patient's home. For non-hospice patients, commercial insurance prescription plans should cover medications, but the availability of opiates or benzodiazepines in the community may be limited in certain geographic areas.[5]
- The primary provider and/or palliative care team should identify one or more area pharmacies that can supply the appropriate medications in a timely fashion, ideally with home delivery services.
- Medications for symptom management should be in the home for use on an urgent basis, even before the patient exhibits symptoms. Medications should be prescribed and dosed to make in-home administration convenient, always considering ease of route, frequency of dosing, and cost. (See Chapter 19: Last Hours of Living.)
- Conversion of opioids to long-acting oral or transdermal preparations reduces the need for frequent dosing by caregivers. When patients nearing death are no longer able to safely and reliably take medications orally, long-acting opioids must be converted to another form because time-release medications cannot be crushed.
- As a patient is nearing the end of life, medications prescribed for comorbid conditions should be reassessed (e.g., antihypertensives, hypoglycemic agents). Liquid or rectal preparations may be preferred over tablets in those with dysphagia, decreased cognition, or disease progression.

EQUIPMENT

- Provision of appropriate home medical and personal care equipment will guarantee an efficient, safe, and comfortable environment in the home. A thorough home evaluation and knowledge of the patient's care needs can help determine what equipment should be ordered and put in place prior to patient's discharge from hospital. Equipment should be reviewed if there is a change in the patient's condition and care needs.

- Most equipment and supplies are provided by hospice agencies under the hospice benefit. Home oxygen must meet established eligibility criteria for reimbursement. Under the hospice benefit, oxygen can be provided for symptom relief regardless of oxygen saturation level.
- For non-hospice patients, some durable medical equipment and supplies are covered by medical insurance and may require a provider prescription.

CAREGIVER SUPPORT AND EDUCATION

- To be effective, the home treatment plan should involve both the patient and the family caregivers, with the interdisciplinary team providing caregiver support and education that is proactive and ongoing.[6]
- The following four caregiver concerns are very common and should be acknowledged and addressed by all members of the clinical team:
  1. Lack of confidence about medication administration
  2. Fear of unintentionally hurting or harming the patient
  3. Uncertainty about what to expect in terms of disease course and dying process
  4. Anxiety about their own coping skills as a caregiver
- Additional topics for education include patient's disease process, trajectory of illness, what complications or warning symptoms to expect, how to manage symptoms, and when to call hospice/palliative care staff or primary MD.
- Explicit instructions and explanations should be provided for all medications and care tasks, with reinforcement during every visit by nurse or physician. Medication charts and a list of care tasks will help guide caregivers in times of stress and during periods when substitute or respite care is in place.
- Offering information about available community resources can also support patients and caregivers in the home

(e.g., faith-based organizations, volunteer/doula programs, meal delivery services, and available friends/family).

- Private pay caregivers in the home setting should be included in all educational and supportive measures. Their participation is a key factor in achieving the patient/family goal to die at home, and their role should be respectfully acknowledged.

MANAGING EMERGENCIES IN THE HOME

- The management of emergencies in the home can be challenging. Depending on the primary disease process, the possibility that the emergency conditions listed below can occur should be anticipated by the care team.
- Caregivers should be prepared with proper medications and supplies in the home to manage these conditions with the support and supervision of nurses and physicians. (See Chapter 14: Palliative Care Emergencies.) Potential emergencies include:
  - Pain crises
  - Increased intracranial pressure/herniation
  - Spinal cord compression
  - Pathologic or traumatic fracture
  - Hemorrhage
  - GI obstruction
  - Superior vena cava (SVC) syndrome
  - Delirium
  - Anxiety, panic attack
  - Hypercalcemia
  - Urinary retention
  - Fecal impaction
- Home hospice programs are equipped to respond to home emergencies on a 24-hour basis, providing an important safety net to both patient and family. In some communities, a palliative care "Rapid Response Service" is available to provide emergent care for emergencies in the home.[7]
- If an emergency situation arises and a family member in crisis calls 911, the hospice, Palliative Care Program, or primary physician managing the patient's care should be notified so that the established goals of care will be identified and maintained.

- Even with a well-coordinated home care or home hospice team, emergency conditions may require transfer to a hospital setting. To optimize patient care and safety, communication between the home care clinicians and inpatient care team will ensure efficient and coordinated medical treatment that is aligned with the patient's preferences and goals for care. (See Chapter 11: Care Transitions.)

ETHICAL ISSUES

When family members are also primary caregivers in the home, ethical issues may arise in the context of managing symptoms, maintaining confidentiality, and responding to family wishes to control the dying process.

1. **Symptom Management:** As death approaches, requests for clinical interventions are often based on caregiver distress rather than patient discomfort. One such example occurs when the family asks for lab work and blood transfusions for management of weakness associated with disease progression or the dying process. Another example is a request for artificial nutrition or hydration when the patient is nearing death and unable to take food or fluid by mouth.

   In these situations, clinicians must weigh the benefits of treating the caregiver distress against the possible burden for the patient, and determine if the proposed interventions remain consistent with the goals of care. These situations provide an opportunity to counsel and educate the family about expected physiologic changes during the dying process and to assess what additional emotional supports the family may require.

2. **Confidentiality:** Confidentiality can be jeopardized when family caregivers and close friends in the home can readily hear medical information shared by the care team with the patient, health care proxy, or surrogate. While it may be assumed that all persons in the home have standing to be aware of protected health information, this should be confirmed with the patient or an appointed representative whenever possible.

3. **Responding to Family Requests:** Families may ask the clinician if "anything can be done" either to maintain life longer than is expected or to hasten death in the hope of maintaining dignity and relieving suffering. The family should be advised that palliative care will neither hasten nor slow death, and also should be given assurances that excellent symptom control will be provided so that suffering is minimized, comfort is enhanced, and dignity preserved. The team should also explore with the patient or caregivers if there are underlying concerns that are motivating these requests, e.g., depression, anxiety, worry about the possibility of uncontrolled pain, or fear of death. (See Chapter 23: Responding to Requests for Hastened Death.)

PALLIATIVE CARE ISSUES

- In-home palliative care significantly increases patient and family satisfaction by providing essential clinical expertise and around-the-clock support so that patients and their families can achieve the goal of dying at home.[8]
- Patient and caregivers should be counseled, educated, and supported so that they feel safe, competent, and comfortable with the plan of care and its implementation.
- On every visit to the home, team members should "check in" with caregivers to see how they are feeling and coping. Encouragement and support should be offered to family members for the important role they have assumed in the care of the patient.
- Members of the interdisciplinary palliative care team—nursing, physical therapy, occupational therapy, speech therapy, chaplaincy, and social work—are trained to address patient and caregiver questions and offer reassurance and reinforcement about areas of concern. For example, the physical therapist can educate caregivers on proper use of lifts, transfers, turning, and repositioning techniques that empower the caregiver to provide safe and competent care. Chaplaincy and social work can address unresolved and painful family dynamics.

Please also see:
Chapter 21: Spirituality
Chapter 24: Assistive Aids and Devices
Chapter 108: Nursing

TAKE-HOME POINTS

- Patients nearing the end of life often express the wish to die at home. Before offering care at home as an option at the end of life, clinicians must evaluate the patient's clinical condition, determine the availability and ability of a designated caregiver, and identify services and resources that are adequate to meet the patient's care needs.

- Careful assessment, planning, and coordination of end-of-life care in the home will ensure that the medical, practical, emotional, spiritual, and educational needs of the patient and caregivers will be met.

- The interdisciplinary team providing care for patients at the end of life must anticipate issues that may arise, provide essential education, and be prepared to manage complex symptoms and medical emergencies that may occur in the home setting.

- All patient and caregiver needs and concerns about home as the place of death should be identified and addressed. Adequate caregiver education, support, and counseling should be provided, including when and how to contact emergency clinical support, mastering proper medication administration, and managing care tasks.

REFERENCES

1. Weitzen S, Tena JM, Fennell M, et al. Factors associated with site of death: a national study of where people die. *Med Care.* 2003;*41*:323–35.
2. Hays JC, Galanos AN, Palmer TA, et al. Preference for place of death in a continuing care retirement community. *Gerontologist.* 2001;*41*:123–128.
3. Doyle D. Palliative medicine in the home: an overview. In:Doyle D, Hanks G, Cherny N, Calman K, eds. *Oxford Textbook of Palliative Medicine, 3rd ed.* New York: Oxford University Press; 2005: 1097–1116.
4. Jencks SF, Williams MV, Coleman EA. Rehospitalization among patients in the Medicare fee-for-service program. *N Engl J Med.* April 2, 2009; *360*:1418–1428.
5. Morrison RS, Wallenstein S, Natale DK, et al. "We don't carry that,"—failure of pharmacies in predominantly nonwhite neighborhoods to stock opioid analgesics. *N Engl J Med.* 2000; *342*(14):1023–1026.
6. Bee PE, Barnes P, Luker KA. A systematic review of informal caregivers' needs in providing home-based end-of-life care to people with cancer. *J Clin Nurs.* 2009;*18*(10):1379–1393.
7. King G, Mackenzie J, Smith H, et al. Dying at home: evaluation of a hospice rapid-response service. *Int J Palliat Nurs.* 2000;*6*:280–287.
8. Brumley R, Enguidanos S, Jamison P, et al. Increased satisfaction with care and lower costs: results of a randomized trial of in-home primary care. *J Am Geriatr Soc.* 2007;*55*:993–1000.

16

Cultural Considerations

INTRODUCTION

Culture can be defined as an integrated pattern of human behavior that is based on shared knowledge, beliefs, values, attitudes, rules of behavior, and world view. It includes social, religious, linguistic, dietary, geographical, and historical factors. It is a synergistic force that shapes behavior yet also interacts with and is influenced by personal history, work experience, education, and economic status.

Culture is the way of life of a group of people. It includes the behaviors, beliefs, values, and symbols that they accept, generally without thinking about them, and that are passed along by communication and imitation from one generation to the next. It includes the roles, rituals, communication, languages, relationships, thoughts, courtesies, beliefs, practices, customs, manners of interacting, and expected behaviors of a group.

CULTURE IS DYNAMIC

- Culture is active and dynamic and applicable to all peoples. It can change over time because of migration, to meet new challenges to the group, through interactions with other groups, or even to adapt to climate. It is a multilayered concept consisting of personal, family, and community levels, at home, school, and in the workplace.
- Culture organizes perceptions and shapes behavior. It tells group members how to behave and provides their identity. Culture is difficult to quantify because it frequently exists at an unconscious level, or at least tends to be so pervasive that it escapes everyday thought. Like an iceberg, very often only the "tip" of complex cultural perceptions is evident on the surface (Figure 16.1).[1] Specific components of culture include ethnic identity, gender, age, differing abilities, sexual orientation, religion and spirituality, financial status, place of residency, employment experience, and education level.

CULTURE AND ETHNICITY

The concepts of culture and ethnicity are often confused because they overlap, but they can be distinguished as follows:

- Culture can be broadly understood as the totality of what a group of people think, what they value and how they behave, and what is passed on to future generations.
- An ethnic group is bound together by a shared heritage based upon a common geographical origin, ancestry, history, religion, language, and frequently a shared territory or nationality. Ethnicity is a term used to describe such a group's identity and perception of themselves.
- An ethnic group may share a common culture, but not all cultural groups are based on ethnicity. Examples of other types of "cultures" include those formed around religious, social, or political traditions and behaviors.

ETHNIC DIVERSITY IN THE UNITED STATES[2]

- Ethnic heterogeneity and diversity within the population creates a more complex cultural environment for health care providers. According to the 2010 census, the U.S. population is approximately 66% non-Hispanic White, 13% Black, 15% Hispanic, 5% Asian, and 1% American Indian/Alaska Native.
- The U.S. Census Bureau projects that by 2050, "minorities" will become the majority. The biggest increase will be seen in the Hispanic population, with an expected doubling between 2000 and 2050.
- Approximately 20% of the elderly population in the United States belongs to minority groups, including African Americans, Asians, Hispanics, and those of Pacific Island descent. Minority elders are expected to account for 50% of the elderly population by 2050.

An Iceberg Concept of Culture

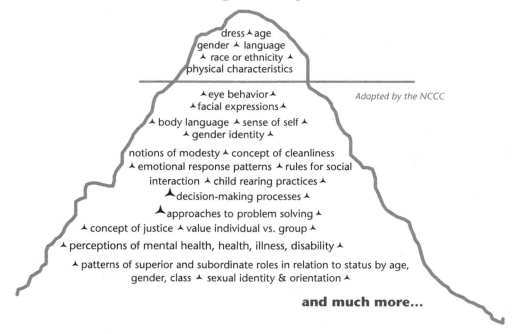

FIGURE 16.1: An iceberg concept of culture.

Source: The National Center for Cultural Competence, 2008.

WHY DOES CULTURE MATTER IN HEALTH CARE?

There is evidence to suggest that health care disparities exist for racial and ethnic minorities in the United States, even when they are insured to the same degree and when other health care access-related factors are taken into account. The Institute of Medicine (IOM) report *Unequal Treatment: Confronting Racial and Ethnic Disparities in Healthcare* concluded that bias, prejudice, and stereotyping by providers may contribute to differences in care.[3]

CULTURAL COMPETENCE IN HEALTH CARE

- Culturally competent heath care has been defined as care that incorporates the importance of culture, assessment of cross cultural relations, vigilance toward the dynamics that result from cultural differences, expansion of cultural knowledge, and adaptation of services to meet culturally unique needs.[4]
- The goal of a culturally competent health care system is to deliver the highest quality of care to every patient, regardless of race, ethnicity, cultural background, or English language proficiency.

LINGUISTIC COMPETENCY

- As a part of cultural competency, linguistic competency provides health care professionals with additional skills and knowledge. The National Center for Cultural Competence has defined linguistic competency as the capacity of an organization and its personnel to communicate effectively and convey information in a manner that is easily understood by diverse audiences including persons of limited English proficiency, those who have low literacy skills or are not literate, and individuals with disabilities.[5]
- Language is one of the critical barriers in caring for a culturally diverse older population. Currently the U.S. population consists of 11% foreign born, 18% who speak a language other than English at home, and 8% who speak English less than "very well."[6]

- Limited English proficiency has been associated with adverse health status, less use of health care services, negative health outcomes, decreased rates of preventive care, less ability to understand care, increased risk of unethical care, and less satisfaction with care.[7,8]

ROLE OF CULTURE IN PALLIATIVE CARE DECISION-MAKING

- Although providers in all areas of health care should demonstrate culturally competent behaviors and attitudes, the treatment of patients with life-threatening illnesses and their families calls for extreme sensitivity to cultural attitudes and beliefs.
- There is also a compelling need to communicate critically important and complex medical information in a language and manner that patients and families can understand. If the patient and family members do not speak or understand English, all reasonable efforts should be made to use professional interpreter services. When professional interpreters are not available, other health care providers or family members may serve as translators, with the agreement of the patient.[9]
- Cultural factors strongly influence a patient's reactions to advanced illness and also have a significant impact on decisions concerning goals for care. Being knowledgeable and sensitive about the role of culture in health care beliefs and attitudes can help clinicians successfully elicit and honor patient values and preferences for treatment (Table 16.1).

DEVELOPING CULTURAL COMPETENCY

- Health care professionals must learn and develop skills to respond to the increasing demographic changes in their patient population and to fully comply with regulatory and quality of care requirements.

TABLE 16.1: ROLE OF CULTURE IN PALLIATIVE CARE PLANNING

Palliative Care Domain	Issues Affected by Culture
Management of pain and distressing symptoms	Suffering and pain Role of nutrition Alternative medicine
Advance care planning	Patient autonomy vs. dependence Withdrawal vs. withholding Role of family in caring Designating a health care proxy Attitudes about postmortem and organ donation
Establishing goals of care	Family decision-making Key participants Quality of life vs. quantity of life Religious practices and beliefs Socioeconomic influence Preferred location of death Place of death (home, hospice, or hospital)
Psycho-social-spiritual support	Meaning of illness/suffering Meaning of the dying process and death Religious practices and beliefs Death and dying rituals, funeral and burial practices Bereavement and expression of grief Self-care
Communication	Disclosure/truth telling Preferred language Language taboos

- Cross-cultural education programs for health care trainees have been instituted to enhance awareness of cultural and social factors and their influence on the delivery of health care.[10]
- Tools for cross-cultural communication have been developed that clinicians may incorporate into the normal structure of their therapeutic encounters. The two models below can improve communication, heighten awareness of cultural issues affecting health care decisions, and facilitate collaborative treatment planning.

The Explanatory Model[11]

This model is a culturally sensitive approach designed to elicit information about the patient's perception of the health problem, his/her therapeutic goals, and the psychosocial and cultural meaning of the illness. Suggested questions to help explore these issues include:

What do you call your problem?

What do you think caused your problem?

Why do you think it started when it did?

What does your sickness do to you? How does it work?

How severe is it? How long do you think you will have it?

What do you fear most about your illness?

What are the chief problems your sickness has caused you?

Anyone else with the same problem?

What have you done so far to treat your illness? What treatments do you think you should receive? What important results do you hope to receive from the treatment?

Who else can help you?

The LEARN Model[12]

This cross-cultural communication tool is based on the mnemonic L-E-A-R-N.

Listen to the patient's perception of the problem

Elicit the health beliefs of the patient

Assess priorities, values and supports

Recommend treatment

Negotiate treatment

TABLE 16.2: "LEARN" TO BE CULTURALLY SENSITIVE IN PATIENT ENCOUNTERS[9]

Listen actively with empathy and respect	Identify yourself and greet the patient Determine if there is a need for interpreter services Set the tone by asking open-ended questions and being patient
Elicit the health beliefs of the patient, as they relate to the reason for the visit as well as the patient's health behaviors	"What worries you the most?" "Have you started any treatment on your own or gotten advice from others?" "What do you think has caused the problem and what do you think started it?" "How can I be of most help to you?"
Assess priorities, values, and supports in the patient's life that may impact health and health behaviors	"I'd like to get to know you more today. Could you tell me about yourself?" "With whom do you live? Where do you work?" "What brought you to this country? How does medical care differ here?" "Do you have family and friends that help you with decisions or give you advice?" "Do you have any trouble reading medicine bottles or appointment cards?" "Is transportation a problem for you?"
Recommend a plan of action with adequate explanation and understanding	Use language the patient can easily understand (avoid jargon) Be guided by the patient about how much information to provide Check to make sure has understood by asking him/her to paraphrase For example: "To be sure that we understand each other, would you please tell me what I just explained to you?"
Negotiate by involving the patient in next steps and decisions	"Now that we understand each other, let's come up with a plan that works for you." "What do you think should be the next steps?"

This model is not intended to replace the structure of the medical encounter but is rather a supplement to the history-taking process. The aim is to elicit the patient's theoretical explanation of the reason for the problem. Table 16.2 outlines the steps of the L-E-A-R-N model and suggests strategies and language that may helpful.

TAKE-HOME POINTS

- Increasing ethnic heterogeneity and diversity within the U.S. patient population creates a complex cross-cultural environment for health care providers.
- The goal of a culturally competent health care system is to deliver the highest quality of care to every patient, regardless of race, ethnicity, cultural background, or English language proficiency.
- Clinicians should strive to understand the patient as a whole person, including background, birth, immigration, family illness experiences, and other important ethnic and cultural data.
- Caring for patients from different cultural backgrounds in situations of serious illness or at the end of life can be an especially challenging and complex endeavor.
- If the patient and family members do not speak or understand English, all reasonable efforts should be made to use professional interpreter services. Other health care providers or family members may serve as translators in an emergency.
- Tools for cross-cultural communication have been developed that clinicians may incorporate into the normal structure of their therapeutic encounters.

REFERENCES

1. National Center for Cultural Competence. A closer look at culture. http://www11.georgetown.edu/research/gucchd/nccc/documents/ppt-culture.pdf. Accessed April 29, 2013.
2. Byrd L, Fletcher A, Menfield C. Disparities in health care: minority elders at risk. *The ABNF Journal.* Spring 2007;*18*(2):51–55.
3. Unequal treatment: understanding racial and ethnic disparities in health care. In: Smedley BD, Stith AY, Nelson AR, eds. *Committee on Understanding and Eliminating Racial and Ethnic Disparities in Health Care, Board on Health Sciences,* Institute of Medicine. 2002. http://www.iom.edu/Reports/2002/Unequal-Treatment-Confronting-Racial-and-Ethnic-Disparities-in-Health-Care. Accessed June, 2012.
4. Betancourt JR, Green AR, Carrillo JE, Ananeh-Firempong O. Defining cultural competence: a practical framework for addressing racial/ethnic disparities in health and health care. *Public Health Reports* July-August 2003:*118*:293–302.
5. The National Center for Cultural Competency. Conceptual Frameworks/Models, Guiding Values and Principles. http://nccc.georgetown.edu/foundations/frameworks.html accessed July 20, 2012.)
6. Language use in the United States. American Community Survey Reports. April 2010. U.S. Census Bureau. http://www.census.gov/hhes/socdemo/language/data/acs/ACS-12.pdf. Accessed July 2012.
7. Woloshin W, Bickell NA, Schwartz LM, Gany FG, Welch HG. Language Barriers in Medicine in the United States. *JAMA.* 1995;*273*(9):724–728.
8. Ponce NA, Hays RD, Cunningham WE. Linguistic Disparities in Health Care Access and Health Status Among Older Adults. *J Gen Int Med.* July 2006; *21*(7):786–791.
9. National Consensus Project for Quality Palliative Care. Clinical Practice Guidelines for Quality Palliative Care, Second Edition, 2009. http://www.nationalconsensusproject.org/guideline.pdf. Accessed July, 2012.
10. Kripalani S, Bussey-Jones J, Katz MG, Genao I. A prescription of cultural competence in medical education. *J Gen Intern Med.* 2006;*21*:1116–1120.
11. Kleinman A, Einseberg L, Good B. Culture, illness, and care: clinical lessons from anthropologic and cross-cultural research *Ann Intern Med.* 1978;*88*:251–258.
12. Berlin EA, Fowkes WC. A teaching framework for cross-cultural healthcare, *West J Med.* 1983; *12*(139):934–938.

17

Complementary and Alternative Medicine

INTRODUCTION

The field of complementary and alternative medicine (CAM), more recently termed *"integrative health,"* describes not only the integration of complementary therapies with traditional Western medicine, but also the idea of attention to patients' combined physical, mental, and spiritual needs, a focus particularly appropriate in the palliative care patient. In addition, the nonauthoritarian, partnership role of the CAM healer with the participant may be particularly appealing to patients experiencing loss of control due to the consequences of a serious illness.

Studies on the prevalence of CAM in cancer patients are indicative of the surge in popularity of CAM therapies. They suggest that 40–85% of cancer patients use CAM in hopes of improving healing response, reducing side effects of standard treatments, and improving their quality of life.[1]

EVIDENCE BASE

- Research evidence exists to support the role of some CAM therapies; for others, additional studies are needed. The extremely widespread use of dietary supplements provides a cautionary tale for the appropriate use of CAM. No well-done clinical trials support the use of the many dietary supplements commonly used by cancer patients, including echinacea, shark cartilage, grape seed extract, milk thistle, and numerous others.
- Since dietary supplements are not regulated under the same Food and Drug Administration (FDA) category as food and drugs, product content and safety are not guaranteed. Some products have been associated with toxicities, such as hepatotoxicity from chaparral, comfrey, and kava kava; other products may affect cell proliferation (Dong quai, ginseng) or interfere with cancer treatments (e.g., St. Johns Wort's effect on the cytochrome P450 system, altering levels of chemotherapeutic agents, or antioxidants interfering with the oxidative mechanism of radiation therapy).
- Most importantly, patients who turn to CAM for their primary therapy may forgo conventional treatment, hastening suffering and death in some cases.[1] Therefore, until evidence becomes available, it is prudent to advise against the use of dietary therapies for cancer patients.
- There are, however, numerous integrative health modalities that are supported by research evidence or empirical evidence and that have demonstrated or theoretical efficacy in palliative care patients.[2,3]

Acupuncture

Acupuncture is one of the ancient practices of Oriental medicine. It is based on the theory that good health results from the free flow of life energy, called chi or qi, along pathways in the body called meridians. Diseases and ill health are treated by stimulating points along the meridians with fine needles to restore a balanced flow of energy.

- There is evidence that acupuncture is effective for certain palliative care indications:

  Nausea and vomiting: The NIH Consensus Statement on acupuncture concluded that acupuncture is effective in reducing adult chemotherapy-related and postoperative nausea and vomiting.[4]

  Pain: Uncontrolled studies have demonstrated the effectiveness of acupuncture in controlling cancer pain, as well as pain related to procedures and chronic pain such as headaches.[5] It may also be effective in reducing dyspnea.

  Others: Acupuncture has also been used to treat xerostomia, hot flashes, and depressed mood, but more studies need to be done to support its use for these symptoms.[5,6]

- Potential adverse reactions: When practiced by licensed providers, acupuncture is quite safe, and significant adverse events are rare. Most common minor adverse events are needle pain, tiredness, and minor bleeding. Acupuncture should be avoided in patients with a bleeding diathesis, neutropenia, or lymphedema.
- Patients should ask their insurance company whether acupuncture treatments are covered in their plan.

Mind-Body Therapies

The National Center for Complementary and Alternative Medicine (NCCAM) defines mind-body therapy as "behavioral, psychologic, social and spiritual approaches to medicine not commonly used."[7] These approaches include meditation, relaxation, guided imagery, hypnosis, and biofeedback. These and other, more conventional behavioral and psychosocial therapies have been applied with increasing frequency to numerous palliative care-related conditions, including pain, anxiety and depression, symptoms of stress, and insomnia. As with other CAM therapies, more studies are needed to evaluate the efficacy of these mind-body therapies.

- A number of meditation techniques have been utilized in patients with pain and psychological distress. One of the most widely studied techniques is Mindfulness-Based Stress Reduction, which teaches awareness of the moment by focusing the mind to reduce physiological and psychological reactions to stress. Studies of its use in cancer patients support benefits in mood and sleep quality, and lower levels of stress.[8] Other studies support its use for headache and chronic pain in the general population.[9,10,11]
- Mind-body therapies have been suggested for the following possible uses in palliative care patients:
  - Progressive muscle relaxation as an adjuvant to antiemetics for chemotherapy-related nausea and vomiting
  - Relaxation and guided imagery for acute treatment-related pain and psychological distress
  - Relaxation for anxiety and depression
  - Mind-body therapies for cancer-related fatigue
  - Relaxation and self-hypnosis for mood and sleep

- Group CAM support offering meditation, affirmation, imagery, and ritual for quality of life and mood
- Tai chi and yoga (see below), hypnosis, and progressive muscle relaxation for pain control
- Because strong evidence of benefit is lacking for many of these therapies, clinicians should base decisions for use on available research evidence, clinical judgment, risk/benefit assessment, and patient preferences.[2]
- Many different types of therapists offer mind-body therapies, some of them licensed and with graduate degrees, others not licensed and with various forms of training and experience. Patients should be encouraged to ask about training, and ideally obtain referrals from health care professionals or others who are familiar with the therapist's record of working with clients with serious illness.
- Most of the mind-body therapies are not covered by insurance unless delivered by an MD, PhD, or MSW, but patients should nevertheless be encouraged to ask insurers whether treatments are covered.

Yoga

Yoga, with roots in ancient Hindu spiritual practice, combines breathing exercises (pranayama), physical postures (asana), and meditation. Its benefit lies in its purported ability to balance mind, body, and spirit, and support the flow of life energy (qi). Benefits are thought to occur via upregulation of the parasympathetic nervous system and increase in brain gamma aminobutyric acid (GABA).

- Yoga for palliative care patients must be carefully tailored to the patient's endurance, with consideration of individual factors such as bony pathology. Limited evidence supports its efficacy in improving sleep in cancer patients.[12] Studies in general population groups have demonstrated effectiveness for low back pain.[13]
- Yoga is also thought to be beneficial in reducing stress, depression, anxiety, and fatigue, but studies are needed to document this efficacy. Restorative postures and pranayama (breathing) exercises may be both energizing and relaxing. Yoga Nidra, a meditative/guided imagery exercise, may be used for stress, anxiety, and insomnia.

- Yoga teachers are registered with the Yoga Teachers Alliance; palliative care patients are advised to seek out teachers who offer classes or individual sessions specifically tailored to patients with serious or chronic illness.
- Insurance plans do not cover yoga therapy.

Tai Chi

Tai chi is a form of Chinese martial art that can also be considered a mind-body therapy, as it combines a flow of physical movements, or forms, with self-exploration.

- Some uses of Tai Chi relevant to palliative care patients include proposed benefits for cardiovascular health, balance, mood, bone strength, stress reduction, sleep, and relief of fibromyalgia and musculoskeletal pain.[14,15]
- Tai chi teachers are not licensed. Participants are encouraged to inquire about the teacher's experience and knowledge of working with patients with serious illness.
- Tai Chi is not covered by insurance.

Massage Therapy

In basic massage therapy, practitioners use their hands and fingers to manipulate muscles for a variety of therapeutic reasons. The difference between massage types or techniques is determined by how massage is applied. Variations in the speed, pressure, intensity, and intent of the massage will yield different therapeutic results. Slower massage techniques tend to be more relaxing, while vigorous massage techniques are stimulating.[16]

- Research indicates that massage therapy may help reduce stress and tension, bolster the immune system, improve mood, and reduce chronic muscle tension and postural imbalances. Certain types of massage therapy may also confer benefit in areas such as pain control, sleep disturbances, anxiety, depression, physical discomfort, stress reduction, and mood.[17,18]
- Geriatric patients may benefit from massage, especially for chronic muscle pain, tension, and discomfort due to lack of adequate exercise, disuse, atrophy, poor body awareness and biomechanics, and degenerative changes such as osteoarthritis and spinal stenosis.
- In the palliative care setting, where the focus of care is on pain and symptom reduction, patient comfort, and quality of life, modified massage techniques can improve patients' experience of their illness and enhance satisfaction with their hospital stay.
- Massage techniques must be adapted for palliative care patients due to the complex interaction of the patient's illness, the medical therapies involved, and the constraints of the hospital environment. The massage intervention for seriously ill hospitalized patients aims to reduce symptoms and to help the patient feel more comfortable and composed.
- After reviewing relevant clinical information about a patient, an experienced and skilled licensed massage therapist should be able modify standard techniques to accommodate a wide variety of therapeutic needs for the palliative care population.
- Massage therapists should be licensed in the state where they practice; this ensures that they are adequately trained. Different states have varying recommendations for the amount and type of training required.
- Some insurance companies will pay for medical massage and manual lymph drainage with a prescription from a doctor.

Useful Websites for Information on CAM

1. National Center for Complementary and Alternative Medicine (NCCAM) http://nccam.nih.gov/health
2. American College of Physicians (ACP) http://www.acponline.org/acp_press/comp_alt_med
3. Mayo Clinic: Complementary and Alternative Medicine http://www.mayoclinic.com/health
4. National Cancer Institute (NCI) http://www.cancer.gov/cancertopics/treatment/cam

REFERENCES

1. Jacobs BP, Gundling K. *The ACP Evidence-Based Guide to Complementary and Alternative Medicine*. ACP Press; Philadelphia, 2009.
2. Deng G, Cassileth BR. Integrative oncology: Complementary therapies for pain, anxiety and

mood disturbance. *CA Cancer J Clin.* 2005;*55*: 109–116.

3. Pan CX, Morrison RS, Ness J, et al. Complementary and alternative medicine in the management of pain, dyspnea, and nausea and vomiting near the end of life: A systematic review. *J Pain SymptomManage.* 2000;*20*:374–387.

4. Acupuncture. NIH Consensus Statement. 1997;*15*: 1–34.

5. Pfister DG, Cassileth BR, Deng GE, et al. Acupuncture for pain and dysfunction after neck dissection: results of a randomized control trial. *J Clin Oncol.* 2010;*28*(15):2565–2570.

6. Dean-Clower E, Doherty-Gilman AM, Keshaviah A, et al. Acupuncture as palliative therapy for physical symptoms and quality of life for advanced cancer patients. *Integr Cancer Ther.* 2010;*9*(2): 158–167.

7. National Center for Complementary and Alternative Medicine. http://nccam.nih.gov/health/whatiscam. Accessed February 1, 2012.

8. Smith J, Richardson J, Hoffman C, et al. Mindfulness-based stress reduction as supportive therapy in cancer care: systematic review. *J Adv Nurs.* 2005;*52*:315–327.

9. Kabat-Zinn J, Lipworth L, Burney R, Sellers W. Four-year follow-up of a meditation-based program for the self-regulation of chronic pain: Treatment outcomes and compliance. *Clin J Pain.* 1986;*2*(3):159–173.

10. Morone NE, Greco CM. Mind-body interventions for chronic pain in older adults: A structured review. *Pain Med.* 2007;*8*(4):359–375.

11. Sierpina V, Astin J, Giordano J. Mind-body therapies for headache. *Am Fam Phys.* 2007;*76*(10): 1518–1522.

12. Bower JE, Woolery A, Sternlieb B, Garet D. Yoga for cancer patients and survivors. *CA Control.* 2005;*12*(3):165–171.

13. Sherman KJ, Cherkin DC, Erro J, et al. Comparing yoga, exercise, and a self-care book for chronic low-back pain. *Ann Intern Med.* 2005;*143*:849–856.

14. Kuramoto AM. Therapeutic benefits of Tai Chi exercise; research review. *WMJ.* 2006;*105*(7): 42–46.

15. Wang C, Schmid CH, Rones R, Kalish R et al. A randomized control trial of Tai Chi for fibromyalgia. *N Engl J Med.* 2010;*363*(8):743–754.

16. National Center for Complementary and Alternative Medicine. http://nccam.nih.gov/health/backgrounds/manipulative.htm#def. Accessed February 1, 2012.

17. Moyer CA, Rounds J, Hannum JW. A meta-analysis of massage therapy research. *Psychological Bulletin.* 2004;*130*(1):3–18.

18. Cassileth BR, Vickers AJ. Massage therapy for symptom control: outcome study at a major cancer center. *J Pain Symptom Manage.* 2004;*28*:244–249.

CROSS-REFERENCES WITH OTHER CHAPTERS IN THIS BOOK

Pain Management

(See Chapter 29: Pain Management.)
Integrative health, or complementary and alternative medicine (CAM), interventions that have shown efficacy in treatment of pain include acupuncture, mediation, Mindfulness-Based Stress Reduction, relaxation, guided imagery, and yoga.[3]

Headache

(See Chapter 38: Headache.)
Meta-analyses of randomized controlled trials demonstrate that mind-body therapies such as biofeedback, cognitive behavioral therapy, hypnosis, meditation, and relaxation training significantly reduce symptoms or migraine, tension, and mixed-type headaches.[11]

Shortness of Breath; Dyspnea

(See Chapter 41: Dyspnea.)
One study demonstrated the effectiveness of acupuncture in reducing dyspnea in patients with severe COPD.

Nausea and Vomiting

(See Chapter 53: Nausea and Vomiting.)
Acupuncture and mind-body therapies have shown some efficacy in cancer patients with surgery- and chemotherapy-related nausea and vomiting

Depression

(See Chapter 64: Depression.)
Mind-body therapies including Mindfulness-Based Stress Reduction, relaxation, hypnosis, yoga, and tai chi have shown effectiveness in the treatment of depression.

Anxiety

(See Chapter 65: Anxiety.)
Mind-body therapies including Mindfulness-Based Stress Reduction, relaxation, hypnosis, yoga, and tai chi have shown effectiveness in the treatment of anxiety.

Osteoarthritis

(See Chapter 86: Osteoarthritis.)
Current studies suggest some evidence for the use of acupuncture to treat osteoarthritis of the knee.[1]

Osteoporosis and Fractures

(See Chapter 88: Osteoporotic Fracture.)
Evidence suggests the efficacy of tai chi in maintaining bone mineral density in postmenopausal women, as well as improving muscle strength and reducing falls.[1]

Breast Cancer

(See Chapter 97: Breast Cancer.)
Support groups for breast cancer patients offering complementary and alternative medicine (CAM) interventions including meditation, affirmation, imagery, and ritual have been shown to be effective in improving quality of life and mood.

18

Clinician Self-Care

INTRODUCTION

All health care professionals can experience the substantial personal and professional pressures that come with taking care of patients in today's U.S. health care system. Palliative care professionals face the added challenges of providing care to seriously ill patients and their families who are navigating a very emotional and stressful time in their lives.[1]

Given the physical, emotional, and spiritual demands of offering compassionate care for seriously ill patients and their families, combined with the organizational and administrative challenges of the health care work environment, palliative care clinicians must develop a strategy for self-care. Whether it is a structured formal practice or an informal collection of self-awareness techniques, all palliative care professionals should integrate practical and effective self-care strategies into the fabric of their personal and professional lives.

CONSEQUENCES OF NEGLECTING SELF-CARE

- Many commentators have pointed to the paradox of health care professionals dispensing advice to others yet personally ignoring advice about leading a balanced life. This is not a new problem for medical practitioners.[2] Some providers are just not familiar with the early warning signs and symptoms of unhealthy personal and professional pressures that may be overwhelming them. Or they may know that they are profoundly stressed, but may not be familiar with self-care strategies that can help restore the balance in their lives and help manage the pressures they are coping with in their job.
- Lack of awareness and/or inability to establish an effective self-care practice can eventually progress to the deep physical and emotional exhaustion of burnout or compassion fatigue.

BURNOUT AND COMPASSION FATIGUE

- Burnout and compassion fatigue are related conditions. But although they are frequently used interchangeably in the literature, they are not equivalent concepts.
- **Burnout** is defined by Maslach as "a syndrome of emotional exhaustion and cynicism that occurs frequently among individuals who do people-work of some kind."[3] Emotional exhaustion has been identified as the first stage of burnout, followed by depersonalization employed as a coping strategy, and eventually resulting in feelings of reduced personal accomplishment.[4]
- **Compassion fatigue** (CF) is a more recent construct, first used in 1992, and defined as a "deep, physical, emotional, and spiritual exhaustion accompanied by acute emotional pain."[5] Because CF is associated with helping or wanting to help a traumatized or suffering person, it is also referred to as secondary or vicarious traumatization. One theory explains compassion fatigue in the health care professional as the result of extended exposure to the suffering and trauma of others while simultaneously receiving little or no emotional support for oneself in the workplace, and with no self-care practices in place.[6]

PREVALENCE

- Extensive research has confirmed that nurses are particularly susceptible to burnout.[7] One study found that 40% of hospital nurses have burnout levels that exceed the norms for health care workers, and that their job dissatisfaction is four times greater than the average for all U.S. workers.[8]

- In a large national sample of physicians from several specialties, 46% of responders reported at least one symptom of burnout. Rates of burnout differed according to specialty, with the highest prevalence occurring in "front line" physicians (family medicine, general internal medicine, and emergency medicine).[9]
- In a study of students at seven U.S. medical schools, burnout was reported by 49.6% of students, with 11% reporting suicidal ideation within the past year.[10]
- Palliative care practitioners have a number of personal and job-related stressors, and the prevalence of burnout is significant. The literature is conflicting, however, as to whether palliative care clinicians have higher or lower rates of burnout than other health professionals.[11]

CAUSES, RISK FACTORS, AND SYMPTOMS

Table 18.1 compares the causes, risk factors, signs, and symptoms of burnout and compassion fatigue.

CONSEQUENCES OF UNADDRESSED BURNOUT AND COMPASSION FATIGUE

Many studies on the impact of burnout on the health care system have suggested that physician burnout may erode professionalism, influence quality of care, increase the risk for medical errors, and promote early retirement.[9]

DIAGNOSIS

The standard assessment tool for burnout is the Maslach Burnout Inventory (MBI), available from Consulting Psychologists Press, http://www.cpp.com. The MBI is a validated instrument consisting of 22 questions that measures the three classic signs and symptoms of burnout:

1. **Emotional exhaustion**: measures feelings of being emotionally overextended and exhausted by one's work
2. **Depersonalization**: measures an unfeeling and impersonal response toward recipients of one's service, care treatment, or instruction
3. **Reduced accomplishment**: measures feelings of competence and successful achievement in one's work

- The length of the MBI can limit its utility in surveys of health care professionals.

Responses to just two questions from the MBI ("I feel burned out from my work" and "I have become more callous toward people since I took this job") have been shown to help assess burnout in medical professionals when the MBI cannot be used.[12]
- Assessment tools for compassion fatigue include the Professional Quality of Life Scale (http://proqol.org/ProQol_Test.html) and the compassion fatigue self-test (http://www.compassionfatigue.org/pages/selftest.html).

PREVENTIVE STRATEGIES

- All health care professionals must attend to self-care and renewal for the sake of themselves, their family, friends, colleagues, and their patients and families. The following recommendations for preventing burnout are based on suggestions from palliative care experts.[1,11,13]
- Self-awareness, self-reflection, and self-monitoring: Pay attention to stress level and understand what the triggers are; be aware of personal limits; be clear about reasons for working in the field of palliative care.
- Techniques for developing self-awareness include journaling, regular conversations with a trusted colleague, and setting time aside for personal reflection.
- Take advantage of supportive colleagues on the interdisciplinary team to discuss complex cases and explore difficult emotions. Find peers who understand the work and can serve as a sounding board.
- Utilize regularly scheduled support mechanisms, e.g., formal supervision for practicing therapists or social workers.
- For new palliative care practitioners, mentoring from a more experienced practitioner can be especially helpful. Experienced palliative care professionals frequently have achieved enhanced appreciation of the existential and spiritual domains of their own life as a result of caring for patients who are nearing the end of life. Rewarding and deeply satisfying benefits include a reciprocal healing process; inner self-reflection; closer connection with colleagues, family, and friends; and a heightened sense of spirituality.

TABLE 18.1: BURNOUT VS. COMPASSION FATIGUE: CAUSES AND RISK FACTORS

	Burnout	Compassion Fatigue
Definition	State of mental and/or physical exhaustion caused by excessive and prolonged stress Mental distress manifested in individuals who experience decreased work performance resulting from negative attitudes and behaviors	"Cost of caring" for others in emotional pain Sometimes known as secondary or vicarious traumatization
Cause	Stress arising from interaction with work environment Result of: Frustration Powerlessness Inability to achieve work goals	Stress arising from clinician/patient relationship
Risk Factors	***Individual risk factors***: Early in career Being single Lack of openness to change Triad of doubt, guilt, and exaggerated sense of responsibility ***Job risk factors***: Time pressure Solo practice Inadequate resources Lack of social and supervisor support Lack of information and control ***Organizational risk factors***: Lack of reciprocity/loyalty not rewarded Human services job Must display or suppress emotion on the job Must be emotionally empathic on the job ***Other risk factors:*** Previous mental health problems (especially depression) Low "hardiness" or resilience External locus of control Avoidant or passive/defensive coping style Type A personality	***Individual risk factors***: High expectations/idealism Perfectionism Lack of self-awareness ***Job risk factors:*** Short intervals between caring for patients No debriefing process ***Other risk factors***: Personality traits of compassion and empathy Personal history of trauma or victimization Working with traumatized and/or victimized people
Signs and Symptoms	Overwhelming exhaustion Feelings of cynicism and detachment from the job Sense of ineffectiveness or lack of personal accomplishment	Similar to PTSD Hyperarousal Disturbed sleep Irritability or outbursts of anger Hypervigilance Avoidance Desire to avoid thoughts, feelings, conversations associated with patient's pain and suffering Re-experiencing Intrusive thoughts or dreams Psychological or physiological distress in response to reminders of work

TABLE 18.2: CONSEQUENCES OF UNADDRESSED BURN-OUT OR COMPASSION FATIGUE

Domain	Consequence
Physical	Fatigue Sleeping problems Somatic complaints
Emotional	Irritability Anxiety Depression Guilt Helplessness
Personal	Depletion of emotional and physical resources Negative self-image Self-neglect Mental illness (anxiety, depression, substance abuse, suicide)
Behavioral	Aggression Callousness Pessimism Defensiveness Cynicism Avoidance of patients Acting out (verbally or physically) Poor concentration
Interpersonal	Poor communication Social withdrawal Lack of sense of humor Feelings of anger and frustration toward patients, families, colleagues Neglect of family and social obligations Poor patient interactions
Job-Related	Quitting Poor work performance Absenteeism Lateness Compromised patient care (increased use of technology, goals of care not discussed, increased length of stay) Loss of boundaries

- Developing a personal support system (family, friends, a supportive primary relationship) helps to maintain the balance between work and other aspects of one's life.
- Develop a personal self-care practice as a source of serenity and balance, possibly with a spiritual element such as meditation, yoga, or tai chi.
- Physical release is just as important as mental activity. Be sure to find time to include exercise in the daily routine.

IMPORTANCE OF TEAM SUPPORT[1,12,14]

A core function of the interdisciplinary palliative team is to provide meaningful support to team members. Results from studies showing that palliative care clinicians do not experience a higher level of stress and burnout than other health care professionals have been attributed to the support that palliative care team members offer to each other.[11]

- Team leaders should facilitate excellent team communication and consistently reinforce the importance of team building, support, and renewal. Specific strategies include:

- Continual monitoring for sustainable workload
- Promotion of choice and control for team members
- Recognition and reward for job well done
- Facilitating a supportive work community
- Promotion of fairness and justice in workplace
- Regular times should be set aside for the team to address difficult situations (patient-related, team-related, system-related) and to engage in problem-solving together.
- Support groups for medical professionals should be available for team members.
- Schwartz Center rounds are multidisciplinary rounds where health care professionals discuss difficult emotional and social issues that arise during patient care (http://www.theschwartzcenter.org/programs/rounds.html).
- Team processes and rituals acknowledge losses and help mourn patients who have died (e.g., memorial services, patient recognition rounds, staff debriefings).
- Teams should also celebrate their achievements, even in the context of difficult or unsuccessful cases, and find satisfaction in having tried to do the right thing.

WHEN TO SEEK TREATMENT

- The self-help strategies described above, combined with discussion with colleagues and mentors, can help address common stressors encountered by palliative care professionals.
- For more complex or troublesome symptoms, it is essential to seek professional counseling. Symptoms indicating need for follow-up with a mental health professional include:
  - Continued feelings of sadness, exhaustion, anger, worthlessness, hopelessness, suicidal ideation, or anxiety that interferes with work and relationships
  - Self-prescribing of medications (particularly sedative-hypnotics)

- Substance abuse (alcohol, prescription drugs, illegal drugs)
- Excessive or addictive behaviors (gambling, exercise, eating, shopping)
- Continued sleep disturbance (nightmares, insomnia)
- Loss of professional boundaries

TAKE-HOME POINTS

- All health care professionals experience substantial personal and professional pressures and stresses. Palliative care professionals face the added challenges of providing care to seriously ill patients and their families at a very emotional and stressful time in their lives.
- Lack of awareness or inability to practice self-care can eventually put palliative care clinicians at risk for the deep physical and emotional exhaustion of burnout or compassion fatigue.
- Palliative care practitioners have a number of personal and job-related stressors, and the prevalence of burnout is significant. The literature is conflicting, however, as to whether palliative care clinicians have higher or lower rates of burnout than other health professionals.
- Whether it is a structured formal practice or an informal collection of self-awareness techniques, all palliative care professionals should integrate practical and effective self-care strategies into the fabric of their personal and professional lives.
- Self-help strategies described above, combined with discussion with colleagues and mentors, can most likely address the common symptoms of burnout. For more complex or troublesome symptoms, it is essential to seek professional counseling.

REFERENCES

1. Meier DE, Beresford L. Preventing burnout. *J Palliat Med.* 2006;9(5):1045–1048.
2. Hatem CJ. Renewal in the practice of medicine. *Patient Education and Counseling.* 2006;62:299–391.
3. Maslach C, Jackson SE. The measurement of experienced burn-out. *J Occup Behav.* 1981;2:99–113.
4. Payne N. Occupational stressors and coping as determinants of burnout in female hospice nurses. *J Adv Nurs.* 2001;33(3):396–405.
5. Pfifferling J, Gilley K. Overcoming compassion fatigue. *Fam Pact Manage.* 2000;7(4):1–6.

6. Radley M, Figley C. The social psychology of compassion. *Clin Soc Work J.* 2007;*35*:205–214.

7. Leiter MP, Maslach C. Nurse turnover: the mediating role of burn-out. *J Nurs Manage.* 2009; *17*:331–339.

8. Aiken LH, Clarke SP, Sloane DM, et al. Hosoitak nurse staffing and patient mortality, nurse burnout, and job dissatisfaction. *JAMA.* 2002;*288*(16):1987–1993.

9. Shanafelt TD, Boone S, Tan L, et al. Burnout and satisfaction with work-life balance among US physicians relative to the general US population. *Arch Inter Med.* 2012; doi:10.1001/archinternmed.2012.3199.

10. Dyrbye LN, Thomas MR, Massie FS, et al. Burnout and suicidal ideation among U.S. medical students. *Ann Intern Med.* 2008;*149*:334–341.

11. Kearney MK, Weininger RB, Vachon MLS, et al. Self care of physicians caring for patients at the end of life. *JAMA.* 2009;*301*(11):1155–1164.

12. West CP, Dyrbye LN, Sloan JA, Shanafelt TD. Single item measures of emotional exhaustion and depersonalization are useful for assessing burnout in medical professionals. *J Gen Intern Med.* 2009;*24*(12):1318–1321.

13. Vachon MS. Staff stress in hospice/palliative care: a review. *Palliat Med.* 1995;*9*:91–122.

14. Vachon MLS. Caring for the caregiver in oncology and palliative care. *Seminars in Oncology Nursing.* 1998;*14*(2):152–157.

19

Last Hours of Living

INTRODUCTION

Terminally ill patients are cared for in a variety of settings, and death may therefore take place at home with hospice or traditional home care, or in a residential hospice, an extended care facility, or a hospital. Regardless of setting, the last hours of living can be managed to minimize burdensome and distressing symptoms and to maximize quality of life for patients, their families, and other caregivers. (See Chapter 15: Dying at Home.)

WHAT ARE SOME PHYSIOLOGIC CHANGES DURING THE DYING PROCESS?

Offering appropriate support to family members during this process will allow them to make the best possible use of the remaining time with their loved one and will make the bereavement period easier. Fear and anxiety about the dying process can be relieved by giving patients and families clear guidance about what to expect during the normal dying process. Recognizing and understanding some of the normal bodily changes that most patients go through near the end of life can make this time easier for patients, families, and caregivers.

1. Bodily changes:
   Increasing weakness, fatigue, sleepiness
   Decreasing appetite and fluid intake
   Decreasing blood perfusion: hypotension, mottling
   Neurologic signs: lethargy, confusion, restlessness, delirium
   Pain: stiffness, contractures, pre-existing painful conditions
   Loss of ability to close eyes (loss in periorbital fat pads)
2. Changes in respiratory pattern:
   Altered breathing patterns
   Diminishing tidal volume
   Periods of apnea
   Cheyne-Stokes respirations

   Accessory muscle use
   Respirations with mandibular movements
   Last reflex breaths
   Gurgling in back of throat ("death rattle")
3. Loss of ability to swallow

WHY IS IT IMPORTANT TO NOTE THE SIGNS AND SYMPTOMS OF LAST HOURS OF LIVING?

- Psychologically prepares clinical staff for impending death and allows interdisciplinary team members to counsel and support family
- Psychologically prepares family for impending death
- Allows family members to gather if so desired
- Ensures availability of appropriate medications to treat end-of-life symptoms ("Comfort Pack")[1]
- Allows discussion of plans concerning what should be done if/when patient dies
- Gives an indication of time frame for funeral planning

MANAGEMENT OF THE DYING PROCESS

- In a national survey of patients, families, physicians, and other health care providers, all four groups shared the same priorities for what is important at the end of life, citing pain and symptom management, preparation for the end of life, opportunity to gain a sense of completion and say goodbye, and preference for strong relationships between patients and their health care professionals.[1]
- Table 19.1 describes the expected physiologic changes that take place at the end of life, and offers management considerations to minimize distressing

TABLE 19.1: MANAGEMENT OF THE DYING PROCESS[2,3,4]

Physiologic Change	Findings	Possible Distress for Patient/Family	Management Considerations	Strategies for Counseling
Increasing weakness, fatigue	Decreased ability to perform even limited activities	Decreased ability to function normally Increased risk of falls	Education Trial of methylphenidate, dexamethasone Review meds and discontinue unnecessary ones	Normalize; avoid false reassurances
Decreasing appetite and fluid intake	Patient refusing food, pocketing food, or aspirating	Fear of dehydration, thirst, starvation	Education Oral rehydrating fluids IV fluids Trial of dexamethasone	Normalize; teach that decreased eating and drinking are a natural part of dying process Remind families, caregivers that dehydration does not cause patient distress and may be protective IV fluids may be harmful, causing fluid overload, breathlessness, cough, secretions, incontinence, skin breakdown Focus on mucosa and conjunctiva care with artificial saliva/tears
Decreasing blood perfusion	Cool or mottled extremities Lowering BP Confusion	Patient feeling cold or cool to touch Blue tinge to skin	Education Discontinue blood pressure meds, diuretics	Describe how organ system function deteriorates as death approaches
Neurologic dysfunction	Lethargy; confusion; delirium with restlessness, agitation, or stupor	Inability to communicate with patient Unable to assess symptoms	Gentle reorientation Antipsychotic meds to treat delirium Review meds and d/c if unnecessary	Emphasize patient can hear and feel touch even if unable to talk Encourage life review and sharing good memories Play music if appropriate Reduce unnecessary stimuli/visits Keep the room quiet
Pain	Signs of pain in unconscious patient include persistent vs. fleeting expression Grimacing Incident vs. rest pain Distinct from terminal delirium	Fear of increased pain Unable to assess due to inability to communicate	Use WHO strategies for pain control Titrate all pain meds to renal and liver function	Teach how to use scales to assess pain in nonverbal patients Identify potential/common sources of pain: contractures, stiffness, wounds, pre-existing painful conditions Teach safe use of standing dose and rescue opioids Continue counseling to dispel fears and misconceptions about opioids

Loss of ability to close eyes	Eyes open	Why does this happen? Cultural interpretations of dying with eyes open	Education Reassurance	Explain loss of periorbital fat pads Eye masks if desired Use artificial tears or ointment
Changes in respiratory pattern	Altered breathing patterns Diminishing tidal volume Apnea Cheyne-Stokes respirations Accessory muscle use Respirations with mandibular movements Last reflex breaths Gurgling in throat	Fear of patient suffocation Fear of patient discomfort Apprehension re: "death rattle"	Oxygen vs. air by nasal canula Fan with air across face Low-dose opioids for dyspnea Anticholinergic meds for secretions or gurgling	Family support Educate that gurgling or "death rattle" is not uncomfortable for patient but is distressing for family Describe "death rattle" as air moving across a thin membrane of fluid in trachea
Loss of ability to swallow	Loss of gag reflex Pooling of saliva, secretions, causing "death rattle"	Fear of patient choking, suffocation	Aspiration precautions Scopolamine or atropine to dry up secretions Postural drainage Positioning Suctioning	Explain active dying process: -Not swallowing is protective -Avoid force feeding

symptoms, and outlines strategies for educating and supporting the patient, family members, and other involved health care providers.

KEY MEDICATIONS TO ENSURE COMFORT AT END OF LIFE[2]

It is important to have medications on hand in easily absorbed tablets, highly concentrated liquid formulations, or rectal suppositories in case patient cannot swallow effectively (Table 19.2). These medications should include:

Opioids for pain/dyspnea
Antianxiety agents, especially
    benzodiazepines, haloperidol
Antiemetics (e.g., prochlorperazine or
    haloperidol)
Antipyretics (e.g., acetaminophen)

Anticonvulsants (benzodiazepines)
Anticholinergics (glycopyrrolate, atropine eye
    drops, scopolamine patch)
Bowel regimen agents (dulcolax
    suppositories, enemas)

SUPPORTING THE PATIENT AND FAMILY

If a patient or family member becomes anxious or begins to question their prior decisions, arrange to a have "G-O-O-D" discussion to review the following:

G = Goals of Care
O = Options of care
O = Opinion/recommendation from medical
    or health care professional
D = Documentation in chart of above
    discussions

TABLE 19.2: MEDICATIONS AND DELIVERY MODALITIES AVAILABLE FOR THE HOME CARE SETTING

Modality	Examples	Indications	Result
Topical/Transdermal	Anaesthetics (lidocaine)	Neuropathy, post-herpetic neuralgia	Temporary, local pain relief
	Opioids (fentanyl)	Chronic stable pain, unable to take oral opioids	Sustained systemic pain relief
	Anticholinergics (e.g., scopolamine patch)	Excessive oropharyngeal secretions; nausea; visceral pain	Reduced oral and gut secretions
Thermal	Heat	Muscle spasm, chronic inflammation, joint stiffness/pain	Relax local muscles and increase blood flow
	Cold	Sprains, strains, inflammation	Reduce local edema and blood flow
Subcutaneous Infusion	Opioids	Pain, dyspnea	Quick onset pain relief, easily titrated to comfort
Sublingual	Liquid morphine, soluble morphine tablets	Dysphagia	Concentrated solutions absorb quickly for fast pain relief
	Benzodiazepines (e.g., lorazepam, diazepam)	Anxiety related to dyspnea, agitation, nausea, opioid-related myoclonus	Anxiolytic and relief of myoclonus
Rectal	Acetaminophen	Pain, fever	Relief of pain and fever
	Compazine Haldol	Nausea	Useful for opioid-related nausea
	Corticosteroids (e.g., hydrocortisone or prednisolone foam)	Pain, increased intracranial pressure, nausea	Reduce inflammation and intracranial swelling

COMMUNICATION WITH THE LETHARGIC OR UNCONSCIOUS PATIENT

- Lethargy or lack of consciousness is distressing to family.
- Patient awareness is frequently greater than the ability to respond.
- Assume that the patient hears everything and is able to feel touch.
- Create a familiar and quiet environment for patient; reduce stimuli.
- Include patient in conversations, but do not expect patient to speak.
- Give assurances of presence, safety.
- Avoid false or unrealistic assurances or promises.
- Give permission to die.
- Offer gentle touch, e.g., hand massage.
- Five things to say:
  - I love you.
  - I forgive you.
  - Please forgive me.
  - Thank you.
  - Goodbye.

AS EXPECTED DEATH APPROACHES

- Discuss the status of patient with family and caregivers; establish realistic and achievable care goals.
- Describe role of physician and the interdisciplinary team.
- Reinforce that what the patient experiences is not what onlookers see.
- Reinforce indications, signs, and events of normal dying process.
- Ask about and encourage personal, cultural, religious rituals; encourage funeral planning.
- Identify importance of the family support system throughout the process.

SIGNS THAT DEATH HAS OCCURRED

- Absence of heartbeat, respirations
- Pupils fixed and dilated
- Color turns to a waxen pallor as blood settles
- Body temperature drops
- Muscles, sphincters relax:
  - Release of stool, urine
  - Eyes can remain open
  - Jaw falls open
  - Body fluids may trickle internally

WHAT TO DO WHEN DEATH OCCURS

Options for next steps depend on place of death.

1. If death occurs at home
   - Advise the family not to call 911.
   - If patient was receiving home hospice care, the family is strongly encouraged to call hospice first. Hospice personnel can make death pronouncement.
2. If death occurs in a facility (hospital, nursing home, etc.)
   - Call a physician to pronounce death.
   - Review the protocol for death pronouncement and how to inform the family of a patient's death.
3. Things to consider:
   - Funeral provider should be contacted at the time of death.
   - Make a list of family and friends who should be notified.
   - There are no specific "rules" for what should happen.
   - There is rarely any need for a coroner.
   - Consider organ donation.
   - Traditions, rites, and rituals are important and meaningful.

AFTER EXPECTED DEATH OCCURS[5]

- The focus of care shifts from patient to family and caregivers.
- Invite those who were not present to be at the bedside.
- Create a peaceful, accessible environment.
- Coping with loss is different for everyone; family members time to "process" what has happened.
- Work with the interdisciplinary team, especially bereavement counselors, for grief and bereavement follow-up.
- Assess acute grief reactions.
- Express sorrow for the loss and thank the family for the privilege of caring for their loved one.

FOLLOW-UP

- Notify other involved physicians and caregivers of the death.
- Stop services (e.g., hospice, home health, aides, etc.).
- Arrange to remove equipment/supplies.
- Secure valuables with executor.
- Dispose of medications, biologic wastes.

TAKE-HOME POINTS

- As the end of life approaches, priorities for patients, families, and physicians include pain and symptom management, preparation for death, opportunity to gain a sense of completion, and preference for strong relationships between patients and their health care providers.
- There are normal and predictable physiologic changes that occur during the last hours of living. Preparing family and caregivers to recognize and understand these changes can make this time easier for patients, families, and caregivers.
- The last hours of living can be managed to maximize quality of life and minimize burdensome and distressing symptoms.
- A well-managed and peaceful dying process with an involved and prepared family is associated with improved bereavement outcomes and facilitates family members' ability to recover and go on with their lives.
- Key medications to ensure comfort at the end of life should be available in easily absorbed tablets, intensols, or rectal suppositories in case the patient cannot swallow effectively.

- After the patient's death, the focus of care shifts to family and caregivers. Interdisciplinary team members, especially bereavement counselors, should be notified for grief and bereavement assessment and follow-up.

REFERENCES

1. Steinhauser KE, Christakis NA, Clipp EC, et al. Factors considered important at the end of life by patients, familiy, physicians, and other care providers. *JAMA*. 2000;*284*(19):2476–2482.
2. Clary PL, Lawson P. Pharmacologic pearls for end-of-life care. *Am Fam Physician*. June 15, 2009;*79*(12):1059–1065.
3. Wildiers H, Dhaenekint C, Demeulenaere P, et al. Atropine, hyoscine butylbromide, or scopolamine are equally effective for the treatment of death rattle in terminal care. *J Pain Symptom Manage*. July 2009;*38*(1):124–133.
4. Wildiers H, Menten J. Death rattle: prevalence, prevention and treatment. *J Pain Symptom Manage*. Apr 2002;*23*(4):310–317.
5. Midland D. *Fast Fact and Concept #64: Informing Significant Others of a Patient's Death*. 2nd Edition. http://www.eperc.mcw.edu/fastFact/ff_64.htm. Accessed September 27, 2009.

20

Grief and Bereavement

INTRODUCTION

Grief is a universal and normal emotional response to a loss. **Mourning** is the psychological process of gradually incorporating a loss into one's life; mourning also refers to the external manifestation of loss, which may be influenced by culture, family background, and individual personality. **Bereavement** is the experience of losing to death a person to whom one is attached; it is characterized by feelings of grief for an indefinite period of mourning, usually followed by a gradual adjustment to life without the deceased.

PREVALENCE[1]

- Death of family and close friends is a universal life experience that becomes more frequent as a person ages. In the U.S., 75% of deaths occur in persons over 65. Approximately 45% of U.S. women and 14% of men aged 65 and older are widowed.

IMPACT OF BEREAVEMENT

- Bereavement is associated with increased mortality due to many causes, including suicide. Contributing factors that have been identified include psychological stress, loneliness, and changes in social ties, living arrangements, eating habits, and economic support. Bereaved individuals also have higher rates of disability, medication use, and hospitalization than non-bereaved population.
- Data are inconclusive as to whether elderly vs. younger bereaved individuals experience poorer bereavement outcomes. Older adults may be at greater risk because of their increased incidence of:
  - Widowhood
  - Chronic medical problems
  - Functional impairments that may make the physical and emotional demands of caregiving for a seriously ill loved one more burdensome
  - Social isolation and limited social supports often caused by declining health, increased debility, death of friends, and protracted period of caregiving

TYPES OF GRIEF AND TREATMENT OPTIONS

Anticipatory Grief

- Grief and bereavement are not always experienced within the context of death. People with advanced illness may also grieve the loss of good health, functional ability, one's social network, and activities and relationships that previously helped define the individual and gave "meaning" to his/her life.
- Grief can also sometimes be experienced over a period of years by patients with chronic and/or advanced illness, and by their loved ones. This process has been referred to in the literature as "anticipatory" grief. Anticipatory grief is a painful experience; however, it is not inherently pathologic. Common manifestations of anticipatory grief include:
  - Anxiety and multiple illness-related fears
  - Sadness
  - Depression
  - Anger or hostility
  - Guilt
  - Withdrawal from loved ones (by ill person)
  - Withdrawal from ill person (by loved ones)

Treatment/Support for Anticipatory Grief

- When patients are approaching the end of life, it is important to address their own as well as their family's concerns, and also to evaluate their respective psychological functioning. Focusing on physical symptoms such as pain, energy level, sleep, and appetite may distract providers from signs of anticipatory grief, existential distress, anxiety, or depression.

- Open-ended questions can help distinguish, for example, between "normal" anticipatory mourning and clinical depression, as well as provide insight about patient and family risk factors and coping resources.[2] Sample questions include:
  - "How are you doing with all that has been happening?"
  - "I notice that you seem (sad, upset, angry, irritable, etc.), and that's certainly understandable given what's going on. Can you tell me more about what you are thinking and feeling?"
  - "Given what we know about the course of your illness, what are you hoping for now?"
  - "What are you most worried about?"
  - "What helps you cope with what's going on? What have you found helpful in the past?"
  - "How can I and the other members of the team best help you?"
- These questions may prompt discussions that will help the health care team to understand the illness-related concerns of the patient and family and may help guide appropriate intervention. Issues commonly raised by seriously ill people and their families include:
  - Worries about the disease course, including what can they expect, symptom and function-wise, as their illness progresses
  - What help will the medical team specifically be able to offer them?
  - Will they be abandoned by their doctors and nurses?
  - Can they count on their health care providers to offer symptom relief as needed and abide by their end-of-life preferences?
  - Worries about leaving their family behind and how their loved ones will manage without them; there may be particular unease about a family member with medical, psychiatric, substance abuse, or other psychosocial difficulty who might, in fact, have trouble "surviving" after the patient's death

When to Refer for Psychosocial Intervention

- Addressing "anticipatory grief" issues with patients and their families is a critical element of any plan for the seriously ill. Doing so gives assurance that they will not be abandoned by the health care team despite the lack of curative medical interventions.
- Talking with patients about issues related to the expected course of their disease process is likely to be within the skill set and "comfort zone" of most physicians. Patient concerns that have less straightforward "solutions," however, may call for ongoing and skilled psychosocial intervention. A clinician who has access to an interdisciplinary team should call upon social work, psychology, and chaplaincy colleagues for assistance. Other options include palliative care consultations or referral of patient and families to community-based organizations that can provide counseling and support.

Uncomplicated Grief

- Uncomplicated grief is a term used to describe the range of feelings, behaviors, and other reactions that occur after a death that are socially and culturally defined as "normal." There is wide acceptance of the theory that normal grief progresses through five stages: disbelief or shock; separation distress or yearning; angry protest; depressed mood or despair; and ultimate acceptance and recovery from the loss.[3]
- The term "uncomplicated" is something of a misnomer because even this normative grief can be quite complex. The symptoms are often the same as those seen in more pathologic grief reactions and can be experienced as powerfully and be as subjectively distressing as more pathologic grief reactions. Manifestations of post-death grief can occur in multiple domains:
  1. **Physical**: changes in sleep and appetite patterns, somatic complaints such as fatigue, generalized weakness, palpitations, chest tightness, headaches, GI disturbances, and decreased immune system functioning
  2. **Emotional**: bereaved individuals often feel a mix of feelings such as sadness,

anger, anxiety, loneliness, irritability, guilt, and relief.

3. **Cognitive**: decreased concentration, confusion, disbelief at times that the loss has occurred, and intrusive thoughts about the deceased. "Ghosting," or a sense of the presence of the lost loved one, is common. Grieving individuals may find that they are often tearful and report crying spells or recurrent dreams of the deceased.

4. **Behavioral**: carrying objects belonging to their lost loved one, or wearing an article of their clothing. Conversely, some people avoid any reminders of the deceased by refusing to talk about them or by staying away from persons or places associated with their loved one.

5. **Substance abuse**: increased risk for self-destructive behavior, including alcohol or substance abuse, attempts to self-medicate with prescription and over-the-counter drugs, antisocial conduct, and suicide.

6. **Social**: withdrawing from usual routines and activities, including those previously enjoyable, or curtailing contact with family and friends. In contrast, some deal with grief by devoting their time to a single activity such as work to the exclusion of others.

7. **Spiritual**: expression of grief through a heightened or diminished religiousness; some individuals voice anger with God, question their previous religious beliefs, or develop an altered view of life's meaning.

Treatment/Support for Uncomplicated Grief

- Most bereaved survivors adapt to the reality of their loss over time and resume their daily activities and relationships. The intensity and acuity of uncomplicated grief gradually decreases over time as the attachment to the deceased loosens, thereby freeing up the person's emotional energy to be reinvested in the present and future.
- Those who effectively adjust to the death of a loved one never fully "get over" the loss or totally sever their bonds to the deceased; rather, they continue to maintain a connection through memories and rituals that permit them to accommodate the loss and move forward with their lives despite it.

When to Refer for Psychosocial Intervention

Some survivors may find it helpful to participate in bereavement support groups and/or bereavement-related workshops. Try to link family with community bereavement resources that are often offered by local hospices or faith-based organizations and are usually open to the public.

Bereavement Follow-Up Suggestions for the Health Care Provider[4]

- Make a condolence phone call and/or send a condolence letter to family. This acknowledges the patient's "personhood" and the significance of the loss to the family. It also offers family support and comfort and can potentially help with the grieving process.
- Some bereavement experts advise that a handwritten note or letter is the preferred method, as it provides the loved ones with something tangible that they can hold onto and refer back to over time. The basic elements of a phone call or handwritten expression of condolence are:
  1. An expression of condolence regarding the loss ("I am sorry for your loss." "I was saddened to learn of John's death.")
  2. A personal remembrance of the person ("I will always remember his strong spirit despite the many challenges he faced.")
  3. Recognition of the importance of the caregiving relationship to the physician ("It was a privilege to help care for John.")
  4. Words of comfort to the family, including acknowledgement of their care/support of the patient, if appropriate ("You took excellent care of John." "You were such a good advocate for him.")
- If requested by the family or otherwise indicated, arrange to meet with the family to answer any remaining questions regarding the illness and death and to provide closure.

Prolonged Grief Disorder (Complicated Grief)[5]

- For some people, bereavement may be characterized by grief reactions that don't subside over time and often result in long-term functional impairments, including persistent bereavement-related anxiety, depression, and/or other adjustment disorders including prolonged grief disorder.

- This problematic adjustment to loss of a loved one has been associated with several factors, including death of a spouse/partner, high levels of burden including caregiving responsibilities, physical exhaustion, and lack of social support during the pre-bereavement and post-death period.
- Other risk factors for prolonged grief disorder (also referred to as complicated grief) include:[3]
  - History of prior significant losses
  - Nature of relationship with deceased
  - Maladaptive coping skills
  - Psychiatric and/or substance abuse history
  - Concurrent stressors and burdens
  - Circumstances surrounding the death: expected vs. unexpected; cause of death: suicide, homicide, death from a "stigmatized" illness
    Perception of death as preventable
    Perception that deceased "suffered" prior to death
    Perception that medical care received was inadequate
- Prolonged grief disorder may coexist with other mental health problems; however, it constitutes a distinct set of symptoms that clinicians should be able to identify and then determine how to appropriately intervene. Boelen and Prigerson propose the following diagnostic criteria for prolonged grief disorder:[6]
  - *One* of three symptoms of "separation distress":
    Intense memories/thoughts about the lost relationship
    Severe recurrent episodes of distress related to the lost relationship
    Persistent intense yearning re: the loss
  - *Five* of the following loss-related "cognitive, emotional, behavioral symptoms":
    Feeling that part of the self has died, feelings of emptiness
    Avoidance of reminders of the loss
    Difficulty trusting others
    Extreme bitterness/anger
    Difficulty accepting the reality of the loss
    Absence of emotion, or "numbness"
    Feeling that life is unfulfilling and lacks meaning
    Feeling stunned or shocked

Treatment/Support for Complicated Grief

- Persons experiencing prolonged grief disorder require professional intervention and should ideally be referred to a mental health professional who specializes in working with the bereaved.
- A meta-analysis of controlled trials for prevention or treatment of complicated grief determined that treatment interventions can effectively diminish short- and long-term complicated grief symptoms, but preventive interventions do not appear to be effective.[7] Recent studies have shown that a form of cognitive behavioral therapy specifically targeted to prolonged grief disorder was more effective than traditional interpersonal therapy in helping those who are grieving.[8] Other promising approaches include brief dynamic psychotherapy, crisis intervention, and support groups.
- Therapeutic interventions may be more effective in conjunction with administration of selective serotonin reuptake inhibitors (SSRIs), but randomized trials are needed to confirm the efficacy of pharmacologic agents in the treatment of complicated grief.[9]
- Local hospices or mental health associations are good resources for locating experienced bereavement professionals. Many health insurance plans do offer coverage for therapeutic interventions provided by in-network mental health providers.

TAKE-HOME POINTS

- Bereavement is the experience of losing to death a person to whom one is attached; it is characterized by feelings of grief for an indefinite period of mourning, usually followed by a gradual adjustment to life without the deceased.
- Anticipatory grief is a term used to describe the feelings that may engulf a patient and family members after there is a diagnosis of a terminal illness. It occurs during the interval when there is knowledge that death is impending, but before the death actually happens.
- Uncomplicated grief describes the range of feelings, behaviors, and other reactions that occur after a death that are culturally defined as "normal."

- Most bereaved survivors adapt to the reality of their loss gradually and go on to resume their daily activities and relationships. For some people, however, the grief reactions do not subside over time, and these people may suffer from long-term functional impairment known as "complicated grief" or "prolonged grief disorder."
- Persons experiencing prolonged grief disorder require treatment and should ideally be referred to an experienced mental health professional. A variety of treatment interventions can effectively diminish complicated grief symptoms. These include cognitive behavioral therapy, brief dynamic psychotherapy, crisis intervention, and therapeutic support groups.

REFERENCES

1. Stroebe M, Schut H, Stroebe W. Health outcomes of bereavement. *Lancet*. 2007;*370*:1960–1973.
2. Clukey L. Anticipatory mourning: processes of expected loss in palliative care. *Int J Palliat Med*. 2008;*14*(7):316–325.
3. Zhang B, El-Jawahri A, Prigerson HG. Update on bereavement research: evidence-based guidelines for the diagnosis and treatment of complicated bereavement. *J of Palliat Med*. 2006;*9*(5):1188–1203.
4. Prigerson H, Jacobs SC. Caring for bereaved patients: "All the doctors suddenly just go." *JAMA*. 2001;*286*(11):1369–1377.
5. Prigerson HG, Bierhals AJ, Kasl SV, et al. Traumatic grief as a risk factor for mental and physical morbidity. *Amer J Pyschiatry*. 1997;*154*(5):616–623.
6. Boelen PA, Prigerson HG. The influence of symptoms of prolonged grief disorder, depression, and anxiety on quality of life among bereaved adults: a prospective study. *Eur Arch Psychiatry Clin Neurosci*. 2007;*257*:444–452.
7. Wittouck C, Van Autreve S, De Jaegere E, et al. The prevention and treatment of complicated grief: a meta-analysis. *Clin Psychol Rev*. 2011;*31*:69–78.
8. Wetherell JL. Complicated grief therapy as a new treatment approach. *Dialogues Clin Neurosci*. 2012;*14*(2):159–166.
9. Bui E, Nadal-Vicens M, Simon N. Pharmacological approaches to the treatment of complicated grief: rationale and brief review of the literature. *Dialogues Clin Neurosci*. 2012;*14*(2):149–157.

21
Spirituality

INTRODUCTION

Spirituality can be defined as the aspect of humanity that refers to the way individuals seek and express meaning and purpose and the way they experience their connectedness to the moment, to self, to others, to nature, and to the significant or sacred.[1]

Although religion has historically been identified as the organized system of beliefs, practices, and rituals designed to express spirituality, an increasing number of Americans define themselves as spiritual while simultaneously reporting that they are not members of a particular religious affiliation.[2,3]

WHY IS SPIRITUALITY IMPORTANT IN HEALTH CARE?

- Numerous studies have documented uncontrolled suffering in patients with advanced illness, and increasing attention is being paid to the realm of spiritual suffering for patients with serious illness.[4,5,6] Rates of spiritual distress are very high, regardless of the patients' underlying illness, as has been demonstrated in patients with cancer, HIV, heart failure, liver failure, and lung disease.[7,8,9]
- Not only does spirituality play a role in the existential distress that can afflict patients with serious illness, but it also can have an impact on their overall health and suffering. Spiritual distress has been associated with poor outcomes including anxiety, depression, and increased mortality.[6,10,11] Conversely, spiritual support has been associated with increased use of hospice and fewer burdensome treatments at the end of life.[12,13]
- Although many clinicians are hesitant to address spiritual and religious matters with their patients, it has been demonstrated that patients with spiritual distress do want to discuss their existential fears and concerns with their health care team.[14] Patients'

spirituality and religion, as well as that of their families, often play an important role in complex treatment decisions and discussions about the goals of care during the course of an advanced illness.

AN INTER-PROFESSIONAL MODEL OF SPIRITUAL CARE

- In response to the evolving understanding of the role of spirituality in health care, national guidelines and regulatory agencies have urged adoption of standards of spiritual care for patients with advanced illness. One of the core precepts of clinical palliative care is that patients' spiritual and existential concerns should be identified, documented, and addressed with the best evidence-based interventions.[15,16]
- In recent years, providing spiritual care for patients with advanced illness has shifted away from community-based clergy to clinically trained, multi-faith chaplains.[17] Indeed, the health care chaplain is no longer "just" a religious figure but has clearly emerged as a core member of the health care team. As the role of the chaplain has become much more important, however, it has become apparent that there are not enough chaplains to meet the complex needs of the increasing numbers of patients with serious illness, especially in the acute care hospital setting.[18]
- One solution to the chaplain shortage is to utilize the health care provider as the "generalist" in spiritual care, and to engage the chaplain/clergy as the specialist or consultant for more complicated or acute spiritual issues. This "triage" approach has been proposed by a recent consensus panel of experts in health care chaplaincy.[1] In this inter-professional model of spiritual care, palliative care clinicians perform an initial spiritual screening to explore and understand every patient's spiritual

symptoms, values, and beliefs. Relevant religious and spiritual information is then documented and integrated into the overall plan of clinical care. If a patient or a family member displays signs of complicated, unresolved, or stressful spiritual suffering or conflict, a referral is made to a board-certified chaplain or other appropriate spiritual care professional.

CORE COMPETENCIES OF SPIRITUAL CARE

- In the inter-professional model of spiritual care, all clinical team members share responsibility for the spiritual care. Physicians, nurses, and other clinical team members should be able to discuss and respond to spiritual concerns within a scope appropriate for a clinician-patient relationship. Core competencies of this "generalist" approach to spiritual care include:[19]

  1. Understanding that the spiritual dimension of a patient's life is an avenue for compassionate caregiving
  2. Being able to apply an understanding of a patient's spirituality and cultural beliefs and behaviors to appropriate clinical contexts (e.g., in disease prevention, care plan formulation, treatment interventions, or challenging clinical decision-making scenarios)
  3. Appreciating and respecting the role of health care clergy and other spiritual leaders, and understanding how to communicate and collaborate with them on behalf of a patient's physical and/or spiritual needs
  4. Developing an understanding of one's own spirituality or existential dimension and how it can be nurtured as a part of personal and professional growth (Understanding how one's own beliefs can affect the care that is delivered is also a core competency related to spirituality in medicine.)

SPIRITUAL SCREENING

- There are no simple, well-validated screening tools for spiritual distress in patients with serious illness. Clinicians should encourage patients to freely and openly express their spiritual beliefs and needs, and should also help them to identify sources of support from

their spiritual or religious community. The relevant information elicited from taking this "spiritual history" should then be documented in the patient's chart, integrated into the plan of care, and reassessed on a regular basis. Special attention should be paid to honoring any patient and family wishes about rituals at any point during the illness or at the time of death.

- If the patient and family reveal that their faith-based or personal spiritual practice is an important source of support, the plan of clinical care should also include a referral to a chaplain, pastoral counselor, or other spiritual care providers, including clergy or other community resources, for spiritual counseling and support.

- **FICA** is an acronym for a framework that health care clinicians can use to identify the needs of seriously ill patients and how their spiritual beliefs, practices, and concerns might be relevant to their health care.[19] Unlike medical history taking, spiritual assessment guides like FICA are not limited to a single set of fixed questions. Rather, FICA offers an open-ended and interpretive approach that allows the clinician to better understand the patient's personal experience of spirituality and to explore individual needs. Sample questions are provided below for each step of the discussion.

  F—Faith (assessment of patient's faith and belief)
  What is your faith and belief? Do you consider yourself spiritual or religious?
  What things do you believe in that give meaning to your life?

  I—Is that faith or belief **Important** in the patient's life?
  What influence does it have on how you take care of yourself?
  How have your beliefs influenced your behavior during this illness?
  What role do your beliefs play in regaining your health?

  C—Community (an assessment of the patient's spiritual community)
  Do you have a community that supports you, and how?
  Is there a person or group of people you really love, or who are really important to you?

  A—Address (a determination of how the patient would like the provider or health care team to address these spiritual domains in their medical care) *How would you like me and your health care team to address these issues in your health care?*

TAKE-HOME POINTS

- Spirituality is the aspect of humanity that refers to the way individuals seek and express meaning and how they experience their connectedness to the moment, to self, to others, to nature, and to the significant or sacred. An increasing number of Americans define themselves as spiritual while simultaneously reporting that they are not members of a particular religion.
- Patients with advanced illness have unmet needs, especially in the realm of spiritual distress. Although many clinicians are reluctant to address spirituality with their patients, patients with spiritual distress do want to discuss these types of concerns with their health care team.
- Providing spiritual care for patients with advanced illness has become the domain of clinically trained, multi-faith health care chaplains. As the role of the chaplain has become more important, however, it has become apparent that there are not enough chaplains to minister to the increasing numbers of patients with serious illness, especially in the hospital setting.
- One solution to the chaplain shortage is to use the health care provider as the "generalist" in spiritual care, and to engage the chaplain/clergy as the specialist or consultant for more complicated or acute spiritual issues. In this inter-professional model of spiritual care, palliative care clinicians perform an initial spiritual screening and integrate relevant spiritual information into the plan of clinical care.
- When a patient or a family member displays signs of complicated, unresolved, or stressful spiritual suffering, a referral should then be made to a board-certified chaplain or other appropriate spiritual care professional.

REFERENCES

1. Puchalski C, Ferrell B, Virani R, et al. Improving the quality of spiritual care as a dimension of palliative care: the report of the Consensus Conference. *J Palliat Med.* Oct 2009;*12*(10):885–904.
2. Health Care Chaplaincy. Literature Review—Testing the Efficacy of Chaplaincy Care. http://www.healthcarechaplaincy.org/templeton-research-project/literature-review.html. Accessed March 4, 2012.
3. Newport F. In U.S. increasing number have no religious identity. 2010. http://www.gallup.com/poll/128276/Increasing-Number-No-Religious-Identity.aspx.
4. Mako C, Galek K, Poppito SR. Spiritual pain among patients with advanced cancer in palliative care. *J Palliat Med.* Oct 2006;*9*(5):1106–1113.
5. Desbiens N, Wu A. Pain and Suffering in Seriously Ill Hospitalized Patients. *J Am Geriatr Soc.* 2000;*48*(5):S183–S186.
6. Fitchett G, Murphy PE, Kim J, Gibbons JL, Cameron JR, Davis JA. Religious struggle: prevalence, correlates and mental health risks in diabetic, congestive heart failure, and oncology patients. *Int J Psychiatry Med.* 2004;*34*(2): 179–196.
7. Yi MS, Mrus JM, Wade TJ, et al. Religion, spirituality, and depressive symptoms in patients with HIV/AIDS. *J Gen Intern Med.* Dec 2006;*21* (suppl 5): S21–27.
8. Murray SA, Kendall M, Grant E, Boyd K, Barclay S, Sheikh A. Patterns of social, psychological, and spiritual decline toward the end of life in lung cancer and heart failure. *J Pain Symptom Manage.* Oct 2007;*34*(4):393–402.
9. Hui D, de la Cruz M, Thorney S, Parsons HA, Delgado-Guay M, Bruera E. The frequency and correlates of spiritual distress among patients with advanced cancer admitted to an acute palliative care unit. *Am J Hosp Palliat Care.* Jun 2011;*28*(4):264–270.
10. Johnson KS, Tulsky JA, Hays JC, et al. Which domains of spirituality are associated with anxiety and depression in patients with advanced illness? *J Gen Intern Med.* Jul 2011;*26*(7):751–758.
11. Pargament KI, Koenig HG, Tarakeshwar N, Hahn J. Religious struggle as a predictor of mortality among medically ill elderly patients: a 2-year longitudinal study. *Arch Intern Med.* Aug 13-27, 2001;*161*(15):1881–1885.
12. Balboni TA, Paulk ME, Balboni MJ, et al. Provision of spiritual care to patients with advanced cancer: associations with medical care and quality of life near death. *J Clin Oncol.* Jan 20, 2010;*28*(3):445–452.
13. Phelps AC, Maciejewski PK, Nilsson M, et al. Religious coping and use of intensive life-prolonging care near death in patients with advanced cancer. *JAMA.* Mar 18, 2009;*301*(11): 1140–1147.
14. Williams JA, Meltzer D, Arora V, Chung G, Curlin FA. Attention to inpatients' religious and

spiritual concerns: predictors and association with patient satisfaction. *J Gen Intern Med.* Nov 2011;*26*(11):1265–1271.

15. National Quality Forum. *A National Framework and Preferred Practices for Palliative and Hospice Care Quality.* Washington, DC; 2006.

16. National Consensus Project for Quality Palliative Care. Clinical Practice Guidelines for Quality Palliative Care, Second Edition. 2009. http://www.nationalconsensusproject.org.

17. Handzo G, Wintz S. Professional chaplaincy: establishing a hospital-based department. *Healthc Exec.* Jan-Feb 2006;*21*(1):38–39.

18. Wintz S, Handzo G. Pastoral care staffing & productivity: More than ratios. *Chaplaincy Today.* 2005;*21*(1):3–10.

19. Puchalski CM, Lunsford B, Harris MH, Miller T. Interdisciplinary spiritual care for seriously ill and dying patients: a collaborative model. *The Cancer Journal.* 2006;*12*(5):398–416.

22

Palliative Sedation

INTRODUCTION

Palliative sedation (PS) is the use of medication to cause a reduced level of consciousness in order to relieve intractable symptoms experienced by an imminently dying patient. Palliative sedation is employed only when other symptom-targeted treatments, short of sedation, have failed. Relief of distress is the goal, not hastening death. **Respite sedation** is a form of palliative sedation used for a predetermined period of time to give a patient relief from refractory symptom(s). Sedation is reduced at the end of a period of time to allow the patient to awaken, and a decision is made whether sedation is still required to mitigate the patient's suffering.[1]

PREVALENCE

The literature reveals a wide variability in the use of palliative sedation (2%–52%).[2] The actual frequency of palliative sedation is difficult to determine, as there is no standard definition accepted by all clinicians. Ethical and moral considerations may affect treatment decisions.

INDICATIONS

Physical Symptoms

Patients who are nearing the end of life may experience one or more refractory symptoms as death approaches. These symptoms can include pain, dyspnea, agitation, restlessness, nausea, and myoclonus that have not responded to conventional treatments such as opioids, benzodiazepines, and neuroleptics.

Psycho-Existential Suffering

- It is important to recognize and acknowledge that significant suffering can occur even when physical symptoms are well controlled. There is, however, no consensus on the utilization of palliative sedation for psycho-existential suffering as the sole intolerable, refractory symptom in an imminently dying patient.[1]

- Psycho-existential suffering is generally understood to be caused by a loss of meaning or purpose in life, or a death anxiety that may have elements of fright, dread, terror, anguish, or regret.
- As with all psychological or spiritual distress, clinicians should assure the patient that the appropriate clinical professionals have assessed the patient and that all recommended treatments and interventions have been employed.
- Ethics committee involvement may be warranted in some cases.

DECISION-MAKING PROCESS

- Identify the clinical problem (e.g., uncontrolled symptoms; intractable suffering). Utilize all appropriate expertise and exhaust all treatment options to manage symptoms before considering palliative sedation. An interdisciplinary meeting will help to assure that the goals of care and the intent of palliative sedation are understood by clinical staff, patient, and family, and that ethical concerns and misconceptions are addressed.
- If the symptom burden remains uncontrolled, meet with the patient (assuming he/she has capacity) and family to discuss prognosis, treatment options, alternatives to, and goals of, palliative sedation. The discussion should include a review of the patient's wishes regarding treatment options, assignment of a health care proxy (HCP), and/or clarification of the patient's surrogate decision-maker if patient does not have capacity to appoint a HCP. (See Chapter 9: Communication Skills.)
- Obtain informed consent to sedate for relief of refractory symptoms. See Table 22.1 for a sample palliative sedation consent form.
- Determine if the patient would like to be awakened at a later time to see if symptoms

TABLE 22.1: SAMPLE CONSENT FORM: PALLIATIVE SEDATION FOR
REFRACTORY SUFFERING

Patient name: _____

Documentation of refractory suffering:

_____

_____

_____

_____

Palliative measures previously attempted:

_____

_____

_____

_____

Outcomes of previously attempted palliative measures:

_____

_____

_____

Patient _____ Health Care Proxy/Patient Representative _____ (check one)

_____ Able to respond intelligibly to queries

_____ Able to articulate the decision

Information presented:

_____ Nature and progress of stage of terminal illness (prognosis)

_____ Nature and possible impact of proposed controlled sedation

_____ Limitations, side effects, and risks of the proposed controlled sedation

_____ Issues related to hydration and nutrition during sedation

☐ I am aware that Dr. _____ (primary physician) agrees with the plan to initiate palliative sedation. With knowledge of the risks discussed by the physician(s), I consent to controlled sedation for refractory suffering.

Date: _____

_____   _____
Patient or authorized representative signature   Relationship

Physician Signature _____   Date _____

can be controlled without sedation. Patient and family must be made aware that there is a chance that the patient may not be able to be awakened.

- If feasible, create a plan allowing the patient and family time to prepare. The patient may wish to spend time with loved ones and/ or a chaplain, if time and symptom distress permits.

- Discussion and preparation with the family as well as members of the interdisciplinary team is essential. Maintaining close communication, with 24/7 access to an experienced clinician, is imperative.

IMPLEMENTATION OF PALLIATIVE SEDATION

Pre-Sedation Considerations

1. Clarify goals of care and prognostic information with the various members of the medical team, including the primary physician, relevant specialists, and the palliative care consultant.

2. Discuss sedation plans with the clinical staff, including nurses, nursing assistants, social worker, physicians, and chaplain. Set aside time to discuss in depth, if necessary, the need for sedation and the ethical principles on which the intervention is based (e.g., a patient's right to relief from suffering, professional duty to relieve suffering, the principles of autonomy and beneficence, and the use of informed consent). Create a safe environment in which all concerns and conflicts can be discussed.

3. Document that the appropriate DNR form is in the medical record.

4. Document discussions and planning in the patient's chart. Be sure to include indications for palliative sedation, who participated in discussions, patient or surrogate wishes (where applicable), goals, and prognosis.

5. Assure ongoing communications and arrange 24/7 access to an experienced clinician for the clinical team and the patient's family.

6. Prepare for initiation of sedation with the goal of titrating the medication only to the level necessary to achieve symptom relief. Order medications and dosages, including a basal rate with rescue dose for breakthrough symptoms. Be sure to include indications for using rescue doses.

7. Review current orders and eliminate interventions that do not contribute to patient's comfort (i.e., discontinue compression devices, subcutaneous heparin, blood glucose monitoring via finger stick, pulse oximetry, etc.). Include in the treatment plan specific interventions such as frequency of vital signs, nutrition and hydration, mouth care, and hygiene as the patient's condition dictates.

8. Create a calm, quiet environment by eliminating extraneous noise, reducing glare from overhead lighting, providing unobtrusive clinical care and monitoring, and keeping phones and beepers on vibrate.

9. Encourage family to keep visitation and conversations consistent with the goals of care.

Procedure

1. Full participation of the patient's primary physician should be encouraged during the decision to initiate palliative sedation. Once the determination is made that palliative sedation will be used, consider transfer of the patient's care to the palliative care service or hospice, if available. This will allow for provision of the specialized skills, support, and oversight necessary for palliative sedation.

2. Sedation can be instituted using one of the medications listed on the Drug Protocol for Palliative Sedation (Table 22.2).

3. Sedation may be monitored with the Richmond Agitation Sedation Scale (RASS).[4]

4. A registered nurse, nurse practitioner, or physician should be available to assess the patient continuously during the initiation of therapy. Thereafter, hourly assessments by a registered nurse should be performed until a stable dose is reached.

5. Once the patient is sedated, medication is not to be increased unless there is evidence of distress.

6. Decrease in sedatives *can* be initiated at the discretion of the physician or at the request of the health care proxy or surrogate.

7. Goal of sedation is to provide relief of symptoms/suffering, and medications should be titrated carefully to achieve this goal. However, *gradual* deterioration of respirations is expected in imminently dying patients and should not alone constitute a reason for decreasing sedation.

8. Sedation should not be attempted by increasing opioid dosages. However, opioids should be continued at the previous level in order to ensure pain control and to prevent opioid withdrawal.

After Care

- The goal of palliative sedation is to alleviate suffering. When properly administered,

TABLE 22.2: SAMPLE DRUG PROTOCOL FOR PALLIATIVE SEDATION [5]

Drug Name/Class	Midazolam/Versed/benzodiazepine	Lorazepam/Ativan/benzodiazepine	Pentobarbital/Nembutal/Long acting barbiturate	Phenobarbital/Long acting barbiturate	Chlorpromazine/Thorazine/antipsychotic
Suggested starting dose	Infusion IV or SQ 0.5–2 mg/hr after a load of 1–5 mg	IV/SC: infusion 0.5–1 mg/hr PO: 1–10 mg/day in 2–3 divided doses Usual 2–6 mg/day in divided doses	IV: 100 mg. Repeat every 1–3 minutes, up to 200–500 mg total dose	IV or SC: 200 mg bolus	IV or IM: 12.5 mg q 4–12 h or 3–5 mg/hr IV PR: 25–100 mg q 4–12 h
Usual maintenance dose	30% of induction dose	IV: 12–24 mg/day PO: 12–24 mg/day	IV: 1mg/kg/hour infusion. May increase to 2–3 mg/kg/min	Infusion IV: 0.5 mg/kg per hour via continuous SC injection or IV	12.5–25 mg q 2–4 hours PO, PR, or IV Parenteral: 37.5–150 mg/day PR: 75–300 mg/day
Onset of action	IV: 1–5 minutes Half-life: 1–4 hours but prolonged with cirrhosis, CHF, obesity or elderly	IV: 5–20 minutes Half-life: Adult 13 hours. Elderly 16 hours. ESRD: 31–70 hours	IV: about 1 minute Half-life: 15–50 hours	IV: about 5 minutes Peak: IV about 30 minutes Half-life: 53–140 hours	IM: 15 minutes Oral: 30–60 minutes Half-life: initial 2 hours Terminal 30 hours
Drug interactions	CNS depressant, so use cautiously with opiates or CNS depressants—decrease midazolam dose by 30%	CNS depressants and psychoactive medications Decreased metabolism of lorazepam with phenytoin and valproic acid	Multiple drug interactions CNS depression potentiated by opioids	Incompatible with hydromorphone	May increase hypotensive effects of opioids; multiple drug interactions

(continued)

TABLE 22.2: (CONTINUED)

Drug Name/Class	Midazolam/Versed/benzodiazepine	Lorazepam/Ativan/benzodiazepine	Pentobarbital/Nembutal/Long acting barbiturate	Phenobarbital/Long acting barbiturate	Chlorpromazine/Thorazine/antipsychotic
Side effects or adverse reaction	Decreased respiratory rates, variations in BP and pulse, paradoxical behavior or excitement	Sedation, respiratory depression, hypotension, and paradoxical agitation	Lethargy, drowsiness, bradycardia, hypotension, CNS excitation or depression	Can cause hemodynamic instability[3] hypotension, bradycardia, syncope, lethargy, CNS depression or excitation, hypoventilation	May cause EPS symptoms, anticholinergic effects, cardiac conduction abnormalities, sedation hypotension, neuroleptic malignant syndrome and urinary retention and paradoxical agitation
Incremental dose for titration	Bolus is equal to hourly rate every two hours	Titrate dose in increments of 0.5–1 mg q 15 minutes times three. IV or SQ push, titrate by 1 mg q 2 hours	Increase by 1 mg/kg increments per hour to maintain sedation		
Issues to consider/incompatibilities	Has short half-life. Drug of choice for respite sedation. May be mixed with morphine, fentanyl, hydromorphone, atropine, scopolamine, dopamine, lorazepam, haloperidol	Compatible with morphine, fentanyl and hydromorphone, haloperidol. IV: do not exceed 2 mg/min. Dilute with equal volume of compatible diluent (D5W or NS)	IV pushes can be given undiluted but should not be given faster that 50 mg/minute; solution is highly alkaline—avoid extravasation	Has long half-life and reversal of sedation is difficult; No analgesic effect	Has long half-life and reversal of sedation is difficult. No analgesic effect

Note: Drug selection will vary according to institutional policies and patient profile.

it does not cause death and may actually prolong life.[1] Education should be provided to the entire team in order to help identify and address family and clinician emotions related to intense suffering.

- Opportunities for debriefing and self-care resources should be offered to all team members before, during, and after the sedation process. (See Chapter 18: Self-Care.)

TAKE-HOME POINTS

- Palliative sedation (PS) is the use of medication to cause a reduced level of consciousness in order to relieve intractable symptoms experienced by an imminently dying patient.
- There is no consensus on the use of palliative sedation for psycho-existential suffering as the sole intolerable, refractory symptom in an imminently dying patient.
- Utilize all appropriate expertise and exhaust all treatment options to manage symptoms before considering palliative sedation. Ethics committee involvement may be warranted in some cases.

- The goal of palliative sedation is to alleviate suffering. When properly administered, it does not cause death and may actually prolong life.
- Opportunities for debriefing and self-care resources should be offered to all team members before, during, and after the sedation process.

REFERENCES

1. Kirk T, Mahon M. National Hospice and Palliative Care Organization (NHPCO) Position Statement and Commentary on the Use of Palliative Sedation in Imminently Dying Terminally Ill Patients. *J Pain Symptom Manage.* 2010;39(5):914–923.
2. Bruce S, Hendrix C, Genrty J. Palliative sedation in end-of-life care. *Journal of Hospice and Palliative Nursing.* 2006;8(6):320–327.
3. Claessens P, Menten J, Schotsmans P, Broeckaert B. Palliative sedation: a review of the research literature. *J Pain Symptom Manage.* 2008;36(4):310–333.
4. Cherney N, Radbruch L. The Board of the European Association for Palliative Care. European Association for Palliative Care (EAPC) recommended framework for the use of sedation in palliative care. *Palliat Med.* 2009;23(7):581–593.
5. Lynch M. Palliative sedation. *Clin J Oncol Nurs.* 2003;7(6):653–667.

23

Responding to Requests for Hastened Death

INTRODUCTION

A direct request for some form of hastened death from a patient or family member because of physical or existential distress and suffering is not uncommon in the setting of progressive debilitation from a terminal disease. Receiving such a request is not a new phenomenon for health care professionals, but it always presents a challenge to the clinical team.

Such requests are best understood as expressions of despair and are often about something other than a settled rational conviction that it is time to die. It is not the purpose of this chapter to discuss the moral and ethical dimensions of this issue, but rather to offer guidance to the clinician who must formulate an appropriate response to a request for hastened death.

TERMINOLOGY[1]

- **Request for hastened death** is defined as a request for voluntary termination of one's own life by self-administration of a lethal substance, with the direct or indirect assistance of a physician. The clinician does not administer the medication but assists by providing the means with which a patient can end his/her life (for example, by giving information, a prescription, or directions).
- Request for a hastened death must be distinguished from a decision to **withhold or withdraw life-sustaining therapy**, which honors the refusal of treatments that a patient does not desire, that are burdensome to the patient, or that will provide no benefit.
- **Physician-assisted suicide (PAS)** is a term used to describe the actions of a physician who assists a patient who acts to bring his/her life to an end. In the United States, PAS is currently legal in only three states, Oregon, Washington, and Montana.
- **Euthanasia** is the administration of a medication with the intention of causing death in the context of an incurable or painful disease. Euthanasia is illegal in the United States.
- **"Double effect"** describes the clinical scenario where a patient receives medications such as opioids or benzodiazepines with the intent of treating severe and distressing symptoms; the unintended side effect, however, may be to indirectly and unintentionally contribute slightly to a hastened death.

PREVALENCE

- Several studies have reported that 17% to 40% of critical care, oncology, and hospice nurses surveyed had received at least one request for assisted death from a patient or family member.[1]
- Empirical studies of patients with advanced cancer and AIDS found that 8% to 15% of patients may have thought about a hastened death.[2] In one study of terminally ill cancer patients, 17% of patients reported a high desire for hastened death.[3]

LEGAL PERSPECTIVES

- In the United States, the Supreme Court has ruled that the act of requesting assistance from a health care provider to end one's life is not a constitutionally protected right. As a result, decisions and legislation on physician-assisted suicide have essentially been delegated to the states.
- Currently, Oregon, Washington, and Montana have laws allowing physician-assisted suicide to occur in accordance with guidelines and procedures that strictly limit access. The Washington law is based closely on the Oregon Death with Dignity Act (DWDA).

THE OREGON EXPERIENCE[4]

- Under DWDA, cognitively intact adults with prognosis of six months or less may request a prescription for PAS. Required steps in the process include:

1. Patient must make two verbal requests (separated by at least 15 days), and one written request to physician.
2. Both prescribing and consulting physician must confirm the diagnosis, prognosis, and capacity determination; the patient must also be informed of feasible alternatives including comfort care, hospice care, and pain management.

- Cumulative data from the Oregon DWDA (1998 to 2007) reveal that 541 people were given prescriptions, and 341 died from ingesting the prescribed medications. More than one-third of those receiving prescriptions did not ingest the prescribed medication, suggesting that maintaining control over the timing and manner of one's death may be sufficient for a significant number of patients in distress.[5]

FACTORS UNDERLYING A REQUEST FOR HASTENED DEATH

- A request to hasten death is a phenomenon that does not necessarily reflect a wish to die, but rather may be a response to overwhelming physical, emotional, or spiritual/existential distress among patients in the advanced stages of illness.
- Commonly cited reasons for requesting hastened death include:[6]
  - Fear of intractable pain
  - Inadequately controlled physical symptoms (e.g., dyspnea, anorexia, nausea, insomnia, anxiety), or the fear that these symptoms may develop
  - Difficulties in relationships with family and significant others (e.g., caregivers feeling overwhelmed or frustrated, patient feeling the family is inattentive and uncaring, worry about being a burden)
  - Wish for greater attention from the physician
  - Psychological disorders (e.g., grief, depression, anxiety)
  - Organic mental disorders (delirium, dementia)
  - Personality and substance abuse disorders

- Personal values (e.g., desire for death with dignity, self-determination, autonomy, need for control and self-reliance, intolerance for suffering, disability, or dependency)
- A systematic literature review and meta-ethnography from the perspective of patients identified major themes underlying the wish to hasten death[7] as a response to:
  - Physical/psychological/spiritual despair
  - Loss of sense of self
  - Fear
  - A desire to live, but "not in this way"
  - As a way of ending suffering
  - As a method of reasserting control over life

RESPONDING TO A REQUEST FOR HASTENED DEATH

- A request for hastened death should always be addressed as an urgent clinical matter and "a cry for help." Such a request is often made subtly, with ambiguous language, while at other times a request may be clear, direct, and offered verbally or in writing.
- Regardless of the style of the communication, and before responding directly to the request, the first step is to conduct a multidimensional evaluation:[8]
  1. **Clarify what is meant by the request**: Listen with compassion and openness to the patient's concerns. The request may in fact be a plea to address undermanaged physical symptoms, spiritual or existential suffering, or a desire for reassurance that severe pain and fears of abandonment will be adequately managed. See Box 23.1 for suggested language.[9,10]
  2. **Support** the patient: Affirm your professional commitment and the continued support of the health care team. Reassure the patient of your ongoing involvement no matter what lies ahead, but be honest and direct about personal and professional boundaries that limit the honoring of the request.
  3. **Evaluate** the patient's decision-making capacity: Assess for confusion or delirium; also for depression, anxiety, grief. Review for past history of suicidal attempts, psychiatric issues, alcohol

---

BOX 23.1   CLARIFYING THE REQUEST: SUGGESTED LANGUAGE

"I would like to clarify what you are asking about....Can you tell me more?"
"Sometimes when people have been sick, they can feel lonely and like they are on their own. Do you feel this way?"
"What has led you to this request?"
"Do you feel this (desire to die) more so at any particular time of day or night, for example, when your visitors have left, or when you first wake up in the morning?"
"Is this feeling with you all the time, or does it come and go?"

---

or drug abuse, or recent significant bereavement.

4. **Explore** the underlying physical, emotional, and existential factors that may be contributing to the patient's suffering and distress. See Box 23.2 for suggested language.[9,10]

5. **Acknowledge** and respond to the patient, family, and provider emotions that may be associated with the request for hastened death. Clinicians should also attempt to identify and explore their own emotional and psychological reactions to the patient's request for hastened death and should actively seek support and assistance from colleagues.

6. **Intensify** treatment of the root causes of the request when possible, identifying untreated physical, psychological, social, and spiritual symptoms. Review for any reversible symptomatic issues, and clarify the plan of care. Discuss potential solutions with multidisciplinary team members. Consult and involve other health care professionals with the expertise to address patient and family needs.

7. **Respond** directly to the request for hastened death after completing this comprehensive evaluation. Most requests for hastened death will be resolved if unmet physical, emotional, and spiritual needs are identified, validated, and managed with a program of high-quality palliative care.

- In the event of repeated and persistent requests for hastened death that cannot be resolved with these recommendations, continue to work in partnership with patient and family. Options include seeking expert consultation and seeking assistance from community-based resources such as Compassion & Choices (http://www.compassionandchoices.org).

TAKE-HOME POINTS

- A direct request for hastened death because of physical or existential distress is not uncommon in the setting of progressive debilitation from a terminal disease.

BOX 23.2   EXPLORING PATIENT DISTRESS: SUGGESTED LANGUAGE

"What are the hardest things for you right now, or the things that cause you the greatest worry?"
"Can you tell me more about the things that frighten or concern you the most at this moment?"
"What do you feel could be improved in your treatment?"
"Some people give a lot of thought to their death and how it might be for them as that time draws closer—have you been thinking about this?"
"Can you tell me about how others have reacted to your being ill like this?...Who would you say best understands what you are going through?"
"Sometimes people going through such times can feel disappointed in their beliefs or faith....Have you felt this way?"

- Such requests are best understood as an expression of despair and are often about something other than a settled rational conviction that it is time to die.
- A request for hastened death should be addressed as an urgent clinical matter, with immediate steps taken to clarify the request, followed by assessment and treatment of possible underlying causes of the request.
- Clinicians should identify and explore their own emotional and psychological reactions to the patient's request for hastened death and actively seek support and assistance from colleagues.
- Most requests for hastened death will be resolved if unmet physical, emotional, and spiritual needs are identified, validated, and managed with a program of high-quality palliative care.
- In the event of repeated and persistent requests for hastened death that cannot be resolved, partnership with patient and family should be continued while seeking expert consultation.

REFERENCES

1. Ersek M. The continuing challenge of assisted death. *Journal of Hospice and Palliative Nursing.* 2004;6(1):46–59.
2. Hudson PL, Kristjanson LJ, Ashby M, et al. Desire for hastened death in patients with advanced disease and the evidence base of clinical guidelines: a systematic review. *Palliat Med.* 2006;20:693–701.
3. Breitbart W, Rodenfeld B, Pessin H, et al. Depression, hopelessness and desire for hastened death in terminally ill patients with cancer. *JAMA.* 2000;284(22):2907–2911.
4. Abrahm JL. Patient and family requests for hastened death. *Hematology American Society of Hematology Education Book.* 2008;1:475–480.
5. "Death with Dignity Act Annual Reports" March 3, 2009. http://www.oregon.gov/DHS/ph/pas/ar-index.shtml.
6. Block SD, Billings A. Patient requests to hasten death: evaluation and management in terminal care. *Arch Intern Med.* 1994;154:2039–2047.
7. Monforte-Royo C, Villavicencio-Chavez C, Tomas-Sabado J, et al. What lies behind the wish to hasten death? A systematic review and meta-ethnography from the perspective of patients. *PloS one.* 2012;7(5):1–16.
8. Quill T, Arnold R. Evaluating requests for hastened death. Fast Facts and Concepts. May 2006; 156. http://www.eperc.mcw.edu/fastFact/ff_156.htm.
9. Hudson PL, Schofield P, Kelly B, et al. Responding to desire to die statements from patients with advanced disease: recommendations for health professionals. *Palliat Med.* 2006;20:703–710.
10. Emanuel LL, von Gunten CF, Ferris FD, Hauser JM, eds. The Education in Palliative and End-of-Life Care (EPEC), Module 5 Physician Assisted Suicide, The EPEC Project 2003.

24

Assistive Aids and Devices

INTRODUCTION

Assistive technologies (AT) include devices, equipment, or technology used to improve, maintain, or slow decline in the function of a disabled patient. Examples include durable medical equipment, modified devices used for ADLs, and electronic items including computer interface devices.

DEMOGRAPHICS[1]

As the population ages, the rate of disability is declining, but because the geriatric population is growing dramatically, the absolute number of disabled Americans is rising.

- In 2007, 42% of people over age 65 reported a functional limitation; 14% had difficulty performing one or more IADL (Independent Activities of Daily Living).
- Women have higher levels of functional limitations than men. In 2007, 47% of female Medicare enrollees aged 65 and over had difficulty with ADLs or IADLs or were in a facility, compared with 35% of male Medicare enrollees.

PURPOSE

- Assistive technology and devices serve to maintain independence and function for older or seriously ill patients, and they also decrease caregiver burden.[2]
- Patients report that use of assistive devices can improve confidence and feelings of safety, encouraging increased activity levels and independence.[3]
- Maintenance of function is a prognostic indicator in serious illness and may improve response to curative therapies, as well as help prevent secondary infections and skin breakdown.

BARRIERS TO USE[2]

- Elderly patients may resist the "disabled" label and refuse to acknowledge any loss of function. These patients and their

caregivers can benefit from education on how assistive technologies help preserve function, maximize quality of life, encourage independence, and reduce caregiver burden. Other barriers include:

- Patients, family, and health care providers are often unaware of what devices and technology are available.
- Devices and technology may be perceived by patients as complicated or difficult to use.
- There is often a learning curve before AT can be utilized effectively; physical or occupational training may be required.
- Patient may experience feelings of embarrassment or shame caused by appearing disabled, dependent, or "old" in public.
- Patients may fear losing current personal assistance or attention if assistive technology is successful.
- Cost of equipment may be prohibitive.

SELECTING THE APPROPRIATE ASSISTIVE TECHNOLOGY[4]

- Clinicians should be acquainted with the range of assistive devices and technology available for their elderly or seriously ill patients (Tables 24.1, 24.2, and 24.3).
- Selecting the appropriate device or technology begins with an assessment of what type of assistance is needed, with referral to specialists for evaluation when necessary.
- Other key factors in the process include determining whether the patient is motivated to use the device that is indicated and assuring that the patient or caregiver receives adequate training on how to use the device/technology safely and effectively.
- Some assistive devices are simple and may be ordered by the nonspecialist or even purchased from a medical supply store by the patient or caregivers. Other devices

TABLE 24.1: ASSISTIVE DEVICES AND TECHNOLOGY IN THE HOME[5,6,7]

Category	Indication	Examples
Home and environment modifications	Fall prevention	Wireless doorbell with adjustable volume (patient has the doorbell button; caregiver has the wireless receiver) Clear floor rugs, electric cords Night lights +/-motion sensors Electric fall detectors
	Wandering	Door alerts signal movements of cognitively impaired patients at risk for wandering Pressure mats Emergency response systems Signal transmitting devices alert caregiver and give location Baby monitor: increased supervision while allowing caregiver more independence

may require referral to a specialty durable medical equipment (DME) clinic in a Department of Rehabilitation Medicine.

REIMBURSEMENT
- There is currently no universal method of reimbursement that covers the broad range of assistive technologies and devices available to elderly or disabled patients.
- If prescribed by a physician, some durable medical equipment is covered by Medicare Part A or B, depending on the disability and the type of equipment ordered. The provider/clinician must describe and document the rationale and need for the equipment.
- Depending on the patient's eligibility, assistance may also be available from state Medicaid programs, the VA Health Benefits Service Center, or private health insurance policies.
- For smaller devices, and especially when time is a factor, families may choose to pay out of pocket than await insurance procedures.
- Rental and purchase at secondhand stores can significantly lower cost for some items. Durable medical equipment may also be loaned to home hospice patients at no cost to patient.

PALLIATIVE CARE ISSUES
- Assistive technology helps older or disabled adults to continue the activities they have always mastered and enjoyed but must now manage differently. These devices may be as simple as a walker for easier ambulation or perhaps an amplification device to make it possible to watch television or talk on the telephone.
- For chronically or terminally ill patients at home, the use of assistive technology changes over time from supporting independence and maintenance of ADLs to comfort care and providing family members with strategies to ease the caregiver burden.
- Assistive technologies available for bed-bound patients include:
  - Electric hospital bed: repositioning and sitting patient up, elevation for lower extremity edema, turning for hygiene, etc
  - Adding handrails or trapeze to conventional bed to increase bed mobility
  - Hoyer lift for transfers
  - Mobile hospital table: ease of serving meals, organizing personal effects
- Adaptive equipment and positioning devices should be used when indicated to provide comfort and pain relief:
  - Specialized mattress for skin protection
  - Body, neck pillows
  - Specialty cushions for various conditions, e.g., post-mastectomy cushions
  - Heel, elbow protectors
  - Communication strategies or devices that help patient express discomfort, pain

TABLE 24.2: ASSISTIVE DEVICES/TECHNOLOGIES FOR SUPPORT OF ADLS[4-8]

Category	Indication	Examples
Tools to assist with Activities of Daily Living (ADLs)	Personal hygiene/ grooming	Large grips on toothbrushes; electric razor in lieu of blade
	Dressing/undressing	Velcro closures in lieu of shoelaces/buttons; elastic shoelaces Zipper pulls, trouser pulls Long-handled shoehorns; sock aid; reachers
	Self-feeding	Large grips on cutlery, kitchen utensils Spoon/fork combinations Plates and bowls with suction cups for stability while eating; rubberized place mats Kitchen cupboards fitted with self-lowering racks Lowered sinks and countertops
	Toileting/bathing	Raised toilet seat for greater ease in arising Toilet frame: greater ease in arising, arm supports help if lower extremity (LE) weakness Bedside commode, bedpan, urinal: may be required if ambulation decreases or urge incontinence or diarrhea develops A "3-in-1 toilet seat" can transition from toilet frame to bedside commode Grab bars: installed adjacent to commode for stability, ease of arising from commode Grab bars, bench in tub/shower for lower fall risk Bathtub transfer bench: straddles tub and floor, reduces fall risk if LE weakness or balance problems Handheld shower head for ease of showering while seated on bench
	Transfers	Slide board: from car to wheelchair Slide board, bedside rails: from wheelchair to bed Hoyer lift: for patient unable to sit up
	Ambulation/mobility	Canes, walkers, wheel chairs (Table 24.3) Leg lifter For stairs: non-slip treads; adequate lighting; handrails; chair lift "Riser" electric chair: maintain independence if proximal muscle weakness
Sensory impairment	Hearing loss Vision loss	Hearing aids; amplifiers Glasses and magnification aids Books on tape Talking wrist watches and mobile phones Large-button devices, e.g., TV remote, telephone, calculators Tablet devices both as easier to see screens and as remote controls for other devices
Computer access	Allow disabled, homebound, older patients to enjoy social interaction, educational programs, connection to family and friends	Special software allowing access to Internet for vision- or hearing-impaired patients Modified keyboard and/or mouse, voice-recognition and/or read-aloud devices, e.g., hands-free communication devices Specialized devices allowing disabled patients to use computer

TABLE 24.3: AMBULATION AIDS[3,7]

STRAIGHT CANES (standard vs. aluminum)	Provide support, redistribute weight from a weak leg; increase confidence and balance, spread center of gravity over a broader base, increase proprioception to the ground/floor. Carried in the hand contralateral to lower extremity deficit	
Indication	Type	Comment
Poor balance, ataxias, peripheral neuropathies Little to no weight-bearing	Standard wooden cane	Least expensive; must be cut to correct height; typically trimmed to greater trochanter or ASIS or wrist crease, elbow flexed 15–30 degrees when in use
	Aluminum cane	Adjustable and lightweight; lightly more expensive but easier to adjust
Partial weight-bearing (PWB): painful arthritis, CVA, patients with metastatic lesions who are allowed PWB	Offset cane	Adjustable and enhanced weight-bearing as hand is centered over long axis of the cane
Partial weight-bearing: painful arthritis, CVA, patients with metastatic lesions who are allowed PWB	Quad cane	Increased base allows more weight-bearing for antalgic (painful) gait but slows gait
Hemiplegia, patients with metastatic lesions who are non-weight-bearing	Sidestepper/ hemi-walker/walk cane	Allows continuous weight-bearing, e.g., hemiplegia
WALKERS	**Provide increased base of support, lateral (side-to-side) stability, and weight-bearing**	
Indication	Type	Comment
Useful for severe ataxia patient but not for cognitively impaired	Standard walker	Four legs in simultaneous contact with ground Most stable but slower. More difficult than a cane
Good for moderate ataxia or balance deficits	Front-wheeled walker	Patients who cannot lift standard walker Permit more normal gait but less stable Allow some weight-bearing
For patients with mild ataxia, "cautious gait" Deconditioned patients must be cognitively intact to control	Four-wheeled walker (Rolator™)	For balance, not for weight-bearing. Least stable, i.e., highest fall risk Readily equipped with seats for rest breaks, hand brakes, larger wheels Not for weight-bearing or balance
Good for moderate ataxia or balance deficits	Platform walker	Allows partial weight-bearing for patients who are NWB on one upper limb (e.g., due to amputation, metastatic lesions, pain)

(continued)

TABLE 24.3: (CONTINUED)

WHEELCHAIRS	**Useful for patients who are not yet bedbound but able to walk only short distances** **Most patients are required to have PT/OT evaluation before insurance will reimburse, but hospice patients may be given non-customized loaner units**	
Indication	Type	Comment
Standard wheelchair	Self-propelled Most commonly have removable armrests and leg rests, depending on disability	Available in a variety of heights and widths with varying wheel types The most energy-efficient means of ambulation (lowest metabolic demand) Vendors and/or PT/OT can advise the prescribing physician
Pulmonary and cardiac disorders, paraplegia, and tetraplegia; patient must have intact vision and cognition	Motorized wheelchair, scooters	Very limited number of patients are eligible Usually, detailed letter of medical necessity describing every detail of the equipment required before insurance will cover Surprisingly heavy and may not be feasible in all homes

TAKE-HOME POINTS

- Assistive technologies and devices serve to maintain independence and function for older or seriously ill patients, enable patients to better tolerate curative therapies, and decrease caregiver burden.
- Clinicians should be acquainted with the range of assistive devices and technology available for their elderly or seriously ill patients.
- When considering the use of assistive devices, clinicians should determine whether the patient is motivated to use the device and also make sure that the patient or caregiver receives adequate training on how to use the device/technology safely and effectively.
- Expert consultation about available assistive devices and technology may be indicated for complex patient and family needs.

REFERENCES

1. Older Americans 2010: Key indicators of well-being. *Federal Interagency Forum on Aging-Related Statistics*. Washington, DC: U.S. Government Printing Office. July 2010.
2. Skymne C, Dahlin-Ivanoff S, Claesson L, Eklund K. Getting used to assistive devices: ambivalent experiences by frail elderly persons. *Scandanavian Journal of Occupational Therapy*. Mar 2012;*19*(2): 194–203.
3. Bradley S, Hernandez C. Geriatric assistive devices. *Am Fam Physician*. Aug 2011;*84*(4):405–411.
4. Brummel-Smith K, Dangiolo M. Assistive technologies in the home. *Clin Geriatr Med*. 2009;*25*(1): 61–77.
5. Meyer MM, Derr P. *The Comfort of Home: An Illustrated Step-by-step Guide for Caregivers*. Portland, OR: Care Trust; 1998.
6. Berry BE, Ignash A. Assistive technology: providing independence for individuals with disabilities. *Rehabil Nurs*. 2003;*28*(1):6–14.
7. Choi H, Sugar R, Fish DE, Shatzer M, Krabak B, eds. *Physical Medicine and Rehabilitation Pocketpedia*. Philadelphia, PA: Lippincott Williams and Wilkins; 2003.
8. Miskelly FG. Assistive technology in elderly care. *Age and Ageing*. 2001;*30*:455–458.

25

Rehabilitation

INTRODUCTION

Palliative care is specialized medical care for people with serious illness that is focused on providing patients with relief from the symptoms, pain, and stress of a serious illness, with the goal of improving quality of life for both the patient and the family. The specialty of physical medicine and rehabilitation (PM&R) deals with the prevention, diagnosis, and treatment of functionally limiting disease or injury. Rehabilitation specialists use physical and pharmacologic regimens to help patients restore function due to impairments, disabilities, and illness.[1]

PALLIATIVE CARE REHABILITATION

While the goals of these two specialties have not traditionally been seen as intersecting, there is a growing understanding of their compatibility, especially for older adults who struggle with the symptom burden of one or more chronic illnesses.

Proponents of palliative care rehabilitation point to three key areas of commonality: emphasis on enhancing quality of life in the context of serious illness; importance of an integrated focus on mind, body, and spirit; and delivery in a model of collaborative partnership between patients, families, and the interdisciplinary care team.[1]

DEMOGRAPHICS

- The U.S. population is aging, and the number of people with chronic comorbidities is rising, even as the incidence of those comorbidities falls.[2] The population born between 1947 and 1963 will be the healthiest generation in history as they enter their geriatric years, but because of their large numbers the demand for rehabilitation care for them will be increased.
- As a result of these evolving demographics and recent diagnostic trends in hospice

care, emerging opportunities for PM&R involvement now extend to palliative care in the hospice setting. At the beginning of the hospice movement in the United States, 90% of hospice patients had a primary diagnosis of cancer. By 2005, however, the percent of hospice admissions with a cancer diagnosis dropped below 50%. By 2010, only 35.6% of hospice admissions were cancer-related.[3]

- As more patients enter hospice with impairments and disability associated with non-cancer chronic diseases (heart failure, lung disease, stroke, and general debility), palliative rehabilitation interventions can help reduce pain, optimize function and comfort, and maximize quality of life.[4]

RESTORATIVE VS. PALLIATIVE REHABILITATION

- Rehabilitation therapy is divided into three categories, each addressing a range of functional activities:[5]
  1. Physical therapy (PT) is concerned with gross functional mobility, defined as a change in body position, and includes any physical states or limitations that affect the ability to change position. Another term used for gross functional mobility is "transitional movements."
  2. Occupational therapy (OT) is the area of rehabilitation that includes Activities of Daily Living (ADLs), including self-care and home management.
  3. Speech therapy deals with tasks involving the oral-pharyngeal-laryngeal function, as well as cognitive components involved in the process of communication.
- Traditional rehabilitation medicine focuses on maximizing quality of life and function based on a patient's physical limitations. The

restorative approach to rehabilitation fosters the patient's independence and autonomy by offering new ways to perform ADLs and/or direct a caregiver. Treatment is often focused on healing as well. In the case of permanent disability, emphasis is placed on helping the patient and family cope with and adapt to the new limitation caused by a stroke, spinal cord injury, or amputation.

- In palliative rehabilitation, this standard restorative continuum is reversed. Rather than working to return to a pre-morbid level of function, palliative care patients are supported as they face the prospect of disease progression accompanied by functional decline over time.

- The clinical goals of geriatric palliative rehabilitation are to maintain as much functional independence as possible, provide emotional support to patient and family members, mitigate uncomfortable or distressing symptoms, and reduce the caregiver burden of serious illness. Strategies to accomplish these goals are pursued in a step-wise manner during the progression from the early to late stages of a serious illness as follows:[6]

  1. **Preventive**—preventing the symptoms and complications of the underlying disease process.
  2. **Restorative**—the patient is expected to be free of restrictive disease or symptoms for an appreciable time, and the goal is to regain as much as possible of the function and strength that may have been lost due to disease process or treatment side effects.
  3. **Supportive**—where persistent residual disease is expected, the focus of rehabilitation is to maintain function at new baseline for as long as possible.
  4. **Palliation**—for patients with advanced disease, rehabilitation aims to increase functional independence, reduce pain and discomfort, maximize quality of life, and reduce the burden of care for family members.

- Core principles of palliative rehabilitation practice include patient and caregiver education and communication, realistic and individualized patient-centered goals for care, continuity of care, and supporting the whole family throughout the disease trajectory.[7, 8]

PATIENT BENEFITS

- Palliative rehabilitation, can alleviate a patient's fears of being a burden on caregivers reduces feelings of helplessness, increase the patient's sense of competence and control, and contribute to an improved mood and sense of well-being.

- Studies indicate that rehabilitation contributes to improved function and quality of life for cancer patients. Improved functional status as a result of rehabilitation may also help improve cancer patients' tolerance of burdensome treatments such as chemotherapy or radiation.[9]

- Palliative rehabilitation can help identify and manage shifting care priorities and goals in the face of advancing illness:
  - Early in disease, the goal is preserving function and reducing dependency.
  - As illness progresses, priorities will include safety, environment assessment, assisted mobility, fall prevention measures, transfer techniques, and instruction and use of assistive devices; emphasis remains on vocational adjustment, psychological support, and enhancing patient's sense of mastery and control.
  - When the patient is closer to the end of life, the focus will shift to quality of life and maximal comfort for the patient (e.g., bed positioning to preserve skin integrity, pain relief techniques, attention to hygiene, gentle massage).

CAREGIVER BENEFITS

- Instruction, teaching, and support is offered to caregivers as they learn how to perform physically taxing or complex care routines. This caregiver education improves quality of care and reduces risk of caregiver injury.

- Maintaining patient capacity and function may provide physical relief and extra free time for caregivers; it may also help minimize or delay the need for costly patient care such as increased home health aide hours, equipment, home modification, crisis intervention, respite care, etc.

REFERRAL FOR PALLIATIVE REHABILITATION

- Palliative rehabilitation emphasizes realistic and achievable goals of care, strategies to control pain and distressing symptoms, and helping patients and caregivers adjust to the discouraging loss of independence and function while maximizing quality of life for both patient and family.

- Rehabilitation programs typically begin with light activity and gradually progress to moderate activity under the supervision of a trained practitioner (Table 25.1).
- Rehabilitation programs must be individualized to each patient's limitations and goals. After therapists discuss the risks and benefits with patient and family, the parameters of the prescription or recommendations may be liberalized. For example, a COPD patient may want to ambulate to bathroom. In most health care settings, this patient's pulse oximetry would be monitored closely; at home or in the hospice environment, however, the patient's autonomy and self-esteem are prioritized over the digital readout.
- As the patient progresses through the disease trajectory, therapies become gradually less aggressive or demanding. When the patient is closer to the end of life, emphasis will shift to quality of life and comfort, including pain-relief techniques such as desensitization, gentle massage, healing touch, vibration, visualization, and relaxation.

UNDERUTILIZATION OF PALLIATIVE REHABILITATION

In spite of palliative rehabilitation's potential benefits for controlling distressing symptoms (e.g., pain, skin breakdown, lymphedema) and its potential for advancing two key goals of care identified by palliative care patients (improving quality of life and not being a burden on others), palliative rehabilitation remains an underutilized care modality.[10] Reasons that referrals are not made to palliative rehabilitation include:

- Clinician perception that rehabilitation is not appropriate for the older or seriously ill adult population, based on the assumption that geriatric patients are more accepting of physical limitations as "only to be expected," and that seriously ill patients will not benefit.
- Restorative bias of rehabilitation professionals when they formulate

treatment plans, goals of care, and outcome evaluation for palliative care patients. There is a widespread perception that patients who are frail and debilitated, or possibly near the end of life, are not appropriate candidates.

- Health care system and delivery barriers include shortage of subspecialty-trained PT, OT, and speech pathologists[7] and lack of availability and access. Also, although Medicare and most insurance plans cover outpatient rehabilitation evaluation and treatment when need is certified by a health care provider, deductibles and copays still apply, and there may be a cap on services in a single year.

TAKE-HOME POINTS

- There is a growing understanding of the importance of palliative rehabilitation, especially for older adults who struggle with the symptom burden of one or more chronic illnesses.
- Geriatric palliative care and rehabilitation medicine share three key areas of commonality: emphasis on enhancing quality of life in the context of serious illness; importance of an integrated focus on mind, body, and spirit; and delivery in a model of collaborative partnership between patients, families, and the interdisciplinary care team.
- While traditional rehabilitation programs focus on restoration of function, palliative rehabilitation supports patients as they face the prospect of disease progression accompanied by inevitable functional decline over time.
- Palliative rehabilitation contributes to improved function and quality of life for cancer patients. Improved functional status due to rehabilitation intervention may help improve cancer patients' tolerance of burdensome treatments such as chemotherapy or radiation.
- Rehabilitation leading to improved patient capacity and function may provide physical relief and extra free time for caregivers, and it also may delay the need for additional costly patient supports such as increased home health aide hours, equipment, home modification, crisis intervention, respite care, etc.

TABLE 25.1: PALLIATIVE REHABILITATION THERAPIES

Symptom or Disability	Prescription and Possible Interventions	Benefits/Comments
Lymphedema	Manual lymphedema decompression (MLD) Congestion decompression techniques/ physiotherapy (CDT/CDP) Compression stockings/garments and instruction in donning/doffing (See Chapter 58: Lymphedema)	Prevent pain Preserve motion and function Minimize and prevent disfigurement Psychosocial adjustment Foster emotional well-being Prevent secondary infection
Ambulation training Musculoskeletal pain	Isometrics Passive range of motion (PROM) and/or Assistive/ Active range of motion (A/AROM) physical therapy Progressive resistive exercises (PRE) Joint preservation techniques Restriction release Assistive devices evaluation as appropriate Modalities such as collator packs, ultrasound, cold laser (See Chapter 24: Assistive Aids and Devices)	Increased autonomy and dignity May require orthopedic clearance if there are bony metastases Modalities that enhance blood flow must be restricted from areas of tumor
Skin breakdown	Bed mobility: Supine-to-sit, roll, scoot, positioning Instruct caregivers in "back school" techniques: bed height, positioning/posture (See Chapter 59: Pressure Ulcers)	Increased autonomy and dignity Caregiver education leading to improved care
Dyspnea	Airway clearance techniques: cough, autogenic and postural drainage, paced and pursed lip breathing, chest percussion, vibration (See Chapter 41: Dyspnea)	Better function, quality of life Decreased anxiety
Dysphagia, poor PO intake, cachexia Communication difficulties	Swallow/Barium Swallow evaluation Modified consistency, discussion of artificial nutrition for select diagnoses Explore supplements, appetite stimulants, medication adjustments for motor neuron disease (See Chapter 49: Dysphagia) Speech therapy Oromotor skills (e.g., tongue coordination, pocketing, chin tuck) Auditory, visual, reading comprehension	Prognostic value; may help guide decision-making Determine appropriate calorie intake Improved family understanding of benefits and burdens of artificial nutrition
Anxiety/depression	Relaxation, visualization, massage therapy, Reiki, healing touch (See Chapter 17: Complementary and Alternative Medicine)	Mood is frequently improved with improved physical function and independence
ADLs: Self-care Transfers Home safety	Assistive device evaluation and training Adaptive techniques Energy conservation techniques Home modifications (See Chapter 24: Assistive Aids and Devices)	Increase feelings of self-worth Independence is frequently enhanced with improved functional status

REFERENCES

1. Wu J, Quill T. Geriatric rehabilitation and palliative care: opportunity for collaboration or oxymoron? *Topics in Geriatric Rehabilitation.* 2011;*27*(1):29–35.

2. Hung WW, Ross JS, Boockwar KS, Siu A. Recent trends in chronic disease, impairment and disability among older adults in the United States. *BMC Geriatr.* 2011;*11*:47. http://www.biomedcentral.com/1471-2318/11/47.

3. NHPCO. *Facts and Figures: Hospice Care in America.* Alexandria, VA: National Hospice and Palliative Organization, January 2012. http://www.nhpco.org/files/public/Statistics_Research/2011_Facts_Figures.pdf. Accessed September 1, 2012.

4. Mueller K. Impact of physical therapy intervention on patient-centered outcomes in a community hospice. *Topics in Geriatric Rehabilitation.* 2011;*27*(9):2–9.

5. Frost, M. The role of physical, occupational, and speech therapy in hospice: patient empowerment. *Am J Hosp Palliat Care.* 2001;*18*(6):397–402.

6. Dietz J. Adaptive rehabilitation of the cancer patient. *Curr Probl Cancer.* 1980;*5*(5):1–56.

7. Briggs RW. Models for physical therapy practice in palliative medicine. *Rehabilitation Oncology.* 2000;*18*(2):18–21.

8. American Occupational Therapy Association Statement: the Role of Occupational Therapy in End-of-Life Care. http://www.aota.org/Practitioners/Official/Statements/End-of-Life-Care.aspx. Accessed December 2011.

9. Huang ME, Sliwa JA. Inpatient rehabilitation of patients with cancer: efficacy and treatment considerations. *PM&R.* 2011;*3*:746–757.

10. Quill T, Norton S, Shah M, et al. "What is most important for you to achieve?" *J Palliat Med.* 2006;*9*(2):382–388.

26

Mechanical Ventilation

INTRODUCTION

Mechanical ventilation (MV) is an intervention that uses machines to help patients breathe when they are unable to breathe sufficiently on their own. The goal of MV is to support a failing respiratory system until improvement can occur either spontaneously or as a result of intervention. Primary objectives of MV include:[1]

- Physiologic
  Support pulmonary gas exchange
  Increase lung volume
  Reduce the work of breathing
- Clinical
  Reverse hypoxemia
  Reverse acute respiratory acidosis
  Relieve respiratory distress
  Avoid iatrogenic lung injury and other
  complications

TYPES OF MV

1. **Invasive ventilation**, historically the cornerstone of ventilatory strategy, requires placement of an endotracheal tube or tracheostomy tube into the windpipe to deliver air directly into the lungs.
2. **Noninvasive ventilation** (NIV) allows respiratory support without the need for endotracheal intubation.
   - Two types of NIV are commonly used: noninvasive continuous positive airway pressure (CPAP) and noninvasive positive pressure ventilation (NPPV).
   - Goals of NIV are to (1) reduce work of breathing; (2) improve gas exchange (oxygenation and ventilation), and (3) reduce left ventricular load.[2]
   - NIV is usually delivered with oronasal, nasal, or full face mask. Benefits include decreased use of sedatives and endotracheal tubes, fewer nosocomial pneumonias, and improved patient communication and neurofunctional status.[2]

- Ideally, NPPV will be used if the underlying cause of the respiratory failure is thought to be reversible; in the event that the desired response is not achieved, or if the patient is not tolerating the NPPV, it should be stopped.[3]

MAKING DECISIONS ABOUT MECHANICAL VENTILATION

Overview

- Mechanical ventilation is usually initiated in the hospital setting with the expectation that it will be discontinued when the patient recovers the ability to breathe on his or her own. Weaning the patient from the ventilator is not always successful, however. In this case, choices about continuing with prolonged MV will have to be made that have complex clinical, emotional, and quality-of-life implications for all concerned.
- If the decision is made to continue with prolonged MV, the patient will be ventilator-dependent. Respiratory failure requiring prolonged dependence on MV is the hallmark of chronic critical illness, a term used to describe the status of patients who survive an initial episode of critical illness but do not fully recover and therefore remain dependent on intensive care. The mortality rate for chronic critical illness exceeds that for most malignancies, and functional dependence persists for most survivors.[4]

Clinical Considerations

- For older patients and those with chronic illnesses that compromise respiratory function, the use of ventilator support should ideally be explored in advance, before the actual decision must be made about the initiation and or continuation of MV.

- Clinicians should use these advance care planning discussions to help patients and families identify their goals for care, including preferences for prolonged respiratory support, if such a clinical scenario should develop. Patients with advanced COPD, for example, may at some point require intubation and MV to sustain life. For these patients and their families, advance care planning about MV can be explored simultaneously with curative treatment.[5] Topics that should be considered include prognosis and trajectory of illness, treatment options, expectations for MV use, risks and benefits, and clarification of personal values and preferences concerning life-sustaining treatments.
- In the event of hospitalization for an acute situation, advance directives are frequently not available, and there is often no time for careful decision-making. In these situations, the patient will typically be intubated to allow for clarification of clinical status and identifying treatment goals.

Note on Communication

Establishing a method of communication for a patient who is on ventilator support is essential for patient and family quality of life, for interactions with professional caregivers, and to allow the patient to participate in critical decision-making discussions.

- Verbal communication is possible on a ventilator with modifications to the trach cuff and to vent settings. In the presence of a tracheostomy and vent dependence, devices such as a one-way speaking valve can facilitate verbal communication.
- Nonverbal communication techniques may include writing, communication card, and eye gaze board. A speech and language pathologist can assess the clinical conditions and determine the best means of communications and suggest appropriate devices.

Options for Mechanical Ventilation

Identifying the goal of respiratory support is the first step to creating an effective treatment plan that is consistent with patient and family preferences for care. There are four possible options for mechanical ventilation: (1) temporary MV; (2) time-limited trial of MV; (3) withdrawal of MV; and (4) prolonged MV.

1. **Temporary MV**: The patient is expected to make a full recovery from acute respiratory decompensation and will be successfully weaned from the ventilator.
2. **Time-limited trial of MV**: When the patient is seriously or chronically ill, and the prospect for recovery is not clear, mechanical ventilation may be used for a time-limited trial, i.e., for a predetermined time to allow physical recovery, with a plan to reevaluate treatment options if goals for care are not achieved within a certain time frame.[6]
3. **Ventilator withdrawal**: For some patients (or their surrogates who are aware of the patient's previously stated wishes), chronic mechanical ventilation is not consistent with their agreed-upon values, preferences, and goals of care. As a result, the decision is made to discontinue ventilator support.

   - To effectively manage discontinuation of mechanical ventilation, planning is essential. (See Appendix 1, Guidelines for Ventilator Withdrawal). Careful discussions between the medical team and patient/family must occur prior to removal of any therapies. All questions regarding the ventilator removal procedures should be carefully explored to ensure full patient/family comprehension. If discontinuing the ventilator is being considered, other treatment modalities such as artificial nutrition, hydration, blood draws, and invasive testing should be reassessed to ensure that these therapies are consistent with the goals of care.
   - Family consensus is important. If, after discussing withdrawal of MV, the family is not in agreement with the next step, it is important to allow time for resolving differences so that a unified decision can be reached. Conflict resolution is an important consideration.
   - If a decision is made to discontinue MV, managing expectations is essential. Families should be aware that the patient may not die immediately, and

that movement or sound from the patient does not necessarily equate with discomfort or suffering. Families should also be assured that opioids and benzodiazepines will be used to control the any symptoms of breathlessness and anxiety during the withdrawal of ventilator support. (See Appendix 2, Symptom Management During Withdrawal of Mechanical Ventilation.)

- Spiritual concerns should be explored, particularly if cultural or religious tradition require specific rituals.[7] (See Chapter 16: Cultural Considerations.)
- Family members should receive all the support they require during and after ventilator withdrawal.[8] Examples include:
  - Give thoughtful consideration to the location of extubation. Careful attention should also be given to adequately prepare families for what they may witness and experience during extubation.
  - Determine if family members prefer to be present during the removal of the ventilator and at the time of death.
  - Managing realistic expectations of the dying process is important. Counsel families that life expectancy is not predictable and that patient comfort will remain the focus and goal of care. Also, discontinuing MV does not always result in death, and families should be prepared for this possibility.
  - When a patient is stable after withdrawal of MV, transfer to a hospice facility may be appropriate. It is best to discuss this option prior to discontinuation of MV so that families understand the rationale and benefits of a change in care setting. The goal is to avoid families feeling that they and the patient are being unexpectedly moved out of the hospital at such a critical time.

4. **Prolonged mechanical ventilation**: If it becomes clear that the patient is unlikely to ever become independent of the ventilator, the patient or a surrogate must decide whether prolonged respiratory support is consistent with the established goals for care. Personal preferences, societal or family values, and religious beliefs may influence this choice.

- The information that patients and families require for informed discussion and decision-making about maintaining prolonged ventilator support includes[9]:
  - The nature of the patient's illness and treatments
  - Prognosis for outcomes, including ventilator independence, function quality of life, and mortality
  - Impact on patient experience, including symptom burden (e.g., noninvasive ventilation may be also be experienced as burdensome by patients, and may not be consistent with care goals)
  - Potential complications
  - Expected care needs after hospitalization
  - Alternatives to continuation of MV or noninvasive ventilation when patient cannot be weaned
- When the decision is made to maintain chronic ventilator support, the patient is transitioned out of the ICU onto a medical unit, and eventually transferred to a nursing home. Discharge to care at home is typically not an option for these patients because of underlying comorbid conditions, residual organ dysfunction, and increased risk of complications.
- Management considerations for prolonged MV will apply whether the patient is cared for in a hospital, in a skilled nursing facility, or at home. (See Appendix 3, Management Considerations for Prolonged Mechanical Ventilation.)

TAKE-HOME POINTS

- The goal of mechanical ventilation is to support a failing respiratory system until improvement can occur either spontaneously or as a result of intervention.
- If a patient is unlikely to recover the ability to breathe on his or her own, decisions about continuing with prolonged MV will have to be made that have complex clinical, emotional, and quality-of-life implications for all concerned.
- Careful exploration of patient's and family's achievable goals for care is an important part of creating a long-term care plan.
- If the prospect for recovery is not clear, MV may be used for a time-limited trial to allow

physical recovery, with a plan to reevaluate treatment options if goals for care are not achieved within a certain time frame.

- If a decision is made to discontinue mechanical ventilation, family members should receive the support they require before, during, and after ventilator withdrawal.
- Opioids and benzodiazepines are used to control the symptoms of breathlessness and anxiety during the withdrawal of ventilator support.
- Chronically critically ill patients who are maintained on prolonged ventilator support are eventually transitioned out of the ICU onto medical units, and eventually discharged to a long-term care facility. Discharge to home is usually not feasible for these patients due to comorbid illnesses, residual organ dysfunction, and increased risk of complications.
- The mortality rate for chronic critical illness exceeds that for most malignancies, and functional dependence persists for most survivors.
- Care of a ventilator-dependent patient in the home is time consuming, requires an advanced level of problem solving ability and technical support, and is mentally and physically taxing for families.

REFERENCES

1. Slutsky AS. Mechanical ventilation. American College of Chest Physicians Consensus Conference. *Chest.* 1993;*104*:1833–1859.
2. Jaber S, Michelet P, Chanques G. Role of non-invasive ventilation (NIV) in the perioperative period. *Best Pract Res Clin Anaesthesiol.* 2010;*24*:253–265.
3. Yeow M, Mehta RS, White DB, Szmuilowicz E. Using non-invasiove ventilation at the end of life. Fast Facts and Concepts. May 2010;230. Available at http://www.eperc.mcw.edu/fastfact/ff_230.htm. Accessed August 30, 2012.
4. Nelson JE, Cox CE, Hope AA, Carson SS. Chronic critical illness. *Am J Respir Crit Care Med.* 2010;*182*:446–454.
5. Patel K, Janssen DJA, Curtis JR. Advance care planning in COPD. *Respirology.* 2012;*17*:72–78.
6. Quill TE, Holloway R. Time-limited trials near the end of life. *JAMA.* 2011;*306*(13):1483–1484.
7. Rubenfield G, Crawford S. Principles and practice of withdrawing life-sustaining treatment in the ICU. In: Curtis JR, Rubenfield, G, eds. *Managing death in the intensive care unit. The transition from cure to comfort.* New York: Oxford University Press; 2001:127–147.
8. Von Gunten CF, Weissman DE. Information for patients and families about ventilator withdrawal, 2nd edition. Fast Facts and Concepts. July 2005;35. Available at http://www.eperc.mcw.edu/fastfact/ff_035.htm. Accessed July 3, 2012.
9. Nelson JE, Kinjo K, Meier DE, Ahmad K, Morrison RS. When critical illness becomes chronic: informational needs of patients and families. *Journal of Critical Care.* 2005;*20*:79–89.
10. Von Gunten CF, Weissman DE. Ventilator Withdrawal Protocol, 2nd Edition. Fast Facts and Concepts. July 2005;33. Available at http://www.eperc.mcw.edu/fastfact/ff_033.htm. Accessed July 3, 2012.
11. Puntillo K, Stannard D. The intensive care unit. In Ferrell B, Coyle N, eds. *Textbook of Palliative Nursing. 2nd ed.* New York: Oxford University Press: 2006;817–833.
12. Von Gunten CF, Weissman DE. Symptom Control for Ventilator Withdrawal in the Dying Patient, 2nd Edition. Fast Facts and Concepts. July 2005;34. Available at http://www.eperc.mcw.edu/fastfact/ff_034.htm. Accessed July 3, 2012.
13. "Mechanical Ventilation: Beyond the ICU." American College of Chest Physicians. 1999. http://www.chestnet.org/accp/patient-guides/mechanical-ventilation-beyond-icu. Accessed July 3, 2012.

APPENDIX 1

Guidelines for Ventilator Withdrawal

1. Clinical documentation is critically important and should include:
   - Patient prognosis both with and without life-sustaining interventions
   - Consideration of alternatives to withdrawal
   - Written documentation of the patient's wishes recorded and a copy included in the medical record
   - Evidence of clear and convincing wishes, in lieu of advanced directives, entered into the medical record in order to satisfy ethical and legal issues
2. Once the decision has been made to withdraw MV, careful consideration should be given to the method of discontinuation. There are two methods of withdrawing ventilator support: immediate extubation and terminal weaning (Table 26.1).[10,11]
3. In addition to the physiological issues of removing the tube or ventilator, other issues that need to be addressed include:
   - A physician or nurse practitioner, nurse, and respiratory therapist should be present at the time of extubation. The patient will need to be monitored closely after ventilator withdrawal regardless of which mode of removal is utilized.
   - Neuromuscular blockade should be stopped prior to removal of the ventilator and return of neuromuscular function should be achieved.
   - Medication for dyspnea and anxiety need to be drawn up and ready for immediate bedside administration.
   - Bedside alarms should be turned off or minimally silenced. Families tend to be distracted by monitors, waiting for the moment of cardiac arrest. Monitors and alarms can also be a barrier to meaningful interaction with the patient.
   - Families should be asked about special rituals and customs and the presence of chaplain or clergy. Families also should be helped with arrangements and accommodations.

TABLE 26.1: WITHDRAWING VENTILATOR SUPPORT[10,11]

Immediate Extubation	Terminal Wean
Technique	**Technique**
Removing ETT abruptly after suctioning Humidified air or oxygen (O2) is applied to maintain lip, mouth and throat moisture	Ventilatory support is gradually reduced over time to mimic room air prior to extubation Fio2, respiratory rate, mode and positive end expiratory pressures (peep) are reduced in a step-wise approach Humidified air or O2 is applied to maintain lip, mouth and throat moisture
Advantages	**Advantages**
Swift removal of patient from unnecessary machinery and technology Intentions of action clear—remove artificial life support to allow death	Allows for anticipation of and treatment of symptoms Artificial airway may be left in place to facilitate removal of secretions Allows family to separate removal of artificial life support and death, thereby reducing perception of cause and effect
Disadvantages	**Disadvantages**
Patient may experience preventable symptoms (tachypnea, dyspnea, death rattle). Increased distress to family	Possibly prolonged death, which may be distressing to family

APPENDIX 2

Symptom Management During Withdrawal of Mechanical Ventilation[12]

There are several medications available to decrease or eliminate distressing symptoms during withdrawal of MV (Table 26.2):

Shortness of Breath
- Opioids may be utilized to quell the sensation of air hunger.
- Starting dose can vary from morphine sulfate 5 mg IV (or equivalent) upward depending on patient size, opioid tolerance and level of distress.
- Dose can be given every 10 minutes and increased by as much as 100% with each dose, if the symptom persists.
- An opioid infusion may be necessary to ensure patient comfort.
- The literature does not support the use of nebulized opioids; this treatment is not likely to reduce respiratory symptoms.

Anxiety-related Respiratory Distress
- A benzodiazepine infusion may be necessary, but often around-the-clock dosing is sufficient.
- It is important to be clear with families that these medications are given to prevent or treat signs or symptoms of respiratory distress or pain. The intent is not to hasten death or suppress respirations.

Oropharyngeal Secretions (Death Rattle)
- Pooling of oropharyngeal secretions at the end of life causes rattling during the respiratory cycle commonly referred to as "death rattle."
- Although "rattling" effect is not thought to be uncomfortable to the patient, it can be very distressing to family members.
- Repositioning of the patient is the most useful tool to manage secretions that have already accumulated.
- Anticholenergic medications such as glycopyrrolate, scopolamine, or atropine can be used to arrest the production of these secretions.
- Suctioning can be used if the secretions appear to be in the mouth or throat.
- Deep tracheal suction should be minimized, unless an artificial airway is in place.
- Nasotracheal suctioning should be avoided as it can be painful.

TABLE 26.2: WITHDRAWAL OF MV: SYMPTOM MANAGEMENT

Symptom	Goal/Purpose of Management	Medication/Intervention
Tachypnea/SOB	Quell sensation of air hunger	Opioids
Anxiety-related respiratory distress	Prevent/treat shortness of breath	Benzodiazepine
Pooling of oropharyngeal secretions ("death rattle")	Most likely not uncomfortable to patient, but helps to relieve family distress	Anticholenergics, e.g., glycopyrrolate, scopolamine, atropine Repositioning patient Suctioning of mouth and throat Avoid deep or nasotracheal suction; if it becomes necessary, use nasal trumpet to minimize nasophryngeal trauma
Airway constriction (wheezing)	Alleviate symptoms	Bronchodilators

APPENDIX 3

Management Considerations for Continuing Ventilator Support

CARE SETTING

- After treatment for chronic critical illness, patients maintained on prolonged ventilator support are eventually transitioned out of the ICU onto medical units and then, if they are stable, typically discharged to a long-term care facility where their complex care needs can be addressed.
- For stable patients with neurological deficits, care at home may be possible, but a number of logistical and clinical issues must be considered before a discharge to home is attempted. The expense of this care is significant and financial resources must be a factor in care planning.
- Competent and highly motivated family members can be trained to provide ventilator care in the home, but this commitment is not to be taken lightly. Care of a ventilator-dependent patient is time intensive, requires an advanced level of problem-solving ability and technical support, and is mentally and physically taxing for families. These caregiving issues are likely to contribute significantly to caregiver burden, and this possibility should be included in the discussions to identify the goals of prolonged ventilator use.

CARE TRANSITION AND COORDINATION

- A written discharge plan should include provider contact information, responsibilities of patients and caregivers for daily care, itemized list of all required equipment, resources in the community for health, social needs, and contingency plans for emergency situations.[13] (See Chapter 11: Care Transitions.)
- Community-based agencies offer assistance with care coordination for ventilator-dependent patients at home. Licensed Respiratory Care Practitioners provide pre-discharge evaluation, caregiver training and education, home safety assessment, home equipment, and regularly scheduled follow-up assessment.

CAREGIVING ISSUES

Before a ventilator-assisted individual is discharged from the hospital to home, the patient and all caregivers must be trained in aspects of long-term mechanical ventilation and should demonstrate to the health care team that they have learned to carry out appropriate care techniques, including:

- Frequent assessment to assure safety and comfort
- Sedation to control anxiety or agitation, if necessary
- Assistance with (or complete performance) of ADLs such as bathing, toileting, dressing, and possibly eating
- Attention to nutritional needs: options include percutaneous gastrostomy tube (PEG), nasogastric (NG) tube, or careful oral feeding with close monitoring for aspiration.
- Routine assessment of ventilation:
  - Endotracheal tube (ETT) is a temporary measure and should be checked for proper positioning.
  - Tracheostomy tubes require cleaning two to three times daily.
  - Suctioning may be needed multiple times per day.

EQUIPMENT AND SUPPLIES[13]

- Equipment and supplies that must be on hand include power sources, ventilator circuits, humidifiers, oxygen as needed and for emergencies, suctioning machine and supplies, and alarms to signal vent malfunction, air pressure problems, power failure, and need for patient assistance.
- The firm that supplies mechanical ventilation equipment should offer 24-hour emergency repair and maintenance service, and must have an equipment inventory adequate to service equipment failure.

27

Artificial Nutrition and Hydration

INTRODUCTION

Artificial nutrition and hydration (ANH), also referred to as nutritional support, is medical treatment given to persons who are unable to eat or drink enough to sustain life. The historical purpose of ANH was to serve as a "bridge" to recovery during a critical illness. ANH is delivered as a solution consisting of a medically balanced mix of nutrients and fluids administered through a nasogastric or gastrostomy tube, or intravenously. There are two types of nutritional support:

1. **Enteral** (tube feeding): A special liquid food mixture is given through a tube into the stomach or small bowel. A nasogastric tube is placed through the nose into the stomach or bowel, or a tube is surgically inserted through the skin into the stomach or the bowel (gastrostomy or jejunostomy).
2. **Parenteral**: Nutritional support is provided through a large vein in the chest or the arm, bypassing digestion in the stomach or bowel. This method should be used only when enteral route is not an option.

GOALS OF THERAPY

Malnutrition, defined as the imbalance between food intake and requirements, is a common problem in patients with chronic or severe illness.[1] Patients and families of malnourished patients hope that ANH will prolong life, improve quality of life, improve energy level, and decrease morbidity. They often expect that proper nourishment will lead to weight gain, improved strength, and a return to the patient's previous functional state.

POTENTIAL COMPLICATIONS

While there is considerable debate over the value of ANH in various clinical situations, it is clear that parental/enteral nutrition is not risk-free. Numerous complications have been described, including sepsis, catheter occlusion, and catheter dislocation. Gastrostomy tubes are associated with leakage, aspiration, cellulitis, infections, and morbidity arising from patient transfer to hospitals for treatment of complications. Complication rates as high as 17% and procedure-related mortality of 0.5% have been reported.[2]

THE ROLE OF ANH IN SERIOUS ILLNESS

- To date, randomized controlled trials have not convincingly demonstrated that artificial nutrition has a beneficial impact on clinical outcomes. While some data suggest that ANH may be helpful for selected cancer patients,[3, 4] the use of ANH in other situations shows no benefit.[5] It has also been established that, despite widespread belief to the contrary on the part of clinicians, tube feeding does not decrease incidence of aspiration pneumonias in demented patients.[6,7] (See Chapter 77: Feeding Tube Management.)
- Despite lack of evidence showing benefit, ANH is nevertheless routinely offered to patients with serious disease. In practice, the decision to institute nutritional support is usually based on factors other than evidence-based considerations. These contributing factors include social and cultural norms, religious beliefs, moral values, economic considerations, patient and family preferences, and lack of provider training or opportunity for timely discussion and counseling with the patient and family caregivers.
- Choice of care setting may also have a significant impact on whether or not nutritional support is implemented. For example, a nursing home may not be equipped to care for a patient receiving parenteral nutrition (TPN) or who requires time-consuming hand-feeding. Most long-term care facilities will accept dysphagic patients without feeding tubes

only if there are clear advance directives in place. If the patient is at home, a family caregiver must be available to assist with nutritional support if self-care is not feasible. The lack of a caregiver to support ANH may necessitate a change in care setting.

MAKING THE DECISION ABOUT ANH

Given the complex issues underlying the choice to use enteral or parenteral feeding, making the decision about initiating nutritional support is a challenging process. As outlined above, discussions about ANH should be based on medical evidence, while also considering the hopes and wishes of the patient or surrogate decision-maker. The process described below will help clinicians, patients, and families to make an appropriate decision and will assure that the plan of care is implemented and honored.

1. **Gather the facts**: A clinician must gather clinical and psychosocial information from several important sources. In addition to available evidence and disease-specific practice guidelines, the following considerations must be weighed:
   - Prognosis of the underlying disease processes
   - Route available (oral, enteral/tube, parenteral/IV)
   - Functional and cognitive status (Is patient bed- or chair-bound? If delirious, will patient pull out tube or IV?)
   - Resources (Are there sufficient financial resources, e.g., are copays affordable? Is a caretaker available and trained to support ANH?)
   - Family and patient preference (Religious beliefs, cultural traditions, goals and values, and prior experience of family with ANH must be considered.)
2. **Determine patient/family preferences**: In order to elicit patient and family preferences, the issues must be identified and explored together by patients and families and the involved clinician(s), ideally during one or more family meetings. Important issues to explore when counseling patients and families about ANH, with suggested language for exploring some of the topics, include:[8]

- What are patient and family hopes and goals for ANH? Are they the same/ different? Are these goals achievable? (*"What are you hoping we can accomplish with a feeding tube?"*)
- How can unachievable goals be reframed to ones that are more realistic? (*"I wish that were possible. It sounds like all of us would be happier if that were so."*)
- Identifying and understanding the cultural, social, and personal factors that underlie the reasons for or against ANH (*"Tell me more about that...."*)
- How can the evidence (or lack of it) help to facilitate the conversation?
- Explore concerns, spoken or unspoken, about withholding/withdrawing ANH. For example, families are often concerned that they may be starving their loved to death. (*"What is the hardest part?"* or *"As you look to the future, what is your biggest worry?"*)
- Explain the loss of appetite or refusal to eat that accompanies serious illness as a normal part of the disease progression. Patients are rarely hungry.
- Respond to the emotions around the decision regarding ANH as family members identify the meaning of food and feeding as a measure of caring for a loved one.
- Review the consequences of tube feeding (risks, adverse events), the fact that underlying disease(s) will continue to progress, and that ANH may lead to complications that may hasten death or lengthen a difficult dying process.
- Describe to the family the expected clinical course without nutritional support, and explain comfort measures that will be employed. (See also: Chapter 6: Ethical Decision-Making, Chapter 8: Advance Care Planning, Chapter 9: Communication Skills, and Chapter 10: Managing Conflict.)
3. **Conduct a benefit vs. burden analysis**: After the clinical and psychosocial facts have been gathered and the patient/family wishes have been determined, a benefit/burden analysis should be conducted in order to reach an informed decision regarding ANH (Table 27.1). This analysis should include

TABLE 27.1: BENEFITS VS. BURDENS OF ANH TREATMENT OPTIONS

Treatment Option	Benefit	Burden
Artificial nutrition and hydration	May prolong life Patient gets more nutrition Patient may improve enough to be able to eat again Caregiver reassurance that patient is "not starving"	Risk of infection Enteral-discomfort from enteral food bolus Parenteral-fluid overload Morbidity associated with hospitalizations for treatment-related side effects Requires active family involvement to achieve the treatment plan Patient may become agitated because of tube/line May limit where patient can receive care
Forego artificial nutrition and hydration	May allow improved quality of life Increases the options for settings of care Treatment is aligned with patient goals, interventions Hand-feeding may be possible	Providing food is a social activity and a universal symbol of caregiving; may be difficult to forego for emotional, cultural, religious reasons. Families may be disturbed by a perception that patient is "starving."
Time-limited trial of artificial nutrition and hydration	Temporary nutritional support may facilitate healing Allows an opportunity to see if patient's condition will improve Requires advance agreement about hoped-for milestones and decision to stop treatment if it is not meeting agreed-upon goals	See risks and burdens of ANH above

the points of view of patient, family, and in some situations the clinician provider(s). The process should be one of negotiation, consensus-building and shared decision-making, with the final decision made by the patient/family after receiving provider guidance and input.

4. **Document and communicate the decisions concerning ANH**: It is essential to document the decisions that have been made about ANH and then to take steps to ensure that this information is communicated across all care settings so that goals for care remain clearly established and decision-makers are supported.

FREQUENTLY ASKED QUESTIONS ABOUT ANH[9]

1. **Will artificial nutrition and hydration (ANH) increase the patient's chance of survival?** There are no randomized trials comparing patients with and without feeding tubes to determine who lives longer. Therefore there is no definite answer to this question.

2. **Once started, can ANH be discontinued?** Yes, a feeding tube can be removed at any time. Reasons for discontinuing tube feeding may include:
   - Patient may have improved and can now eat normally.
   - Patient may not have improved as expected and the feeding tube may no longer be in patient's best interest.
   - Often a decision to discontinue is made after a time-limited trial of ANH, i.e., after clinicians and patient/family have agreed to a defined period of nutritional support to see if there is improvement or deterioration based upon agreed-upon clinical outcomes.

3. **Will the withdrawal of ANH lead to a long and painful death?** No. For patients

who are approaching the end of life, death normally occurs in weeks or months, depending on continued oral intake and amount of edema and third-space fluid in the body. For patients who are unconscious, the process is quite peaceful. Caregivers of conscious patients, and the patients themselves, report that those who are near death are seldom hungry. The most common complaint is dry mouth, which can be alleviated with ice chips, lubricants for the lips, and other appropriate oral care.[10]

4. **Does avoiding ANH contribute to a more comfortable death?** Yes. Hospice workers and others who care for the dying report that patients who are not tube-fed seem more comfortable. When ANH is discontinued, caregivers frequently note that symptoms of abdominal discomfort, nausea, vomiting, incontinence, and shortness of breath are decreased.[10]

TAKE-HOME POINTS

- Artificial nutrition and hydration (ANH) is medical treatment given to persons who are unable to eat or drink enough to sustain life.
- ANH is not a risk-free intervention. Complications include sepsis, catheter occlusion, and catheter dislocation.
- Randomized controlled trials have not convincingly demonstrated that artificial nutrition has a beneficial impact on clinical outcomes for seriously ill patients.
- Despite lack of supporting evidence, ANH is nevertheless routinely offered to patients with serious disease. Factors that contribute to the decision to institute nutritional support include social and cultural norms, religious beliefs, moral values, economic considerations, and patient and family preferences.
- Decisions about ANH should be based on a careful benefit/burden analysis of many

relevant factors, including prognosis, achievable goals of care, choice of care setting, social and cultural norms, religious beliefs, economic considerations, and patient and family preferences.

REFERENCES

1. Norman K, Pichard C, Lochs H, Pirlich M. Prognostic impact of disease-related malnutrition. *Clin Nutr.* 2008;*27*:5–15.
2. Potack JZ, Chokhavatia S. Complications and controversies associated with percutaneous endoscopic gastrostomy: report of a case and literature review. *Medscape J Med.* 2008;*10*(6):142.
3. Bachmann P et al. Practice guideline. Summary version of the Standards, Options and Recommendations for palliative or terminal nutrition in adults with progressive cancer (2001). *BJC.* 2003;*89*(suppl 1): S107–S110.
4. Mirhosseini N et al. Parenteral Nutrition in Advanced Cancer: Indications and Clinical Practice Guidelines. *J Palliate Med.* 2005;*8*(5): 914–918.
5. Koretz R. Do data support nutrition support? Part II. Enteral artificial nutrition. *J Am Diet Assoc.* 2007;*107*:1374–1380.
6. Gillick M. Rethinking the role of tube feeding in patients with advanced dementia. *N Engl J Med.* 2000;*342*:206–210.
7. Finucane TE, Christmas C, Travis K. Tube feeding in patients with advanced dementia: a review of the evidence: *JAMA.* 1999;*282*(14):1365–1370.
8. Quill T. "I wish things were different": expressing wishes in response to loss, futility and unrealistic hopes. *Ann Intern Med.* 2001;*135*:551–555.
9. Making Choices: Long term feeding tube placement in elderly patients. 2008 http://decision-aid.ohri.ca/docs/Tube_Feeding_DA/PDF/TubeFeeding.pdf. Accessed December 4, 2011.
10. Artificial Nutrition and Hydration and End of Life Decision-making. 2009. Pamphlet#QA200; Partnership for Caring at http://www.partnershipforcaring.org. Accessed December 4, 2011.

SECTION III

Caregivers

28

Caregivers

INTRODUCTION

For the geriatric patient living with severe or life-threatening illness, it is usually the caregiver who is the primary contact for the health care provider, and also the decision-maker for the patient.

A survey by the National Alliance for Caregiving and AARP in 2004 found that 21% of people over 18 in the United States were caregivers, representing 44.4 million people. Many of these caregivers may be "sandwiched" between the needs of their own children and the needs of aging parents. Or the caregiver can be an elderly spouse or a relative who may be only marginally healthier or more able to cope than the patient. This person might also be a neighbor or close friend, or in some cases a paid caretaker.

UNDERSTANDING THE ROLE OF THE CAREGIVER

- When an 80-year-old patient with heart failure is admitted to the hospital for the third time in one month, there may be a need to adjust his medical regimen, but it is just as likely that there is a problem with the caregiving arrangement. The caregiver is an integral and essential component of the care plan. More than any single medication prescribed, caregivers help to keep the patient healthy and out of the hospital or nursing home. It can be helpful to think of the caregiver as an additional organ system, just as crucial to the patient's well-being as any other. If the caregiving system fails, it will put the patient's health at risk.
- It is the clinician's role to understand the caregiver, just as he would be knowledgeable about the medications or treatments that he prescribes. While many practice settings will have the support of social workers, it is critical for all clinicians to have some understanding of what benefits and resources are available to support caregivers, and how caregivers

can find and access these resources in the community.
- Medical professionals receive training about the many needs their patients have: medical, social, emotional, and spiritual. But physicians and nurses are less likely to have training about the specific needs of those who care for the patient between medical visits: their caregivers.
- This chapter is designed to help health care providers to assess the caregivers of older patients and their needs. What is their relationship to the patient? How is their relationship with the rest of the patient's family? What are their capabilities? And, most importantly, are they healthy enough (mentally and physically) to care for this person?

CAREGIVER BURDEN

- Caregivers often report their confusion and frustration when dealing with the medical community and health professionals. They cite a lack of communication, caring, and availability as major areas that need improvement. Being a caregiver has also been shown to increase health problems and even mortality. Caregivers providing more than nine hours a week of care have a greater risk of myocardial infarction (MI) and cardiac death, and those reporting emotional strain as a result of caregiving experience increased mortality. Caregivers also have higher rates of depression, which often goes undiagnosed.
- Unfortunately, caregivers may not tell involved health care providers that they are overwhelmed. In fact, caregivers may not even realize how stressed they are. In some cases, the primary care physician or geriatrician may be the only person in caregivers' lives who will recognize their need for additional support and point them in a direction to get help.

IMPROVING CAREGIVER-PROVIDER COMMUNICATION

- Many difficulties that arise for caregivers can be traced back to poor communication. Whether the patient is at home, in rehab, or in the hospital, inadequate communication with the caregiver will cause medical errors, complications, and avoidable stress for everyone.
- Poor communication can also result in complications for the patient, from receiving the wrong medication to lack of proper follow-up, to delayed discharge or hospital readmission (which itself can cause many additional complications).
- When caregivers are polled about what improvements could be made in the health care system, better communication with their doctors is always high on the list. The checklist below, based on the acronym C-A-S-E, will help clinicians to think systematically about what caregivers need, how to communicate with them effectively, and how best to support them.
  C—Communicate
  A—Assess
  S—Support
  E—Educate

C—Communicate

1. **Clarify the goals of the care plan.**
   - Prepare caregivers for the future. Take a few moments to give caregivers a sense of what the natural course of a chronic illness will be. This is particularly crucial in the case of dementia. (See Chapter 67: Dementia.)
   - Write down any changes made, new medications, tests ordered, as well as follow-up instructions.
   - For an inpatient, explain in layman's terms what needs to be done and what to expect for the next 24 to 48 hours.
   - Make sure the caregiver knows who to call at all times (especially after hours) with concerns or questions, so that the default plan is not the emergency department.
   - To assure that the caregiver has understood what has been said, have him or her repeat it back, and encourage questions. Repetition is key. When stressed, a caregiver may need to hear things more than once to assimilate information.
   - Understand patient/family preferences so that the goals of care and the plan are clear and consistent for all parties.

2. **Explain the care team.**
   - For outpatients, give caregivers a list of team members, what role they play in patient care, and how best to reach them.
   - For inpatients, the involvement of hospitalists and consultants with whom most patients will have no prior relationship can cause fear and mistrust. To combat this, a clinician should introduce him- or herself (and any learners present) and explain his or her role in the patient's care. The primary care physician should make sure that the caregiver knows who the admitting attending will be, and that the primary care physician will be in touch with these physicians.

3. **Clarify how team members can be reached** and who should be contacted in which circumstances (i.e., for lab results, refills, questions/updates about treatment etc.).

A—Assessment

1. **Ask about the caregiver or caregivers** (whether they are present or not) during the review of systems or social history.
   - Make a point of asking caregivers how they are doing, what help they are getting, and how their own health is. Sometimes one glimpse at the caregiver will indicate that he or she is not coping well, but many are stoic and say nothing until they are depressed and overwrought. Caregivers can be so focused on the health of another that they neglect themselves.
   - If the caregiver seems sad or depressed, ask "Are you depressed?" It may be surprising how honest people will be. Be sure to have some names on hand for referral if the caregiver does express a need for help, or refer the caregiver back to his or her own primary care physician for evaluation and referral. (See Chapter 64: Depression.)
   - Ask an open-ended question about the caregiver's understanding of the

patient's current state of health. If the caregiver's view seems completely at odds with reality, this person will likely need more support as the patient's illness/condition progresses.

2. **Explore the home situation**.
   - Can the patient still perform any IADL/ADLs, and if not, who assists him or her? What additional help is needed to make this situation workable and safe now? (This is particularly crucial when the caregiver is also elderly.) (See Chapter 24: Assistive Aids and Devices.)
   - What additional help will be needed in the next six months, and how will this be achieved? It is always better to help the caregiver anticipate needs in advance rather than to respond to crises.
   - What are the finances of the patient/caregiver, and what services can be provided by Medicare, Medicaid, or their private insurance? Exploring these questions before an acute need arises is always better. An early referral to a social worker, hospital benefits office, or eldercare attorney can save time, money, and grief later on and can expedite transfer to the next level of care. (See Chapter 13: Health Insurance.)

3. **What is the plan if the caregiver should become or be hospitalized?**
   - Are there family or friends who could be relied on to take over in an emergency? Is there a plan to hire a private caregiver, perhaps through a licensed nursing agency? Note that respite programs normally cannot accommodate emergency/unplanned admissions. Long-term care facilities and assisted living facilities are among those that can manage a planned respite. For an enrolled hospice patient, respite care may be an option.
   - If there is no safe way to keep someone in the community, what are the long-term care (LTC) options? If the patient needs LTC and does not already have Medicaid or long-term care insurance, the patient should be referred to a social worker and/or elder care attorney. Let the caregiver know that long-term care is sometimes the right answer and best for the patient

because of the availability of medical and nursing care in these settings. It does not mean the caregiver has failed.

4. **Does the patient qualify for hospice?**
   - Even if the caregiver (and/or patient) do not want hospice, they may reconsider if they understand the additional benefits it provides. (See Chapter 12: The Hospice Model of Palliative Care.) For example, enrolling in hospice (when the patient qualifies) is the only way to get ongoing nursing visits and some supportive care (home aides) through Medicare.
   - Hospice can be an excellent way for a caregiver to feel supported and connected to a community. Enrolling in hospice can also avoid unnecessary (and unwanted) hospitalizations because resources are available 24/7 to address questions and concern or a change in the patient's condition. If indicated, inpatient care is available as well. Hospice can provide short respite for the caregiver by bringing the patient to an inpatient unit for a few days.
   - Studies suggest that hospice actually improves survival for some patients, as well as reducing caregiver distress and reducing the risk of complicated bereavement.

S—Support

1. **Validate the caregiver's work and experience**.
   - Having a medical professional ask about and acknowledge the challenging job of caregiving can be very empowering. In many cases, one caregiver shoulders most of the burden of caregiving—in most cases a daughter. Ask what other family is available and how they might be asked to help.
   - Remind the caregiver that it is sometimes not possible to convince loved ones to do what we think is best for them. Unless the courts declare the patient incompetent, the caregiver is dealing with an autonomous adult, who may choose to make bad (or even dangerous) decisions.

2. **Empathize with the caregiver**.
   - Caregiving brings up all kinds of emotions, and the health care provider

may be one of the few outlets the caregiver has. Listening intently and mirroring back what is said ("I hear that you are frustrated, angry, sad, overwhelmed," etc.) can help make the caregiver feel understood. Keep in mind not to take it personally when the caregiver expresses anger.

- The child-caregiver is often someone who feels good when caring for others, but may do so even to his or her own detriment. Encourage caregivers to accept help from others. (A number of community resources can be contacted easily online to solicit help where needed. Two of these resources are www.carecircle.com and www. caringbridge.org.)

3. **Refer the caregiver to a support group.**
   - Many hospitals or community centers have support groups.
   - Other resources include www. wellspouse.com and www. caps4caregivers.org.

4. **See other chapters in this volume**
   - Chapters that may offer helpful insights on supporting the caregiver include: Chapter 4: Special Issues in Caregiving, Chapter 9: Communication Skills, and Chapter 10: Managing Conflict.

E—Educate

1. **Encourage caregivers to explore resources.** There are many places for caregivers to turn for help. Some caregivers already know what benefits and resources their loved ones are entitled to; others will need help understanding how and where to begin. (Just searching "caregiver" on Google will produce an exhaustive list of options, which can be overwhelming to many caregivers.)

2. The following websites and publications will help caregivers get started and find additional help in their local area:

Government Sites

1. www.eldercare.gov—Nationwide eldercare locator links by zip code to state and local agencies (U.S. Administration on Aging)
2. www.medicare.gov—General information on Medicare
3. www.medicare.gov/caregivers

National Not-for-Profit Sites

1. www.alz.org—Alzheimer's association website
2. www.uja.org—United Jewish Association: allows search for community resources by zip code
3. www.unitedway.org/programs—United Way provides community resources by zip code.
4. http://www.aarp.org/families/legal_issues—Legal services at reduced fees for AARP members

Sites for Advance Directives

1. www.caringinfo.org—National Hospice and Palliative Care Organization website for caregivers: well organized information for caregivers; living will/health care proxy for all states
2. www.agingwithdignity.org/5wishes.html—Five Wishes form will help to think through preferences for end-of-life care.

Sites for Caregivers

1. www.caregiver.org—National Family Caregiver Alliance: thorough, well-designed site with information, resources, and advice for caregivers
2. www.nfcacares.org—National Family Caregivers Association: information and resources for caregivers
3. www.caremanager.org—To find geriatric care managers in all states
4. http://www.ama-assn.org/ama1/pub/upload/mm/433/caregiver_english.pdf—Caregiver self-assessment questionnaire: enables caregivers to assess their level of stress
5. www.benefitscheckup.org—Site designed to help individuals determine what benefits can be claimed for patient or caregiver.

Resources for Better Communication with Health Care Professionals

1. National Transitions of Care Coalition (NTOCC): *Taking Care of My Health Care:* A guide for patients and their family caregivers to use so they can be better prepared when they see a health care professional and can ask the right kind of questions to elicit the information they need. http://www.ntocc.com/

Portals/0/Taking_Care_Of_My_Health_Care.pdf

2. NTOCC's *Guidelines for a Hospital Stay*: This brochure helps guide the patient, family, and caregiver on how to obtain safe and successful health care at the hospital. http://www.ntocc.com/Portals/0/Hospital_Guide.pdf

3. *Transitions Toolkit* by Consumers Advancing Patient Safety (CAPS): This toolkit provides patients with the tools and information they need to make a smooth transition from the hospital to their next destination. http://www.patientsafety.org/page/transtoolkit

4. *Tools for Family Caregivers*: The National Family Caregivers Association has developed a number of tools and educational materials ranging from national educational campaigns to Tips and Tools for family caregivers. http://www.thefamilycaregiver.org/caregiving_resources

Recommended Reading for Caregivers

Uncertain Inheritance: Writers on Caring for Family, edited by Nell Casey. HarperCollins, NY 2007.

My Mother, Your Mother: Embracing "Slow Medicine," the Compassionate Approach to Caring for Your Aging Loved Ones, by Dennis McCullough, MD. HarperCollins, NY 2009.

How to Care for Aging Parents, by Virginia Morris. Workman Publishing, NY 1996.

Eldercare for Dummies, by Rachelle Zukerman, PhD. Wiley Publishing, NY 2003.

Doing the Right Thing: Taking care of your elderly parents even if they didn't take care of you, by Roberta Satow, PhD. Penguin Group, NY 2005.

Learning to Speak Alzheimer's, by Joanne Koenig Cost. Houghton Mifflin, NY 2004.

A Dignified Life," by Virginia Bell. Health Professions Press, Baltimore, MD 2002.

The Caregiver's Survival Handbook: How to care for your aging parent without losing yourself, by Alexis Abramson with Mary Anne Dunkin. The Berkley Publishing Group, NY 2004.

The Eldercare Handbook: Difficult Choices, Compassionate Solutions, by Stella Mora Henry, R.N., with Ann Convery. Harper Paperbacks, NY 2006.

SPECIAL CAREGIVER SITUATIONS

The Frail or Very Elderly Caregiver

One of the side effects of increased life expectancy is the old caring for the *very* old. This may mean a frail spouse caring for a husband or wife who is even more disabled—or an elderly child caring for a parent who has reached the 90s or even 100 years. Figuring out how to support these caregivers can present additional challenges. Table 28.2 lists some of the relevant considerations.

The "Difficult" Caregiver

All health professionals have encountered caregivers who can be a challenge to deal with. Interactions with them may feel overwhelming, especially if there is a perception that they complicate or interfere with offering the best care to their loved one.

Consider the following example:

Mrs. G. is an 80-year-old woman with stage III colon cancer and COPD. She underwent surgery and chemotherapy when her cancer was diagnosed six months ago. Since the chemotherapy, her energy has not been good and she is mainly homebound. Before this diagnosis, she had lived alone in her own home and was able to drive. She now depends on her daughter for all of her IADLS but is independent for most of her ADLs. She has hired an aide a few hours a day to help with bathing and cooking, which is rapidly diminishing her small savings.

She is admitted with a COPD flare. The palliative care service is called because, although the patient has clear Do Not Resuscitate and Do Not Intubate orders in place, the daughter is insisting that the patient be intubated. The patient is on BiPAP due to a rising CO_2 level and is becoming more somnolent. She is also taking off the mask due to delirium. The daughter exclaims, "This is a hospital—you are supposed to cure people—not let them die!" The clinical staff is frustrated. They want to respect the wishes of the patient, and they feel the daughter is being selfish and unreasonable.

When a caregiver is upset, it can be helpful to explore potentially relevant (but frequently unexpressed) emotional and family issues by asking open-ended questions, such as:

TABLE 28.1: C-A-S-E CHART

Tool	What to Do
Communication	Clarify care plan Discuss prognosis and disease progression Write down changes in meds, tests, what to expect, etc. Have caregiver repeat back instructions Clarify team structure and contact mechanism, particularly for unfamiliar roles such as hospitalist
Assessment	Take note of caregiver appearance Does caregiver seem sad or depressed? Overwhelmed? Familiarize yourself with home situation. Who assists with ADL/IADL? What additional help is needed to make this situation workable and safe now? Is the caregiver frail or with chronic health issues? What resources are available for emotional/financial support? What gaps or deficiencies may impinge on the care plan? What will happen if caregiver is not available? Is there backup? Would hospice be available to provide additional support? Is the caregiver realistic about prognosis? Will caregiver need bereavement support?
Support	Acknowledge the difficult job the caregiver is doing Reinforce that there is no way to do things perfectly Reassure caregiver that needing help does not mean he/she has failed Encourage advocacy for patient Explore available benefits and financial resources Encourage creation of advance directives (or implementation of directives already in place) Refer to support groups or private therapy when needed Refer to primary care physician if concerned about caregiver mental/physical health Listen to feelings expressed and mirror back so caregiver feels heard
Education	Provide disease-specific information Refer to community resources Refer to useful websites for caregiver information, benefits, support groups, etc. Recommend books

- How have things been going for you?
- What's hard about the situation?
- Tell me a little bit about your family.
- What are you hoping we can accomplish for your loved one?

During further discussions with Mrs. G's daughter, the clinical staff is able to understand that the anger she is expressing is really misplaced (i.e., transference), and that the decisions she is making are motivated by the very strong emotions she is experiencing:

- *Anger with her mother for choosing to pursue the chemotherapy that the daughter had been against, which she sees as the reason for this rapid decline*

- *Anger with her mother's doctors for not predicting how functionally dependent her mother would become*
- *Frustration at not being able to prevent her mother's suffering*
- *Fear that her mother is so sick and she cannot do anything to cure her*
- *Guilt for sometimes thinking it would be better if her mother died before she has to move from her home*

After meeting with the palliative care team, who helped her explore and start to come to terms with some of these feelings, the daughter was reassured that her mother was getting good care. She also began to understand and appreciate how much the staff was

TABLE 28.2: SUPPORTING THE ELDERLY OR FRAIL CAREGIVER

Consideration	Possible Intervention
Home situation unsafe but caregiver refuses help	Enlist family See if the caregiver needs medical or psychiatric evaluation If safe, start slowly and gradually introduce home care services and/or increase the hours of care Consult social worker, hospital lawyer or local Adult Protective Services about next steps to ensure patient safety and possible guardianship
Caregiver is hospitalized	Are there family or friends to step in? Can they afford short-term paid care in the home? Can they qualify for sub-acute rehab? Patient may need hospitalization for safety
Caregiver relies on income from patient, but patient needs long-term care	Enlist social work or benefits office to see if patient or caregiver qualifies for additional benefits
Caregiver unwilling to be separated from patient who needs long-term care	Could caregiver and patient remain home with additional help? Could caregiver and patient go to long-term care together? Could caregiver and patient move in with family?
Caregiver is neglectful	Try to figure out whether there is neglect—and why. Is the caregiver overwhelmed, physically or mentally impaired, etc? If neglect is malicious or cannot be corrected, follow specific state and institutional protocols and laws regarding reporting elder abuse and neglect.

helping her mother and honoring her wishes regarding treatment.

TAKE-HOME POINTS FOR DEALING WITH "DIFFICULT CARETAKERS"

Caregiving can trigger strong emotions. It is the nature of all human relationships that we experience a range of emotions when interacting with one another, particularly those closest to us. Caring for another human being during a period of serious illness and disability is apt to magnify these feelings.

1. Emotional issues faced by caregivers may cause difficulty and even be disruptive for the involved health care providers. Some of the feelings that caregivers report are:

Guilt:
- For not being able to save the person
- For not having spent more time with the person
- For not wanting to be caregiver in the first place
- From feeling inadequate for the job
- For being resentful of the person and their needs
- From not being able to protect a parent (or loved one) from making choices that leave them in danger

Anger:
- For being robbed of time and opportunity for closure
- Because of perceived problems with medical care
- For the role reversal—having to care for someone who can now no longer care for them (for child/caregivers)
- At losing the parental figure/spouse before the person is physically gone
- For having to care for someone who was never a good parent to them

Sadness/Depression:
- Due to feeling alone and isolated (particularly problematic when patients require 24-hour care and there is no one else to care for them)

- Because there is no one to speak with about it and no one understands
- As a result of overwhelming needs of the patient
- Caused by feelings of inadequacy or inability to do the job as well as they would like

2. The appropriate use of open-ended questions can be very helpful for exploration of complicated caregiver feelings and emotions. The answers to these questions often reveal previously unidentified issues and may suggest potential solutions.

SECTION 4 ————————————

Symptoms

29

Management of Pain in Older Adults

CASE
Mr. C is an active 84-year-old man with a history of prostate cancer and atrial fibrillation who lifts weights in a gym several times a week. He presents to the emergency department with low back pain that began suddenly three days ago. He says it is severe (10/10), sharp, worse with movement, and improves with rest. It does not radiate and is not associated with any numbness or tingling. He reports no change in his ability to urinate or have bowel movements. He has no motor weakness, but the severity of the pain has immobilized him.

DEFINITION
Pain is a subjective experience with both sensory and emotional aspects. Acute pain ceases after the injury that caused it has healed. Chronic pain persists longer than expected (or, somewhat arbitrarily, beyond three months).

PREVALENCE
The annual prevalence in older adults of any pain is 70% to 85%. Chronic or persistent pain is 20% to 50%.

CONSEQUENCES OF UNTREATED PAIN
- Only 66% to 80% of older adults with pain seek health care for their symptoms. Many of those who do seek care are undertreated.[1]
- Inadequate pain management puts older adults at risk for the complications shown in Table 29.1 below.

LIKELY ETIOLOGIES
There are several important pain etiologies, each of which is treated somewhat differently. Older adults may experience pain in any of the following categories:

Nociceptive Pain:
- Caused by a painful stimulus transmitted along normally functioning nerve fibers from the peripheral nervous system to the central nervous system. Two main subtypes of nociceptive pain are:

- **Somatic pain (musculoskeletal)** is transmitted by peripheral nociceptors. Well-localized; often constant; described as "sharp," "throbbing," or "aching." Examples include osteoarthritis, fracture, bruise, skeletal muscle spasm.
- **Visceral pain** arises from the abdominal or thoracic viscera. It is poorly localized; often episodic; described as "deep," "cramping," or "aching." Examples include renal colic, bowel obstruction, cardiac ischemia, pancreatitis.

Neuropathic Pain:
- Pain originating from injury or disease in the peripheral or central nervous system.
- Can be constant or episodic; often described as "burning," "shooting," "electric shocks." Examples include diabetic or alcoholic peripheral neuropathy, sciatica, post-stroke pain, and chemotherapy-induced peripheral neuropathy.

LOCATION
The four most frequently reported sites of pain in older patients are knee, hip, hand, and lower back. Other common sites include chest (nonspecific), neck, pelvis, and foot.

Mr. C's pain is well-localized, sharp, lacks features commonly associated with visceral or neuropathic pain, and is therefore likely to be somatic pain. He also has several Pain Red Flags (Table 29.2) that raise the level of suspicion for serious underlying pathology.

DIAGNOSIS
- Management of pain in the older patient begins with identifying the likely cause. In particular, it is very helpful to differentiate neuropathic from somatic pain.
- The etiology of pain is determined through history, assessment of the pain, physical examination, and selective use of laboratory tests or radiologic exams.

TABLE 29.1: CONSEQUENCES OF POORLY MANAGED PAIN

Domain	Consequence
Behavioral	Depression, anxiety, substance abuse, social isolation, suicidal ideation
Cardiovascular	Hypertension, increased incidence of DVTs
Cognitive	Delirium
Constitutional	Sleep disturbance, fatigue, anorexia, weight loss, functional impairment, falls
Immune	Reduced immune function
Musculoskeletal	Impaired mobility, muscle spasm
Respiratory	Decreased volume, atelectasis
Societal	Increased health care utilization, increased cost

History

- The patient's self-report remains the gold standard for assessment of pain.
- However, there are special challenges to taking an accurate history from older patients, as they may be more reluctant to report pain, believe that pain is a normal part of aging, or think that reporting pain is tantamount to complaining. They may underreport pain out of fear that it is a harbinger of serious illness. Older patients can also have an exaggerated fear of becoming addicted to opioid medications.
- Age-associated physical changes in visual acuity and hearing may also make assessment of pain more difficult in the older adult. Be sure to use eyeglasses, hearing aids, and input from family members or caregivers to increase the likelihood of an accurate assessment.
- The question "Are you having pain now?" will be sufficient for pain assessment in most patients. Older adults may use different terminologies for pain, so clinicians should also ask patients if there are any areas that ache, hurt, are sore or uncomfortable, or bother them.

Assessment

Assess at the time of the initial interview and every eight hours thereafter. When pain is moderate to severe, ideally assess at least every hour. Important elements of pain assessment include:

- Location: Because location of the pain is so important for determining etiology and thus therapy, the clinician should verify location by asking patients to "point to where it hurts" or verify by conducting a body survey during physical exam while asking "does it hurt here?" while palpating each region of the body. A drawing of the body (pain map) can also be used to further clarify location of all pains.
- Intensity: Measure with a rating scale such as:
  Numeric Rating Scale (NRS)—Ask "On a scale of 0 to 10, with 0 being no pain at all and 10 being the worst pain imaginable, how would you rate your pain right now?"
  Verbal Descriptor Scale (VDS)—Ask if the patient has no pain, mild pain, moderate pain, severe pain, extreme pain, or the most intense pain imaginable.
- Quality
- Onset, duration, pattern
- Exacerbating and relieving factors
- Impact on physical and social function: self-report or report by caregivers
- Medication history: Obtain information on current and past history of prescription and over-the-counter medications, including complementary and alternative treatments. It can be very helpful to request that all of these medications be brought in for comprehensive review.
- Substance use or misuse history
- Assess for depression, anxiety, social support, and coping strategies

Assessment of pain in patients with cognitive impairment

- There is no evidence that older adults with dementia have reduced pain processing, but they currently receive less analgesia than those without cognitive impairment.[2]

- In cognitively impaired persons, pain is often manifested by agitation, restlessness, irritability, striking out at caregivers, or emotional withdrawal. Self-report (using NRS and VDS described above) should nevertheless always be attempted, regardless of degree of cognitive impairment, and should be corroborated with observational scales and surrogate reports.
- Mild or moderate cognitive impairment can make pain assessment challenging. Evaluation may require considerable patience while giving a patient with cognitive impairment time to respond and repeating the questions as necessary. Assessment strategies include: Assessing pain during movement (active and/or passive), rather than relying on memory; asking yes/no questions; and focusing on the present.
- Severe cognitive impairment can make it almost impossible to get an accurate sense of how a person is experiencing pain. If a patient is unable to communicate, pain assessment should be based on behavioral cues such as moaning, grimacing, agitation, confusion or restlessness, withdrawal, and physiologic cues such as tachycardia or tachypnea.[3] Behavioral expression of pain has considerable variation, but family members and other caregivers can help the clinician to understand what a particular behavior is likely to mean.
- If a patient with dementia shows physiologic or behavioral cues indicative of pain, it is safe to assume that the patient is experiencing severe pain. A trial of analgesics accompanied by a reduction in pain behaviors can be considered a positive indicator of pain, and a reason for continuing the analgesics.
- With dementia there can be a reduction in physiologic and behavioral responses to pain. Therefore in the absence of such cues one cannot assume that the patient is not experiencing pain. In the presence of pathology that is known to be painful in cognitively intact individuals, or when the patient is undergoing a usually painful procedure, clinicians should assume that the patient is experiencing pain.
- There is no consensus on use of a particular scale for patients with cognitive impairment

or the nonverbal patient, but the PACSLAC and Doloplus 2 hold promise.[2,4] Even the most widely used or recommended scales still require the clinician to choose the scale most appropriate for the patient and clinical setting.

- Behavioral symptoms such as agitation, vocalization, restlessness, and withdrawal should be treated with a trial of opioid analgesics before resorting to antipsychotics and anxiolytics.[5]

Exam

- Conduct an initial physical exam focusing on the musculoskeletal and neurological systems, with particular emphasis on the most frequently reported sites of pain in the elderly (listed above under "location"). Note any area of reproducible pain.
- If a plausible reason for pain behavior cannot be identified, proceed to the following domains of a comprehensive physical exam. (See Chapter 2: Principles of Geriatric Palliative Care.)

Musculoskeletal:

- Assess for signs of orthopedic injury and inflammation (redness, swelling, heat)
- Active and passive range of motion
- Examine spine for evidence of deformity and tenderness.

Neurological:

- Assess for pain from normally nonpainful stimuli
- Heightened pain from normally painful stimuli
- Unpleasant abnormal sensations
- Trophic changes (e.g., hair loss, nail changes)
- Autonomic signs (e.g., hyperhidrosis)
- Diminished strength
- Reflexes (hyperreflexia, hyporeflexia, loss of reflexes)

Cognitive:

- Evaluation using the Mini Mental Status Exam, or more detailed neuropsychological testing, may help select a reliable assessment technique as well as an appropriate treatment plan. For example, if a patient is found to be moderately to severely cognitively impaired, behavioral or physiologic indications of pain will be important assessment clues.

- Cognitively impaired patients will also benefit from treatment with standing doses of medication, rather than prn (as needed) dosing.

Function:

- Performance-based functional assessment, which may include elements such as range of motion testing and the Timed "Up and Go" or Short Physical Performance Battery, should be considered in order to understand the pain's impact on function.[6]

Tests

- Renal and hepatic function should be assessed at least at the initiation of treatment because results will influence choice of therapeutic agents.
- Vitamin D deficiency is associated with bone loss, increased falls, and fractures. Many older adults will need supplementation to maintain adequate vitamin D stores. Routine screening should be considered.
- Routine serology should be avoided unless an inflammatory disorder is suspected.
- Arthrocentesis may be indicated for suspected gout or septic arthritis.

Imaging

- Imaging should generally be reserved for ruling out serious pathology when something other than osteoarthritis is suspected.
- Overreliance on imaging in the absence of red flags (Table 29.2) may lead to overdiagnosis, as many older adults have degenerative disease even in the absence of pain.

Although Mr. C's pain is likely to be somatic, he does have a history of cancer, and his back pain is a new symptom. A comprehensive evaluation of the spine, including imaging, is therefore ordered.

TREATMENT OPTIONS

- The cause of the pain must always be properly addressed. When appropriate for patient's diagnosis, functional status, quality-of-life preferences, and goals of care, an attempt should first be made to

---

TABLE 29.2: PAIN RED FLAGS

Pain Red Flags: New pain in an elderly patient associated with any of the following features warrants comprehensive evaluation to rule out serious disorders

Back pain for the first time or following an injury

Presence of osteoporosis

Falls

History of cancer (rule out metastatic disease)

Substance abuse

Pain that wakes patient up

Constitutional symptoms (fever, anorexia, weight loss)

Immunosuppression

Recent history of infection

Back pain that is worse at night or when lying on back (rule out metastatic disease)

Severe or progressive neurologic deficit

Cold, pale, cyanotic, or mottled limb

New dysfunction of bowel or bladder

New onset headache (rule out temporal arteritis)

Severe abdominal pain or signs of shock or peritonitis

---

correct any underlying disease process that may be causing the pain.
- If this approach is not feasible, or if correction is only partially successful, then nonpharmacologic strategies and/or pharmacologic intervention should be considered.

Nonpharmacologic

- Physical activity should be considered for all older adults with chronic musculoskeletal pain. Any physical therapy program should be individualized, and careful attention paid to prescribing for intensity, frequency, and progression. (See Chapter 25: Rehabilitation.)
- Complementary and alternative medicine (massage, acupuncture, tai chi) may offer relief of chronic pain for some patients. (See Chapter 17: Complementary and Alternative Medicine.)
- Cognitive Behavioral Therapy (CBT) may help cognitively intact older adults manage their chronic pain through the substitution

of constructive approaches and positive coping strategies for maladaptive belief systems and negative attitudes about pain.

Pharmacologic

- Treatment usually begins with acetaminophen for mild pain and NSAIDs (with or without adjuvants) for mild to moderate pain. Warning: Due to the increased risk of gastrointestinal, renal, and cardiovascular toxicity, NSAIDs should be used with extreme caution in the elderly and avoided altogether in very frail elders.
- For moderate to severe pain, consider opioids with or without adjuvants.[2,7]

OPIOID THERAPY FOR PAIN

General Principles

- No ceiling effect
- No role for placebos
- Initiate therapy at a low dose and titrate dose slowly to effect or side effects
- Give orally when possible
- Intravenous route is preferred in cases of acute pain or when oral option is not feasible. If intravenous is not an option, then subcutaneous is preferable to intramuscular administration.
- May also use transdermal, rectal, or transmucosal route for opioids, but transdermal should never be used for acute pain
- Treat constipation prophylactically
- Administer analgesics regularly *and* prn if pain is present most of the day[8]
- Reassess frequently to monitor analgesia and side effects.

Patient and Family Education

- Education is essential to address patient and family concerns and misconceptions about opioids, as these widely held beliefs can be major barriers to the successful treatment of pain.

Dosing Considerations

- Individual patients may require a different dose or a different treatment approach. For example, patients who are already taking opioids will require higher doses to control new or worsening pain.
- When the pain is not expected to resolve shortly, medications should be administered "around the clock," and additional prn or rescue doses should be available for breakthrough pain.
- May be given q4h, prn (or q6h, prn for renal impairment), but consider standing doses if patient is not likely to request prns due to reluctance or cognitive impairment.
- Prescribe the standing medication based on its half-life (3–4 hours for short-acting opioids) and the rescue dose based on the time to onset (15–30 minutes for parenteral and 1 hour for oral).

Starting Doses of Pain Medications for Opioid-Naive Patients

Mild Pain:
- Non-opioids: acetaminophen 650–1000 mg PO q6h and/or ibuprofen 200–800 mg PO q6h.
- NSAIDs, including COX-2 inhibitors, should be avoided in the elderly. In some instances, however, the benefits of use may outweigh the risks.
- Daily acetaminophen dose should not exceed 4 g/day in healthy adults, 3 g/day in older frail adults, or 2 g/day in those with underlying hepatic dysfunction.
- Topical NSAIDs for OA
- Glucocorticoids and disease-modifying anti-rheumatic drugs (such as methotrexate) for RA

Moderate/Severe Pain:
- Opioid +/– a co-analgesic. Starting doses are morphine 5–15 mg PO q4h, oxycodone 5–10 mg PO q4h, hydromorphone 2–4mg PO q4h
- Parenteral opioids should be strongly considered; starting doses are morphine 2–5 mg IV/Subcut. or hydromorphone 0.4–0.8 mg IV/Subcut. every 15–30 minutes until the pain is controlled.
- Co-analgesics such as acetaminophen, NSAIDs (see warning above), anticonvulsants, antidepressants, and corticosteroids should be considered.

Selecting the Appropriate Medication

Additional factors to consider when choosing an appropriate opioid medication include:

- Cost
- Setting of care

- Cognitive status and available family and caregiver support
- Patient adherence and reliability
- Patient's ability to swallow long-acting medications

Equianalgesic Opioid Conversions

- If converting between opioids when pain is well-controlled, decrease the dose of the new opioid by 25% to 50% to allow for incomplete cross-tolerance. Be prepared to titrate up rapidly for analgesia in the first 24 hrs.
- If pain is not controlled, you may choose not to decrease the dose.
- Equivalent doses of different opioid analgesics can be calculated as demonstrated in Tables 29.3, 29.4, and 29.5.
- Special consideration must be given to the use of opioids in kidney and liver disease[2,7] (Table 29.6).

Fentanyl Patch Considerations

- Fentanyl patches must not be prescribed to opioid-naive patients. Short-acting opioids should be used to titrate to pain control and then converted to the appropriate fentanyl patch dose.
- For conversion between fentanyl patch and fentanyl IV, assume a 1:1 ratio (e.g.,

a 75 mcg/h fentanyl patch is equivalent to a 75 mcg/h fentanyl IV infusion).

- If converting to or from a fentanyl patch when pain is well-controlled, decrease the dose of the new opioid by 25% to 50% to allow for incomplete cross-tolerance. You may need to titrate up rapidly for analgesia in the first 24 hrs. If converting to the fentanyl patch, titrate up with short-acting opioids. If pain is not controlled, you may choose not to decrease the dose.
- Since the fentanyl patch takes three days to achieve steady state, it is never appropriate to use fentanyl patches to titrate patients with moderate or severe pain.
- Although there is technically no maximum dose, it is usually not practical to prescribe more than four 100 mcg/h patches (400 mcg/h).
- PRN dosing for fentanyl patches:
  - The breakthrough dose of oral morphine for a patient on a fentanyl patch is roughly 1/3 fentanyl patch dose (e.g., if the patient is prescribed a fentanyl patch 75 mcg/h q72h, the breakthrough dose is short-acting morphine 25 mg PO q1h, prn).
  - As always, when starting an opioid-tolerant patient on a new opioid, you may need to decrease the calculated

TABLE 29.3: OPIOID ANALGESIC EQUIVALENCES[2,7]

Opioid Agonists	IV/Subcut./ IM[a] (mg)	PO/Rectal (mg)	Ratio IV to PO IV: PO	Duration of Effect
Morphine	10	30	1 : 3	4 hours
Long-Acting Morphine		30		12 hours
Hydrocodone (Vicodin, Lortab)		30		4 hours
Oxycodone		20		4 hours
Long-Acting Oxycodone		20		12 hours
Oxymorphone (Opana)	1	10	1 : 10	4 hours
Long-Acting Oxymorphone		10		12 hours
Hydromorphone (Dilaudid)	1.5	7.5	1 : 5	4 hours
Fentanyl[b]	0.2 (200mcg)			1–2 hours
Methadone[c]				
Codeine	130	200	1 : 1.5	4 hours

Note: a. Intramuscular administration is discouraged because subcutaneous administration is as effective and less painful; b. See Tables 29.4 and 29.5 for conversions involving fentanyl patches; c. Methadone has a complex pharmacokinetic and pharmacodynamic profile that makes equianalgesic dosing particularly difficult. Consult with an experienced clinician before initiating or adjusting the dose of methadone.

TABLE 29.4: CONVERTING THE CURRENT OPIOID TO A FENTANYL PATCH

Morphine IV/ Subcut./IM mg/24h	Morphine PO/Rectal mg/24h	Oxycodone PO mg/24h	Hydromorphone IV/Subcut./IM mg/24h	Hydromorphone PO/Rectal mg/24h	(2) Then replace the current opioid with the fentanyl patch at the following dose (q72h):
10–19	30–59	20–39	1–2	8–14	12 mcg/h*
21–44	60–134	40–89	3–6	15–33	25 mcg/h
45–74	135–224	90–149	7–11	34–55	50 mcg/h
75–104	225–314	150–209	12–15	56–78	75 mcg/h
105–134	315–404	210–269	16–20	79–100	100 mcg/h
135–164	405–494	270–329	21–24	101–123	125 mcg/h
165–194	495–584	330–389	25–28	124–145	150 mcg/h
195–224	585–674	390–449	29–33	146–168	175 mcg/h
225–254	675–764	450–509	34–37	169–190	200 mcg/h
255–284	765–854	510–569	38–42	191–213	225 mcg/h
285–314	855–944	570–629	43–46	214–235	250 mcg/h
315–344	945–1034	630–689	47–51	236–258	275 mcg/h
345–374	1035–1124	690–749	52–55	259–280	300 mcg/h
375–404	1125–1214	750–809	56–60	281–303	325 mcg/h
405–434	1215–1304	810–869	61–64	304–325	350 mcg/h
435–464	1305–1394	870–929	65–69	326–348	375 mcg/h
465–494	1395–1484	930–989	70–74	349–370	400 mcg/h

(1) If the total daily dose (in mg/24h) of the current opioid is:

prn dose by 25% to 50% to account for incomplete cross-tolerance.

- Do not apply external heat to a fentanyl patch, or prescribe fentanyl patches to patients with temperature over 39°C (102°F), as this can accelerate drug absorption and cause overdose.
- Use caution in cachectic patients, as absorption may be impaired and patients may not achieve adequate analgesia.

Opioid Titration

- For moderate pain, increase the opioid dose at least every 24 hours. For severe pain, titrate more frequently.
- Increase the dose by 25% to 50% for mild to moderate pain, or by 50% to 100% for moderate to severe pain.
- Short-acting strong opioids (morphine, hydromorphone, and oxycodone) should be used to control moderate and severe pain. Long-acting preparations (e.g., sustained-release preparations of morphine

TABLE 29.5: CONVERTING A FENTANYL PATCH TO ANOTHER OPIOID

(1) If the fentanyl patch dose (q72h) is:

(2) Then replace the patch(es) with one of the following opioids 8–12 hrs after patch removal (total mg/24h):
[Note: Divide recommended doses below (in mg/24h) into 6 equal doses given q4h]

	Morphine IV/Subcut./IM mg/24h	Morphine PO/Rectal mg/24h	Oxycodone PO mg/24h	Hydromorphone IV/Subcut./IM mg/24h	Hydromorphone PO/Rectal mg/24h
12 mcg/h	15	45	30	2	11
25 mcg/h	30	90	60	4	22
50 mcg/h	60	180	120	9	45
75 mcg/h	90	270	180	13	67
100 mcg/h	120	360	240	18	90

TABLE 29.6: GUIDELINES FOR OPIOIDS IN KIDNEY AND LIVER DISEASE[2,7]

	Kidney Disease[1]		Liver Disease	
	Renal Failure	Dialysis	Stable Cirrhosis	Severe Disease
Morphine	Do not use	Do not use Not dialyzed	Caution ↓ dose ↓ frequency*	Do not use
Oxycodone	Caution ↓ dose ↓ frequency*	Caution	Caution ↓ dose ↓ frequency*	Caution↓ dose ↓ frequency*
Hydromorphone	Preferred ↓ dose ↓ frequency*	Preferred Not dialyzed, but minimal toxicity	Caution ↓ dose ↓ frequency*	Caution ↓ dose ↓ frequency*
Fentanyl	Preferred	Preferred Not dialyzed, but minimal toxicity	Preferred	Preferred
Codeine	Do not use	Do not use	Do not use	Do not use
Methadone [2]	Preferred—with consultation only	Preferred—with consultation only Not dialyzed, but minimal toxicity	Preferred—with consultation only	Preferred—with consultation only

* ↓ dose means reduce dose by 25–50%. ↓ frequency means reduce standing orders for short-acting opioids from q4h to q6h.
1. Avoid sustained-release oral opioids and fentanyl patches in kidney disease. Note that even the "safest" opioids are not dialyzable.
2. Consult with an experienced clinician before initiating or adjusting the dose of methadone.

or oxycodone or transdermal fentanyl) should be started after the pain is controlled on short-acting opioids. Never use long-acting opioids to control acute pain.

- PRN dosing for breakthrough pain (i.e., acute pain in patients with otherwise controlled pain): give short-acting opioids using approximately 10% of the total 24-hour standing opioid dose, available q 1–2 h (e.g., patient on long-acting morphine 60 mg PO q 12h, breakthrough dose = short acting morphine 15 mg PO q1h prn).
- Patient Controlled Analgesia (PCA) is a safe and effective method for delivery of opioids for pain that is expected to resolve (e.g., post-operative pain) and for acute exacerbations of chronic pain (e.g., pathologic fracture in a patient with chronic pain from bone metastases). Advantages include:
  - The patient self-delivers fixed doses of opioid by pressing a button.
  - A continuous (basal) infusion may also be ordered.
  - Overdose is very infrequent because the patient must be alert in order to press the button.

OPIOIDS AND OLDER ADULTS

Opioid Medications to Avoid

The following opioid medications are not recommended for use by older adults:[9]

- Meperidine (Demerol) is not recommended because its toxic metabolite, normeperidine, has no analgesic effect and is likely to cause myoclonus, seizures, and psychomimetic adverse effects in older adults.
- Propoxyphene (Darvon, Darvocet) is not recommended because it provides analgesia that is no better than acetaminophen, but can cause neuroexcitatory side effects, ataxia, and dizziness.
- Tramadol (Ultram, Ultracet) may be as effective as opioids such as morphine or oxycodone but also may cause seizures or serotonin syndrome.
- Mixed agonist-antagonists, such as pentazocine, butorphanol, and nalbuphine, can cause severe opioid withdrawal when given to patients tolerant to opioids; they are also not recommended as first-line therapy for patients who are opioid-naïve.

Management of Opioid Side Effects

Constipation

- Patients on opioid therapy need an individualized bowel regimen prescribed prophylactically at the beginning of treatment and continued for the duration of the opioid therapy.
- Maintain a high index of suspicion for bowel obstruction or fecal impaction. Rule out impaction with digital rectal exam or abdominal X-ray if clinically suspicious. Rectal disimpaction must occur before treating with an oral laxative.
- **Suggested bowel regimen**:
  - STEP 1: Senna 2 tabs PO at bedtime, plus docusate 100 mg PO tid for stool softening, if necessary. (Can titrate up to 8 senna/day)
  - STEP 2: Add polyethylene glycol 3350 (PEG) powder (17 mg/8 oz of water); for patients with hepatic failure, lactulose is preferred—30 ml PO q24h. (Can titrate up to every 6 hours)
  - STEP 3: If constipated for 3 or more days, add bisacodyl suppository (10–20 mg q24h), docusate mini-enema at bedtime (docusate, PEG, glycerine), mineral oil retention enema. If no results, add a high colonic tap water enema (nursing order). (See Chapter 45: Constipation.)
- **Sedation**:
  - May occur with start of opioids or with increase in dose (precedes development of respiratory depression)
  - Distinguish from exhaustion due to pain
  - Tolerance develops within days; fatigue resolves
  - Psychostimulants may be useful, e.g., methylphenidate (Ritalin)
- **Respiratory depression**:
  - Rarely clinically significant
  - Tolerance to respiratory depression develops much faster than to analgesia.
  - Pain is a potent stimulus for respiration.
  - If respiratory depression is clinically significant, management options include:
    - Identify and treat contributing causes
    - Reduce opioid dose and observe
    - Use naloxone for life-threatening respiratory depression only (See "Opioid Overdose" below)

- **Nausea/vomiting**: (See Chapter 53: Nausea and Vomiting)
  - Onset with start of opioids
  - Tolerance usually develops within days
  - Prevent or treat with antiemetics
- **Delirium**: (See Chapter 34: Delirium.)
  - Almost always multifactorial
  - Presentation: Acute onset (hours to days); disturbance of arousal (hypo- or hyper-; change in cognition; medical etiology likely based on history, physical, and labs
  - Delirium is more likely caused by untreated or undertreated pain than by administration of opioids.[10]
- **Myoclonus**: (See Chapter 39: Myoclonus.)

Addiction

Addiction should be distinguished from chemical dependence, tolerance, and pseudo-addiction.

- Dependence is the development of a withdrawal syndrome following dose reduction or administration of an antagonist.
  - Often develops after only a few days of opioid therapy
  - Not a clinical problem if drug is tapered before discontinuation
  - Taper by no more than 50% of the dose per day; avoid opioid antagonists
- Tolerance is a change in the dose-response relationship induced by exposure to the drug and manifests as a need for a higher dose to maintain an effect.
  - Analgesic tolerance is rarely a problem
  - Opioid doses remain relatively stable in the absence of worsening pathology
  - Increased opioid requirements after stable periods is often a signal of disease progression
- Addiction can be defined as compulsive use in spite of harm, craving, or impaired control over use of the substance.
  - It is important to recognize aberrant drug-related behaviors and understand the differential diagnosis for this behavior.
  - Pseudo-addiction: Behaviors that suggest possibility of addiction but are driven by pain and disappear with adequate analgesia.
  - Risk of iatrogenic addiction in older medically ill patients with pain and

no prior history of substance abuse is extremely small (far less than 1%).

Management of Substance Abuse

- Managing patients with a history of substance abuse can be particularly challenging. Patients with a prior history of substance abuse can be particularly reluctant to risk recurrent addiction. Patients with a prior history of opioid use may also have higher opioid dosage requirements for adequate analgesia.
- Multiple assessments, frequent monitoring and honest communication are essential. These must be implemented with firmness and compassion to assure the clinician that responsible use of medication is occurring, and to reassure the patient that, with monitoring, effective analgesic therapy will be provided. (See Chapter 66: Alcohol Abuse and Dependence.)

Opioid Overdose

- Naloxone (Narcan) should be used only for life-threatening opioid-induced respiratory depression, an exceedingly rare occurrence in patients on chronic stable opioid doses.
- In order to minimize symptoms of opioid withdrawal (agitation, fever, emesis, and pain) when naloxone is needed, dilute 1 ampule (0.4 mg) with normal saline to a total volume of 10 ml (1 ml = 0.04 mg) and administer 1 ml IV q 1 min prn. This careful titration will reverse respiratory depression without causing withdrawal.
- The half-life of naloxone (1 hour) is shorter than the half-life of opioid agonists; therefore additional doses or a continuous infusion of naloxone may be needed.

NEUROPATHIC PAIN MANAGEMENT[9,11]

- For patients with neuropathic pain, obtaining satisfactory relief is often a challenge. Patients should be advised that, even with medication, they may continue to have some level of discomfort, and that achieving effective dosing may take time.
- Because the evidence supporting treatment of many painful neuropathic disease processes is not conclusive, clinicians should carefully select from the following therapies based on a benefit/burden analysis that includes safety, tolerability, and drug interactions.
  - Topical analgesics: Topical lidocaine is effective for localized neuropathic pain in older adults, e.g., post-herpetic neuralgia (PHN) and allodynia.
  - Antidepressants: Tricyclic antidepressants (TCAs) can help relieve peripheral neuropathies; advantages include cost-effectiveness, possible relief of depression, and once-a-day dosing. Must be titrated slowly, and consideration should be given to anticholinergic and cardiac side effects. Selected SSRIs are also effective (citalopram, escitalopram, paroxetine).
  - Antiepileptics: Gabapentin and pregabalin are approved for neuropathic pain; they have few drug interactions and may enhance sleep. Pregabalin has a simpler dosing regimen and fewer side effects; gabapentin can cause sedation and dizziness.
  - Opioid agonists: While not the primary treatment choice for neuropathic pain, opioids can serve as a bridge while first-line medications are being titrated; they may also be necessary for some patients with chronic neuropathic pain. Because of their quick onset, opioids are also effective for acute neuropathic pain and for breakthrough dosing.

INTERVENTIONAL PAIN MANAGEMENT

- The evidence supporting the long-term efficacy of interventional pain management techniques in older adults remains mixed.
- For patients who have not benefitted from optimal medical management, clinicians may offer interventional options such as epidural steroid injections for radicular pain, kyphoplasty for vertebral compression fractures, and spinal cord stimulation for a variety of chronic pain syndromes.[12]

CHRONIC PAIN MANAGEMENT

- In addition to the above pharmacologic and interventional treatment strategies, chronic pain management should include physical exercise, complementary and alternative medicine, and cognitive behavioral therapy (see nonpharmacologic treatment options, above).

TAKE-HOME POINTS

- Pain in the elderly is prevalent and continues to be undertreated.
- Assessment and frequent reassessment, using tools appropriate for cognitively intact or impaired older adults when necessary, is the first step in recognizing pain and a key component of effective clinical management.
- Older patients may be reluctant to report pain for a variety of reasons, including belief that pain is a normal part of aging, suspicion that it is a harbinger of serious illness, or fear of becoming addicted to opioid medications.
- Careful selection of analgesic drugs based on evidence of benefit and risk of harms to older adults is essential.
- Once an appropriate analgesic is selected, it is advisable to start at lower doses and to titrate up more slowly than is the case for younger adults.
- Nonpharmacologic approaches to pain management can be effective and may help reduce drug toxicity and the risk of polypharmacy.
- Patients with neuropathic pain may continue to have some level of discomfort even with medication, and achieving effective dosing may take time.
- Chronic pain management should include physical exercise, complementary and alternative medicine, and cognitive behavioral therapy.

REFERENCES

1. Herr, K. Pain in the older adult: an imperative across all health care settings. *Pain Manag Nurs.* Jun 2010;*11*(2 Suppl):S1–10.

2. Pasero C, McCaffery M. *Pain Assessment and Pharmacologic Management.* St. Louis, MO: Mosby; 2010.

3. American Geriatrics Society Panel on Pharmacological Management of Persistent Pain in Older Persons. Pharmacological Management of Persistent Pain in Older Persons. *J Am Geriatr Soc.* 2009;*57*(8):1331–1346.

4. Zwakhalen S, Hamers J, Berger M. Improving the clinical usefulness of a behavioral pain scale for older people with dementia. *J Adv Nurs.* 2007;*58*(5):493–502.

5. Husebo BS, Ballard C, Sandvik R, Nilsen OB. Efficacy of treating pain to reduce behavioral disturbances in residents of nursing homes with dementia: cluster randomized clinical trial. *BMJ.* 2011;*343*:d4065.

6. Hadjistavropoulos T, Herr K, Turk DC, et al. "An Interdisciplinary Expert Consensus Statement on Assessment of Pain in Older Persons." *Clin J Pain.* 2007;*23*(1)Suppl:S1–43.

7. Fine PG, Portenoy RK. A clinical guide to opioid analgesia. New York: McGraw-Hill; 2004.

8. American Pain Society (APS). *Principles of analgesic use in the treatment of acute pain and cancer pain*, 6th Edition. Glenview, IL: APS; 2008.

9. Chai E, Horton JR. Managing pain in the elderly population. *Curr Pain Headache Rep.* 2010;*14*:409–417.

10. Morrison RS, Magaziner J, Gilbert M, Koval KJ, McLaughlin MA, Orosz G, Strauss E, Siu AL. Relationship between pain and opioid analgesics on the development of delirium following hip fracture. *J Gerontol A Biol Sci Med Sci.* Jan 2003;*58*(1):76–81.

11. McGeeney BE. Pharmacological management of neuropathic pain in older adults: an update on peripherally and centrally acting agents. *J Pain Symptom Manage.* 2009;*38*(2):S15–27.

12. Christo PJ, Li S, Gibson SJ, Fine P, Hameed H. Effective treatments for pain in the older patient. *Curr Pain Headache Rep.* Feb 2011;*15*(1):22–34.

30
Fatigue

CASE

Mrs. S, an 84-year-old woman, comes to your office accompanied by her daughter, with the complaint of feeling increasingly tired over the past several months. Her medical history is significant for hypertension, osteoarthritis, chronic kidney disease (Stage 3), and NYHA Class III congestive heart failure. She tells you that she now takes naps during the day but still does not feel well rested. She has gradually had to limit her activities during this time period but notes that despite these changes she continues to lack energy. Mrs. S has also become more dependent on her daughter for help with shopping, cleaning, and meal preparations, activities she previously performed independently. She feels extremely guilty about the burden she is placing on her daughter and is tearful as she speaks with you.

DEFINITION

Fatigue is a complex concept and is often used interchangeably with terms such as asthenia, lassitude, prostration, lethargy, exercise intolerance, lack of energy, and weakness. Even in the medical literature, there is no universally accepted definition of fatigue. However, most definitions of fatigue, particularly in the medical context of cancer and multiple sclerosis, encompass the following characteristics:

- Subjective sense of tiredness or exhaustion
- Lack of physical and/or mental energy
- Related to underlying illness or treatment
- Not proportional to level of recent activity
- Interferes with usual and desired level of function
- Not relieved by rest
- Not due to comorbid psychiatric illness

CANCER-RELATED FATIGUE

- The definition of *cancer-related fatigue* by International Classification of Diseases-10 (ICD-10) criteria requires "significant fatigue, diminished energy or increased need to rest, disproportionate to any recent change in activity level" to be present every day or nearly every day for two consecutive weeks out of the last month. Five out of 10 additional symptoms—such as generalized weakness, diminished concentration, insomnia, and marked emotional reactivity—are required for the diagnosis.
- Along with these symptoms, the fatigue must cause significant distress or impairment, must be a consequence of cancer or cancer treatment, and must not be due to a comorbid psychiatric disorder.[1]

FATIGUE IN PALLIATIVE CARE

In 2008 the European Association for Palliative Care (EAPC) steering committee suggested a working definition of fatigue as "a subjective feeling of tiredness, weakness or lack of energy." The group found this broader definition to be more relevant for the palliative care setting.[2]

PREVALENCE

- Fatigue is one of the most common symptoms of chronic illness, cancer, and cancer treatment. The prevalence in the palliative care setting has been reported in the range of 48–78%.[3] In an American palliative care program of 1000 patients, fatigue was one of the five most common symptoms (84%).[4]
- Fatigue has been reported in up to 99% of patients following radiotherapy or chemotherapy.[2] More than half of patients with multiple sclerosis and the majority of patients with COPD and congestive heart failure (CHF) describe fatigue as one of their most troubling symptoms.

CONSEQUENCES OF UNTREATED FATIGUE

Despite its prevalence, fatigue is often an under-recognized, under-assessed and under-treated symptom. It is frequently considered a natural trait of aging and advanced disease that should be tolerated. However, fatigue is associated with significant physical, psychosocial, and spiritual consequences:

- Prevents participation in preferred activities, by impeding Activities of Daily Living and affecting cognitive function
- Limits social interaction
- Leads to changes in self-esteem and social roles
- Often associated with mood disturbances—feeling listless, depressed, irritable

LIKELY ETIOLOGIES

Advanced diseases of any type may cause fatigue, and multiple factors are likely to contribute. The pathophysiology is not fully understood, but several hypotheses exist. Differentiating primary fatigue from secondary fatigue is a useful approach to understanding the underlying mechanism.[2]

- **Primary fatigue:**
  - Directly associated with the disease and/or its therapy
  - Likely related to high cytokine load
  - Includes both peripheral and central mechanisms
  - Central mechanisms may involve changes in neural function of HPA (hypothalamo-pituitary-adrenal) axis and neuronal systems underlying arousal and fatigue.[5]
  - Peripheral mechanisms may be related to energy imbalance.[5]
- **Secondary fatigue:** The following causes of secondary fatigue are particularly prevalent in the geriatric population due to the increased number of comorbidities, the tendency toward polypharmacy, and the under-recognition of depression in this population:
  - Concurrent syndromes or diseases such as anemia, cachexia, fever, infections, or metabolic disorders
  - Pro-inflammatory cytokines that play a major role in cachexia, anemia, fever, and infection.[6]
  - Drugs with sedative properties (opioid analgesics, benzodiazepines, antidepressants, or anticonvulsants)
  - Ineffective coping strategies and prolonged stress response
  - Depression, both situational and major depressive disorder

DIAGNOSIS

Exam

- Whether fatigue is defined as a symptom or a clinical syndrome, addressing the subjective experience of the patient is the most important part of the assessment.
- It is imperative to remember that a palliative care approach focuses on the subjective experience of the patient, and this assessment should be the indicator for treatment. When the patient is unable to self-assess, the substituted estimation of caregivers can be useful.
- A comprehensive assessment of fatigue recognizes both a physical and a cognitive dimension. Additionally, consistent evaluation of other symptoms like pain, breathing difficulties, sleep disturbances, and depression is necessary while planning a treatment strategy. Many instruments have been developed to assess fatigue:[3]
  1. Single-item scales ("Do you get tired for no reason?")
  2. Questionnaires and checklists, including the Functional Assessment of Cancer Therapy-Fatigue (FACT-F), Functional Assessment of Chronic Illness Therapy-Fatigue (FACIT-F), Fatigue Assessment Questionnaire, and Multidimensional Fatigue Inventory, are used in fatigue research.
  3. The Brief Fatigue Inventory (BFI) and Edmonton Symptom Assessment Scale (ESAS) are important tools due to their ease of use and reproducibility.
- For geriatric patients, the single-item scale is a simple question that most practitioners can incorporate into their practice to screen for fatigue. Once fatigue is identified, the BFI is a useful tool to explore the degree to which fatigue impacts the patient's life and allows for monitoring of symptom improvement or progression over time. Most of the scales do require a degree of cognitive function, and may or may not be useful with the substituted judgment of a caregiver.

Tests

Secondary causes of fatigue can be identified through laboratory evaluation:

- CBC, iron studies for evaluation of anemia
- Chemistry including calcium, albumin, magnesium, and phosphate to evaluate electrolyte disturbances

- Creatinine and bilirubin to evaluate organ dysfunction
- TSH, free T3, and T4 to rule out hypothyroidism
- Vitamin D, B1, B6, and B12 for vitamin deficiency

After further questioning, it becomes clear that the fatigue Mrs. S is experiencing not only interferes with her general activity but also affects her relationships with her family and her overall quality of life. You use the Geriatric Depression Scale to screen for depression, and her score is 4 (negative for depression). A review of her medications does not identify any medications known for sedation. You check basic lab tests to look for secondary causes of fatigue that might be reversible. As expected, Mrs. S has an anemia of chronic disease and an elevated creatinine. The rest of her lab tests are within normal limits. Mrs. S wonders if you have any recommendations that will alleviate her fatigue.

TREATMENT OPTIONS

Treating Secondary Causes

If the burden of treatment does not outweigh the benefit and is consistent with the patient's goals, secondary causes of fatigue should be identified and treated (Table 30.1).

- Manage pain through individually tailored regimens and dose modifications
- Correct the underlying problem, e.g., treat anemia through repletion of iron, folate, and/or vitamin B12, transfusion of red blood cells or erythropoietin administration in conditions like chronic renal insufficiency
- Address metabolic disorders, electrolyte, and hormonal imbalances
- Treat depression with antidepressants; selective serotonin reuptake inhibitors (SSRIs) and atypical antidepressants

TABLE 30.1: TREATMENT OF FATIGUE IN PALLIATIVE CARE PATIENTS

Treating Cause of Fatigue		Treating Symptom of Fatigue	
Cause	Treatment	Treatment	Examples
Anemia	Erythropoietin Transfusion	Stimulant drugs	Modafinil, Methylphenidate
Infection	Antibiotics	Steroid	Dexamethasone (for 1-2 weeks)
Fever	Antipyretic drugs		
Dehydration	Hydration		
Electrolyte imbalance	Bisphosphonate, correction	Diary	
Cachexia	Nutrition, Anabolics	Physical training	
Hypothyroidism Hypogonadism	Hormone substitution	Energy conservation	Prioritization, delegation of tasks
Depression	Anti-depressant	Energy restoration	Relaxation, enjoyable activities
Sleep disturbances	Sleep hygiene, sedatives		
Pain	Pain management		
Sedative Polypharmacy	Reduce dose or rotate drugs		

Adapted from Radbruch L. *Palliative Medicine.* 2008;22:13–22.

preferred over tricyclics due to their side effect profiles.

- Treat symptoms such as shortness of breath.
- Reduce dosing or rotate sedating medications.

Symptomatic Treatment

- For many geriatric palliative care patients, treating the underlying causes of primary or secondary fatigue may take too long, not be effective, or prove to be too burdensome. For these patients, providers should focus on symptomatic treatment through pharmacologic and nonpharmacologic means.
- Most management strategies have been developed for the treatment of fatigue arising as a side effect of cancer treatment. These treatment approaches can be adapted to provide relief of fatigue in the geriatric and palliative care population as well.

Nonpharmacologic

1. **Establish realistic expectations.**
   - Educate patients and caregivers on symptoms and expected course.
   - Prepare caregivers for the potential need for assistance with activities of daily living.
   - Encourage patients to conserve energy by setting limits on exertion, prioritizing and delegating tasks.
   - Counsel patients to participate in energy restoration strategies including relaxation and enjoyable activities.
   - These measures often reduce feelings of anxiety and guilt related to the patient's experience of fatigue.
2. **Encourage exercise**
   - Effective in reducing symptoms of fatigue.
   - Activity level should be adapted to performance status.
   - Patients frequently try to combat fatigue with extended periods of rest that do not restore energy. In fact, the reduction of physical activity may worsen fatigue.
3. **Recommend stress management**
   - Therapy: brief psycho-educational group interventions, cognitive behavioral therapy, individual psychotherapy

- Complementary and alternative approaches: acupuncture, mind-body techniques, music and art therapy, massage, spiritual counseling. Of these complementary and alternative therapies, massage has been shown to have a direct effect on patient's experience of fatigue.[7]

Pharmacologic[3]

1. **Methylphenidate:**
   - Effective in several trials for the treatment of opioid-induced sedation and for fatigue in advanced cancer patients
   - Useful in depression in palliative care settings
   - Usual prescribed daily dose: 5–10 mg (can be titrated up to 40 mg per day as tolerated)
   - Dose-limiting side effects: loss of appetite, slurring of speech, nervousness, and cardiac symptoms
   - Geriatric considerations: Methylphenidate is contraindicated in patients with glaucoma and/or cardiac arrhythmias
2. **Modafinil:**
   - Used in trials for the treatment of fatigue in advanced neurologic diseases such as MS and ALS and in patients with HIV/AIDS.
   - Recommended dose: 200–400 mg orally per day, but in the geriatric population, clearance may be reduced, especially in those with diminished renal and/or hepatic function. Use of reduced doses should be considered in this patient population (100 mg daily).
   - Adverse effects: GI upset, headache, dizziness, rhinitis, and (rarely) cardiac arrhythmias
3. **Megestrol acetate:**
   - FDA approved for cachexia related to HIV/AIDS and cancer-related fatigue.
   - Improves appetite, increases activity, and contributes to overall well-being in advanced cancer patients.
   - Dose range: 400–800 mg, but the lower dose of 400 mg appears to be as effective as the 800 mg dose in AIDS-related cachexia. If considering use in the geriatric population, advise starting with the lower dose.
   - Common side effects: hypertension, sweating, weight gain, hot flashes, mood swings, and GI upset

4. **Low-dose corticosteroids (methylprednisolone or dexamethasone):**
   - Limited data from controlled trials and some anecdotal support for use in the treatment of fatigue in patients with advanced disease and multiple symptoms.
   - Useful in relieving fatigue for a short period of time or for a specific event (usually one or two weeks).
   - Side effects: infection, mood swings, insomnia, myalgias, and elevated blood glucose

PALLIATIVE CARE ISSUES

- An important consideration when treating fatigue is the recognition that, at the very end of life, fatigue is an expected development and may actually serve a protective role.
- Family members and caregivers will benefit from education about disease progression and the normal dying process.

TAKE-HOME POINTS

- Fatigue is often an under-recognized, under-assessed and undertreated symptom in the geriatric population.
- Fatigue can impact a patient's functional performance and psychosocial well-being.
- Health care providers should understand the difference between primary and secondary fatigue and know how to assess fatigue via screening tools and diagnostic tests.
- Counseling patients and caregivers about fatigue and setting realistic expectations help to alleviate feelings of anxiety and guilt.
- Exercise and some complementary therapies may improve the patient's experience of fatigue.
- Medications can be used cautiously in the geriatric population for fatigue that is related to chronic illness.

REFERENCES

1. Cella D, Davis K, Breitbart W, Curt G. Cancer-related fatigue: prevalence of proposed diagnostic criteria in a United States sample of cancer survivors. *J Clin Oncol.* 2001;*19*:3385–3391.
2. Radbruch L et al. Fatigue in palliative care patients—an EAPC approach. *Palliat Med.* 2008; *22*:13–22.
3. Narayanan V, Koshy C. Fatigue in cancer: A review of literature. *Indian J Palliat Care.* 2009;*15*:19–25.
4. Walsh D, Donnelly S, Rybicki L. The symptoms of advanced cancer: relationship to age, gender, and performance status in 1000 patients. *Support Care Cancer.* 2000;*8*:175–179.
5. Gutstein HB. The biologic basis of fatigue. *Cancer.* 2001;*92*:1678–1683.
6. Kurzrock R. The role of cytokines in cancer-related fatigue. *Cancer.* 2001;*92*:1684–1688.
7. Davies, RD, Gabbert SL, Riggs PD. Anxiety Disorders in Neurologic Illness. *Current Treatment Options in Neurology.* 2001;*3*:333–346.

31

Failure to Thrive

CASE

Mrs. C, a 96-year-old woman with peripheral vascular disease, hypertension, and hypothyroidism, arrives at the ER accompanied by her daughter. Ms. C reports that her mother does not eat any more; Mrs. C picks at her food, but does not eat much other than a few bites of puddings and ice cream. Mrs. C has lost five pounds in the last two to three weeks. She keeps to her room and does not seem interested in visitors, even missing her grandson's birthday party a few weeks ago. Physically, she has declined; she now requires help to move from the bedroom to a chair in the living room. A month ago, she walked back and forth to the bedroom using a walker, and would stand in the shower to bathe. Today, she stopped walking completely, and her daughter brought her to the ER. She asks what can be done to help her mother.

DEFINITION

Internists imported the term *"failure to thrive"* from the pediatric literature in the 1980s. Failure to thrive (FTT) in the elderly describes a syndrome of "gradual decline in physical and/or cognitive function, accompanied by weight loss, reduced appetite, and social withdrawal, that occurs without immediate explanation."[1]

- Overlap exists with the concept of debility, and the two terms may be used interchangeably. Debility, in context of hospice admission in particular, evokes the combination of multiple cumulative medical comorbidities with declining functional status to indicate a terminal condition.[2] Both reflect the challenge of prognostication in the absence of a single anatomic disease driving an older adult's decline. In contrast with FTT, debility more specifically addresses the combination of multiple organ system failures and highlights the primacy of central nervous system disease (that is not advanced dementia). However, they share featured criteria for weight loss, poor nutrition,

dependence in ADLs, and an overall functional decline.[2]

- The term "failure to thrive" intersects with descriptions of frailty, and the literature in recent years has moved away from its use. In a clinical context, FTT describes a combination of changes that correlate with functional loss and nutritional abnormalities, sometimes referred to as the final stages of frailty, an irreversible process presaging decline and death.[3,4]
- The Institute of Medicine defines FTT as follows:

Weight loss >5% of total body weight		Dehydration
		Depressive symptoms
Decreased appetite	**AND**	Impaired immune function
Poor nutrition		Low cholesterol
Inactivity		levels

- Other authors cite a combination of biopsychosocial failure and malnutrition, without immediate explanation for the decline.[5] To summarize these multiple theories and definitions, failure to thrive:

1. Represents a poorly defined syndrome marked by malnutrition and its sequelae and characterized by cognitive (depression/dementia) and functional decline.
2. Is not part of the normal aging process; nor should the term be used to describe the final stages of a known terminal illness.
3. Invites focused exploration of possible reversible etiologies, while acknowledging FTT as a herald of the end of life.[3,6]

Ms. C reports that her mother's doctor diagnosed dementia several years ago, but that her mother's decline has been slow. She continues to be verbal and has been declining food, stating she is not hungry or (falsely) that she has already eaten. She has seemed to withdraw from activity and does not move willingly from bed or chair. Ms. C expresses her frustration, wondering if this is common for older adults.

PREVALENCE

Broad ranges appear in the literature; in general, prevalence increases markedly with age and dependence. For community-dwelling older adults, 5% to 35% is quoted; 25% to 40% for nursing home residents; and 50% to 60% for hospitalized veterans.[6]

On exam, Mrs. C is attentive and answers some questions, mostly inappropriately. She is very thin. She has no focal findings on her exam, no suprapubic or CVA tenderness, no abdominal distention, tenderness, or masses, and no pain on passive motion of her lower extremities, including internal and external rotation. She has a small stage I sacral pressure ulcer.

EXPECTED DISEASE COURSE

- FTT is associated with hip fractures, decubitus ulcers, decreased immune function (particularly cell-mediated immunity) and increased infection.[6] Depending on the discoveries during evaluation, some aspects of FTT respond well to treatment and support; nutritional interventions, physical and occupational therapy, care support, and social service utilization can lead to stabilization of an elderly person in his or her environment.
- However, the FTT does carry a grim prognosis. When related to a hip fracture, up to 80% of those with FTT after fracture die within a year.[7] A study exploring outcomes for hospitalized patients with weight loss showed that 75% died within a year of their hospitalization.
- Providers noting FTT should initiate a focused evaluation and set of interventions to attempt stabilization. There should also be discussion with the patient and patient's family to explore the goals of care and prepare them for what to expect in the future.

Ms. C feels overwhelmed at Mrs. C's decline. You explain that she does not seem to have only one, but several medical problems causing her decline. You review her medical conditions: coronary artery disease, peripheral vascular disease, hypertension, and chronic renal insufficiency. Ms. C notes that she's become more withdrawn, declining medications, food, and interaction with her loved ones.

LIKELY ETIOLOGIES

- The cause of FTT is most often multifactorial, representing decline in many spheres. With early intervention in multiple areas, hope exists for reversal or stabilization.[5] FTT challenges the provider to explore for reversible or modifiable causes, while acknowledging that many cases will not respond to therapeutic interventions. Common medical conditions associated with failure to thrive in elderly patients include organ failure, chronic infections, chronic inflammation, malnutrition, major depression and cognitive loss, and functional impairment. These conditions are typically caused by underlying disease processes including tuberculosis, cancer, diabetes, heart disease, rheumatological diseases, and stroke.[7]
- Four major domains of FTT represent the areas that "fail": impaired physical function, malnutrition, depression, and cognitive impairment. Some authors argue that each of these influences the others, and it is difficult to sort the etiology from the phenotype of the syndrome.[8]
- After clinical counseling about realistically achievable medical outcomes, the goals of care established with patient and family members will help determine the balance between the benefits and burdens of a diagnostic evaluation.[5,6]

DIAGNOSIS

History

- A comprehensive medical history, including medication history, guides the provider to common medical conditions leading to the FTT syndrome, such as infection, organ failure, malignancy, or depression.[6] Substance use/abuse and sensory deficits may also precipitate FTT.[5]
- Early involvement of other disciplines (nutrition, social work) assists in finding alternate reasons for a patient's decline (difficulty eating, neglect, abuse).

Exam

- Comprehensive history-taking will include assessment for chronic diseases, as well as a thorough medication history, nutritional evaluation, cognitive assessment, depression screen, social and sexual history,

functional evaluation (including ADLs, IADLs, and physical function assessment such as a Timed Up and Go).
- Providers should explore the chronicity of complaints as well in order to determine if decline results from a recent change, or if deficits have been longstanding.

Tests
- No specific tests exist for FTT, but traditional markers of dehydration (BUN, creatinine) and malnutrition (hypoalbuminemia, hypocholesterolemia) may help with diagnosis and prognosis.[3]
- By focusing on those aspects that arise from a careful history and physical exam,

providers may avoid subjecting patients to a fruitless, burdensome workup.

You find no reversible cause of Mrs. C's decline on history or physical exam; she is mildly dehydrated by labs. Her LDL is 40, and her albumin is 2.5. You request a physical therapy consult and start nutritional supplementation. In discussing your results with Ms. C, she asks you if her mother is dying from "old age." She asks if hospice care would be appropriate, since she had great support during her father's illness several years before.

TREATMENT OPTIONS
- Treatment options are determined by the outcomes of initial workup (Figure 31.1).

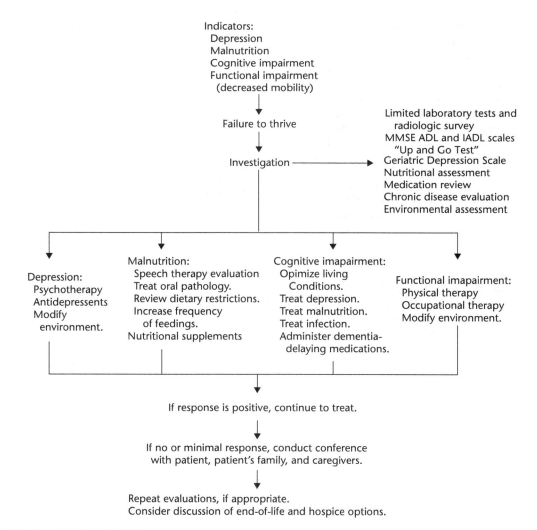

Indicators:
Depression
Malnutrition
Cognitive impairment
Functional impairment
(decreased mobility)

Failure to thrive

Investigation

Limited laboratory tests and
radiologic survey
MMSE ADL and IADL scales
"Up and Go Test"
Geriatric Depression Scale
Nutritional assessment
Medication review
Chronic disease evaluation
Environmental assessment

Depression:
Psychotherapy
Antidepressents
Modify
environment.

Malnutrition:
Speech therapy evaluation
Treat oral pathology.
Review dietary restrictions.
Increase frequency
of feedings.
Nutritional supplements

Cognitive imapairment:
Opimize living
Conditions.
Treat depression.
Treat malnutrition.
Treat infection.
Administer dementia-
delaying medications.

Functional imapairment:
Physical therapy
Occupational therapy
Modify environment.

If response is positive, continue to treat.

If no or minimal response, conduct conference
with patient, patient's family, and caregivers.

Repeat evaluations, if appropriate.
Consider discussion of end-of-life and hospice options.

FIGURE 31.1: Treating FTT.

Note. Robertson RG and Montagnini M. Geriatric failure to thrive. *American Family Physician.* 2004;70(2):343–350.

- Focused interventions in the following domains have been shown to assist in FTT:
  - Nutritional assessment and dietary supplementation[7]
  - Physical therapy and resistance exercise
  - Treatment of depression and other recognized disease processes
  - Cessation of abuse/neglect[3]
- The majority of cases of FTT are not attributable to a single reversible cause; efforts to reverse decline are met with variable success. Individual prognosis can be difficult to determine, given the multifactorial nature and interaction of etiologies and outcomes.

PALLIATIVE CARE ISSUES

- The provider has a duty to recognize the FTT syndrome as a key marker for end of life. Given the prognosis, patients with FTT not responding to the interventions noted above would benefit from an open discussion of what to expect in the future (i.e., continued decline) and a recommendation for interventions designed to maximize comfort and quality of life. For most patients, a referral to hospice care is appropriate.[6]
- Under hospice eligibility criteria for non-cancer patients, those with FTT would be eligible. Criteria include unintentional progressive weight loss of >10%, functional decline, and increase in ER visits or hospitalizations.

TAKE-HOME POINTS

- FTT arises from a complex multifactorial process, marked by malnutrition and cognitive and physical functional decline.

- Failure to thrive carries a grim prognosis; over 75% of patients with irreversible symptoms die within one year.[3]
- Failure to thrive marks an advanced disease state and should trigger advanced care discussions, which then determine the benefits and burdens of further diagnostic evaluation.
- Patients and families should be informed about the natural history of the disease and the prognosis. A focus on quality of life should be encouraged, and referral to hospice should be made if appropriate.

REFERENCES

1. Braun JV, Wylde MH, Cowling WR III. Failure to thrive in older persons: a concept derived. *Gerontologist*. 1988;*28*:809–812.
2. Kinzbrunner BM, Weinreb NJ, Merriman MP. Debility, unspecified: A terminal diagnosis. *Am J Hosp Palliat Care*. 1996;*13*:38–44.
3. Verdery RB. Failure to thrive in old age: follow-up on a workshop. *Journal of Gerontology*. 1997;*52A*: M333–M336.
4. Hammerman D, Toward an understanding of frailty. *Ann Intern Med*. 1999;*130*(11): 945–950.
5. Egbert AM. The dwindles: failure to thrive in older patients. *Nutr Rev*. 1996;*54*(1):S25–S30.
6. Robertson RG, Montagnini M. Geriatric failure to thrive. *Am Fam Physician*. 2004;*70*(2):343–350.
7. Verdery RB. Clinical evaluation of failure to thrive. *Clin Geriatr Med*. 1997;*13*(4):769–778.
8. Sarkisian CA, Lachs MS. "Failure to thrive" in older adults. *Ann Intern Med*. 1996;*124*:1072–1078.

32

Fever and Sweating

CASE

You are visiting one of your elderly patients who is receiving palliative care at home. He is a 72-year-old male with hypertension and severe, debilitating osteoarthritis that leaves him bed-bound and subject to recurrent respiratory and urinary infections. He has had multiple cases of c-diff diarrhea associated with antibiotics, and he now refuses further antimicrobial treatment. The goals of care for your patient include comfort and avoiding hospital admission. His daughter, the primary caregiver, reports that he has been having intermittent fever for the past three days, accompanied by occasional profuse sweating. She tells you that she is quite concerned that her father may have an infection.

PART A: FEVER

DEFINITION

- *Fever* is the elevation of core body temperature above normal. Should be considered in patients with:
  - Persistent elevation of body temperature of at least 2°F [(1.1°C)] over baseline values
  - Oral temperatures of 99°F (37.2°C) or greater on repeated measurements
  - Rectal temperatures of 99.5°F (37.5°C) on repeated measurements
  - Axillary temperature of 99° F (37.2° C) or higher
- Fever of an unknown origin (FUO): febrile illness lasting >3 weeks, with temp >38.3°C on several occasions, and lacking a definitive diagnosis after 1 week of evaluation in the hospital.
- Hyperthermia: a medical emergency of significant elevation in body temperature without an associated pathological process.

PREVALENCE

Older patients with serious infections have 20% to 30% prevalence of fever and lower febrile responses than younger patients.

CONSEQUENCES OF UNTREATED FEVER

- There is little or no evidence suggesting that fever puts older adults at risk for long-term complications or neurological symptoms, although it may add to physical discomfort and patient/caregiver distress.
- There is little clear benefit seen in reducing body temperature, except for patients with severe or unstable coronary artery disease (CAD). Increased metabolic rate can contribute to increased myocardial oxygen consumption in elderly patients, particularly those with CAD.

LIKELY ETIOLOGIES

- Infection
- Tumor (paraneoplastic fever)
- Allergic or hypersensitivity reaction to drugs
- Blood transfusions
- Graft-versus-host disease
- Thrombosis

Less common causes include malignant bowel syndrome, tumor embolization, central nervous system hemorrhage, and coexisting connective tissue disorders

DIAGNOSIS

Exam

Requires taking careful history, medication review, and a thorough physical examination of all major body systems, including meticulous evaluation of the skin and all body orifices (mouth, ears, nose, throat, urethra, vagina, rectum, venipuncture sites, biopsy sites, and skin folds: breasts, axillae, abdomen, and groin).

Tests

- Depending on the results of the history and exam, relevant blood work such as complete blood count with differential, cultures of blood or urine, CXR, and other tests of bodily fluid may be necessary.

- If no obvious source is located, and if complete workup is consistent with overall goals of care, consider seeking occult sources of infection in the CNS or any hardware or appliance the patient may have, such as pacemaker leads, joint replacements, and others.

TREATMENT OPTIONS

The underlying medical condition should be treated. Symptomatic treatment of fever is described below.

Nonpharmacologic

- Increase cool fluid intake to prevent dehydration
- Remove excess clothing and linens
- Keep clothes and sheets dry
- Bathing or sponging with tepid water
- Application of a lubricant to dried lips
- Keeping mucous membranes moist with ice chips
- Convective cooling via increasing air circulation using fans or an airflow blanket

Pharmacologic

Pharmacologic treatment of fever is presented in Table 32.1.

- Pure antipyretics: acetaminophen, NSAIDs, and corticosteroids
- Goal of antipyretics is to decrease the discomfort that fevers may cause, especially when unable to identify or treat the underlying illness.
- Aspirin and NSAIDs, especially in the setting of an inflammatory response to an infectious etiology for fever, should be used with caution in patients with or at risk for thrombocytopenia due to antiplatelet effect.

SPECIAL CONSIDERATIONS

- Paraneoplastic fever:
  - Treat underlying neoplasm with definitive antineoplastic therapy
  - More responsive to NSAIDs than are infectious fevers
- Transfusion-associated fever:
  - Use leukocyte-depleted or irradiated blood products
  - Premedication with acetaminophen and diphenhydramine and use of steroids
- Drug-associated fever:
  - Cessation of the offending agent, when possible
  - Acetaminophen, NSAIDs, and steroid premedication

TABLE 32.1: PHARMACOLOGIC TREATMENT OF FEVER

Class	Medication	Doses	Side Effects
Antipyretics			
Acetaminophen	Acetaminophen	1,000 mg per single dose and up to 3,000 mg per day for geriatric adults	High doses can lead to liver damage, and the risk is heightened by alcohol consumption.
NSAIDs	Salicylates Aspirin Propionic acid derivatives Ibuprofen Naproxen	325–650 mg PO every 4h prn (max: 4 gm/day PO) 200–400 mg PO every 4–6h (max: 1200 mg/day)	The two main adverse drug reactions are GI toxicity and reduction in blood flow leading to renal insufficiency. These effects are dose-dependent and in many cases lead to dyspepsia, ulcer perforation, and upper gastrointestinal bleeding. Consider using with misoprostol or proton pump inhibitor to reduce GI risks in appropriate patients.
Corticosteroids	Prednisone Methylprednisolone	5–60 mg PO daily 4–48 mg/day PO divided daily-QID	Hyperglycemia, weight gain, facial swelling, depression, bone loss, mania, psychosis, or other psychiatric symptoms, unusual fatigue or weakness, blurred vision

Your patient's daughter tells you that she can manage the fever with acetaminophen suppositories, but that she is more concerned about the profuse sweating. She says that during his fever episodes, his clothes and bed sheets become quite drenched with sweat. She asks you whether he should receive some medications to control the sweating. She really does not want to bring her father to the hospital.

PART B: SWEATING

DEFINITION

Sweating (or perspiration) mediates core body temperature by producing transdermal evaporative heat loss. Sweating occurs when fever, exercise, or warm environments require increased heat loss to maintain or return to normal core body temperature.

PREVALENCE

Occurs in 14% to 28% of advanced cancer patients receiving palliative care, is frequently nocturnal, with severity typically rated as moderate to severe.

LIKELY ETIOLOGIES

- Idiopathic
- Tumors: neuroendocrine tumors, gonadotropin-releasing hormones (GNRH), secretory carcinoid, pheochromocytoma
- Hypothalamic disturbances
- Surgery leading to hormonal changes/imbalance (e.g., oophorectomy, orchiectomy)
- Drugs: estrogen, tamoxifen, tricyclic antidepressants, opioids (morphine, fentanyl), nifedipine, ACE inhibitors, corticosteroids, neuroleptics, anticonvulsants (topiramate), antidepressants (fluoxetine, citalopram)

TREATMENT OPTIONS

Nonpharmacologic

Treatment consists of therapy directed at the underlying cause combined with nonspecific palliative interventions.

Pharmacologic

Anecdotally, low-dose thioridazine and the H2 receptor-blocker cimetidine have been reported to have clinical efficacy in the management of malignancy-associated sweating.

TAKE-HOME POINTS

Fever

- Fever is an elevation of body temperature due to adjustment of the hypothalamic set point, usually in response to a pathological stimulus.
- Adverse consequences of fever are rare in older adults; alleviation of uncomfortable constitutional symptoms should be a priority.

Sweating

- Excessive sweating can cause significant difficulties in palliative care management, and its suppression depends on the underlying disease.
- Optimal management of fever and sweating is contingent on meticulous patient assessment, with implementation of appropriate treatment interventions concordant with patient-determined goals of care.

REFERENCES

1. Dalal S, Zhukovsky DS. Pathophysiology and management of fever. *J Support Oncol.* Jan 2006;4(1): 9–16.
2. Outzen M. Management of fever in older adults. *J Gerontol Nurs.* May 2009;35(5):17–23; quiz 24–5.
3. Zhukovsky DS. Fever and sweats in the patient with advanced cancer. *Hematol Oncol Clin North Am.* Jun 2002;16(3):579–588, viii.

33

Behavioral Disorders in Dementia

CASE

Mrs. G is a 78-year-old woman with mild Alzheimer's disease (MMSE 23 out of 30), hypertension, osteoarthritis, and urinary incontinence. Her daughter brings her to your office because she has been "acting up" for the past two weeks. Daughter reports that Mrs. G repeats stories and packs her bags several times a day, stating that she is "going home." She is up frequently at night, pacing and wandering. The other day, she struck her home attendant. Mrs. G's daughter pre-pours her medications, which include donepezil 5 mg daily, hydrochlorothiazide 25 mg daily, lisinopril 10 mg daily, baby aspirin, tolterodine LA 2 mg, and acetaminophen 500 mg once daily.

DEFINITION

The term *"behavioral and psychological symptoms in dementia"* (BPSD) refers to the noncognitive manifestations of dementia. BPSD encompasses the behavioral symptom described as "agitation" (characterized as physical or verbal, aggressive or nonaggressive) that is often related to resistance to care. Psychological symptoms include mood and psychotic symptoms, as well as sleep disturbances.

PREVALENCE

80% to 90% of patients with dementia develop at least one distressing symptom during the course of illness. Lifetime risk is nearly 100%.

CONSEQUENCES OF UNTREATED BPSD

Untreated BPSD causes distress to the patient and caregiver, and often leads to nursing-home placement.

LIKELY ETIOLOGIES

The reversible causes of BPSD are more readily treatable than the underlying dementia. Reversible causes include:

1. Organic causes:
   - Acute medical conditions such as infections (e.g., pneumonia and UTI), pain, angina, constipation, urinary retention, endocrine and electrolyte abnormalities.
   - Medication toxicity or adverse effects of new or existing medications. High-risk medications include psychotropics, opioids, and anticholinergics.
2. Environmental precipitants:
   - Unmet physical needs, e.g., hunger, thirst, fatigue, cold, hot, pain, bowel or bladder incontinence or urgency, constipation, urinary retention.
   - Known environmental triggers such as:
     - Disruption in routine. This can occur with a new caregiver, or when the familiar caregiver is sick or stressed; also due to time zone changes.
     - Overstimulation: crowded and noisy environments may cause a patient to become agitated.
     - Understimulation: may cause boredom and sleep disturbances.

DIAGNOSIS

Evaluation requires a comprehensive history, physical exam, and investigation to identify possible underlying etiologies. Only after medical, environmental, and caregiving causes are excluded can it be concluded that the primary cause of the behaviors is progression of the dementia.

History

Elicit a clear description of the behavior from the patient and/or caregivers about:

Temporal onset and course
Associated circumstances
Relationship to key environmental factors
Precipitants and relievers

Exam

- Perform a comprehensive physical examination to help identify possible

organic cause of BPSD (e.g., dehydration, infections, heart failure, pain, constipation).
- Assess mental status and rule out delirium via Confusion Assessment Method.[1] (See Chapter 34: Delirium.)
- Pay close attention to:
  - Appearance and behavior
  - Speech
  - Mood, thoughts, and perceptions
  - Cognitive function
  - Attention

Mrs. G's history was clarified, and a careful physical and neurologic exam was performed to look for reversible causes of BPSD. Her daughter reported that Mrs. G has been more incontinent these days but has had no fevers, chills, flank pain, or hematuria. Mrs. G has been eating a little less but reports no nausea, vomiting, diarrhea, or constipation. ROS is otherwise negative. There are no new medications and no changes in the caregiving environment.

Physical exam showed a low-grade fever of 100.1, blood pressure 110/70, pulse 98, RR12. Exam is negative except for some suprapubic tenderness, but no guarding, rebound or CVA tenderness. Neurological exam is nonfocal, good strength. Patient is oriented only to person and does not know why she is in your office. She can answer simple questions but is easily distracted. She recalls 0/3 items at 1 minute. She is unable to name the days of the week accurately backward.

Tests
- Tests for new cases of BPSD should include CBC, electrolytes, calcium, drug levels, urinalysis.
- Decision to pursue brain imaging, EKG, chest X-ray, and other studies should be based on history and examination.

TREATMENT OPTIONS
Always treat any organic causes of delirium. Address the underlying medical condition and/or eliminate precipitating, offending medications. Once organic causes have been excluded, numerous guidelines recommend initial trial of nonpharmacological interventions based on the following considerations:[2,4–9]

- 40% of BPSD symptoms spontaneously resolve.
- Placebo response can be substantial.
- There is no FDA-approved medication for treatment of BPSD.

Nonpharmacologic
General nonpharmacologic strategies to minimize development of BPSD include:[2,4–9]

1. Maintain a structured daily routine as predictability of daily routines is reassuring:
   - Encourage independence in ADLs.
   - Perform all ADL/IADLs in a patient-centered manner.
   - Encourage daily exercise.
2. Utilize appropriate communication skills:
   - Speak slowly and clearly in a calm and nonconfrontational manner.
   - Use simple sentence structure and repeated reminders about conversation content.
   - Follow the 3 Rs: Repeat, Reassure, Redirect.
3. Environmental modifications:
   - Keep environment comfortable, calm, and safe.
   - Home-like, familiar surroundings will maximize existing cognitive functions.
   - Conspicuously display clocks, calendars.
   - Links to the outside world through newspapers, radios, and televisions may benefit some mildly impaired patients.
   - Create meaningful activities such as pet or art therapy.
   - Have preferred music playing in the background.
   - Employ soothing aromatherapy.
   - Consider light therapy to encourage proper sleep-wake cycles.
4. For agitation or aggression that is NOT harmful to self or others:
   - **AVOID** physical restraints.
   - Identify and address precipitating factors.
   - Minimize known triggers.
   - Do not confront patient about unwanted behaviors.
5. Employ alternate strategies for agitation or aggression:
   - Distraction techniques.
   - Positive reinforcement to encourage desirable behaviors.
   - Nonpharmacological techniques described above.

6. Nonpharmacologic strategies for sleep disturbances in dementia:[2,4,10]
   - Follow structured sleep and rising times that do not deviate more than 30 minutes. Encourage patients to limit naps to 30 minutes or less, and avoid naps after 1 p.m.
   - Optimize sleep environment by reducing light/noise levels and keeping temperature comfortable.
   - Walk or exercise for 30 minutes daily.
   - Use relaxation, stress management, breathing techniques to promote natural sleep.
   - Modified massage approaches such as hand massage have been found to be helpful in reducing agitation and other distressing behaviors; these can be easily administered by caregivers. (See Chapter 17: Complementary and Alternative Medicine.)
   - Eliminate triggers for nighttime awakenings, i.e., control nighttime pain, give evening snack, administer activating medications in the morning.
   - Reduce or eliminate caffeine, alcohol, and nicotine. Switch to decaffeinated drinks and reduce evening fluid consumption.
   - If nocturia affects sleep, exclude urinary tract infections. Encourage toileting schedules at night, and use of incontinence pads.

Pharmacologic

If nonpharmacological interventions fail, or if "agitated" behaviors become harmful or distressing to patient or others, consider pharmacological agents. Targeted symptoms should be matched to relevant drug class.[2-4,9]

1. **For depression in dementia:**
   - For depression of two weeks' duration resulting in significant distress or sustained depressive features lasting more than two months, use SSRIs.[2-4,7] (Table 33.1) Consider sertraline and citalopram first, given favorable side effect profile and evidence-based studies.[4]
   - If SSRIs are not effective or if the patient is unable to tolerate, consider other classes of antidepressants (i.e., SNRI, TCAs). Tricyclic antidepressants should be avoided because of their cardiac and anticholinergic side effects.

- Though mood stabilizers and psychostimulants may have a theoretic benefit, the use of valproate is not supported by evidence,[11] and the effectiveness of carbemezepine is equivocal for treatment of BPSD.[4]
- If psychostimulants are used to accelerate the treatment of apathetic depression, use them with caution, as this class may worsen delusion and hallucinations.

2. **For sleep disturbances in dememtia**
   - For sleep disturbances unrelated to depression or other psychiatric conditions, and that do not resolve with nonpharmacologic strategies, use time-limited trials of FDA-approved hypnotics. (Table 33.2)
   - Underlying conditions should be investigated carefully before introduction of any drug therapy. Clinicians should note the following:
     - Current guidelines on pharmacologic treatments apply only for primary sleep disorders.
     - Randomized controlled trials of newer agents have not been tested in this population.
     - Benzodiazepine receptor agonists should not be used more than three times a week, given risk of tolerance and development of paradoxical insomnia when the agent is stopped.
   - Avoid benzodiazepines and antihistamines.

3. **For agitation and aggression in dementia**
   - For distressing agitation/aggression or intermittent distressing delusions or hallucinations persisting for at least one month, guidelines suggest time-limited trial of antipsychotics after nonpharmacologic attempts have failed (Table 33.3).[2-4,9]
   - If a patient is unable to tolerate antipsychotics, consider cholinesterase inhibitors or SSRIs for controlling agitation.[4]

A check of CBC differential, chemistries, UA, and urine culture reveals UA with positive nitrites and leukocyte esterase, mild leukocytosis with left shift but otherwise normal chemistries. Bactrim is prescribed, and Mrs. G's incontinence resolves and her behavior returns to baseline.

TABLE 33.1: TREATMENT OF DEPRESSIVE FEATURES OF BPSD (MEDICATIONS LISTED ARE NOT FDA-APPROVED TO TREAT BPSD AND ARE OFF-LABEL RECOMMENDATIONS.[4,9])

Class	Daily Dose	Comments
Selective serotonin reuptake inhibitors		**Target symptoms:** Depression and anxiety; limited studies on efficacy
		Watch for: GI upset, hepatotoxicity, bleeding, insomnia, asthenia, strokes, seizures, QTc prolongation, SIADH hyponatremia, serotonin syndrome, pancytopenia, glaucoma, impotence.
		Black Box Warning: Children and young adults have a higher suicide risk
		Avoid: Monoamine oxidase inhibitors for 2 weeks; abrupt withdrawal Generics available unless otherwise indicated
Citalopram (Preferred)	10–20 mg	Class effect as above Significant improvement in agitation, aggression, psychosis Avoid doses > 20 mg in patients > 65 year given dose-dependent QTc prolongation Available as tablet and solution
Escitalopram	5–10 mg	Class effect as above **Avoid:** Doses > 10 mg in patients > 65 year given dose-dependent QTc prolongation Available as tablet and solution No generics available
Fluoxetine (Avoid)	10–40 mg	Class effect as above Tendency to avoid because of many cytochrome P-450–related drug interactions Available as tablet, capsule, and sustained release, solution
Paroxetine (Avoid)	10–40 mg	Class effect as above Tendency to avoid because of many cytochrome P-450–related drug interactions Available as tablet, controlled release, and solution
Sertraline *Preferred	25–100 mg	Class effect as above Sertraline (25–50 mg) showed significant improvement in the agitation behaviors Available as tablet or solution
Trazodone	25–150 mg	Class effect as above. Watch especially for sedation, falls, hypotension Used especially for insomnia Available as tablet
Serotonin norepinephrine-mediated		
Bupropion	75–225 mg	**Target symptoms:** Depression More activating, relative lack of cardiac effects
		Watch for: Irritability, insomnia, increased seizure risk (especially in patients with opiate, stimulant, alcohol use), rash, HTN, QTc prolongation, anaphylaxis
		Black Box Warning: Children and young adults have a higher suicide risk
		Avoid: Concurrent use of MAOI x 2 weeks Available as tablet, extended release Generics available

(continued)

TABLE 33.1: (CONTINUED)

Class	Daily Dose	Comments
SNRI's		**Target symptoms:** Depression
		Watch for: GI upset, hepatotoxicity, bleeding, insomnia, strokes, seizures, QTc prolongation, orthostatic hypotension, SIADH hyponatremia, serotonin syndrome, pancytopenia, glaucoma, impotence
		Black Box Warning: Children and young adults have a higher suicide risk
		Avoid: Monoamine oxidase inhibitors for 2 weeks; abrupt withdrawal Generic available for all
Duloxetine	20–60 mg	Class effect as above but watch especially for nausea, dry mouth, dizziness Useful for diabetic neuropathy Available as capsule
Mirtazapine	7.5–30 mg	Class effect as above. Watch especially for sedation, hypotension, hypertriglyceridemia, ALT transaminitis Useful for depression with significant insomnia and anorexia Available as tablet, disintegrating tablet
Venlafaxine	25–150 mg	Class effect as above but watch especially for hypertension, insomnia Useful in severe depression Available as tablet, capsule, extended release
Tricyclics Avoid amitryptyline		**Target symptoms:** Depression and anxiety
		Watch for: GI upset, hepatotoxicity, bleeding, strokes, seizures, cardiac arrhythmias, QTc prolongation, anticholinergic side effects, sedation, hypotension, SIADH hyponatremia, serotonin syndrome, pancytopenia, glaucoma, impotence
		Black Box Warning: Children and young adults have a higher suicide risk
		Avoid: Monoamine oxidase inhibitors for 2 weeks; abrupt withdrawal Generics available for all
Desipramine	10–100 mg	Class effect as above Available as tablet
Nortriptyline	10–75 mg	Class effect as above High efficacy for depression if side effects are tolerable Check nortriptyline level to monitor for toxicity Therapeutic range 50–150 ng/dL Available as tablet, capsule, solution
Psycho-stimulants		**Target symptoms:** Depression and fatigue
		MOA: Activates brainstem arousal
		Black Box Warning: May cause chronic abuse, especially in patients with prior drug dependence or alcholism
		Watch for: Agitation, akathesia, insomnia, seizures, strokes, seizures, hypertension, cardiac arrhythmias, pancytopenia, eosinophilia, rash
		Avoid: Monoamine oxidase inhibitors for 2 weeks; abrupt withdrawal Generics available
Methylphenidate	10–60 mg (divided 2–3 times daily)	Class effect as above Available as tablet, capsule, chewable tablets, extended release, solution, transdermal
Modafinil	200–400 mg	Class effect as above Available as tablet

TABLE 33.2: TREATMENT OF SLEEP DISTURBANCES IN BPSD (MEDICATIONS LISTED ARE NOT FDA-APPROVED TO TREAT BPSD AND ARE OFF-LABEL RECOMMENDATIONS.[4,9])

Class	Daily Dose	Comments
FDA approved Hyponotics Benzodiazepine Receptor Agonists		**Target symtom:** Insomnia Risk of dependence
		Associated with: High risk for falls, hip fractures, disinhibition, and cognitive disturbance, amnesia, worsening depression
		Avoid: abrupt withdrawal Generics available
Benzodiazepine		Avoid given side effect profile
Temezepam	7.5–30 mg	Class effect as above Available as capsule
Triazolam	0.125–0.5 mg	Class effect as above Available as tablet
Nonbenzodiazepine		**Watch for:** agitation, hallucination, visual disturbances, dizziness, headaches, anaphylaxis, diarrhea, chest pain, tachycardia Risk of dependence
		Avoid: abrupt withdrawal Generics available unless otherwise indicated
Zolpidem	5–10 mg 6.25–12.5 mg	Class effect as above Available as tablet, extended release, oral spray
Zaleplon	5–20 mg	Class effect as above
		Watch for: in aspirin sensitive, increase risk of tartrazine sensitivity, including bronchial asthma Available as capsule
Eszopiclone	1–3 mg	Class effect as above Available as tablet No generics available
Melatonin Receptor Agonists		
Ramelteon	8 mg	**Target symtom:** Insomnia
		Watch for: anaphylaxis, hallucination, agitation, mania, worsening depression Not recommended in patients with sleep apnea, severe hepatic impairment

TABLE 33.3: TREATMENT OF AGITATION, AGGRESSION, AND PSYCHOTIC SYMPTOMS IN BPSD (MEDICATIONS LISTED ARE NOT FDA APPROVED TO TREAT BPSD AND ARE OFF-LABEL RECOMMENDATIONS.[2-4,9])

Class	Daily Dose	Comments
Antipsychotics		**Watch for:** extrapyramidal effects, tardive diskinesia, neuroleptic malignant syndrome, hypotension, QTc prolongation and torsades de pointes, anticholinergic side effects (i.e., constipation, xerostomia, and somnolence), agranulocytosis, blurred vision; also may lower seizure threshold (*See Black Box warning*[a])

(continued)

TABLE 33.3: (CONTINUED)

Class	Daily Dose	Comments
Haloperidol	0.5–2 mg q2–12 hrs	Class effect as above. Watch esp for extrapyramidal effects can occur with doses >4.5 mg/d More effective for treating aggressive agitation Available as oral, IV, IM, subcutaneous
Aripiprazole	5–15 mg (Max 30 mg/d)	Class effect as above. Watch especially for increased cerebrovascular events in dementia, hyperglycemia, and weight gain Clinical experience suggests better results in hypoactive delirium No adjustment needed with age, renal or hepatic impairment Available as tablet, disintegrating tablet, liquid concentrate, IM (convert to oral ASAP)
Clozapine	12.5–200 mg increase by 25–50 mg/day	Class effect as above. Watch especially for agranulocytosis which requires weekly CBCs and hyperglycemia and myocarditis Poorly tolerated by older adults, so reserved for treatment of refractory cases Do not stop abruptly; taper Available as tablet, rapidly dissolving tablet
Olanzapine	2.5–10 mg	Class effect as above. Watch especially for hyperglycemia and cerebrovascular events in patients with dementia Risperidone and olanzepine effective for aggressive agitation Literature suggests that older age, pre-existing dementia, and hypoactive delirium are associated with poor response Available as tablet, rapidly dissolving tablet, IM injection
Quetiapine	25–200 mg	Class effect as above. Watch especially for hyperglycemia Preferred in patients with Parkinson disease or Lewy body dementia due to its lower risk of extrapyramidal adverse effects Ophthalmologic exam recommended every 6 months Available as tablet
Risperidone	0.5–2/4 mg	Class effect as above and EPS with doses > 1 mg/day Clinical experience suggest better results in patients with hypoactive delirium Risperidone and olanzepine effective for aggressive agitation but risperidone may be more helpful for psychotic symptoms Available as tablet, rapidly dissolving tablet, liquid concentrate, IM
Ziprasidone	40–160 mg	Class effect as above. Watch especially for increased QTc prolongation Evidence is limited to case reports and little published information on use in older adults Least preferred in the medically ill due to risk of QT prolongation vs. other atypical antipsychotics Available in capsule, IM injection

[a] **Black Box Warning for antipsychotic medications:**
Increased risk of mortality. Rate of death was 1.6 to 1.7 times that of placebo.
Mortality: 2.6 vs. 4.5% with just 10–12 weeks of use
Death appeared to be heart-related or from infections (e.g., pneumonia).
Watch for: Diabetes mellitus, hyperglycemia, ketoacidosis, and hyperosmolar states

Note. CBCs = complete blood cell counts
EPS = extrapyramidal symptoms
IM = intramuscular

TAKE-HOME POINTS

- Always obtain a thorough history about disturbing behavioral and psychological symptoms in dementia.
- Rule out delirium and other environmental factors contributing to the behavioral symptoms.
- Nonpharmacologic interventions for BPSD should always be the initial and preferred approach.
- Consider "targeted," time-limited pharmacologic trials for severe or persistent BPSD symptoms. However, given modest evidence of efficacy and moderate level of risk, it is important to choose the agent with the least potential for harm.

REFERENCES

1. Inouye SK. *The confusion assessment method (CAM): training manual and coding guide 2003.* Boston: Yale University School of Medicine; 2003.
2. Salzman C, Jeste D, Meyer RE, et al. Elderly patients with dementia-related symptoms of severe agitation and aggression: consensus statement on treatment options, clinical trials methodology, and policy. *J Clin Psychiatry.* 2008;69(6):889–898.
3. Jeste DV, Blazer D, Casey D, Meeks T, et al. ACNP White Paper: update on use of antipsychotic drugs in elderly persons with dementia. *Neuropsychopharmacology.* 2008;33:957–970.
4. Rabins PV et al. American Psychiatric Association practice guideline for the treatment of patients with Alzheimer's disease and other dementias. Second edition. *Am J Psychiatry.* 2007;164(suppl 12): 5–56.
5. Livingston G, Johnston K, Katona C, et al. Systematic review of psychological approaches to the management of neuropsychiatric symptoms of dementia. *Am J Psychiatry.* 2005;162(11): 1996–2021.
6. Ayalon L, Gum AM, Feliciano L, Areán PA. Effectiveness of nonpharmacological interventions for the management of neuropsychiatric symptoms in patients with dementia: a systematic review. *Arch Intern Med.* 2006;166(20):2182–2188.
7. Gitlin LN, Winter L, Dennis MP, Hodgson N, Hauck WW. A biobehavioral home-based intervention and the well-being of patients with dementia and their caregivers: the COPE randomized trial. *JAMA.* Sep 1, 2010;304(9):983–991.
8. Gitlin LN, Winter L, Dennis MP, Hodgson N, Hauck WW. Targeting and managing behavioral symptoms in individuals with dementia: a randomized trial of a nonpharmacological intervention. *J Am Geriatr Soc.* Aug 2010;58(8):1465–1474.
9. Zec RF, Burkett NR. Non-pharmacological and pharmacological treatment of the cognitive and behavioral symptoms of Alzheimer disease. *NeuroRehabilitation.* 2008;23(5):425–438.
10. McCurry SM et al. Nighttime insomnia treatment and education for Alzheimer's disease: a RCT. *JAGS.* 2005;53(5):793–802.
11. Lonergan E, Luxenberg J. Valproate preparations for agitation in dementia. *Cochrane Database of Systematic Reviews* 2009, Issue 3. Art. No: CD003945. DOI: 10.1002/1465185

34

Delirium

CASE

Mr. Smith is an 83-year-old, cognitively intact male with a past medical history of hormone refractory prostate cancer with metastases to the spine with spinal cord compression. He is on dexamethasone and receiving radiation therapy for pain. On day 3, the nurse found him lying on the floor mumbling to himself. Intermittently, he argues with his nurse and has angrily refused to have blood samples drawn.

DEFINITION

Delirium is a syndrome characterized by an acute change in cognition and attention that fluctuates throughout the day. Clinical criteria used to diagnose delirium include acute onset and fluctuating course, inattention, and either disorganized thinking or altered level of consciousness.[1]

Delirium is a sign of significant physiologic disturbances that may be a symptom of a medical emergency.

PREVALENCE

- Delirium is not commonly found in non-demented individuals living in the community or in long-term care. Prevalence is estimated at <0.5%. It may, however, affect up to 50% of hospitalized patients with risk factors for delirium.[2,3]
- Persistent delirium also affects 23% of patients admitted to post-acute skilled nursing facilities from the hospital. The prevalence of delirium among older patients discharged from the hospital into the community remains unknown.
- Delirium is the most common neuropsychiatric complication experienced by patients with advanced illness, occurring in up to 85% of patients in the last weeks of life.[4]

CONSEQUENCES OF UNTREATED DELIRIUM

Both apathetic and agitated delirium are distressing and frightening for patients and families; episodes are often remembered with anxiety, even after the delirium has cleared. Delirium is associated with:

- Increased caregiver burden and higher rates of nursing home placement
- Increased morbidity and mortality as a harbinger of impending death in patients who are terminally ill; also with adverse outcomes such as aspiration, prolonged immobility, and persistent functional decline[2,3]
- Higher health care costs associated with increase in length of hospital stay and costs per day.

LIKELY ETIOLOGIES

Delirium is often precipitated by multiple organic etiologies, and it is often misdiagnosed or unrecognized, especially the "quiet" or apathetic form of delirium.

Delirium frequently indicates underlying medical problems. Up to 50% of delirium episodes in palliative care patients are potentially reversible.[5] Possible precipitating causes include:

- Infections
- Electrolyte abnormalities, including hypoglycemia, hypercalcemia, hypernatremia, and hyponatremia
- Organ failure, including hypoxia, ischemia, stroke, seizures
- Pain—among the most potent predictors of delirium. Risk of delirium is markedly decreased when pain is treated.
- Medication adverse effects, especially involving high-risk medications such as:
  - Anticholinergics:
    - Histamine H2 blockers (e.g., hydroxyzine, diphenhydramine, ranitidine, famotidine)
    - Antispasmodics (e.g., hyoscyamine)
    - Antiarrhythmics (e.g., digoxin)
    - Diuretics (e.g., furosemide)
    - Antiparkinson (e.g., benzatropine)
    - Overactive bladder treatments (e.g., oxybutnin, tolterodine)

- Bronchodilators (e.g., theophylline)
- Steroids, or abrupt discontinuation of steroids
- Sedatives/hypnotics
- Opioids, especially hyperalgesia from excess opioid doses, or abrupt discontinuation*
- Antidepressants, antipsychotics, benzodiazepines*

(*Note: Despite the risk posed for delirium, medications such as opioids, antipsychotics, and benzodiazepines are often necessary to manage pain and other symptoms which may precipitate delirium if not treated.)

- Withdrawal from alcohol, illicit drugs, or benzodiazepine
- Constipation
- Urinary catheters
- Surgery
- Sleep deprivation due to environmental factors such as excessive noise and interrupted sleep
- New or strange environment

RISK FACTORS
- Age >65
- Cognitive impairment
- Acute illness
- Severe illness
- Infection or hospital admission
- Multiple chronic comorbidities including:
  - Dementia
  - Visual or hearing impairment
  - Functional dependence, immobility, or frailty
  - Acute or chronic renal and hepatic impairment
  - Malnutrition
  - Alcohol excess or withdrawal
- Multiple medications

CLINICAL SUBTYPES OF DELIRIUM
1. Hypoactive subtype (also known as apathetic, quiet, hypoalert, hypoaroused):
   - Most common subtype in the palliative care setting; characterized by psychomotor retardation, lethargy, sedation, and reduced awareness of surroundings
   - Generally occurs with hypoxia, metabolic disturbances, and anticholinergic medications
   - Often mistaken for depression or fatigue and is difficult to differentiate from

sedation attributable to medication side effects, or lethargy in the last days of life
   - Associated with higher mortality than hyperactive delirium. Patients with hypoactive delirium were 1.62 times more likely to die compared with patients who had the hyperactive or mixed subtypes.[4]
   - Associated with significant patient and family distress
2. Hyperactive subtype (also known as hyperalert, agitated, hyperaroused):
   - Characterized by restlessness, agitation, hypervigilance, hallucinations, and delusions
   - Common with alcohol and drug withdrawal, drug intoxication, or medication adverse effects
3. Mixed subtype: a combination of alternating hypoactive and hyperactive delirium states.

DIAGNOSIS

History
History should be focused on risk factors and potentially reversible etiologies listed above, with a thorough review of the medication list for high-risk medications and other drug interactions.

Exam
- Physical examination should assess for signs of infection, dehydration, pain, constipation, fecal impaction, urinary retention, or organ failure. A systematic search for possible reversible etiologies should be conducted.
- Diagnosis of delirium is made clinically. Use the Confusion Assessment Method (CAM).[1] Diagnosis of delirium requires a present or abnormal rating for criteria 1 and 2, plus either 3 or 4.

Criteria:

1. Acute onset and fluctuating course:
   - Is there evidence of an acute change in mental status from the patient's baseline? Corroboration with caregivers and family member is usually required.
   - Did the behavior come and go or wax or wane in severity in the last 24 hours?
2. Inattention:
   - Does the patient have difficulty focusing attention?
   - Is the patient easily distracted?

- Does the patient have difficulty keeping track of what is being said?
- Consider asking the patient to recite the days of the week backward.
3. Disorganized thinking:
    - Is the patient's speech disorganized or incoherent?
    - Does the patient ramble or have irrelevant conversation that is unclear with illogical flow of ideas and unpredictable switching between subjects?
4. Altered level of consciousness:
    - Patients who are calm and alert are considered normal.
    - Patients meet criteria if they are vigilant (hyperalert), lethargic (drowsy, but easily aroused), stuporous (difficult to arouse), or comatose.

Tests

Diagnostic testing will depend upon on history and physical examination findings in the context of patient preferences and goals of care. If results will directly influence treatment, consider the following:

- Laboratory tests such as a CBC with differential, coagulations studies, comprehensive chemistries, drug levels, arterial blood gases, cultures, and EKG
- Brain imaging (to rule out brain metastases, intracranial bleeding, or ischemia), electroencephalogram (to rule out seizures), and lumbar puncture (to rule out leptomeningeal carcinomatosis or meningitis)

TREATMENT OPTIONS

When possible, always treat the underlying medical condition that triggered the delirium.

Nonpharmacologic

- Use of nonpharmacological interventions in the treatment of delirium has resulted in faster improvement of symptoms and cognition scores without adverse effect on mortality or health-related quality of life (level I).[4,6]
- Addressing six risk factors (cognitive impairment, sleep deprivation, dehydration, immobility, vision impairment, and hearing impairment) can reduce the incidence of delirium by 33%.[7]

- All of the prevention and treatment trials with nonpharmacologic interventions were conducted in general medical units or in postoperative patients, not in the palliative care setting. Some of these trials allowed the use of antipsychotics and cholinesterase inhibitors when indicated.[4,6]
- Nonpharmacologic interventions to reduce the risk of delirium include:
    - Place familiar objects (e.g., family photographs), an orientation board, and a clock in patient rooms
    - Reorient patients and encourage cognitively stimulating activities
    - Provide visual and hearing aids when available
    - Facilitate sleep hygiene measures, including relaxation music at bedtime, warm drinks, and gentle massage; avoid waking patients from sleep
    - Minimize noise and interventions at bedtime (e.g., consider minimizing medications after bedtime)
    - Mobilize early, avoid immobility, and avoid indwelling catheters, intravenous lines, and physical restraints
    - Review medications
    - Control pain
    - Monitor nutrition and dehydration, bowel and bladder functioning, and fluid-electrolyte balance

Pharmacologic

- When possible, always try nonpharmacologic interventions for delirium before resorting to pharmacologic strategies.
- Evidence on the safety and effectiveness of antipsychotic medications for the management of delirium symptoms is limited.[8,9] (Box 34.1)
- Despite the lack of sufficient data, the pharmacologic management of delirium in older medical and surgical patients is nevertheless recommended by many experts, especially in situations where adequate care is jeopardized, for patients with severe behavioral or emotional disturbances, and if nonpharmacological methods are not successful.[9]
- Time-limited trials of antipsychotics should be reserved for patients who, despite treatment of the medical

BOX 34.1   BLACK BOX WARNING FOR ALL ANTIPSYCHOTIC MEDICATIONS[10,11]

- Increased risk of mortality. Rate of death was 1.6 to 1.7 times that of placebo.
- Mortality: 2.6 vs. 4.5% with just 10–12 weeks of use.
- Death appeared to be heart-related or from infections (e.g., pneumonia).

condition that triggered the delirium, pose a risk to themselves or others. These medications may prolong or aggravate delirium in some cases and are associated with mortality among dementia patients (Table 34.1).

MANAGEMENT OF DELIRIUM IN TERMINALLY ILL PATIENTS[4]

- The ideal goal of delirium management for a patient in the last days of life is to keep the patient pain-free, awake, alert, calm,

cognitively intact, and able to communicate coherently with family and staff.
- Use haloperidol 0.5–2 mg in divided doses (Level I). Alternative (more sedating) treatment includes chlorpromazine 12.5–50 mg q 4–6 hr.
- May add clonazepam 0.5–1mg every 2 to 4 hr.
- When delirium is a consequence of the dying process, the goal of care may shift to providing comfort through the judicious use of sedatives, even at the expense of alertness.

TABLE 34.1: TREATMENT OF AGITATION AND PSYCHOTIC SYMPTOMS IN DELIRIUM (NONE OF THE MEDICATIONS LISTED IS FDA-APPROVED TO TREAT DELIRIUM; ALL ARE OFF-LABEL RECOMMENDATIONS.)

Class	Daily Dose	Comments
Antipsychotics		**Watch for:** Extrapyramidal effects, tardive diskinesia, neuroleptic malignant syndrome, hypotension, QTc prolongation and torsades de pointes, anticholinergic side effects (e.g., constipation, xerostomia, and somnolence), agranulocytosis, blurred vision. May lower seizure threshold. **Black Box warning:** See Table 2
Haloperidol	0.5–2 mg q2–12 hrs	Class effect as above. Extrapyramidal effects can occur with doses >4.5 mg/d More effective for treating aggressive agitation Remains first-line therapy for terminal delirium[1] A randomized controlled trial of haloperidol and chlorpromazine found that both drugs were equally effective in hypoactive and hyperactive subtypes of delirium[1] May add lorazepam (0.5–1mg every 2 to 4 h) for agitated patients[1] Available as oral, IV, IM, subcutaneous
Chlorpromazine	12.5–50 mg q 4–6 hr	Class effect as above. Watch especially for photosensitivity More sedating and anticholinergic compared with haloperidol A randomized controlled trial of haloperidol and chlorpromazine found that both drugs were equally effective in hypoactive and hyperactive subtypes of delirium Preferred in agitated patients due to its sedative effect[1] Available as oral, IV, IM, subcutaneous (not recommended), per rectum
Aripiprazole	5–15 mg (Max 30 mg/d)	Class effect as above. Watch especially for increased cerebrovascular events, hyperglycemia and weight gain Clinical experience suggests better results in hypoactive delirium. No adjustment needed with age, renal or hepatic impairment Available as tablet, disintegrating tablet, liquid concentrate, IM (convert to oral ASAP)

(continued)

TABLE 34.1: (CONTINUED)

Class	Daily Dose	Comments
Clozapine	12.5–200 mg daily increase 25–50 mg/day	Class effect as above. Watch especially for agranulocytosis, which requires weekly CBCs and hyperglycemia and myocarditis Poorly tolerated by older adults so reserved for treatment of refractory cases Do not stop abruptly. Taper Available as tablet, rapidly dissolving tablet
Olanzapine	2.5–10 mg	Class effect as above. Watch especially for hyperglycemia and cerebrovascular events Risperidone and olanzepine effective for aggressive agitation Literature suggests that older age, pre-existing dementia, and hypoactive delirium are associated with poor response to olanzapine. Available as tablet, rapidly dissolving tablet, IM injection
Quetiapine	25–200 mg	Class effect as above. Watch especially for hyperglycemia Preferred in patients with Parkinson's disease or Lewy body dementia due to its lower risk of extrapyramidal adverse effects Ophthalmologic exam recommended every 6 months Available as tablet
Risperidone	0.5–2/4 mg	Class effect as above and EPS with doses > 1 mg/day Clinical experience suggest better results in patients with hypoactive delirium Risperidone and olanzepine effective for aggressive agitation, but risperidone may be more helpful for psychotic symptoms Available as tablet, rapidly dissolving tablet, liquid concentrate, IM
Ziprasidone	40–160 mg	Class effect as above. Watch especially for increased QTc prolongation Evidence is limited to case reports and little published information on use in older adults Least preferred in the medically ill due to risk of QT prolongation vs. other atypical antipsychotics Available to capsule, IM injection

Note: CBCs = complete blood cell counts; EPS = extrapyramidal symptoms; IM = intramuscular

Mr. Smith has mixed hyper- and hypoactive delirium according to CAM criteria. A careful physical and neurologic examination and review of the medication list suggested dexamethasone, acute spinal cord compression, and environmental changes as key contributors to his delirium. Employing nonpharmacologic interventions as well as administering the lowest effective dose of the steroids may help. Judicious, time-limited use of antipsychotics such as haloperidol or risperidone may be considered if the patient is harmful to self or others, or if delirium is associated with significant patient and family distress and suffering.

TAKE-HOME POINTS
- When possible, treat the underlying medical condition that triggered the delirium.
- Always obtain a thorough history about the "agitated disturbance." Systematically review the history and physical exam to identify common precipitants of delirium.
- Diagnostic testing will depend upon on history and physical examination findings in the context of patient preferences and goals of care.
- After reversible organic causes have been addressed, use nonpharmacologic interventions to treat and/or prevent delirium.
- When nonpharmacologic interventions fail, a time-limited trial of antipsychotics may be used to treat patients with frightening or persistent delirium. However, given that the evidence for these medications is modest at best, it is important to choose the agent with the least potential for harm.

- For terminal patients, judicious use of haloperidol, or chlorpromazine if more sedation is needed, is recommended.
- Lorazepam or another benzodiazepine should be added only if antipsychotics alone are ineffective. Benzodiazepines alone may worsen delirium.

REFERENCES

1. Inouye SK. *The confusion assessment method (CAM): training manual and coding guide 2003.* Boston: Yale University School of Medicine; 2003.
2. Inouye SK. Delirium in hospitalized older patients. *Clin Geriatr Med.* 1998;*14*(4):745–764.
3. Siddiqi N, Holt R, Britton AM, Holmes J. Interventions for preventing delirium in hospitalised patients. *Cochrane Database Syst Rev.* 2007, Issue 2. Art. No: CD005563. DOI: 10.1002/14651858. CD005563.pub2.
4. Breitbart W, Alici Y. Agitation and delirium at the end of life: "We couldn't manage him" *JAMA.* 2008;*300*(24):2898–2910.
5. Leonard M, Raju B, Conroy M, et al. Reversibility of delirium in terminally ill patients and predictors of mortality. *Palliat Med.* 2008;*22*(7):848–854.
6. Pitkälä KH, Laurila JV, Strandberg TE, Tilvis RS. Multicomponent geriatric intervention for elderly inpatients with delirium: a randomized, controlled trial. *J Gerontol A Biol Sci Med Sci.* 2006;*61*(2):176–181.
7. Inouye SK, Bogardus ST Jr, Charpentier PA, et al. A multicomponent intervention to prevent delirium in hospitalized older patients. *N Engl J Med.* 1999;*340*(9):669–676.
8. Michaud L, Bula C, Berney A, et al. Delirium: guidelines for general hospitals. *J Psychosom Res.* 2007; *6*:371–383.
9. Flaherty JH, Gonzales JP, Dong B. Antipsychotics in the treatment of delirium in older hospitalized adults: a systematic review. *JAGS.* 2011;*59*: S269–S276.
10. US Food and Drug Administration. Public Health Advisory: Deaths with antipsychotics in elderly patients with behavioral disturbances. 3/02/10. http://www.fda.gov/Drugs/ DrugSafety/ PostmarketDrugSafetyInformationforPatientsand Providers/DrugSafetyInformationforHeathcare Professionals/PublicHealthAdvisories/ucm053171. htm.
11. US Food and Drug Administration MedWatch Safety Summary. Antipsychotics, Conventional and Atypical. http://www.fda.gov/medwatch/safety/ 2008/safety08.htm#Antipsychotics. June 2008.

35

Terminal Delirium

CASE

Mrs. LS is a 66-year-old female with history of hepatitis C, cirrhosis, end-stage kidney disease requiring hemodialysis (HD), and distant intravenous drug abuse. She was admitted to the hospital after a change in mental status during HD. She was septic and treated with antibiotics. She is lethargic and has difficulty maintaining focus during conversations.

DEFINITION

Terminal delirium refers to the "restlessness" that occurs in patients who are actively dying (with hours to days left to live). While most people die by slipping into deeper and deeper stages of unconsciousness until they are comatose, a small percentage develop agitation, restlessness, and moaning. This cluster of behaviors is often unrecognized as a sign of active dying and is undertreated. The symptom is extremely distressing for patients and families and should be medically managed.[1]

PREVALENCE

While delirium is found in 14% to 56% of hospitalized elderly, terminal delirium occurs in 80% to 90% of dying patients. The overall reversibility rate of delirium is 49% in patients with advanced cancer admitted to a palliative care unit.

CONSEQUENCES OF UNTREATED TERMINAL DELIRIUM

- Patients are often aware of their confusion and agitation, and may feel frightened or paranoid
- Increased family and caregiver distress
- Can contribute to complicated and prolonged grief disorder
- Diminishes the opportunity for closure of relationships at the end of life

LIKELY ETIOLOGIES

- While the causes of delirium are often multifactorial, some contributors such as pain, constipation, and urinary retention can be corrected. The causes of terminal delirium are similar to delirium but occur in the context of terminal illness. (See Chapter 34: Delirium.)
- It is estimated that in 50% of cases, terminal delirium is caused by a reversible etiology.[2] According to recent studies, reversibility of delirium is highly dependent on the etiology.[3] Delirium caused by hypercalcemia was judged reversible in 38% of cases; by medications (37%); by infection (12%); by hepatic failure, hypoxia, disseminated intravascular coagulation, and dehydration each (<10%).
- Irreversibility of delirium was associated with major organ failure and hypoxic encephalopathy.[4]

DIAGNOSIS

History

- If the goal is to attempt to reverse the delirium to give the family potentially more quality time with the patient, then a targeted history and a physical exam focused on reversible etiologies such as pain, constipation, urinary retention, and basic metabolic disturbances may be reasonable.
- If the patient is experiencing terminal delirium, which occurs hours to days before death, extensive workup usually is not in the patient's best interest. Benefit versus burden of workup should be considered.
- If the cause of delirium is thought to be multifactorial, and not likely to be corrected, more attention should be given to controlling the symptoms and supporting the family and caregivers, rather than correcting the cause.

Exam

While the presentation of terminal delirium meets all the criteria of Confusion Assessment Method (CAM), it is often characterized by moans, groans, grimaces, and restlessness that may make the patient appear as if in pain or in distress.

Tests

While an evaluation for readily reversible etiologies should be completed in terminal delirium, extensive testing is often not helpful for the following reasons:

- Patients have a limited life expectancy
- There may be metabolic or disease processes that cannot be reversed
- Diagnostic workup may reveal no precipitant or obvious cause; labs and vital signs may all appear normal

TREATMENT OPTIONS[4]

Treatment of terminal delirium should focus on controlling the symptom, correcting simple reversible causes, establishing support measures, and avoiding complications.

Nonpharmacologic

1. Anticipate terminal delirium by identifying patients who may be at higher risk, and remain vigilant to warning signs or symptoms.
2. Educate family and caregivers as to the nature and cause of the behavior they may observe. Informing families of what to expect may help them to cope with the distressing changes they observe in their loved one. Examples of this approach include:
    - Reassure family that behaviors normally associated as cause and effect may not have such a relationship in delirium. For example, moaning may be caused by pain, but if it does not respond to analgesia, it is most likely due to delirium.
    - Alerting family as to the fluctuating nature of mental status and confusion may help them recognize this pattern.
    - Providing an explanation of the process of delirium and dying may facilitate decision-making about goals for treating the delirium.
    - Explain that controlling the symptom includes manipulating the environment to allow for orientation.

3. Advise that maintaining a quiet and peaceful environment will also help to reduce the stress on family and caregivers.
4. Allow family members to participate in caregiving to the extent that is safe and comfortable for the patient and the family.

Pharmacologic

- Treatment options and choice of medication depend on the goals of the patient and family. Hallucinations that are pleasant and therefore not distressing to the patient and family may not need pharmacologic intervention. Family education and support may be sufficient.
- While neuroleptic or antipsychotic medications may be used initially if the patient's and family's goals are for quality time together, sedating medications are often needed to decrease the agitation that accompanies terminal delirium. (Table 35.1) Benzodiazepines can also be used, only after antipsychotics have been tried without success, but in the event of a paradoxical reaction, higher doses may be indicated. (See Chapter 65: Anxiety.)

HELPFUL LANGUAGE FOR EXPLAINING TERMINAL DELIRIUM TO FAMILIES

"I would like to take a few minutes to explain the behavior you are seeing, if you are interested/able to hear about it..."

"I would be happy to share with you some things that you may see your loved one do or say, if you feel like you can hear it..."

"I know that the moaning/restlessness/groaning you are seeing may seem like your loved one is in pain, but when patients are delirious, the behavior we see isn't always in response to a cause we can identify. We are treating your loved one for any pain he/she may be having, but the moaning/restlessness/groaning could be for a reason we can't identify or for no reason at all..."

"This confusion may be due to several things, and I would like to discuss how much testing we should do in order to identify the actual problem..."

"We hope that we can identify the cause of this confusion. We are treating the symptoms your loved one is exhibiting. At times, even when we correct the problems we can fix, the confusion doesn't improve,

TABLE 35.1: SUGGESTED MEDICATIONS FOR MANAGEMENT OF TERMINAL DELIRIUM (MEDICATIONS LISTED ARE NOT FDA APPROVED TO TREAT DELIRIUM AND ARE OFF-LABEL RECOMMENDATIONS.)

Medication	Dose (PO unless indicated)	Onset of Action	Routes of Administration	Comments
Haloperidol (Haldol)	0.5–4 mg q 6 h and up to q 4 h prn {1mg IV ~ 2 mg PO}	IV: 30–60 min PO: 60–120 min	PO, IV, SC, IM, liquid solution (can use SL)	Typical neuroleptic, antiemetic benefit First-line agent for terminal delirium
Chlorpromazine (Thorazine)	10–25 mg bid {IV and PO dose range the same}	IV: 5–15 min PO: 30–60 min	PO, IV, IM	If IV used, recommend test dose of 1 mg; IM very irritating; preferred for agitated patients due to sedating effects
Lorazepam (Ativan)	0.5–6 mg bid-tid and prn {1mg IV ~ 1mg PO}	IV: 5–20 min PO: 30–60 min	PO, IV, PR, IM	Medium half-life benzo-diazepine, antiemetic benefit (Not to be used without trial of antipsychotic agent)
Diazepam (Valium)	2–10 mg bid-tid and prn {1mg IV ~ 1mg PO}	IV: 5–20 min PO: 30–60 min	PO, IV, PR	Long half-life benzodiazepine, steady plasma concentration (Not to be used without trial of antipsychotic agent)

and that is normally a sign that his/her time is getting short…that he/she is dying.

PALLIATIVE CARE ISSUES

- If a patient has a terminal illness, delirium should be managed with the goal of controlling symptoms, rather than determining the underlying cause.
- It is important to establish realistic goals and expectations with family and caregivers and provide support through this terminal process, because the patient's appearance during an agitated delirium will affect the family's grieving process and may be associated with post-traumatic stress disorder and prolonged grief disorder.
- Families should be advised that some delirious patients see and hear things that may not be there. Often, patients who are dying will make reference to seeing deceased relatives, reliving childhood memories, or will express the need to travel (e.g., "I need to get on the bus"). Misperceptions or hallucinations that

are not distressing or frightening to the patient should not be contradicted or corrected.

Recurrent infection caused Mrs. LS to become agitated, lethargic, and restless. A trial of haloperidol did not improve her symptoms. Hepatorenal failure was diagnosed. After discussion with her health care proxy, she was started on standing chlorpromazine to capitalize on the sedating effects of the medication to calm the restlessness. Mrs. LS expired six days later as a result of sepsis.

TAKE-HOME POINTS

- Treatment of terminal delirium should be initiated immediately upon recognition of the symptom, with or without additional workup for contributing causes.
- Workup may reveal no precipitant or obvious cause—physical exam for constipation, urinary retention, pain, and labs and vitals may all appear normal.
- Terminal delirium may not be responsive to treatment of underlying abnormalities.

REFERENCES

1. Breitbart W, Alici Y. Agitation and delirium at the end of life. *JAMA.* 2008;*300*(24):2898–2910.
2. Forbes C. Management of terminal delirium: a literature review and case study. 2006. http://www.pallcare.ru.en/?p=1178612694. Accessed August 30, 2011.
3. Alvarez-Fernandez B, Formiga F, Gomaz R. Delirium in hospitalized older persons: review. *J Nutr Health Aging.* 2008;*12*:246–251.
4. Leonard M, Raju B, Conroy M, et al. Reversibility of delirium in terminally ill patients and predictors of mortality. *Palliat Med.* 2008;*22*(7):848–854.

36
Sleep Disorders

PART A: INSOMNIA

CASE A

JW is a 65-year-old woman with end-stage meta-static breast cancer. She gets into bed when tired, around 9 p.m., at first to watch television, but then lies awake for several hours worrying about her condition and her family. Once asleep, she wakes frequently with pain and then begins worrying again. She gets out of bed around 9 a.m., estimating her sleep time at 5 hours and feeling unrested. She is tired during the day but rarely, if ever, naps.

DEFINITION

Insomnia refers to difficultly initiating and/or maintaining sleep. Insomnia equivalents may include a complaint of unrefreshing sleep despite adequate (or more-than-adequate) time spent in bed.

PREVALENCE

At least half of elderly patients report difficulties with sleep and, depending on how one screens for it, approximately 20% of the elderly report insomnia, women more frequently than men.[1,2] The prevalence of insomnia in the palliative care setting is quite high, as high as 70% in one study, again somewhat more frequent in women than men.[3]

LIKELY ETIOLOGIES

Causes of difficulty sleeping include:
- Worries, anxiety, and depression
- Conditions that interfere with sleep, such as uncontrolled pain and other burdensome symptoms, and restless leg syndrome (which is often not spontaneously reported)
- Poor sleep hygiene, such as going to bed when tired, though not sleepy, or spending lots of time awake in bed

DIAGNOSIS

History

1. When evaluating sleep difficulties in any patient population, the current and premorbid sleep history and schedule is important. Issues that should be explored include:
   - Bedtime
   - Sleep latency, i.e., the time it takes to fall asleep (patient's estimate)
   - Morning wake time
   - Total sleep time (patient's estimate)
   - Sleep disruptors: environmental (e.g., noise, change in sleeping/living location); sleep-related (e.g., snoring, leg movements); medical conditions disrupting sleep (e.g., pain, nocturia)
   - Level of daytime sleepiness (e.g., frequency and duration of napping/dozing)
   - Habits affecting sleep (e.g., caffeine consumption, exercise, alcohol consumption, bedtime routine, mentation or other wake-promoting activities performed in bed)
   - Medical conditions affecting sleep (e.g., restless legs, thyroid dysfunction, dementia, dyspnea)
   - Psychiatric conditions affecting sleep (e.g., depression, anxiety, fear, spiritual and psychosocial concerns, especially in palliative care patients and their family members)
   - Medications (contributing to insomnia or hypersomnia)
2. Sleep logs and diaries are very helpful in assessing the patient's sleep schedule, both for the clinician and often for the patient him/herself in identifying patterns to be corrected.
3. Questionnaires are also available to aid in the assessment of daytime sleepiness (e.g., the Epworth Sleepiness Scale). Input from the patient's caregiver(s) is useful, especially regarding observations of sleep disruptors. (Sleep log and Epworth Scale are available on American Academy of Sleep Medicine website: http://yoursleep.aasmnet.org/EvaluateSleep.aspx.)

Exam

The physical exam required for the evaluation of sleep disturbances is a general medical one. In the palliative care setting, however, specific emphasis should be placed on determining the causes, locations, and patterns of pain. Additionally, a mental status exam is imperative, including screening for depression, anxiety, dementia, and delirium.

Tests

- In most cases of insomnia, including geriatric and palliative care cases, polysomnographic analysis is not required or pursued. Testing should initially focus on the medical symptoms and conditions suggested by the history and physical examination.
- If symptoms are not controlled with these initial measures, sleep testing should certainly be more strongly considered.
- If sleep apnea is suspected, overnight polysomnography will confirm the diagnosis and guide treatment. Because polysomnographic testing is both rigorous and time-consuming, it may be prudent to pursue empiric symptom control and treatment of the patient's known conditions before sending the patient to a sleep laboratory.

TREATMENT OPTIONS

Nonpharmacologic

1. **Sleep hygiene**: Treatment of any sleep disturbance requires correction of sleep hygiene inadequacies. These recommendations will be tailored to the patient's specific counterproductive practices. Some suggestions include:
   - Reducing caffeine consumption
   - Reducing time spent in bed while awake
   - Establishing a proper bedtime routine
   - Reducing or controlling daytime napping
2. **Cognitive behavioral therapy (CBT)**: The mainstay of treatment for insomnia is cognitive behavioral therapy, which may include elements of relaxation therapy, guided imagery, stimulus control, and more aggressive sleep hygiene modifications, such as sleep restriction.[4] CBT is more effective, long-term, than the chronic use of hypnotic medications. It requires several weeks of participation, and this may be a limiting factor for

some patients with cognitive, mood, or functional impairment.

Pharmacologic[5]

For patients who continue to have insomnia that is distressing enough to require an intervention, several medications are used to treat insomnia (Table 36.1).

PART B: HYPERSOMNIA

CASE B

Mr. B is a 72-year-old obese man with painful diabetic neuropathy. He goes to bed at 11 p.m. and falls asleep readily. He snores loudly and experiences several brief awakenings during the night, often to urinate. He wakes at 6 a.m. feeling unrested. He takes Percocet at bedtime and several times a day. He dozes often when sedentary, which is much of the day.

DEFINITION

Hypersomnia is excessive daytime sleepiness. This may be characterized by planned or inadvertent napping or dozing in inappropriate situations. The term is often used synonymously with "fatigue" or "tiredness," which more accurately describe a low level of physical energy rather than true sleepiness. Hypersomnia can severely impact daytime functioning, including limiting ability to operate a motor vehicle and interact with loved ones.

PREVALENCE

The prevalence of hypersomnia within the palliative care population is not known, though it is believed to be common. The prevalence of fatigue is > 70% in the setting of terminal cancer.[6]

LIKELY ETIOLOGIES

- There may be multiple reasons for daytime hypersomnia, including:
  - Obstructive sleep apnea causing daytime sleepiness
  - Use of short-acting opiates during the day
  - Use of opiates at night, exacerbating the sleep apnea
- For palliative care patients, the life-limiting illness itself, or the treatment used to treat the life-limiting illness, can contribute to hypersomnia. Some common examples include brain tumors, anemia, chemotherapy, radiotherapy, and prescribed medications such as opioids and benzodiazepines.

TABLE 36.1: PHARMACOLOGIC MANAGEMENT OF INSOMNIA

Class	Mechanism of Action	Side Effects
Benzodiazepines	Shorten sleep latency Reduce nocturnal awakenings Increase total sleep time	The longer the half-life, the higher the chance of morning/daytime grogginess Confusion Falls Rebound insomnia upon discontinuation
Non-benzodiazepine sedative hypnotics	Shorten sleep latency Improve perceived sleep quality	Lower risk of confusion Falls (not validated) Less daytime grogginess Zolpidem: parasomnia-like behaviors
Sedating antidepressants	Sedating side effects	Sedation (not evaluated for insomnia)
Antihistamines	Sedating side effect has not been shown to improve sleep quality	Mucous membrane dryness Urinary retention Confusion Avoid in the geriatric, seriously ill, and palliative care settings
Others: Melatonin Valerian	Lack of standardization Minimal study	

DIAGNOSIS

History

In the evaluation of sleep difficulties in any patient population, taking a careful history is the key to identifying the problem(s) and developing a plan of care. (See Part A: Insomnia.)

Tests

Follow guidelines described in Part A: Insomnia.

TREATMENT OPTIONS

Nonpharmacologic

- **Scheduled naps**: In patients with hypersomnia, short naps can be scheduled to coincide with the patient's sleepiest times of day and around activities (including medical treatments/therapy). Napping should be eliminated late in the day (i.e., after 3 p.m.), if at all possible.
- **Medication schedule**: The patient's medication dosing schedule should be altered (if possible) to reduce sedating medications during the day, and avoid stimulating medications in the evening and any medications taken during the night.

Pharmacologic

- There are no studies defining the pharmacologic treatment of hypersomnia in the palliative care setting.

- One recent study suggested that methylphenidate is most effective in controlling fatigue in the chronically ill.[1] However, this medication, even when titrated appropriately, frequently causes the side effects of insomnia, agitation, and palpitations. It is best to begin with a low dose (e.g., 2.5 mg qam or 8 a.m. and no later than 1 p.m.) and increase slowly. Long acting preparations are available as well and can be incorporated if the patient achieves a stable dose.
- While modafinil has not been specifically studied in this patient population and is also expensive, it is considered the first-line treatment for daytime sleepiness of any cause and tends to be better tolerated than methylphenidate.
- Corticosteroids may improve energy level and mood in short courses, but they are fraught with side effects.

PALLIATIVE CARE ISSUES

When hypersomnia is caused by the life-limiting illness and cannot be alleviated by medication, it is sometimes helpful for clinicians to advise patient and family that sleeping more is to be expected in the context of serious illness. Letting them know that this is part of the disease course can alleviate anxiety and fear and can be reassuring both to the patient and family.

TAKE-HOME POINTS

- Insomnia is usually multifactorial and almost always includes elements of inadequate sleep hygiene.
- Always try nonpharmacologic treatments first, and allow sufficient time for improvement.
- Sleep testing is rigorous but can be considered when indicated.
- Hypersomnia can severely limit daytime functioning but may be controlled if it is not related to the underlying life-limiting illness.
- The medical history is key to the evaluation of all sleep disorders.

REFERENCES

1. Stepnawsky CJ, Ancoli-Israel S. Sleep and its disorders in seniors. *Sleep Med Clin*. June 2008;3(2): 281–293.
2. Lichstein KL, Stone KC, Nau SD, McCrae CS, Payne KL. Insomnia in the elderly. *Sleep Med Clin*. June 2006;1(2):221–229.
3. Hugel H, Ellershaw J, Cook L, Skinner J, Irvine C. The prevalence, key causes and management of insomnia in palliative care patients. *J Pain Symptom Manage*. April 2004;27(4):316–321.
4. Hajjar R. Sleep disturbance in palliative care. *Clin Geriatr Med*. Feb 2008;24(1):83–91.
5. Tariq SH, Pulisetty S. Pharmacotherapy for insomnia. *Clin Geriatr Med*. Feb 2008;24(1):93–105.
6. Harris JD. Fatigue in chronically ill patients. *Curr Opin Support Palliat Care*. Sept 2008;2(3):180–186.

37

Dizziness

CASE

An 81-year-old man, Mr. G, presents to the emergency department for dizziness. He is Spanish-speaking. His wife states that after eating breakfast this morning he said he felt "dizzy" and was stumbling as though he were drunk. He has a remote history of "unstable heartbeat" and is on no medication. On exam he is uncomfortable, keeping his eyes closed; he says he feels like he is spinning but denies nausea or vomiting. His speech is dysarthric. He has horizontal nystagmus on bilateral gaze, worse on the left. There may be some diplopia to the left as well. He doesn't withdraw to pinprick on the left side of his face. He has, however, full strength in all four extremities. He is dysmetric on finger-nose testing bilaterally. He is unable to stand even with assistance, or cooperate with a sensory exam.

DEFINITION

Dizziness refers to a variety of abnormal sensations relating to perception of the body's relationship to space. The differential diagnoses for such patients is broad and may include medical, neurological, and otologic causes, and the etiologies can range from benign to life-threatening conditions. Dizziness is thus a challenging symptom, and it is important to develop a framework under which to evaluate each patient. A proposed classification divides dizziness into three main subtypes: vertigo, presyncopal lightheadedness, and other forms of dizziness and disequilibrium (Table 37.1).

PREVALENCE

- Although prevalence studies vary in their definition of the symptom, dizziness is common in all age groups, and its prevalence increases modestly with age. Dizziness is one of the most common reasons older adults visit their doctors.
- Peripheral vestibular etiologies are among the most common causes, with acute labyrinthitis being the most common peripheral vestibular disorder seen in the primary care setting.

- In referral settings, recurrent peripheral vestibular disorders, such as benign paroxysmal vertigo, recurrent vestibulopathy, and Meniere's disease predominate.
- Central vestibular causes are less common. However, as many as 25% of patients with risk factors for stroke who present to the emergency medical setting with vertigo, nystagmus, and postural instability have a stroke affecting the cerebellum.[2]

CONSEQUENCES OF UNTREATED DIZZINESS

- Although dizziness is seldom a sign of any life-threatening disorder, it significantly impairs everyday function and quality of life, causing fatigue, difficulty walking, and avoidance of normal activities.
- Vestibular dysfunction predisposes people to a risk of falls and fractures, which in turn pose a risk of death. Many hip fractures are related to balance disorders.
- Acute vestibular dysfunction may be the only sign of certain stroke syndromes and if unrecognized may put the patient at risk for further neurological deterioration and death.

ETIOLOGIES

The patient in the case presents with an acute vestibular syndrome with facial numbness and ataxia on exam consistent with involvement of the brainstem and cerebellum. This presentation of dizziness is a neurologic emergency. The most likely diagnosis is acute stroke or cerebellar hemorrhage; consider Wallenberg Syndrome (vertebral artery/posterior inferior cerebellar artery (PICA) occlusion).

Immediate brain imaging is indicated in order to confirm the diagnosis. Brainstem strokes confer significant morbidity and disability. In patients with cerebellar hemorrhages or infarctions, compression of the brain stem can develop in the first few

TABLE 37.1: DIZZINESS SUBTYPES[1]

Dizziness Type	Examples
Vertigo A feeling that one's surroundings are moving or spinning Episodic vertigo attacks can last from seconds to days	*Peripheral* Benign paroxysmal positional vertigo Acute labrynthitis/vestibular neuritis Meniere's disease *Central* Cerebellar infarction or hemorrhage Transient ischemic attack Intracranial mass lesion
Presyncope/Lightheadedness Lightheaded, faint feeling, as though one is about to pass out Episodes last seconds to hours	Cardiovascular Metabolic Vasovagal conditions Systemic infection Medication side effects
Disequilibrium and chronic dizziness A sense of unsteadiness that is felt primarily in the lower extremities when walking; feelings of floating or dissociation Usually present, perhaps with varying intensity, for days, weeks, or years	Anxiety or panic disorder Depression Otitis media Sinusitis Visual impairment Post-traumatic vertigo

days after a stroke. These patients require careful monitoring in an intensive care setting, and brain imaging should be repeated. If deterioration occurs, then neurosurgical evaluation for decompression is recommended.

Whereas the above case represents an urgent, "can't miss" diagnosis, most patients with dizziness have less emergent etiologies. The differential diagnosis of dizziness is categorized based on the classification system described above (Table 37.1).

Some of the more common etiologies of peripheral vertigo are described below (Table 37.2).

DIAGNOSIS

History

The most important diagnostic tool is a detailed history to explore the patient's subjective experience of the symptom. This information helps to establish the etiology/classification of the dizziness.

Questions should include:

- Is there a true sensation of movement or spinning?
- Is there a feeling of faintness and lightheadedness?
- Are there vague, persistent feelings of imbalance?

- What are the associated characteristics?
  - Nausea/vomiting may accompany vertigo
  - The sensation of warmth, diaphoresis, and visual blurring may indicate presyncope
  - Palpitations, dyspnea, or chest discomfort to indicate a cardiac cause
- What are the duration, length of the episodes, and exacerbating factors such as head movement?
- Has syncope ever occurred during an episode?
- Do episodes occur only when the patient is upright, or do they occur in other positions?
- Are there persistent sensations of nonvertiginous dizziness or subjective imbalance that is present of most days? Are these associated with anxiety or hyperventilation?

Exam

- The physical exam should include evaluation for orthostatic hypotension. Assessment of the pulse and direct cardiac auscultation may assist in determining if the episode is associated with an arrhythmia.

TABLE 37.2: COMMON ETIOLOGIES OF PERIPHERAL VERTIGO

Disease Process	Pathogenesis	Presentation and Physical Exam	Diagnostic Features and Lab Tests	Treatment
Benign paroxysmal positional vertigo	Otoliths fall into the semicircular canal.	Brief spinning sensation brought on by turning/tilting the head. Each episode of vertigo lasts only 10 to 20 seconds. The dizziness may be quite severe and incapacitating.	The diagnosis can be confirmed by eliciting nystagmus with the Dix-Hallpike maneuver (determines whether vertigo is triggered by certain head movements).	The treatment currently recommended is the bedside Epley maneuver (canalith repositioning maneuver).
Vestibular neuritis	Thought to result from inflammation of the vestibular nerve, presumably of viral origin.	Acute onset of severe, persistent vertigo, nausea, vomiting, and gait instability. When combined with unilateral hearing loss, it is called labyrinthitis.	Electronystagmography will document the unilateral vestibular loss.	Generally resolves spontaneously.
Meniere's disease	Thought to be related to an increase in the volume of fluid in the labyrinth.	Recurrent episodes of spontaneous vertigo lasting for minutes to hours, usually associated with unilateral tinnitus, hearing loss, and ear fullness.	Low-frequency sensorineural hearing loss on audiometry electronystagmography helps to confirm the diagnosis.	Diuretics and salt restriction, plus medications for symptomatic relief as below. In persistent, disabling cases, surgical procedures are available.

- If true vertigo has been indicated by the history, the clinical exam helps to distinguish between peripheral and central vestibular causes.
- Nystagmus is the hallmark finding associated with true vertigo. The Table 37.3 shows features of the neurologic exam that can help to distinguish between central and peripheral causes of vertigo.

Tests
- Labs:
  - Serum electrolytes, glucose, and hematocrit
  - Cardiac enzymes if myocardial ischemia is suspected
  - Blood and urine toxicology screens may reveal the presence of alcohol or other drugs.
- Imaging:
  - CT head if emergent presentation to evaluate for stroke/hemorrhage
  - MRI brain with contrast if non-emergent presentation

- Echocardiogram, telemetry, and event monitoring may help to further establish a cardiac etiology to presyncope.
- Upright tilt table testing is indicated to investigate vasovagal episodes.
- Electronystagmography and audiography may be helpful when evaluating peripheral vertigo.

TREATMENT OPTIONS

Vertigo
- The optimal approach to treatment is to address the underlying problem. However, in many cases of vertigo, the pathophysiology is uncertain and symptomatic therapy is used.
- Treatment for acute vertigo consists of bed rest (1 to 2 days maximum) and symptomatic relief with vestibular suppressant drugs listed in the chart below (Table 37.4).
- It is important to counsel patients that these drugs do not eliminate, but rather reduce, the severity of symptoms.

TABLE 37.3: CENTRAL VS. PERIPHERAL CAUSE OF VERTIGO

Feature	Peripheral (Labyrinth or Nerve)	Central (Brainstem or Cerebellum)
Intensity of vertigo	Severe	Mild
Latency of nystagmus after head movement	3–40 sec	None: immediate vertigo and nystagmus
Fatigability of nystagmus	Yes	No
Type of nystagmus	Unidirectional, often rotatory	Bidirectional or unidirectional
Visual fixation	Can inhibit nystagmus and vertigo	No inhibition
Tinnitus and/or deafness	Often present	Usually absent
Associated CNS abnormalities	None	Extremely common (e.g., diplopia, cranial neuropathies, ataxia, dysarthria)

Presyncope

- The treatment for presyncope is strictly directed toward the underlying cause.
- Certain precautions should be taken regardless of the cause of syncope. At the first sign of symptoms, patients should be placed in a position to maximize cerebral blood flow and offer protection from trauma, such as lying down or sitting with head forward.
- Patients with orthostatic hypotension should be instructed to rise slowly and systematically (supine to seated, seated to standing) from the bed or chair.
- Movement of the legs prior to rising facilitates venous return from the lower extremities.
- Whenever possible, medications that aggravate the problem, such as vasodilators and diuretics, should be discontinued.
- Use of compression stockings may be helpful as well.

VESTIBULAR REHABILITATION THERAPY

- (VRT) is an exercise-based program designed to promote central nervous system compensation for inner ear deficits. The goal of VRT is to retrain the brain to recognize and process signals from the vestibular system in coordination with vision and proprioception.
- Recent evidence suggests that the use of vestibular rehabilitation is a critical component in improving postural stability and decreasing subjective complaints of

TABLE 37.4: PHARMACOLOGIC APPROACH TO SYMPTOMATIC TREATMENT OF ACUTE VERTIGO[3]

Drug	Range of Doses	Use with Caution in	Side Effects
Meclizine	12.5–50 mg every 4–8 hrs PO	Asthma, glaucoma, prostate enlargement	Dryness, drowsiness
Scopolamine	0.1–0.4 mg every 4–6 hrs IM, PO 1.5 mg over 3-day period for transdermal patch	Asthma, glaucoma, prostate enlargement	Dryness, visual blurring, memory loss, confusion
Lorazepam	0.5–2 mg every 4–8 hrs IM, IV, PO	Glaucoma, additive with other CNS depressants	Drowsiness
Diazepam	2–20 mg every 4–8 hrs IM, IV, or PO	Glaucoma, additive with other CNS depressants	Drowsiness

disequilibrium for patients with peripheral vestibular loss.

- Although these studies differ in the specific details of vestibular rehabilitation, common elements include vestibular adaptation and substitution exercises, balance and gait activities, and general conditioning.
- Although VRT does not cure the organic diseases that produce the balance disorder, it improves mobility, prevents falls, and overall has a positive impact on quality of life for the patient.[4]

PALLIATIVE CARE ISSUES

- For most patients, the symptom of dizziness resolves spontaneously, but an important minority of patients can develop chronic, disabling symptoms.
- Chronic dizziness in older persons may constitute a geriatric syndrome—a final common pathway resulting from the interplay of multiple impairments.[1] This view approaches dizziness from functional point of view rather than trying to define a symptom subtype, a single mechanism, and a unifying diagnosis.
- Patients with chronic dizziness may benefit from a comprehensive approach aimed at identifying and managing treatable conditions, whether etiologic or contributory.
- A typical treatment-oriented management program might include: correcting visual impairment; improving muscle strength; adjusting medication regiments; identifying and treating possible psychological comorbidity, such as anxiety or depression; and instructing patients on vestibular exercises.

TAKE-HOME POINTS

- Dizziness has a major impact on a patient's functional capacity and quality of life.
- The most important diagnostic tool is a detailed history focused on the meaning of "dizziness" to the patient.
- It is important to categorize each patient's complaint into a specific subtype of dizziness: true vertigo, presyncope, or disequilibrium and chronic dizziness. This framework will help the physician to narrow the differential diagnoses, which will help lead to a successful treatment or relief of symptom.
- If vertigo is established, a detailed history and physical exam can differentiate between peripheral and central vestibular dysfunction.
- The presence of other neurological symptoms in a patient, or sudden onset of vertigo in a patient with stroke risk factors, should warrant a prompt head CT or stroke-protocol MRI.
- Vestibular rehabilitation should be considered to help improve postural stability for patients with peripheral vestibular loss.

REFERENCES

1. Sloane PD, Coeytaux RR, Beck RS, Dallara J. Dizziness: state of the science. *Ann Intern Med.* 2001;*134*:823–832.
2. Hotson JR, Baloh RW. Acute vestibular syndrome. *N Engl J Med.* 1998;*339*:680–685.
3. Baloh RW. Vestibular neuritis. *N Engl J Med.* 2003;*348*:1027–1032.
4. Hall C, Cox LC. The role of vestibular rehabilitation in the balance disorder patient. *Otolaryngol Clin North Am.* Feb 2009;*42*(1):161–169.

38

Headache

CASE

Mr. C is an 86-year-old man with hypertension, mild dementia, atrial fibrillation on warfarin anticoagulation, hyperlipidemia, and gait instability. He presents to his primary care physician with a week-long history of headaches. The headaches are described as dull and are mainly localized to the right side. The patient has taken acetaminophen without much relief. His wife reports that he has been irritable and increasingly confused over the past few days. The patient denies a history of trauma.

DEFINITION

Headaches occur when mechanical or chemical stimulation causes activation of primary afferent fibers innervating cephalic blood vessels. Most of these nociceptors originate in the trigeminal ganglia.

- Headaches are divided into primary and secondary headache disorders. Primary headache disorders are benign and without an identifiable source, while secondary headache disorders are the result of an underlying illness.

PREVALENCE

Headaches have a lifetime prevalence of 99% in women and 94% in men.[1] Tension-type headache is the most common of the primary headache disorders with a global prevalence of 38%.[2] This is followed by migraine headache with a global prevalence of 10%, and chronic headache with a prevalence of 3%.[2]

CONSEQUENCES OF UNTREATED HEADACHE

- Decreased productivity and efficiency
- Diminished quality of life

CLASSIFICATION AND LIKELY ETIOLOGIES

The International Headache Society classification and diagnostic criteria for headache disorder are presented in Table 38.1.

DIAGNOSIS

History

The evaluation of a patient with headache should include location, quality, frequency, severity, associated features, triggers, and medications.

Exam

- General appearance
- Vital signs including blood pressure, pulse, respiratory rate
- Listen for bruit at the neck, eyes, and head
- HEENT exam (head, ears, eyes, nose, throat)
- Palpation of the head, neck, and shoulders
- Examination of the spine
- Neurologic exam: cranial nerves, motor, sensory, fundoscopy

Tests

The vast majority of headache patients do not require additional testing. When testing is necessary, the following may be helpful: CT Head, MRI, Lumbar puncture, ESR, CBC, EKG.

Mr. C has multiple risk factors for intracerebral hemorrhage, including coumadin anticoagulation, hypertension, and gait instability putting him at risk for falls and head trauma. His confusion and altered level of consciousness are other red flags that neuroimaging is indicated. Mr. C undergoes a non-contrast CT of the head and is found to have a large subdural hematoma. His mental status rapidly deteriorates. Due to his advanced age and comorbidities, surgical intervention is refused by Mr. C's family. He is admitted to the palliative care service and receives symptomatic therapy with steroids and opiates.

TREATMENT OPTIONS

Treatments for headache are dependent on the underlying etiology. Migraine, tension, and cluster headaches make up the vast majority of all benign headaches. Descriptions and pharmacologic recommendations are noted below (Table 38.2).

TABLE 38.1: INTERNATIONAL HEADACHE SOCIETY CLASSIFICATION OF HEADACHE DISORDERS (2004)[3]

Primary Headache Disorders
Migraine
Tension-type headache:
Cluster headache and other trigeminal autonomic cephalalgias
Other primary headaches:
    Cough, stabbing, exertional, orgasmic, hypnic

Secondary Headache Disorders
Head and/or neck trauma
Cranial or cervical vascular disorder:
    Cerebral infarction, TIA, intracranial hemorrhage, arteriovenous malformation, arteritis, carotid or vertebral artery dissection, central venous thrombosis
Nonvascular intracranial disorders:
    High CSF pressure, low CSF pressure, non-infectious inflammatory disease, intracranial neoplasm, carcinomatous meningitis
Substance use or withdrawal:
    Alcohol, food additives, cocaine, cannabis, histamine, medication-overuse
Infection:
    Meningitis, encephalitis, brain abscess, empyema, systemic viral or bacterial infection
Disturbance of homeostasis:
    Hypoxia and/or hypercapnea, dialysis, arterial hypertension
Disorders of the cranium, neck, eyes, ears, nose, sinuses, teeth, mouth or other facial or cranial structures:
    Cervicogenic, acute glaucoma, TMJ
Psychiatric disorder:
    Somatisation, psychosis

SPECIAL CONSIDERATIONS

Use caution when prescribing headache medication for geriatric patients:

- NSAIDS, triptans, and ergot preparations should be used carefully in the elderly. Both triptans and ergotamines cause vasoconstriction and can exacerbate hypertension and underlying vascular disease.
- Elderly patients are also more prone to gastrointestinal bleeding, renal dysfunction, hypertension, and fluid retention caused by NSAID use.
- These medications should also be avoided in presence of CAD, PVD, renal, and liver disease.
- If possible, employ nonpharmacologic methods including avoidance of triggers.

OTHER CAUSES OF HEADACHE RELEVANT TO A GERIATRIC PALLIATIVE CARE POPULATION

Subdural Hematoma

- Frequently seen in elderly patients at risk for falls and head trauma.

BOX 38.1 HEADACHE DANGER SIGNS: CONSIDER SECONDARY CAUSES

- First severe headache
- Worst headache ever
- Altered mental status
- Fever
- Abnormal vital signs
- Focal new neurologic deficit
- New exertional headache
- Onset of headache after age 50
- New headache in immunosuppressed patients
- Change in headache severity or frequency

- Focal neurologic symptoms are less likely because brain tissue damage is often absent.
- No unique or specific headache characteristics. Pain is mild to moderate.

TABLE 38.2: HEADACHE TYPES AND PHARMACOLOGIC TREATMENTS

	Tension Headache	Migraine Headache	Cluster Headache
Description	Pressure or tightening around the head and neck, non-pulsating	Throbbing, pounding, or pulsating	Excruciating pain, centered around one eye
Location	Bilateral	Majority unilateral	Always unilateral
Associated features	None	Nausea, vomiting, photophobia, phonophobia, transient neurologic symptoms	Ipsilateral conjunctival injection, miosis, tearing, nasal congestion
Duration	Minutes to days	4–72 hours[4]	15–180 min[4]
Therapy	NSAIDS, acetaminophen, relaxation, massage	NSAIDS, triptans, ergot preparations	100% oxygen delivered at 10–12 LPM for 15 minutes,[4] triptans, ergotamines

- Often unilateral and ipsilateral to the hematoma.
- May be confusion and fluctuating level of consciousness.

Treatment: Should be patient-specific and based upon goals of care. Neurosurgical consultation, surgical evacuation, steroids to reduce increased intracranial pressure, and opioids for pain.

Giant Cell Arteritis (Temporal Arteritis)

- Most common in patients older than 50;[5] average age of onset is 70 years.[4]
- Headaches are almost always present though their characteristics vary. Local pressure worsens the pain.
- Systemic symptoms include malaise, fever, night sweats, muscle aches, weight loss, jaw claudication.
- Can cause ischemic optic neuropathy and permanent blindness.
- Lab findings: ESR and CRP are increased, hemoglobin is decreased.
- If suspected, the temporal artery must be biopsied.

Treatment: If there is a high index of suspicion, treatment should be started while awaiting biopsy results. Prednisone 1mg/kg per day for one month, followed by a taper of 5% to 10% every 2–4 weeks until discontinued.[5] Maintenance therapy usually for 6–12 months.

Brain Metastases

- Patients with cancer who experience new headache or increased frequency of headache should undergo evaluation for brain metastasis.
- Description of headache: Pain is mild or moderate, often resolves spontaneously. Bifrontal headache is common, but often worse on the ipsilateral side. Frequently associated with nausea and vomiting. Worse with bending.
- Lung, melanoma, renal, breast, and GI tract cancers are most common sources of brain metastases.[6]
- Neoplastic meningitis (NM) or leptomeningeal disease is found in 40% to 50% of patients with hematologic malignancies, mostly acute lymphoblastic leukemia, acute monoblastic leukemia, and high-grade lymphomas.[7]
- Breast cancer, small cell lung cancer, and melanoma are most common solid tumors associated with NM.[7]
- Neurologic signs and symptoms involve multiple levels of CNS (direct brain or spinal cord invasion, obstructive hydrocephalus, cranial nerve palsies).

Treatment: Should be based on functional status, prognosis, and goals of care.

- Single cerebral metastasis—irradiation or surgical excision
- Multiple cerebral metastases or widespread systemic disease— whole-brain radiotherapy, stereotactic radiosurgery

- Leptomeningeal metastases (neoplastic meningitis):
  1. Craniospinal irradiation and systemic high dose chemotherapy (Ara-C or methotrexate)[7]
  2. Intrathecal chemotherapy with repeated lumbar puncture or implanted intraventricular reservoir (i.e., Ommaya reservoir) Methotrexate and Ara-C[7]
  3. Opioids
  4. Dexamethasone if there is increased intracranial pressure >10 mg oral dose followed by 4 mg four times a day[8]

Primary Intracranial tumors

- Headache occurs in about 50% of patients with brain tumors[9]
- Characteristics of headache: Diffuse and often more prominent in the early morning hours; may worsen with bending or valsalva; association with nausea and vomiting

Treatment: Dependent on type and site of tumor, patient's condition, and goals of care.

- Complete surgical removal if extra-axial and not in a critical or inaccessible location of brain
- Shunt to reduce obstructive hydrocephalus
- Radiation therapy
- Corticosteroids are mainstay of treatment of cerebral edema. Dexamethasone: 10 mg orally, followed by 4 mg four times a day[8]
- Opioids
- Emergency treatment of cerebral herniation[10]
  1. Hyperventilation: Decrease PCO2 to 25–30 mm Hg
  2. Osmotherapy: IV mannitol 20% solution 0.5–2.0 g/kg over 15 minutes followed by 25 gm booster doses IV as needed
  3. Corticosteroids: Dexamethasone 100 mg IV push, followed by 40–100 mg every 24 hours based on symptoms

Hypnic Headache

- Age of onset is usually >60 years.
- "Alarm clock" headache that awakens patient from sleep. Duration is typically 15 to 30 minutes.[4]
- Headaches are moderately severe, usually bilateral.
- Hypnic headache syndrome: Headaches occur at least 15 times per month for at least one month.

Treatment

- Bedtime dose of lithium carbonate 200–600 mg[4] (use with caution in the elderly)
- Alternatives are verapamil, caffeine, indomethacin

TAKE-HOME POINTS

- The vast majority of headaches are primary and benign in nature.
- A detailed history and physical exam are necessary to exclude secondary causes of headache that are often life-threatening.
- When a secondary headache is suspected, neuroimaging is essential.
- Diagnostic and treatment interventions should be chosen in the context of prognosis and achievable goals for medical care, which are determined in discussions between patient, family, and medical team.

REFERENCES

1. Rasmussen BK, Jensen R, et al. The epidemiology of headache in a general population: a prevalence study. *J Clin Epidemiol.* 1991;*44*:1147–1157.
2. Stovner L, Hagen K, Jensen R, et al. The global burden of headache: a documentation of headache prevalence and disability worldwide. *Cephalalgia.* 2007;*27*:193–210.
3. The International Headache Society. The International Classification of Headache Disorders, 2nd edition. *Cephalalgia.* 2004;*24*(suppl 1):9–160.
4. Goadsby P, Raskin, N. "Chapter 15. Headache" in Fauci A, Braunwald E, Kasper D, et al. Harrison's Principles of Internal Medicine. 17th Edition: http://www.accessmedicine.com/content.aspx?aid=2890365
5. Shmerling R. An 81-Year-Old Woman With Temporal Arteritis. *JAMA.* 2006;*295*:2525–2534.
6. Barnholtz-Sloan JS, Sloan AE, Davis FG, et al. Incidence proportions of brain metastases in patients diagnosed (1973 to 2001) in the Metropolitan Detroit Cancer Surveillance System. *J Clin Oncol.* July 15, 2004;*22*(14):2865–2872.
7. Siddiqui F, Marr L, Weissman DE. Neoplastic Meningitis. Fast Facts and Concepts. April 2005; #135. Available at: http://www.eperc.mcw.edu/EPERC/FastFactsIndex/ff_135.htm.
8. Fishman RA. *Cerebrospinal fluid in diseases of the nervous system.* 2nd edition. Philadelphia: Saunders; 1992.
9. DeAngelis L. Brain Tumors. *N Engl J Med.* January 11, 2001;*344*:114.
10. Posner JB. Neurologic complications of cancer. *Contemporary Neurology Series.* Philadelphia: FA Davis Co; 1995.

39

Myoclonus

CASE

Ms. CI is a 74-year-old woman who presented to the emergency department after her daughter noticed she was confused and "twitching." She has a history of lumbar spinal stenosis with low back and leg pain, for which she is on long-term opiates. Three days ago her primary care provider started her on gabapentin (Neurontin), 300 mg TID for her pain. Her daughter states that yesterday she was mumbling, and this morning she was nearly nonverbal and "shaking" from time to time. On exam, she is lethargic and incoherent, and she has sudden, jerk-like twitching movements that involve her face, neck, arms, and shoulders. The movements are brief, variable in appearance and distribution, and seem to increase with stimulation and level of alertness.

DEFINITION

Myoclonus refers to quick, sudden, involuntary, lightning-like jerks of a muscle or a group of muscles.[1] Myoclonic jerks may occur alone or in combination, in a repetitive pattern, or seemingly without pattern.

- Myoclonus may be brought about by active muscle contraction (positive myoclonus) or inhibition of ongoing muscle activity (negative myoclonus). The most common example of negative myoclonus is asterixis, which may be seen in liver failure, and to lesser extent in other metabolic encephalopathies, and rarely with focal brain lesions.
- In its simplest form, myoclonus consists of a muscle twitch followed by relaxation. Examples of focal, benign myoclonus in normal individuals are hiccups and "sleep starts" that some people experience while drifting off to sleep.
- When more widespread, myoclonus may involve persistent, shock-like contractions in a group of muscles. Severe cases of myoclonus can distort voluntary movements and severely limit a person's ability to eat, talk, or walk, indicating a possible underlying disorder affecting the central nervous system or peripheral nerves.

PREVALENCE

- Myoclonus is one of the most common involuntary movement disorders. Difficulties exist with identifying the prevalence and incidence of myoclonus, as it is most commonly a symptom of other complex disorders. Therefore, epidemiologic studies often underestimate the prevalence of myoclonus.
- An epidemiologic study examined a defined population of patients in Olmsted County, Minnesota, and found that the annual incidence of all causes of myoclonus was 1.3 per 100,000 person years, and that the population prevalence was 8.6 per 100,000. Secondary myoclonus was the most common type, accounting for 72% of cases, with the majority being associated with episodes of hypoxia, or degenerative diseases such as Alzheimer's. This is the category into which older adults and palliative care patients would fall, although no specific age-related prevalence data exist. Myoclonic epilepsy comprised 17% of cases, with essential myoclonus (i.e., idiopathic) accounting for the remaining 11%.[2]

CONSEQUENCES OF UNTREATED MYOCLONUS

- Highly disabling; interferes with the patient's ability to carry out their ADLs
- Decreases the quality of life
- May be the presenting symptom of a toxic or metabolic disturbance of importance that needs prompt evaluation and correction

LIKELY ETIOLOGIES

The differential diagnosis of myoclonus is broader than that of any other movement disorder and is best organized by use of major clinical syndrome categories. Table 39.1 outlines the diagnoses that may be most relevant to consider in a geriatric or palliative care practice.

In the case of Ms. CI, myoclonus is generalized (affecting multiple regions on both sides of the body) and occurring in a setting of a decline in mental status. Both of these factors suggest "symptomatic" myoclonus as a consequence of a systemic toxic or metabolic derangement. A detailed medication history is relevant, as she was recently started on gabapentin at a relatively high starting dose for the geriatric population, and she takes opioids, both of which can cause myoclonus. Other factors to consider are seizure (less likely with this presentation), electrolyte imbalances, alkalosis or renal failure, and thyroid and liver dysfunction.

DIAGNOSIS

History

- The evaluation of a patient with myoclonus must include a thorough history detailing information about the setting in which the myoclonus is seen, including the duration of the symptom, precipitating and alleviating factors, comorbid illnesses (specifically the presence of other neurological diseases or history of seizures), changes in mental status, and recent changes in medications.

- All drugs, either in isolation or combination, must be scrutinized for a potential role in myoclonus. It is also important to remember that onset of myoclonus secondary to drugs, toxins, and organ failure may be offset by days, weeks, or longer.

- Metabolic disorders due to liver or kidney failure may produce myoclonus by inhibiting drug metabolism. These metabolic derangements may also be manifested by change in mental status, which is another important piece of history that should be investigated.

- It is important to determine if the myoclonus is secondary or a "symptomatic" manifestation of a systemic condition, or an isolated primary neurological phenomenon. Most causes of myoclonus are symptomatic, and particularly in the geriatric population, myoclonus is rarely the manifestation of a de novo neurological condition.

TABLE 39.1: DIFFERENTIAL DIAGNOSIS FOR MYOCLONUS

Physiological
Sleep jerks, anxiety induced, exercise induced, hiccup
Metabolic
Hepatic failure, renal failure, dialysis syndrome, hyponatremia, hypoxia, hypoglycemia, hyperthyroidism
Neurodegenerative
Progressive supranuclear palsy, Huntington's disease, Parkinson's disease, multisystem atrophy, corticobasal degeneration
Dementias
Creutzfeldt-Jakob disease, Alzheimer's disease, frontotemporal dementia
Epileptic myoclonus
Epilepsia partialis continua
Infectious or post-infectious
Herpes simplex, encephalitis, HIV, syphilis, cryptococcus, Lyme disease, progressive multifocal leukoencephalopathy, post-infectious encephalitis
Focal nervous system damage
Post-stroke, trauma, tumor
Medication side effects
Psychiatric medications: tricyclic antidepressants, SSRI antidepressants, monoamine oxidase inhibitors, lithium
Anesthetics: etomidate, propofol
Opioids: especially morphine and hydromorphone
Anticonvulsants: Neurontin, carbamazepine, phenytoin, lamotrigine
Cardiac medications: calcium channel blockers, antiarrythmics
Antineoplastic agents
Contrast agents
Drug withdrawal
Paraneoplastic encephalopathies

Note. Adapted from: Caviness JN, Brown P. Myoclonus: current concepts and recent advances. *The Lancet Neurology.* 2004;3:598–607.

Exam

- When examining a patient with involuntary movements, the clinician must first define the phenomenology of the movements. It is critical to distinguish myoclonus from other abnormal movements such as seizures, tics, chorea, dystonia, and tremor (Table 39.2).
- Considering the varied causes, a wide range of neurological findings may be possible. Alternatively, despite the complaint of abnormal movements, little is revealed during examination of some patients with myoclonus. This is particularly the case for the physiological forms of myoclonus, as well as those associated with epilepsy for which a seizure history is usually apparent.

Tests

Based on the history obtained, one should proceed to evaluate the common disturbances of electrolyte balance and acquired metabolic disorders.
Labs:

- Electrolytes: including Na, K, Mg, Bicarbonate, Phosphorus
- Glucose
- Renal function tests
- Hepatic function tests
- Thyroid antibodies and function
- Paraneoplastic antibodies (if indicated)

Imaging: After reversible causes such as opioid toxicity have been ruled out, neuroimaging can suggest underlying neurologic diagnoses that may explain myoclonus.

- MRI brain with and without contrast may be helpful because findings such as frontal atrophy may be consistent with frontotemporal dementia. In patients with localizing neurological signs in addition to myoclonus, MRI may reveal a focal CNS etiology, such as a tumor or chronic stroke.
- EEG: can rule out epileptic syndromes such epilepsia partialis continua, or findings associated with Creutzfeldt-Jakob disease.
- EMG: can help distinguish fasciculations from myoclonus.
- Genetic testing: may also help identify associated conditions such as Huntington's disease.

TREATMENT OPTIONS

Treatment begins by identifying and resolving the underlying disorder. For example, as in the case of Ms. CI above, drug-induced myoclonus is almost always reversible on withdrawal of the causative agent.

Pharmacologic

- For primary myoclonus treatment, there are few placebo-controlled trials and even fewer double-blind trials. As a result, therapy is empiric, often based on class III evidence. Anti-myoclonic agents are usually used in combination, and multiple drug regimens are sometimes necessary to find the best combination for an individual patient (Table 39.3).

TABLE 39.2: CHARACTERISTICS OF MOVEMENT DISORDERS

Disorders	Movement Characteristics
Myoclonus	Sudden, brief (<100 ms), shock-like, arrhythmic muscle twitches
Seizure	Repetitive, powerful flexion/extension movements, often at a frequency of approximately 2–3 Hz, with lateralized involvement if patient is conscious; a patient cannot be conscious during generalized (bilateral) seizure activity
Athetosis	Slow, distal, writhing, involuntary movements with a propensity to affect the arms and hands
Chorea	Rapid, semipurposeful, graceful, dancelike, nonpatterned involuntary movements involving distal or proximal muscle groups
Dystonia	Involuntary sustained or repeated muscle contractions, often leading to twisting movements and abnormal posture
Tics	Brief, repeated, stereotyped muscle contractions that are often suppressible; can be simple and involve a single muscle group, or complex and affect a range of motor activities including speech
Tremor	Rhythmic oscillating movements of a limb or limbs
Fasciculation	Small, local, involuntary muscle contractions visible under the skin that usually do not bring about movement across a joint

TABLE 39.3: PHARMACOLOGIC TREATMENT FOR MYOCLONUS

Drug Name	Dosing	Contraindications	Drug Interactions	Adverse Events	Comments
Levetiracetam	Start with 500 mg/day with gradual titration by 500 mg per week. The maximum recommended dose is 3000 mg/day	Should be used cautiously in elderly and in those with decreased renal function	Virtually no interactions with other drugs. It is minimally protein- bound and excreted in urine	Generally well tolerated Common: dizziness somnolence asthenia Others: psychosis ataxia	Abrupt withdrawal may precipitate severe worsening of myoclonus
Valproic Acid	Usually started at 125 mg twice daily, and titrated to achieve anti-myoclonic effect, with most patients needing daily doses of 1200–2000 mg	Should not be administered to patients with hepatic disease or significant hepatic dysfunction	Drugs that increase levels of hepatic enzymes may decrease serum levels of valproic acid. Valproic acid may increase levels of warfarin, lamotrigine, phenobarbital, and phenytoin	Fatal hepatic failure may occur in patients taking it within 6 mos. of treatment, even in individuals who have no history of liver disease. Liver function studies therefore need to be monitored frequently Others: • pancreatitis • dose-related thrombocytopenia • action tremor • alopecia • reversible parkinsonism	1st drug specifically used for the treatment of myoclonus[3]
Primidone	Start with 25 mg/day, gradually increasing no faster than 25 or 50 mg/week, with the dose increased to tolerance, with a target of 500–750 mg/day	Use with caution in the elderly because of the risks of sedation, depression, and mental slowness	It is metabolized to phenobarbital and phenyl-ethylmalonamide Phenobarbital induces hepatic enzymes and may decrease the levels of drugs metabolized in the liver. Primidone lowers the levels of warfarin and steroids	Common: • drowsiness with development of tolerance Others: • may exacerbate existing behavioral problems and trigger irritability • impairs memory and tasks requiring prolonged periods of attention	
Clonazepam	Start with 0.5 mg per day and titrate until there is control of symptoms or side effects appear. Large doses may be necessary	Contraindicated in patients with hepatic dysfunction or narrow angle glaucoma	May potentiate the sedative effect of other medications	Common: • drowsiness Others: • ataxia • personality changes	After prolonged use, the dose should be tapered off slowly to avoid withdrawal symptoms

Note. Adapted from: Agarwal P, Frucht SJ. Myoclonus. *Current Opinion in Neurology.* 2003;*16*:515–521.

- As always when prescribing for the elderly, medication should be initiated at lower doses, dose escalation should be managed more slowly, and careful observation is required.

TAKE-HOME POINTS

- Myoclonus describes a symptom and generally is not a diagnosis of disease.
- Workup and evaluation should be targeted to find the underlying medical, metabolic, or toxic cause of the majority of myoclonus cases.
- Treatment begins by identifying and resolving the underlying disorder or precipitating factor.
- Medications must be scrutinized for a potential role in myoclonus, with the symptoms almost always reversible upon withdrawal of the offending drug.

- If the patient has primary myoclonus, or if the underlying disorder cannot be identified, anti-myoclonic agents may be used. These medications are usually used in combination, and it is rare for one agent to achieve complete control of myoclonus.

REFERENCES

1. Caviness JN, Brown P. Myoclonus: current concepts and recent advances. *Lancet Neurol.* 2004;3:598–607.
2. Caviness JN, Alving LI, Maraganore DM, Black R, McDonnell, Rocssa WA. The incidence and prevalence of myoclonus in Olmsted County. *Mayo Clin Proc.* 1999;74:565–569.
3. Agarwal P, Frucht SJ. Myoclonus. *Curr Opin Neurol.* 2003;16:515–521.

40

Cough and Secretions

CASE

Mr. M is a 67-year-old male diagnosed with small cell lung cancer six months ago, with disease progression after chemotherapy. He also has a history of chronic obstructive pulmonary disease (COPD), depression, and anxiety. Mr. M presents to the emergency room with a two-day history of increasing shortness of breath, moist and productive cough with purulent sputum, expiratory wheeze, fever, and severe chest pain upon coughing. This is the patient's third hospitalization for COPD exacerbation in the past 12 months.

DEFINITION

Cough is a sudden and often repetitively occurring defense reflex that helps to clear the large breathing passages from excess secretions, irritants, foreign particles, and microbes.[1] A cough has three phases: an inhalation, a forced exhalation against a closed glottis, and a violent release of air from the lungs following opening of the glottis, usually accompanied by a distinctive sound.[1]

CLASSIFICATION OF COUGH

Duration of cough from the time of presentation indicates likely causes.[2]

- **Acute (sudden onset lasting less than three weeks)**
  - Upper respiratory tract infection
  - Lower respiratory tract infection
  - Pneumonia
  - Exacerbation of COPD, asthma, or congestive heart failure (CHF)
  - Pulmonary emboli
  - Environmental irritant
- **Subacute (lasting three to eight weeks)**
  - Post-infectious: pneumonia, pertussis, bronchitis
  - New onset of upper airway cough syndrome (UACS), asthma, gastroesophageal reflux disease (GERD), chronic bronchitis

- **Chronic (lasting longer than eight weeks)**
  - Upper airway cough syndrome (UACS)
  - Asthma
  - Gastroesophageal reflux disease (GERD)
  - Chronic bronchitis
  - Lung tumor
  - Smoking, aspiration, ACE inhibitors

Mr. M. is experiencing acute type of cough, due to both an exacerbation of COPD and progressive small cell lung cancer.

PREVALENCE

29% to 83% of palliative care patients experience cough.[3] 59% of patients with chronic lung disease and lung cancer report cough in the last year of life.[4]

CONSEQUENCES OF UNTREATED COUGH

The complications associated with untreated cough can have a significant physical and psychosocial impact on patients (Table 40.1).

LIKELY ETIOLOGIES

The most common causes of chronic cough are upper airway cough syndrome (related to postnasal drip), asthma, and gastroparesis. Other etiologies are show in Table 40.2 below.

DESCRIPTION OF COUGHS

Coughs are described according to moisture, frequency, quality, regularity, pitch, and loudness. Type of cough may offer clue to its etiology.

- Moist: possible infection
- Dry: cardiac, allergies, or AIDS
- Infrequent: allergies or environmental irritants
- Acute onset: with fever suggests infection
- Acute onset: without fever suggests foreign body, inhaled irritants
- Irregularly occurring: smoking, CHF, tumor, foreign body, or irritant

TABLE 40.1: COMPLICATIONS OF UNTREATED COUGH[5]

Cardiovascular	Arterial hypotension Brady- and tachy-arrhythmias Dislodgement of intravascular catheters Loss of consciousness Rupture of subconjectival, nasal, and anal veins
Constitutional	Sweating Anorexia Fatigue/exhaustion Sleep disturbance
GI	GERD events Herniation Splenic rupture
GU	Urinary incontinence Inversion of bladder through urethra
Musculoskeletal	Rib fractures Sternal wound dehiscence Diaphragmatic rupture Rupture of rectus abdominus muscles
Skin	Petechiae, purpura, disruption of wound
Neurological	Cough syncope Headache Acute cervical radiculopathy Cerebral air embolism Seizures Stroke Malfunctioning ventriculoatrial shunts
Ophthalmologic	Spontaneous compressive orbital emphysema Rupture of conjunctiva
Psychosocial	Fear of serious disease Lifestyle changes Self-consciousness Decreased quality of life Depression

TABLE 40.2: ETIOLOGY[1]

Pulmonary	Infection (bacterial/viral) COPD Asthma Bronchiectasis Cystic fibrosis Interstitial lung disease Sarcoidosis Benign and malignant lung tumors Mediastinal masses Aspiration Pulmonary embolism/infarction
Cardiovascular	Congestive heart failure Aortic aneurysm
Head & Neck	Postnasal drip Dryness secondary to mouth breathing
GI	Gastroesophageal reflux disease (GERD)
Drugs	ACE inhibitors(dry cough)
Other	Foreign body Smoking Air pollution Dust and other allergens Smoke from wood-burning fireplaces; secondhand smoke Inhaled irritants Anxiety state Occupational exposures

- Postural influence: cough when lying suggests postnasal drip; when erect suggests pooled secretions in upper airway

Mr. M's moist and productive cough with purulent sputum and fever suggests infection.

DIAGNOSIS

Diagnostic workup should be based on the patient's goals of care. A comprehensive history and physical examination reveals the etiology of cough in 80% of patients with advanced illness.

Mr. M's chest X-ray showed emphysematous changes but no evidence of pneumonia. Pulse oximetry showed O_2 saturation of 87%. CBC revealed an elevated white blood count of 16,000. CT scan revealed increase in size of the patient's small cell lung tumor. Pulmonary function tests revealed FEV1 < 50% predicted.

History

The evaluation of a patient with cough should include:

- Primary diseases and comorbidities
- Hemoptysis
- Dyspnea
- Frequency and duration of cough
- Aggravating and relieving factors
- Fevers, chills, myalgias
- Night sweats and weight loss
- Sputum production and color
- Review medication list

- Oral secretions contributing to cough
- Hydration status
- Smoking history
- Allergies
- Sinus conditions
- GERD symptoms
- Subjective measurement using visual analog scale
- Environmental causes: smoking and/or secondhand smoke, wood-burning heat source, air pollution, animals, occupational exposures.

Exam

- Overall appearance
- Level of anxiety
- Vital signs
- Skin color
- Chest and lung exam
- Attention to intensity, pitch, and duration of breath sounds, and if cough clears secretions
- Upper airway assessment of nasal drainage, throat irritation, or sinus congestion
- Use of accessory muscles, retractions, or vein distention
- Attention to rib tenderness
- Abdominal exam: distention, masses, tenderness, enlarged organs, or abnormal sounds.

Mr. M's physical examination revealed decreased breath sounds bilaterally with bilateral crackles. Patient was using accessory muscles and appeared dusky. Patient verbalized feeling anxious.

Tests

Depending on the underlying etiology, the following evaluations may be needed to verify the etiology of the cough: chest X-ray, echocardiogram, CT scan, barium swallow, spirometry, or empiric treatment with proton pump inhibitor to "diagnose" GERD.

TREATMENT OPTIONS

The underlying cause of cough should be treated when possible, especially if it will improve quality of life. Benefits and burdens of diagnostic workup and treatment should be consistent with patient's goals for care.

Nonpharmacologic

General considerations include:

1. Posture/position:
   - It is impossible to cough effectively when lying flat.
   - Elevate head of bed.

2. Breathing techniques:
   - In the sitting position, have patient take a deep breath and hold it for two to three seconds and then cough.
   - Manually or mechanically assisted cough may be helpful with patients who have neuromuscular diseases and expiratory muscle weakness.
   - Huffing may assist patients with COPD and cystic fibrosis.
3. Patients with cystic fibrosis may benefit from chest physiotherapy and drainage.
4. Encourage adequate fluid intake to keep secretions loose.
5. Use throat lozenges for coughs related to irritation of the pharynx, usually due to infection or malignancy.[3]
6. Environmental conditions:
   - Eliminate dusts, allergens, smoke from the environment.
   - Humidify the room.
7. Lifestyle changes:
   - Smoking cessation
   - Dietary recommendations if cough due to GERD: 45 grams of fat/day; eliminate foods and beverages that are acidic or that relax the lower esophageal sphincter tone (coffee, tea, soft drinks, citrus fruit, tomato, alcohol, chocolate, mint); nothing to eat or drink two hours before reclining.
   - Patients with dysphagia should be positioned with head raised to 80 to 90 degrees while eating, and at least 45 to 60 degrees for 30 minutes after meals.
   - Patients should be well rested prior to eating. Keep suction readily available. Consider thickened beverages and dysphagia diet to reduce risk of aspiration.

Pharmacologic

Choice of pharmacologic treatment is based on the identified cause of the cough (Table 40.3).

MANAGEMENT OF COUGH

Additional medications to suppress cough for symptomatic relief include:

1. Guaifenesin 200 mg to 400 mg PO every 4 hours (not > 2400 mg/day)
   - Inhibits cough reflex by increasing sputum production and decreasing viscosity
   - Not for use with ACE inhibitor cough

TABLE 40.3: PHARMACOLOGIC TREATMENT OF COUGH[1]

Cause	Treatment	Example
Ace inhibitor cough	Discontinue ACEI if possible If not, suppress cough	Start different antihypertensive See additional med list below
Asthma	Inhaled bronchodilator + inhaled corticosteroids	Albuterol Beclomethazone diproprionate
Bronchiectasis	Bronchodilator	Albuterol Ipratropium bromide
Acute bronchitis	Antitussive medication B2 agonist bronchodilator (if wheezing)	Dextromethorphan Albuterol
Chronic bronchitis	Acute exacerbation—antibiotics B2 agonist bronchodilator +/− anticholinergic	Albuterol Ipratropium bromide
Bronchitis (non-asthmatic eosinophlic)	Inhaled corticosteroids Bronchodilator Trial of discontinuation of drug product	Bechlomethazone dipropionate Albuterol or ipratropium bromide
Chronic upper airway congestion syndrome (post nasal drip)	Antihistamine + decongestant	Brompheniramine Pseudoephedrine
Common cold	Antihistamine + decongestant +/− anti-inflammatory	Brompheniramine Pseudoephedrine Nonsteroidal anti-inflammatory agents (NSAIDS)
Congestive heart failure	Diuretics Centrally acting medication	Furosemide Opioids
GERD	Proton pump inhibitor and/or H2 Antihistamine +/− prokinetic	Omeprazole Famotidine Metoclopramide
Lung tumors	Centrally acting cough suppressant	Opioids
Post-infectious cough	Bronchodilator	Ipratopium
Superior vena cava syndrome cough	Corticosteroids	Decadron Prednisone
Tamponade-cardiac	At end of life, treat symptomatically	Analgesics Anxiolytics Oxygen

2. Central antitussives: Most effective antitussive agents are opioids of any type.
   - Hydrocodone 5 to 10 mg orally every 4 to 6 hours
   - Codeine 10 to 20 mg orally every 4 to 6 hours
3. Dextromethorphan 10 to 30 mg orally every 4 hours (not > 120 mg/day)
   - Not for chronic cough related to asthma or emphysema since these antitussives raise airway resistance.
   - Dextromethorphan inhibits cytochrome P450.
   - Dextromethorphan may cause serotonin syndrome.
   - Codeine and dextromethorphan available alone or in elixir with guaifenasin.
4. Benzonatate 100 mg orally every 8 hours (not > 600mg/day)
   - Deadens afferent stretch receptor sites in airways.
   - Side effects are GI upset, sleepiness, pruritus, dizziness, rash, headache, and constipation.
   - No published controlled studies confirm its effectiveness, but multiple uncontrolled studies support its use.

Expert opinion confirms adding it to an opioid.[6]

5. Lidocaine 1 to 2 ml of 1% to 2% solution via nebulizer up to 4 times per day
   - There are no clinical trials supporting this intervention.
   - *Patients must not take anything by mouth for 1 hour post nebulized lidocaine to prevent aspiration.*
6. Steroids: reduce inflammation, bronchospasms, or edema
   - Prednisone 40 to 60 mg orally per day for 10 to 14 days with slow taper to lowest dose
   OR
   - Dexamethasone 4 mg/day orally

MANAGEMENT OF SECRETIONS

1. To decrease viscosity:
   - Albuterol 0.5 ml in 2.5 ml of saline via nebulizer
   - Adequate fluid intake
2. To dry secretions—anticholinergics:
   - Hyoscyamine 0.125 to 0.25 mg sublingually every 4 to 6 hours
   - Glycopyrrolate 1 to 2 mg orally 2 to 3 times per day, or 0.1 to 0.2 mg IV every 4 to 6 hours
   - Scopolamine patch 1.5 mg TD (behind ear) every 72 hours
   - Atropine drops: 1 to 2 drops SL q 4 hours PRN
3. Overhydration: Decrease or stop IV fluids or tube feedings if consistent with goals of care.
4. Pneumonia: Give antibiotics if consistent with goals of care.
5. Pulmonary edema: Use diuretic.

OTHER MANAGEMENT OPTIONS

The decision to employ interventional therapies for cough should be based on the patient's prognosis, comorbidities and achievable goals of care.

- Tumor-induced cough: radiation therapy
- Malignant pleural effusion with cough: thoracentesis with pleurodesis or indwelling pleural drainage cathether
- Cardiac tamponade with cough: percardiocentesis. Pericardial window can prevent recurrence if patient is good surgical candidate.[4]

PALLIATIVE CARE ISSUES

- Chronic coughing at the end of life adds to a patient's suffering by causing pain, loss of sleep, fatigue, and shortness of breath.
- Near the end of life, the priority shifts from finding the cause to symptom relief.
- Treatments that are effective for reducing the burden of cough include:
  - Opioids to suppress the cough
  - Diuretics if the cough is due to fluid overload or congestive heart failure
  - Antibiotics to treat infection if this is consistent with the patient's goals of care
  - Bronchodilators to decrease wheezing and cough
  - Steroids to decrease inflammation
  - Anticholinergics (glycopyrolate, scopolamine, atropine drops) to help dry up excessive secretions
  - Limiting intravenous fluid and artificial nutrition to decrease the burden of secretions
  - If cough is due to pleural effusion, positioning the patient on the side of the pleural effusion can help decrease cough[3]
  - Discontinue ACE inhibitor medication if possible

Mr. M's treatment plan included oxygen 2 liters via nasal cannula, morphine 2 mg IV every four hours for chest pain associated with cough and dyspnea, albuterol 0.5 ml in 2.5 ml saline via nebulizer every 6 hours and levofloxacin 750 mg PO daily for five days.

Cough and associated pain decreased by day two of hospitalization, and morphine was switched to hydrocodone 5 mg/5 ml 10 ml q 4 hour PRN for cough, pain, or dyspnea.

An oncology consult was ordered to address the patient's worsening lung cancer. No further cancer-specific treatment options were available. A meeting to discuss goals of care was organized, and the patient decided to enroll in home hospice.

TAKE-HOME POINTS

- Cough can severely impair quality of life for patients and families.
- Interventions are based on the patient's goals of care, prognosis, and risk/benefit analysis.
- Reversible causes should be identified and treated.
- If feasible, treatment should be directed at the underlying cause.

- Treat symptomatically even if waiting for acute therapy to work.

REFERENCES

1. Irwin RS, Baumann MH, Bolser DC, Boulet L, et al. Diagnosis and management of cough. Executive Summary. ACCP evidence-based clinical practice guidelines. *Chest.* 2006;Supplement 1(*129*):1–23.
2. Irwin RS, Madison JM. The diagnosis and treatment of cough. *N Engl. J Med.* 2000;*343*(23):1715–1721.
3. Doyle D, Hanks G, MacDonald N. *Oxford Textbook of Palliative Medicine.* Oxford, England: Oxford University Press; 2004:602–604.
4. Fournier J. Cough. In Kuebler K, Heidrich D, Esper P, eds. *Palliative & End-of-Life Care.* Philadelphia: Elsevier Saunders; 2007:301–313.
5. Irwin RS. Complication of Cough ACCP Evidence-Based Clinical Practice Guideline. *Chest.* January 2006;*129*(Suppl 1):54S–58S.
6. Marks S, Rosielle DA. Non-Opioid Anti-Tussives. Fast Facts and Concepts. March 2008:200. Available at: http://www.eperc.mcw.edu/EPERC/FastFactsIndex/ff_200.htm.

41

Dyspnea

CASE
Mr. M is an 88-year-old male with a history of hypertension, congestive heart failure, and progressive chronic obstructive pulmonary disease (COPD). He is admitted to the hospital with a third viral pneumonia in one year. Mr. M. complains of shortness of breath with any physical exertion, eating, and during conversation. On physical examination, Mr. M is pale, cachectic, with bilateral rhonchi, tachycardia, and 2+ pedal edema. Mr. M and his family understand that his COPD is end-stage and his goal is to be as comfortable as possible and to remain at home. Mr. M appointed his son as his health care proxy and completed a "do not resuscitate/intubate" (DNR/I) order. Mr. M reported having a personal will, and he decided to give his son his financial power of attorney.

DEFINITION
Dyspnea (also commonly referred to as "shortness of breath") is the subjective experience of breathing discomfort caused by interactions between physiological, psychological, social, and environmental factors.[1] Dyspnea can be acute, chronic, or terminal and may result in severe debility and impaired quality of life.[2]

PREVALENCE[3]
- Occurs in 55% to 70% of patients with advanced diseases, especially cancer and end-stage heart or lung disease
- 41% of palliative care patients experience dyspnea, with 46% rating their symptom as moderate to severe. In advanced cancer, dyspnea is an indicator of poor prognosis, whether it occurs alone or in conjunction with other symptoms.

CONSEQUENCES OF UNTREATED DYSPNEA
Untreated dyspnea can contribute to anxiety, increased suffering, decreased quality of life, difficulties with activities of daily living, and increased social isolation.

PREDISPOSING FACTORS

Structural Factors
- Increased chest wall stiffness increases work of breathing.
- Decrease in skeletal muscle, increase in anteroposterior diameter decreases maximum volume expiration.
- Decrease in elasticity of alveoli causes a decrease in vital capacity.

Other Factors[4]
- Allergens
- Anemia
- Anxiety
- Cachexia
- Cancer
- Dehydration increases mucous plugging.
- End-stage organ failure (lung, heart, liver, kidney)
- GERD (gastroesophageal reflux disease)
- Infection
- Immobility increases aspiration risk, deep vein thrombosis, pulmonary embolism.
- Lung disease (COPD, lung cancer)
- Obesity
- Surgery: recent abdominal, pelvic, or chest surgery

DIAGNOSIS
- Diagnostic workup for dyspnea should be determined by patient's goals of care, prognosis, risk/benefit ratio and patient/family wishes.
- Evaluation should include a comprehensive history and physical exam, but testing is not indicated if the results would not change the current plan of care.

History
- Acute onset versus chronic
- Comorbidities and underlying diseases

- Timing, precipitating factors, associated symptoms, and alleviating factors
- Smoking history
- Psychological history including mental health issues, history of anxiety, coping style of patient and family, meaning of the symptom to the patient and family
- Presence of advance directives such as health care proxy, living will, and wishes regarding resuscitation and intubation
- Environmental factors that might contribute to dyspnea, such as air quality, animals, use of oxygen, climbing stairs, distance to bathroom

Exam[5]
- Color of skin, nails, lips, capillary refill, and clubbing
- Examine of head, neck, and chest for presence of nasal flaring, tracheal deviation, jugular venous distention
- Observe chest shape and movement, costal retractions, accessory muscle use, sternal/spinal deformities.
- Observe inspiration/expiration ratio through facial and oral expression.
- Palpate chest to assess for tenderness, masses, nodes, fremitus, and crepitus.
- Percuss the chest to assess resonance or dullness (dullness indicates consolidation; resonance indicates presence of air).
- Auscultate the lungs for adventitious or diminished breath sounds, voice sounds, and pleural friction rubs.
- Observe overall nutritional state.

Since the goals of care for Mr. M are to remain comfortable and be at home, no diagnostic testing is indicated, as results would not change the plan of care.

Tests
If determining the underlying cause is a goal of care, the following diagnostic tests can be considered:

- Chest X-ray
- Pulmonary function tests
- Pulse oximetry
- EKG
- CBC
- Electrolyte profile
- CT scan/MRI
- Arterial blood gases

Measurement of Dyspnea
- *Visual Analogue Scale* (0–100; "not at all breathless" to "severely breathless"). The VAS is a valid and reliable tool that assesses dyspnea by using a 100 mm line that can be either horizontal or vertical. Word anchors are attached at each end to indicate the extremes of the sensation of breathing (zero representing "no breathlessness" and 100 representing "worst possible breathlessness." The patient places a mark along the line that corresponds with the symptom intensity. The clinician measures the distance from the bottom of the scale (vertical) or from the left (horizontal) to the patient's mark.[2]
- *Modified Borg Scale* 0-10. This is a valid and reliable tool for the evaluation of dyspnea severity. Uses a 10-point scale with descriptors, zero for "no breathlessness at all," 5 for "severe breathlessness," and 10 for "maximum breathlessness."[2]
- For nonverbal geriatric patients, assess objective indicators such as tachypnea, gasping, use of accessory muscles, anxiety, restlessness, agitation, grimacing, and tachycardia. Ask family members and/or caregivers to describe patient's baseline behaviors.
- Clinicians should clarify the words and language used by patients to describe their dyspnea, as descriptors may vary due to language and cultural background.

Using the modified Borg Scale for dyspnea assessment, Mr. M rated his dyspnea at a 7.

TREATMENT OPTIONS
- There often is a clear, treatable etiology underlying the dyspnea symptoms (e.g., asthma or COPD). See Table 41.1 for treatment strategies.
- For dyspnea that is not reversible, a comprehensive symptom management plan should utilize nonpharmacologic and pharmacologic measures (Table 41.2).

Nonpharmacologic
Practical/environment modifications:
- Position patient sitting up and support head, neck, arms with pillows.
- If lying on side, position with compromised lung down.
- Use fan or open window for cool air.

TABLE 41.1: TREATMENT OF UNDERLYING ETIOLOGIES

Rales	If fluid overload, reduce artificial feedings and stop IV hydration if consistent with goals of care. Diuretic may be indicated.
Effusions	Thoracentesis. If effusion recurs, consider pleurodesis or indwelling drain based on goals of care. During active dying phase, administer opioids and benzodiazepines as needed.
Anemia	Blood transfusion will improve dyspnea and energy if consistent with goals of care. Erythropoietin for patients with anemia of chronic conditions due to malignancy, chronic renal disease, chronic liver disease, HIV, and diseases of an infectious or inflammatory nature. In actively dying patients, bleeding and bone marrow failure are part of the process and treatment is symptomatic using opioids and benzodiazepines.
Thick secretions	Use nebulized saline and expectorant if patient has strong cough reflex. When cough reflex is weak, dry up secretions with anticholinergics (above).
Bronchospasms	Nebulized albuterol or inhaler. Add corticosteroids as needed.
Anxiety	Sit patient upright and support arms with pillows. If patient on side, have compromised lung down. Fan or open window for cool air Calming music, relaxation techniques, touch, prayer, massage, guided imagery, hypnosis Supportive presence—staff member, family, friend, companion, doula Opioids and anxiolytics (above)
Psychosocial concerns	Family, social, and financial concerns can exacerbate dyspnea as well as underlying psychiatric diagnoses. Calming presence and listening skills Counseling using interdisciplinary team If dyspnea is related to unfinished business, assist patient/family with practical matters (wills, HCP, advance care planning, durable power of attorney for financial matters, guardianship for children under 18 years old, or other dependent individuals). Address patient's fears related to dying.
Religious/ Spiritual concerns	Attentive presence and listening skills Do a spiritual assessment Elicit patient's religious/spiritual concerns. Involve team chaplain, patient's clergy, or rabbi.
Continuity of care concerns	Consistent with patient/family goals of care and clinical status, refer to home health agency and/ or hospice for ongoing symptom management, patient, family support, and 24/7 availability.

- Pulmonary rehabilitation if consistent with goals of care.
- Ask patient "yes" and "no" questions; don't expect patient to talk a lot.
- Plan activities to conserve energy.
- Small, frequent meals
- Noninvasive positive pressure ventilation for hypercapnic patients if consistent with patient's goals of care

Relaxation techniques:

- Massage therapy
- Guided imagery, relaxation exercises

- Pursed lip breathing
- Calming music, distraction
- Hypnosis

Spiritual:

- Listen to psychosocial and spiritual concerns and coordinate appropriate resources.
- Touch, reassurance
- Prayer
- Supportive presence of staff, family, friends, doula
- Address fears related to illness and dying.

TABLE 41.2: PHARMACOLOGIC TREATMENT OF DYSPNEA[2,6]

Treatment	Dose/Med	Mechanism of Action	Comments
Opioids	*Opioid-naive patients* Morphine 2.5–5 mg PO q 4 hours Morphine 0.5 mg–2 mg IV q 4 hours Hydromorphone 1–2 mg PO q 4 hours Hydromorphone 0.1–0.3 mg IV q 4 hours PRN *Patients on opioids*: Increase dose 25–50% in mild-moderate dyspnea, 50–100% in severe dyspnea	Decreases ventilatory response to hypoxia and hypercapnia Reduces metabolic rate and O_2 consumption Alters perception of breathlessness Has cardiovascular effects of vasodilation and decreases peripheral resistance, which improves O_2 supply and reduces lung congestion	In naive geriatric patient, start low and go slow In kidney disease adjust dose and medication; AVOID MORPHINE, use longer dosing intervals Maintain safe environment to reduce risk of falls Titrate dose to symptom relief and monitor patient's response Manage predictable side effects such as nausea, constipation
Oxygen	O_2 2–6 liters if pulse ox < 90% or air hunger continuous or PRN per patient comfort level	Depresses hypoxic drive, reducing demand of ventilation	Use least restrictive device to enable communication and eating (nasal cannula) Humidify O_2 if 4 liters or greater. Avoid high concentrations of O_2 in patients with COPD as CO_2 is retained, which creates drive to breathe Patients at home (with exception of home hospice patients) must meet specific physiological criteria to qualify for home oxygen: a) Stable disease on full medical regimen with Pa O_2 < 55 mgHg and SaO_2 at rest < 88% b) Pt with PaO_2 55–59 mmHg and Sa O_2 89% with tissue hypoxia from pulmonary hypertension, corpulmonale, erythrocytosis, edema from right side heart failure or impaired mental status should receive home oxygen c) Pt with PaO_2 > 60 mmHg and SaO_2 >90% who has exercise desaturation, sleep desaturation not corrected by CPAP or lung disease with severe dyspnea responding to O_2
Anxiolytics: add if opioid alone is not effective	Lorazepam 0.25–1 mg PO/IV q 4 hours Alprazolam 0.25–1 mg PO q 4 hours	Depresses hypoxic/ hypercapnic ventilatory response and alters emotional response Binds to GABA and inhibits neurotransmitters in CNS	Anxiety is often a component of dyspnea When opioids alone are not effective, add anxiolytic Benzodiazepines are most commonly used Maintain safe environment to limit falls

(continued)

TABLE 41.2: (CONTINUED)

Treatment	Dose/Med	Mechanism of Action	Comments
Corticosteroids: add if inflammation is contributing to dyspnea	Prednisone 2.5–5 mg PO every 6 hours Dexamethasone 2–4 mg PO BID Methylprednisolone 10 mg IV every 6 hours	Reduces inflammation by suppressing migration of polymorphonuclear leukocytes and reverses the increased capillary permeability	Risk/benefit of long-term use must be weighed due to side effects (osteoporosis, infection) May increase appetite and sense of well-being
Bronchodilators	Albuterol Ipratroprium 1–2 puffs 4x per day (See Chapter 72: End Stage Lung Disease, for more bronchodilator options.)	Causes smooth muscle dilation of the airways and increases airflow	Useful in reactive airway disease/ bronchospasms Side effects tremors, agitation and anxiety may heighten dyspnea
Diuretics	Furosemide 10–30 mg PO/IV daily or twice a day depending on response	Inhibits reabsorption of sodium and chloride in ascending loop of Henle and distal renal tubule, causing increased excretion of water and electrolytes	Use when dyspnea is associated with fluid volume overload Monitor electrolytes based on goals of care Reduce or stop artificial feeding and IV hydration for symptom relief
Antibiotics	If consistent with goals of care, consider empirical trial of antibiotic based on suspected organism		An empirical course of A/B may be indicated if dyspnea is secondary to infection Evaluate based on goals of care if use is prolonging dying process
Anticholinergics	Glycopyrrolate 0.4mg IV/SQ q 3 hours PRN Scopolamine patch 1–3 patches q 3 days Hyoscyamine (Levsin) 0.125 mg PO or SL q 8 hours Atropine optham sol 1–2 drops SL q 4 PRN	Blocks acetylcholine at parasympathetic sites in smooth muscle, secretory glands, and CNS and inhibits salivary secretions	Useful when secretions build up in posterior oropharynx ("death rattle") due to weak cough Reduce or discontinue artificial feedings and IV hydration if in keeping with goals of care

Mr. M and his family were taught proper positioning of the patient: sitting up with head, neck, and arms supported. A bedside fan and cool air across his face helped to control the perception of breathlessness. Relaxing music and massage therapy were also helpful. The palliative care chaplain met with Mr. M for a spiritual assessment and notes that he copes through prayer and the strength of his family. Mr. M reported "being at peace."

Pharmacologic

Opioids are the standard pharmacological agents for management of distressing dyspnea. See Table 41.1 for additional treatments.

Mr. M is opioid-naive and has chronic renal insufficiency, so low-dose hydromorphone, 0.2 mg IV q 6 hours, is recommended. Oxygen by nasal cannula @ 2 liters is given. Furosemide 20 mg IV resulted in diuresis. Viral pneumonia was suspected, and no antibiotics were ordered. After hydromorphone, oxygen and furosemide, Mr. M reported that his dyspnea had declined to a level of 2.

Mr. M reports some anxiety, especially at night. Lorazepam 0.5 mg PO q 6 hours PRN was recommended. The palliative care chaplain and social worker continued to follow Mr. M and his family for emotional and spiritual support.

REFRACTORY DYSPNEA

- Increase opioid dose 25% to 50% (moderate) or 50% to 100% (severe) every 4 hours as needed. Consider continuous IV or SQ opioid infusion with bolus dosing for breakthrough dyspnea. If no response, add dexamethasone 2 to 4 mg IV/PO twice a day.
- Position patient in the sitting position; support arms on pillows. Address treatable conditions such as pulmonary edema, bronchospasms, fever. If no response and patient/family distress is high, consider palliative sedation. (See Chapter 22: Palliative Sedation.)
- Involve the entire interdisciplinary team. Provide ongoing support for the patient and family. If death is imminent, advise family about what to expect during the normal dying process.

On the third day of hospitalization, Mr. M reported less relief from the hydromorphone 0.2 mg IV. He reported dyspnea at level 7 pre-hydromorphone and 5 post-hydromorphone. Hydromorphone was increased to 0.4 mg IV q 4hours with 0.2 mg IV q 2 hours PRN for breakthrough. Mr. M had a better response to this increased dose, reporting dyspnea at level 2 after hydromorphone 0.4 mg IV.

PALLIATIVE CARE ISSUES

- The entire interdisciplinary team should be involved in treatment, as dyspnea derives from the complex interaction of physical, psychological, social, spiritual/existential, and environmental factors.
- Underlying conditions that may contribute to the dyspnea should be treated when consistent with patient's goals of care and when benefits outweigh the risks.
- If death is imminent, the family should be advised about what to expect during the normal dying process.

Mr. M's symptoms stabilized on the 4th day of hospitalization and he asked to go home with home hospice. The family was in agreement and

supportive. Mr. M was discharged on hydromorphone 2 mg PO q 4 hours with 2 mg PO q 1 hour PRN breakthrough for dyspnea, as well as lorazepam 0.5 mg PO q 4 hour, as needed for anxiety.

TAKE-HOME POINTS

- Dyspnea and fear of dyspnea cause severe disability and impaired quality of life for patients and should be aggressively managed using an interdisciplinary approach.
- The patient's goals of care should determine the extent of the workup and treatment of underlying causes of dyspnea.
- Anxiety often accompanies dyspnea and should be addressed as well.
- Opioids are the first choice of treatment for dyspnea.
- Nonpharmacologic treatments can be effective when used in conjunction with medications.

REFERENCES

1. Lanken PN, Terry PB, DeLisser HM, et al. An official American Thoracic Society clinical policy statement: palliative care for patients with respiratory diseases and critical illnesses. *Am J Respir Crit Care Med.* 2008;17:912–927.
2. Spector N, Connolly M, Carlson K. Dyspnea: applying research to bedside practice. *AACN Adv Crit Care.* 2007;18:45–50.
3. Bruera E, Ripamonti C. Dyspnea in Patients with Advanced Cancer. In Berger A, Portnoy R, Weissman D, eds. *Principles and Practice of Supportive Oncology.* Philadelphia: Lippincott, Williams & Wilkins, 1998;295–308.
4. Balkstra C. Dypsnea. In LaPorte Matzo M, Sherman D, eds. *Gerontologic Palliative Care Nursing.* St. Louis: Mosby, 2004;303–316.
5. Dudgeon D. Dypsnea, Death Rattle and Cough. In Ferrel B, Coyle N, eds. *Textbook of Palliative Nursing.* New York: Oxford University Press, Inc., 2001;164–174.
6. Brown J. Usage and Documentation of Home Oxygen Therapy: Executive Summary Department of Health and Human Services, Office of the Inspector General. 1999; 1–27: http://www.dhhs.gov/progorg/oei.

42

Anorexia/Cachexia

CASE

Mrs. A is an 84-year-old woman with advancing Alzheimer's dementia. She also has underlying hypertension, which has been well controlled. Her family has concerns that the patient seems to have decreased appetite and has lost about 10 lbs in the last year. Her home health aide reports that the patient seems to be pushing food out with her tongue when fed and at times seems to choke and cough when drinking liquids.

DEFINITION

Anorexia is the loss of appetite, while *cachexia* is characterized as loss of weight, muscle atrophy, fatigue, weakness, and significant loss of appetite in someone who is not actively trying to lose weight. Cachexia can be due to decreased caloric intake as a consequence of anorexia but can also be related to a hypermetabolic or hypercatabolic state from the underlying disease process.

- When anorexia and cachexia result from progression of underlying disease, the condition usually cannot be permanently reversed; no treatments have been proven to increase longevity. However, it is important to assess and manage comorbid conditions while educating and supporting the family in distinguishing between the normal progression of disease, over which they have no control, and things they can do to make the patient feel better.

PREVALENCE

Anorexia and cachexia are common to most chronic illnesses, reported in up to 80% of patients with cancer and also in the end stages of most chronic diseases, including dementia, heart failure, and emphysema.

LIKELY ETIOLOGIES

- Underlying disease:
  - Disordered swallowing (stroke, dementia, tumor)
- Inability to remember to eat (dementia, stroke)
- Need for assistance with eating
- Hypercatabolic/metabolic state, in many chronic diseases
- Loss of appetite
- Depression
- Hypothyroidism/Hyperthyroidism
- Due to other symptoms, especially nausea, vomiting, and constipation, altered taste

DIAGNOSIS

Exploration to assess if symptoms are distressing to patient. History and examination to explore reversible causes:

- Screen for depression (Geriatric Depression Scale, http://www.stanford.edu/~yesavage/GDS.html)
- Evaluation of related symptoms
- Tests-TSH

TREATMENT OPTIONS

- Treatment should focus on therapies for reversible causes and education for patients and families regarding the significance of this symptom how it is related to the severity of the underlying illness.
- Although medication therapies can improve appetite and weight, none has been shown to increase longevity. Corticosteroids have been associated with increased appetite and sense of well-being in cancer patients, but there are no studies in older adults, and potential benefits should be weighed against the known adverse effects. Similarly, progesterone use in nursing home residents improved appetite, but side effects limited its use.
- Nonpharmacologic treatment should therefore be the primary approach.

For Mrs. A, her anorexia and weight loss are probably results of her advanced dementia. Nonpharmacological approaches such as offering

TABLE 42.1: TREATMENT OPTIONS

Nonpharmacologic: Primary approach to these symptoms	Offer favorite foods Nutritional supplements Encourage small, frequent meals Determine if assistance with feeding is required Avoid gastric irritants like spicy food and milk Discontinue unnecessary medications that may cause loss of taste/appetite: NSAIDs, antipsychotics, calcium channel blockers, anticholinergics

Pharmacologic*:
*None proven to increase longevity
	Corticosteroids:
	   Dexamethasone 2–20 mg/daily
	   Prednisone 20–40 mg/daily
	Progesterones
	Megestrol acetate 200 mg PO q6–8
	Vitamin supplementation: trial of zinc 20–100 mg daily to restore taste

favorite foods and encouraging small, frequent meals of appropriate consistency are most effective. In situations where the family insists that something be done about the poor PO intake despite a thorough educational process, a trial of the corticosteroids or progesterones can be considered after a conversation about realistic goals even with the use of these medications and the medications' potential side effects. The role of artificial feeding and nutrition may be discussed at this point. (See Chapter 27: Artificial Nutrition and Hydration.)

TAKE-HOME POINTS

- Anorexia and cachexia can be more distressing to families than to the patients themselves.
- Treatment should incorporate education regarding the underlying disease as well as nonpharmacologic interventions to promote comfort and address symptoms.

- Pharmacologic treatments are not proven to extend life but may be considered as a trial of therapy for patients with bothersome symptoms.

REFERENCES

1. Fainsinger R. Pharmacological approach to cancer anorexia and cachexia. In: Bruera E, Higginson I eds. *Cachexia-Anorexia in Cancer Patients.* Oxford, England. Oxford University Press; 1996;128–140.
2. Bruera E et al. A controlled trial of megesterol acetate on appetite, caloric intake, nutritional status and other symptoms in patients with advanced cancer. *Cancer.* 1990;66:1279–1282.
3. Chun A, Morrison RS. Palliative Care. In: *Hazard's Geriatric Medicine and Gerontology.* Halter JB, Ouslander JG et al, eds. New York, NY: McGraw-Hill Companies; 2009;373–384.

43

Ascites

CASE

Mrs. S is a 74-year-old patient with diabetes mellitus, congestive heart failure (EF unknown), and liver disease from alcohol use. She is still drinking almost every day. She comes to your office complaining of increasing abdominal girth and early satiety. She does not have dyspnea, fever, or abdominal pain. On examination she has shifting dullness. What tests do you order and what treatment options are available?

DEFINITION

Ascites is abnormal fluid accumulation in the peritoneal cavity. *Cirrhosis* refers to chronic liver disease. *Compensated cirrhosis* means an anatomically fibrotic liver without clinical complications such as encephalopathy, variceal bleeding, hepatorenal syndrome, hepatopulmonary syndrome, hepatocellular carcinoma, or ascites.

PREVALENCE

- Cirrhosis affects 5.5 million people, or 2% of the U.S. population.[1]Although liver disease is generally not thought of as a geriatric disease because of the association with substance abuse, 60% of all newly diagnosed chronic liver disease occurs in the elderly.[2]
- Ascites is the most common complication of chronic liver disease. Ascites occurs in 50% of patients within 10 years of a diagnosis of compensated cirrhosis.[3]

LIKELY ETIOLOGIES

Listed in Table 43.1 below are all the causes of ascites.

CONSEQUENCES OF UNTREATED ASCITES

- Discomfort due to abdominal distention
- Infection of ascites fluid
- Shortness of breath

- Hernia
- Decreased oral intake due to early satiety
- Decreased mobility if the ascites is massive
- Frequent hospitalizations

DIAGNOSIS

The workup requires a comprehensive history, physical exam, and investigation of the possible underlying etiologies.

History

- Since the most common cause of ascites is cirrhosis, the history should detail risk factors for liver disease:
  - Alcohol use
  - Intravenous or intranasal drug use (hepatitis C and B)
  - Diabetes or obesity (non-alcoholic fatty liver disease)
  - Unprotected sexual activity (hepatitis B)
  - Asian descent (hepatitis B)
- Obtain history suggestive of malignancy:

TABLE 43.1: ETIOLOGIES

Disease Process	Likelihood of Ascites as a Symptom
Cirrhosis	81% (The most common cause of ascites is advanced liver disease.)
Cancer	10%
Heart failure	3%
Tuberculosis	2%
Dialysis	1%
Pancreatic disease	1%
Other	2%

Data from: Runyon BA. *N Engl J Med.* 1994;330:337–342.

- Gynecologic malignancies are particularly associated with ascites.
- Patients with malignancy-associated ascites usually have a high tumor burden, so they usually have cancer-associated symptoms such as weight loss even with the accumulation of fluid.
- Ask about symptoms consistent with advanced congestive heart failure.
- Patients should be asked about tuberculosis risk factors such as HIV or immigration from an endemic area.

Exam
- Check for shifting dullness to determine if patient has ascites (83% sensitivity and 56% specificity).[4] Look for stigmata of chronic liver disease (See Chapter 76: End-Stage Liver Disease):
  - Caput medusa
  - Spider telengiactasias
  - Palmer erythema
  - Gynecomastia
- Check for signs of advanced congestive heart failure.
- Breast, pelvic, and lymph node examination to rule out malignancy as part of the comprehensive examination.

Tests
- Diagnostic paracentesis:
  - Serum-ascites albumin gradient, if ≥1.1 then 97% accuracy that cause is portal hypertension from liver disease.[4]
  - Complete cell count. (White blood cell count less than 500 with less than half polymorphonuclear neutrophils is consistent with ascites caused by liver cirrhosis, heart failure, and renal disease; a white blood cell count greater than 500 is consistent with infection, malignancy, and pancreatitis.)
  - Cultures if infection suspected.
  - Glucose if infection or cancer suspected. (Glucose levels are low with infection or malignancy.)
  - The ascitic fluid/serum (AF/S) ratio of LDH is 0.4 in uncomplicated cirrhotic ascites and close to 1 with infections and cancer.
  - Cytology almost 100% positive in peritoneal carcinomatosis.[5]

- See Figure 43.1 for algorithm indicating the use of the different test of ascites fluid to help identify the cause.
- Ultrasound to evaluate for ascites undetectable by physical exam, hepatic masses, and portal vein thrombosis.
- Blood work including:
  - Comprehensive metabolic panel including liver enzymes
  - Prothrombin time
  - Complete blood count
  - Brain natriuretic peptide (BNP) levels to rule out congestive heart failure

TREATMENT OPTIONS
- See Table 43.2 for etiology-based options for treating ascites.
- Referral to liver disease specialist should be considered early after diagnosis of cirrhotic ascites to help with management or for those in whom transplantation may be an option. Older age is no longer considered an absolute contraindication for transplantation.

Mrs. S's physical exam revealed findings consistent with liver disease including caput medusa, palmar erythema, and jaundice. Her lab tests also indicated liver dysfunction. She was symptomatic from her ascites, so a large volume paracentesis was performed and the patient was started on diuretics. Because she had not had a paracentesis before, the fluid was sent for cell count, albumin, protein, and cultures. The patient was also advised to stop drinking because alcohol decreases portal pressure and increases ascites accumulation.

PALLIATIVE CARE ISSUES
- Even while patients are pursing aggressive life-prolonging treatments such as transplantation, palliative care is appropriate since ascites is associated with significant impairment of quality of life. Palliative care is needed to address goals of care, advance directives, practical support for patient and family, and symptom management.
- Ascites is associated with a poor prognosis, and therefore all treatments should be evaluated in terms of benefits and burdens. In addition, if a hepatologist is involved, he

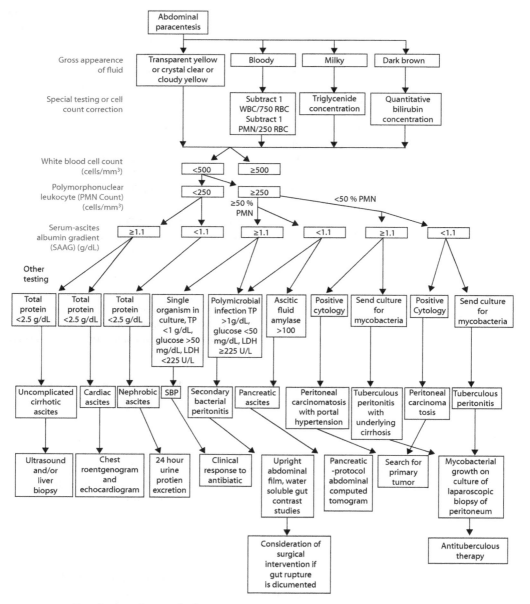

FIGURE 43.1: Classification of ascitic fluid.

or she should be consulted when making treatment recommendations, especially when opioids are considered.

TAKE-HOME POINTS

- The most common cause of ascites is cirrhosis.

- Ascites in the setting of liver cirrhosis or cancer is a harbinger of poor prognosis and is associated with poor quality of life. Palliative care should be offered simultaneously with all other appropriate treatments.

- Paracentesis provides the most immediate relief of symptoms.

TABLE 43.2: ETIOLOGY-BASED TREATMENT OPTIONS FOR ASCITES

Etiology of Ascites	Nonpharmacologic Intervention	Pharmacologic Intervention
Cirrhosis	Sodium restriction of 2 grams a day	Diuretics, either spironolactone (100 mg to 400 mg once a day orally) alone or with furosemide (40 mg to 160 mg once a day orally)[4]
	Water restriction only if severe hyponatremia	
	Stopping alcohol use will reduce portal hypertension	Avoid NSAIDs because of reduced effectiveness of diuretics and increased risk of renal failure and bleeding
	Therapeutic paracentesis	
	Other options if patient is not responsive to maximum doses of diuretics and salt restriction:	Judicious use of low-dose opioid if severe pain due to distention, especially if therapeutic paracentesis is not an immediate option
	If previously responded to diuretics, evaluate for worsening liver disease or a new complication such as portal vein thrombosis or hepatocellular carcinoma	(See Chapter 29: Management of Pain in Older Adults.)
	Consider referral to hospice	Paracentesis: can be performed as an outpatient even while receiving hospice care; immediate symptom relief but can accelerate malnutrition
	Serial large volume paracentesis	
	Indwelling drainage catheter (may not remain patent, is portal for infections)	
	Transjugular intrahepatic portosystemic shunt (TIPS) (can precipitate or worsen encephalopathy and may not remain patent)	
	Liver transplantation	
Malignancy	Salt restriction not helpful	Diuretics can be tried but not effective unless there is portal hypertension
	Other options	
	Therapeutic paracentesis as needed	Opioids for discomfort at reduced dosages and longer intervals
	Indwelling drainage catheter (may not remain patent and is portal for infections)	Morphine 2 mg IV every 6 hours with 1 to 2 mg IV every 15 to 30 minutes for rescues or morphine 5 mg orally every 6 hours with 5mg oral every hour as needed for rescues
	Obtain oncologic input for disease-specific options	
	Poor prognosis, so consider hospice if goals of care are comfort	Oxycodone 5 mg oral every 6 hours with 5 mg every hour as needed for rescues
Other	Treat underlying cause	

REFERENCES

1. Sanchez W, Talwalker JA. Palliative care for patients with end-stage liver disease ineligible for liver transplantation. *Gastroenterol Clin North Am.* 2006;*23*:201–219.
2. Junaidi O, Di Bisceglie AM. Aging liver and hepatitis. *Clin Geriatr Med.* 2007;*23*:889–903.
3. Runyon B. Care of the patient with ascites. *N Engl J Med.* 1994;*330*:337.
4. Runyon B. Management of the adult patient with ascites due to cirrhosis: an update. *Hepatology.* 2009;*49*:2087–2107.
5. Runyon BA, Hoefs JC, Morgan TR. Ascitic fluid analysis in malignancy-related ascites. *Hepatology.* 1988;*8*:1104–1109.

44

Bowel Obstruction

CASE
Mrs. E, a 78-year-old woman, developed nausea, vomiting, abdominal pain, and distention over a two-day period. Her last bowel movement was three days prior, and until then she had fairly regular, daily-to-alternate-day bowel movements. She has a past medical history of hypertension, diabetes, hypercholesterolemia, osteoarthritis, and coronary artery disease. Her surgical history includes an appendectomy and an open cholecystectomy. Her last colonoscopy (15 years ago) revealed two benign polyps.

DEFINITION
Bowel obstruction refers to significant blockage of the passage of luminal contents. Obstruction can be defined by its location (small intestine vs. colon), by acuity, or by the mechanism of obstruction (partial or complete structural compromise of the lumen vs. functional or pseudo-obstruction) (Box 44.1).

PREVALENCE
Small bowel obstruction is one of the most common reasons for surgical intervention and accounts for up to 12 to 16% of surgical admissions for acute abdominal pain annually.[1] Though not as common, the incidence of large bowel obstruction increases with age.

On physical exam, Mrs. E has normal BS and her abdomen is soft and minimally tender. Bowel sounds are present but hypoactive. Vital signs are stable: BP 110/60 with pulse of 90.

DIAGNOSIS
- Symptoms of bowel obstruction may include abdominal pain (cramps centered around the umbilicus), distention, nausea and vomiting (can be fecaloid in colonic obstruction), severe constipation, diarrhea (around obstruction), fever.
- For patients who present with indications of complete bowel obstruction or intestinal strangulation (fever, severe steady pain, tachycardia, obstipation, leukocytosis), prompt surgical exploration is imperative. Clinicians should be aware that a potentially serious bowel obstruction in elderly patients can present atypically (e.g., with delirium, but no fever or leukocytosis).

BOX 44.1 TYPES OF BOWEL OBSTRUCTION

Type	Causes
Mechanical	Postoperative adhesions, fecal impaction, neoplasm (benign or malignant), hernia, stricture. diverticular disease, foreign body (including gallstone), volvulus (twisting of bowel on its mesentery), trauma, and rarely, intussusception
Functional or pseudo-obstruction	Medications, post-surgical ileus, electrolyte imbalance, medications, appendicitis, pancreatitis, diverticulosis, mesenteric ischemia, cholangitis, and sepsis Ogilvie's syndrome: Acute pseudo-obstruction, often associated with pneumonia, sepsis, myocardial infarction, congestive heart failure, Alzheimer's, Parkinson's, and post-operatively after hip fracture surgery; can often lead to metabolic derangements (low potassium)

History

- Severity, character (cramping, sharp, radiating), location, and duration of abdominal pain
- Medication use (opioid analgesics, anticholinergics, calcium channel blockers)
- Characteristics of bowel movement; change in bowel habit
- Blood in stool
- Vomiting
- Severe constipation; inability to pass flatus
- Gastrointestinal surgery or diseases

Exam

- Vitals (febrile, hypo/hypertensive, tachycardic)
- Abdominal exam (mass or dilated loops may be visible and palpable)
- Digital rectal exam (an empty rectum does not rule out bowel obstruction higher up in the GI tract)

IMPORTANT: Fecal impaction in older adults may present initially as possible bowel obstruction. Treatment strategies fecal impaction include:

- Digital disimpaction, together with warm tap water
- Suppositories
- Colonic enema for lower GI impaction

Tests

When bowel obstruction suspected, comprehensive metabolic panel, complete blood count, lactate

Imaging

- If mechanical obstruction suspected on upright abdominal X-ray, then CT abdomen
- If intestinal ischemia suspected: MRI/MRA

A CT of her abdomen revealed that Mrs. E has a colonic mass at the site of the obstruction and multiple metastases to the liver. After discussion with her two daughters, Mrs. E. agreed to surgical resection of the mass.

TREATMENT OPTIONS

The cause, location, severity of obstruction, and goals of care will guide the consideration of surgical vs. nonoperative treatment approach to bowel obstruction.

Nonsurgical management

Patients with small bowel obstruction can be managed with non-operative therapy.[2] Instituting the following treatment measures for geriatric palliative care patients should be based on underlying etiology, prognosis, and patient's goals for care:

- Hospitalization
- Nasogastric suction to decompress the upper gastrointestinal tract
- Urinary catheter to monitor fluid output
- Prompt attention to correction of fluid and electrolyte imbalance, as failure to do so may increase symptom burden
- IV antibiotics if bowel ischemia suspected
- Steroids should be considered to help decrease tumor-related edema. Fever may accompany obstructive symptoms and should be treated with acetaminophen.
- Pain associated with bowel obstruction is significant and should be aggressively managed with an appropriate opioid analgesic regimen.[3] (See Chapter 29: Management of Pain in Older Adults.) Recent evidence has shown that early treatment with opioid analgesics does not contribute to missed or delayed diagnosis.[4]

Surgical Intervention

- IMPORTANT: When a suspected small bowel obstruction is accompanied by signs of strangulation, immediate surgery is indicated.
- When making a decision about surgical intervention in the geriatric palliative care population, factors that should be considered include underlying etiology and mechanism of obstruction, patient and family goals for care, available and appropriate surgical techniques, and likelihood that surgical option will relieve the obstruction or alleviate the symptoms.
- Disease-specific interventional procedures may include:
  1. Diverticulitis: Segmental colonic resection for perforation, abscess or stricture formation
  2. Cecal volvulus: Resection of the involved segment or fixation of the cecum
  3. Sigmoid volvulus: Colonoscopic decompression followed by placement of a rectal tube can often decompress the loop, and if volvulus recurs, segmental resection of redundant colon may be helpful.

4. Malignant bowel obstruction: Metastatic abdominal or pelvic cancer can cause mechanical and/or functional bowel obstruction. If the obstruction is caused by external compression, internal occlusion, or motility disorder, options to alleviate the symptom may include palliative surgery, colonic stenting, and decompressive gastrostomy.

NUTRITIONAL CONCERNS
- Liquid nutritional supplements (oral or via gastrostomy) can be used by patients with partial bowel obstructions.
- If nutritional support is a goal for a patient with complete bowel obstruction, parenteral (peripheral or total) nutrition may be an option. Clinicians should be aware, however, that parenteral nutrition is associated with mechanical, metabolic, and infectious complications. (See Chapter 27: Artificial Nutrition and Hydration.)
- Options for nutrition should be carefully considered when developing a care plan for patients with bowel obstruction. Certain care settings, for example, may not be equipped to care for a patient receiving parenteral nutrition.

PALLIATIVE CARE ISSUES
- When patients are not candidates for surgery, or if surgical intervention is not consistent with goals for care, medical management should focus on aggressive pain management and palliation of burdensome symptoms.
- Support and education on the expected course of disease should also be provided to the patient and family caregivers.
- For opioid-induced constipation in patients with advanced illness, subcutaneous methylnaltrexone can induce rapid laxation. Treatment does not interfere with analgesia and does not cause withdrawal symptoms.[5]

TAKE-HOME POINTS
- When a suspected bowel obstruction is accompanied by signs of strangulation, peritonitis, or sepsis, immediate surgery is indicated.
- Detailed history and physical exam with relevant radiographic tests provide valuable information that will help guide treatment—curative or palliative.
- Prompt attention should be given to correction of fluid and electrolyte imbalance to avoid increased symptom burden.
- Decisions concerning interventions and symptom management should take into consideration underlying etiology, prognosis, and patient and family goals for care. Be sure that comfort is always a priority, regardless of other goals.
- Pain associated with bowel obstruction is significant and should be aggressively managed with an appropriate opioid analgesic regimen.

REFERENCES
1. Hayanga AJ, Bass-Wilkins K, Bulkley GB. Current management of small-bowel obstruction. *Adv Surg.* 2005;39:1–33.
2. Rocha FG, Theman TA, Matros E, et al. Non-operative management of patients with a diagnosis of high-grade small bowel obstruction by computed tomography. *Arch Surg.* 2009;144(11):1000–1004.
3. Delgado-Aros S, Camilleri M. Pseudo-obstruction in the critically ill. *Best Pract Res Clin Gastroenterol.* 2003:17(3):427–444.
4. Ranji SR, Goldman LE, Simel DL, Shojania KG. Do opiates affect the clinical evaluation of patients with acute abdominal pain? *JAMA.* 2006;296(14):1764–1774.
5. Thomas J, Karver S, Cooney GA, et al. Methylnaltrexone for opioid-induced constipation in advanced illness. *N Engl J Med.* 2008;358:2332–2343.

45

Constipation

CASE

Mrs. S is an 88-year-old woman with hypertension, hypothyroidism, and severe, debilitating osteoarthritis that has left her wheelchair-bound. She presents with complaints of constipation, which she describes as difficulty having a bowel movement daily, having to strain to get the stool out, hard stool, having to self-disimpact occasionally, and a sense of incomplete evacuation. She is seeking advice because her constipation is making it hard for her to urinate, making her feel full all the time, and she has occasional rectal bleeding after straining.

DEFINITION

Physicians often define constipation by stool frequency (fewer than three times a week), while patients like Mrs. S often focus on the symptoms that constipation causes. To avoid these discrepancies, the more objective Rome Criteria may be used to define constipation.

PREVALENCE

Prevalence is 2% to 28% in the general population, with a significant increase after the age of 70 years.[1] This compares to 21% to 50% of patients admitted to hospice or a palliative care unit.[2,3]

CONSEQUENCES OF UNTREATED CONSTIPATION

- Delirium
- Abdominal pain or discomfort
- Urinary retention or incontinence
- Fecal impaction
- Overflow fecal incontinence that manifests as diarrhea
- Development of rectocele, enterocele, rectal prolapse, intestinal obstruction
- Stercoral ulceration and intestinal perforation

LIKELY ETIOLOGIES

- Although aging per se does not cause constipation, older adults tend to have decreased mobility, multiple comorbidities, and multiple medications that contribute to constipation, as in the case of Mrs. S.

Prior to initiating workup for functional constipation, it is important to make sure that Mrs. S does not have secondary causes of constipation that may be readily reversed. (Potential contributors to Mrs. S's constipation are highlighted in Table 45.1. Note that even opioids account for only 25% of constipation in cancer patients on opioids.[4])

BOX 45.1 ROME II CRITERIA FOR DEFINING CHRONIC FUNCTIONAL CONSTIPATION IN ADULTS

Two or more of the following for at least 12 weeks in the preceding 12 months:
Straining in more than 25% of defecations
Lumpy or hard stools in more than 25% of defecations
Sensation of incomplete evacuation in more than 25% of defecations
Sensation of anorectal obstruction or blockade in more than 25% of defecations
Manual maneuvers (e.g., digital evacuation, support of the pelvic floor) to facilitate more than 25% of defecations
Fewer than three defecations per week

Drossman DA, Thompson WG, Talley NJ, Funch-Jensen P, Janssens J, Whitehead WE. Identification of subgroups of functional gastrointestinal disorders. Gastroenterol Int. 1990;3:159–172.

TABLE 45.1: SECONDARY CAUSES OF CONSTIPATION

Secondary Cause	Examples
Fluid depletion	Decreased intake Excessive loss
Decreased dietary fiber	
Debility	Immobility Weaknesses leading to inability to increase intra-abdominal pressure
Medications	Antacids with calcium or aluminum Anticholinergics Antidepressants especially tricyclics Antiemetics: ondansetron, granisetron Antihistamines: H2 blockers Anticonvulsants such as dilantin and lamotrigine Antispasmodics Amiodarone Beta blockers Calcium channel blockers Calcium supplements Diuretics Iron Levodopa Opioids
Comorbid disease	Amyloidosis Anal fissures, strictures, hemorrhoids Anxiety Autonomic neuropathy Cerebrovascular disease Colonic strictures Depression Delirium Diabetes Hypercalcemia Hyperparathyroidism Hypothyroidism Inflammatory bowel disease Irritable bowel syndrome Obstructive colonic mass lesions Parkinson's disease Rectal prolapse or rectocele Scleroderma Somatization Spinal cord injury, tumors Uremia

- Primary functional causes (usually requires a GI consultation) include: normal transit constipation, slow transit constipation, and anorectal dysfunction. Secondary causes are listed in Table 45.1.

DIAGNOSIS

The workup for constipation requires a comprehensive history, physical exam, and investigation of the possible underlying etiologies.

Exam

- Determine the cause and eliminate the offending medication or treat the underlying medical condition.
- Look for evidence of systemic diseases.
- Pay attention to bowel sounds and masses on the abdominal exam.
- Perform a rectal exam with attention to stool, masses, strictures, and rectoceles.
- Inspect the perianal area for fissures, hemorrhoids, masses, and evidence of previous surgery.
- Check of perianal reflex and tone of external and internal sphincter.

Tests

- CBC
- TSH
- Electrolytes
- Calcium
- Phosphorus
- Magnesium
- Consider any abdominal plain films to look for evidence of impaction and obstipation.

Further Work-Up

- Evaluate and determine the need for a GI referral for more invasive tests that may include colonoscopy and anal manometry.
- The decision to pursue further workup should be based on prognosis, goals of care, and consideration of whether the stress and discomfort of invasive testing is justified by the clinical need for additional evaluation.
- The overwhelming majority of patients with constipation do not require additional workup.

TREATMENT OPTIONS

Nonpharmacologic

- Massage, exercise, and biofeedback have been suggested, but there is limited evidence on their effectiveness. Among older adults receiving palliative care, mobility is usually limited and exercise is often not an option.

- While the addition of fiber in the diet or as a supplement is often recommended in frail or chronically ill older adults with constipation, these agents increase the likelihood of fecal impaction in the context of decreased mobility and inadequate water intake.
- Patients should be educated on effective toileting habits, including:
  - Going to the toilet at the same time each day
  - Taking advantage of the gastro-colic reflex about 30 minutes after a meal, especially after breakfast
- Ensuring that the toilet seat is the correct height
- Ensuring privacy

Pharmacologic

As there is a lack of evidence-based guidelines based on randomized controlled trials, suggested best practice guidelines are offered in Table 45.2. The choice of laxative depends on patient preference and side effect profiles.

Workup did not reveal any modifiable secondary causes. Nonpharmacological treatments were initiated without success. Mrs. S was then started on senna and colace, without relief despite increasing titration. Polyethelene glycol was then added and colace was removed. With this new regimen,

TABLE 45.2: PHARMACOLOGIC TREATMENT GUIDELINES

Class	Examples	Advantages	Disadvantages
Oral Agents			
Stool softener/ Lubricant	Docusate: 100 mg 2–3 times daily	Can be used with stimulants for synergistic effect Safe to use in resolving intestinal obstruction Helpful in those with fissures or hemorrhoids	Ineffective when used alone in frail older adults or in palliative care patients
Osmotic	*Polyethylene glycol:* 17 g once daily *Lactulose:* 15 to 45 mL (20 grams/30 mL) orally 3 to 4 times daily for 24 to 48 hours; maximum 40 grams/day; *Sorbitol:* 15–30 mL po of 70% solution 1–2 times a day; 120 mL rectally of 25–30% solution; *Magnesium citrate:* 150–300 mL daily; Mg sulfate: 15–30 g 1–2 times daily; *MOM:* 30–60 mL daily; *Sodium phosphate:* 10 g once daily	Causes water retention in the intestinal lumen and thus increasing transit time	Can cause abdominal distention, flatulence, and diarrhea Sweet taste (sorbitol, lactulose) that may not be palatable Sorbitol and lactulose are both very expensive For maximal effect, need to be able to take in large amounts of fluid Associated with electrolyte abnormalities because of high salt content and may precipitate hypokalemia, fluid and salt overload Use with caution in patients with renal insufficiency and CHF
Stimulant/Irritant	Senna: 2 tabs 1–2 times daily; Bisacodyl: 5–15 mg PO daily; Cascara: 325 mg PO daily; Castor oil: 15–60 mL depending on solution (prune juice)	Effective in opioid induced constipation Stimulates peristalsis and increases oro-cecal transit	Can cause abdominal cramps Avoid in intestinal obstruction

(continued)

Class	Examples	Advantages	Disadvantages
Rectal Agents			
Suppositories			
Lubricant	Glycerin: 2–3 g suppository once daily	Soften stools Has some stimulant properties	None
Stimulant	Bisacodyl: 10 mg suppositories every other day	Can be used if oral laxatives are prohibited Can be more convenient and rapid than oral laxatives and rectal enemas	Side effects rare but can cause occasional abdominal cramps and diarrhea Can worsen pre-existing tears in the lining of the rectum and anal fissures
Enemas			
Warm tap water, soapsuds, and mineral oil	Warm tap water: 500 mL rectally; soapsuds: 1500 mL rectally; mineral oil: 100–250 mL rectally	Simple and easily accessible Stimulates the defecating reflex by distending the lumen Soapsuds cause mucosal irritation and can cause more cramping Mineral oil may help stool to remain soft, facilitating expulsion of residual mass	Safe to use but may be a further irritant in patients who already have an irritated or inflamed mucosal membrane
	Phosphate: 60 mL rectally	A prepared formulation is readily available	Should not be used in elderly because it can precipitate water and electrolyte abnormalities with comorbid conditions such as liver failure, inflammatory bowel disease, congestive heart failure, and renal failure
Other			
Methylnatrexone		Effective only for opioid-induced constipation Rapidly induced laxation in patients with advanced illness A mu-opioid receptor antagonist that does not affect central analgesia Does not precipitate opioid withdrawal	SQ delivery Can cause transient abdominal pain, cramping, and flatulence Limited long-term safety information (study population all have life expectancy of 4 months of less) Expensive

and increased fluid intake, the patient was having bowel movements every two days.

FECAL IMPACTION

- Fecal impaction is a medical emergency that often presents with alternating watery diarrhea and constipation, or watery leakage alone. Frequently there is no formed stool because only liquid stool can leak around the area of impaction.
- Fecal impaction cannot be treated with oral laxatives because they are ineffective and may worsen abdominal pain and obstruction. Treatment should include:

- Step 1: Suppositories
- Step 2: Oil retention enema
- Step 3: Phosphate enema
- Step 4: Manual disimpaction (Consider GI consult if the impaction is more proximal and consider use of sedation, i.e., midazolam if extensive disimpaction is anticipated or if the patient is very anxious.)
- Once treatment is successful, start an oral regimen to prevent recurrence of the problem.

PALLIATIVE CARE ISSUES

- Monitoring of bowel movements is important in debilitated palliative care patients, as both bowel distention and fecal impaction can lead to distressing symptoms including depression, delirium, agitation, anorexia, and nausea.
- Because evacuation is not based solely on PO intake, all patients with a life expectancy of at least weeks to a month should have a bowel movement every two to three days. Clinicians should therefore titrate laxatives to prevent constipation and ultimately fecal impaction.

TAKE-HOME POINTS

- Prevention is the key to the management of constipation.
- Consider secondary causes of constipation, as these can guide treatment options.
- Stimulant laxatives should be avoided in patients with intestinal obstruction.
- Fecal impaction is a medical emergency that can lead to life-threatening bowel obstruction, perforation, and death.

REFERENCES

1. Higgins PD, Johanson JF. Epidemiology of constipation in North America: a systematic review. *Am J Gastroenterol.* Apr 2004;*99*(4):750–759.
2. Strassels S, Maxwell T, Iyer S. Prevalence and severity of constipation in patients at admission to hospice. *J Am Med Dir Assoc.* March 2008;*9*(3):B22.
3. Ng K, von Gunten CF. Symptoms and attitudes of 100 consecutive patients admitted to an acute hospice/palliative care unit. *J Pain Symptom Manage.* Nov 1998;*16*(5):307–316.
4. Davis MP. Cancer constipation: are opioids really the culprit? *Support Care Cancer.* May 2008;*16*(5):427–479. Epub 2008 Jan 15.
5. Hsieh C. Treatment of constipation in older adults. *Am Fam Physician.* Dec 1, 2005;*72*(11):2277–2284.

46

Diarrhea and Fecal Incontinence

CASE

Mrs. D is an 80-year-old female brought to the office by her family for recurrent diarrhea of two weeks' duration. She has been having three to six loose, non-bloody bowel movements a day and occasional nocturnal fecal incontinence. She has a history of recurrent frequent loose stools and intermittent constipation. Six months ago she was hospitalized for pneumonia and contracted Clostridium difficile-associated disease. At that time, she was successfully treated with metronidazole.

PART A: DIARRHEA

DEFINITION

Diarrhea is defined as an alteration in normal bowel movement characterized as increase in frequency (>3 per day), decreased consistency, and increased stool weight/volume (>200 gm/day). The following classifications have been suggested according to the duration of diarrhea:

Acute: ≤14 days in duration
Chronic: More than 21 days in duration, or persistent loose/watery stools at least three times a day

PREVALENCE[1,2]

- Acute diarrhea represents one of the five leading causes of death worldwide, especially in children, older adults, and immunocompromised individuals.
- Chronic diarrhea is a common condition and affects approximately 5% of the population worldwide.
- In the United States, rates of 0.7 diarrheal episodes per person per year have been reported, or approximately 200 million episodes per year.
- Although elders may suffer from higher morbidity and mortality when infected with diarrheal disease, rates of infection are no higher than in the general population.

CONSEQUENCES OF UNTREATED DIARRHEA[3]

- Diarrhea is a significant cause of death in older adults and the immunocompromised. Due to abnormalities in water homeostasis, decreased perception of thirst, and the potential for volume depletion, elderly individuals with diarrhea are at a higher risk for multiple complications including delirium, hypolovemia, dehydration, malnutrition, fecal incontinence, de-conditioning, and frequent falls.
- Chronic diarrhea in the geriatric population can also cause social embarrassment and isolation, increased caregiver burden, and more frequent hospitalization.

LIKELY ETIOLOGIES[4]

Acute

- Viral
- Bacterial
- Parasites
- Medication-related

Chronic

In developed countries, principle causes of chronic diarrhea include:

- Irritable bowel syndrome
- Inflammatory bowel disease
- Malabsorption syndromes
- Chronic infections (especially associated with frequent travel, HIV infection, and antibiotic use)
- Miscellaneous factors, e.g., laxative abuse, sugar-free foods, overflow diarrhea caused by chronic constipation/fecal impaction

DIAGNOSIS

History

- Obtaining a careful history may help identify cause and appropriate treatment.

Relevant information includes duration of symptoms, medication use, dietary and travel history, weight loss, abdominal pain, frequency and consistency of stool, characteristics of stool, blood in stool, fever history, and frequency and intensity of associated symptoms (e.g., nausea, vomiting).[4]

- Some patients present with complaint of diarrhea but may be suffering from fecal incontinence. Fecal incontinence is the involuntary loss of feces. It occurs more frequently in older adults and is a leading cause of nursing home placement. (See Part B: Fecal Incontinence.)

Exam

- Vitals, abdomen, skin changes (erythema nodosum, pyoderma), rectal exam for internal/external sphincter tone, fecal impaction, bloody stool.
- Severity of illness suggested by:[4]
  - Profuse watery diarrhea > 6 stool movements per day
  - Signs of hypovolemia
  - Bloody and/or mucousy stool
  - Temperature ≥38.5°C (101.3°F)
  - Duration of illness of >48 hours
  - Severe abdominal pain
  - Recent antibiotic use
  - Diarrhea in the older adult (≥70 years of age)
  - Diarrhea in the immunocompromised

Mrs. D's prior medical history includes diabetes, hypertension, coronary artery disease, obesity, arthritis, and dementia. She has not had any recent sick contacts or recent antibiotic use. She is afebrile, hemodynamically stable and is in no acute distress. Her abdominal exam was benign. She does not show signs of dehydration. On inquiry it is discovered that her niece is a nurse at a community hospital that had a Clostridium difficile outbreak.

Tests

- Because most episodes of acute diarrhea are self-limiting, testing is not necessary for every patient. The decision about whether testing is necessary, and what test to use, should be based on several factors, including:[5]
  - History and physical exam
  - Duration of more than one day that is also associated with bloody stools or fever

- Symptoms of sepsis or evidence of dehydration
- Recent antibiotic use
- Underlying immunocompromised status
- Tests for acute diarrhea:
  - Fecal WBC, ova, parasites
  - CBC, electrolytes
  - C diff toxin assay test
- Tests for chronic diarrhea:
  - CBC, electrolytes
  - TSH
  - Celiac serology
  - CEA
  - Urine 5-HIAA
  - Fecal occult blood
  - Qualitative/quantitative stool fat
  - Colonoscopy with biopsy

Mrs. D's electrolytes and CBC are normal and her stool was negative for WBC, ova, and parasites. She was found to be Clostridium difficile toxin-positive.

TREATMENT OPTIONS

Diarrhea creates a serious risk of dehydration, so critically important initial therapy should include timely fluid repletion and correction of electrolyte abnormality. For noninflammatory illness, continue symptomatic treatment:

- Oral hydration with solutions that contain water, salt, and sugar. Early use of oral rehydration could reduce hospitalizations.
- The composition of the oral rehydration solution (per liter of water) consists of:
  - 3.5 g sodium chloride
  - 2.9 g trisodium citrate or 2.5 g sodium bicarbonate
  - 1.5 g potassium chloride
  - 20 g glucose or 40 g sucrose
- Solution can be made by adding one-half teaspoon of salt, one-half teaspoon of baking soda, and four tablespoons of sugar to one liter of water.[6]
- Management of symptoms when appropriate with loperaminde or bismuth subsalicylate.
- Dietary recommendations: boiled starches and cereals (e.g., potatoes, noodles, rice, wheat, and oats) with salt, crackers, bananas, soup, and boiled vegetables may be consumed. Temporary avoidance of lactose-containing foods can be helpful.
- Empiric antibiotic therapy should be considered for patients with moderate

to severe signs and symptoms of inflammatory/infectious diarrhea, those with immunocompromised status, or when there is a high suspicion of Clostridium difficile.

Mrs. D completed a course of flagyl and her symptoms improved.

PART B: FECAL INCONTINENCE

DEFINITION

Fecal incontinence is the involuntary passage or the inability to control the discharge of fecal material.

TYPES

1. Passive incontinence: Involuntary discharge of feces/flatus without awareness
2. Urge incontinence: Discharge of rectal contents in spite of active attempts to retain these contents
3. Fecal seepage: involuntary seepage with otherwise normal evacuation

PREVALENCE

- Ranges between 1% and 7.4% in otherwise healthy populations, and up to 25% in institutionalized patients.[6]
- Prevalence increases with age; frequency in individuals over 65 increases up to 27%. It is a common cause of institutionalization.[7]

LIKELY ETIOLOGIES

- Causes of fecal incontinence include anal sphincter injury or weakness, impaired anorectal sensation or rectal accommodation, incomplete evacuation, pudendal neuropathy.
- Risk Factors: female gender, diabetes, obesity, stroke, decreased physical activity, older age, episiotomy history, and dementia.

DIAGNOSIS[7]

Workup involves comprehensive history-taking to differentiate fecal incontinence from diarrhea. Patients underreport fecal incontinence, or present with complaints of diarrhea or urgency.

History

- Assess comorbidities, risk factors, duration and progression, characteristics of the incontinence, as well as conditions under which incontinence occurs and impact on quality of life.

- A diary that documents the time of the event, the stool consistency, the urgency, and the need to use pads can be very helpful.

Exam

- Thorough musculoskeletal and neurological exam focused on the back and lower extremities to rule out systemic or neurological disorder.
- Perineal inspection for presence of fecal matter, prolapsed hemorrhoids, dermatitis, scarring.
- Rectal exam can determine whether there is fecal impaction and overflow.
- Check for perianal sensation and anocutaneous reflex.

Tests

Based upon severity of symptom, age, functional status, prognosis, and comorbidities, physiological and imaging studies may include:

- Sigmoidoscopy or colonoscopy, if diarrhea accompanies incontinence.
- Anorectal manometry and anal endosonography with or without a balloon expulsion test, if there is evidence of structural or sensory damage to anorectal region.
- Defecography, if there is suspected rectal prolapse.

TREATMENT OPTIONS[7,8]

Treatment approach should be based upon etiology and severity of the condition. Conservative management is recommended for elderly patients and those with serious illness; more aggressive treatment is recommended only in the event of severe incontinence.

Nonpharmacologic

- Dementia patients can be directed to the toilet, or reminded at intervals.
- Scheduled toileting with a commode at the bedside and supportive measures to improve general health and nutrition of patient may be helpful.
- Environmental barriers that obstruct or limit timely access to bathroom should be eliminated. Assistance should be offered for those who require help with ADLs.
- For ambulatory patients, prompted voiding and habit training can reduce the numbers of incontinent bowel movements.

- Biofeedback can improve the functioning of the external sphincter and also increase anorectal sensation

Pharmacologic

- Loperamide (Immodium) is commonly used to treat fecal incontinence with no underlying infection or inflammation.
- Diphenoxylate/atropine (Lomotil) also reduces stool frequency, but potential for central nervous system side effects should be avoided in the elderly.
- Chloestyramine is helpful if bile acid malabsorption is a possible factor.

Surgery

- Surgical therapy may be considered when conservative treatment has failed in patients with severe fecal incontinence who have specific anatomic defects. Sphincter repair outcomes are variable, but appropriately selected patients do experience improved anal function post-operatively.
- If fecal incontinence persists after resolution of diarrhea or is unrelated to diarrhea, a referral to gastroenterologist for further workup and management is recommended.

TAKE-HOME POINTS

Diarrhea

- A detailed history will help to identify cause of diarrhea. Factors include duration of symptoms, medication use, dietary and travel history, weight loss, abdominal pain, frequency and consistency of stool, characteristics of stool, blood in stool, fever history, and frequency and intensity of associated symptoms (e.g., nausea, vomiting).
- To mitigate risk of potentially dangerous dehydration, initial therapy should include timely fluid repletion and correction of electrolyte abnormality.

- Management is guided by severity and duration of illness, and lab workup when appropriate.
- Empiric antibiotic therapy should be considered for patients with moderate to severe signs and symptoms, those with immunocompromised status, or when there is a high suspicion of Clostridium difficile.

Fecal Incontinence

- Some patients may present with complaint of diarrhea but may be suffering from fecal incontinence.
- Conservative management of fecal incontinence is recommended for elderly patients and those with serious illness, with more aggressive treatment only in the event of severe incontinence.

REFERENCES

1. Pawlowski SW, Warren CA, Guerrant R. Diagnosis and treatment of acute or persistent diarrhea. *Gastroenterology.* 2009;*136*:1874–1886.
2. Herikstad H, Yang S, Van Gilder TJ, et al. A population-based estimate of the burden of diarrheal illness in the United States: Food Net, 1996-7. *Epidemiol Infect.* 2002;*129*:9–17.
3. Trinh C, Prabhakar K. Diarrheal diseases in the elderly. *Clin Geriatr Med.* 2007;*23*:833–856.
4. Guerrant RL, Van Gilder T, Steiner TS, et al. Practice guidelines for the management of infectious diarrhea. *Clin Infect Dis.* 2001;*32*:331–350.
5. Hatchette TF, Farina D. Infectious diarrhea: when to test and when to treat. *CMAJ.* February 22, 2011; *183*(3):339–344.
6. de Zoysa I, Kirkwood B, Feachem R, Linsay-Smith E. Preparation of sugar-salt solutions. *Trans R Soc Trop Med Hyg.* 1984;*78*:260.
7. Tariq SH. Geriatric fecal incontinence. *Clin Geriatr Med.* 2004;*20*:571–587.
8. Rao SS. Diagnosis and management of fecal incontinence: American College of Gastroenterology Practice Parameters Committee. *Am J Gastroenterol.* 2004;*99*:1585–1604.

47

Xerostomia and Oral Mucositis

PART A: XEROSTOMIA (DRY MOUTH)

CASE
Mrs. E is an 82-year-old woman with osteoarthritis, spinal stenosis, and CHF. She presents with complaints of excessive dry mouth that is impairing her appetite and affecting her speech. She has tried artificial saliva, and every over-the-counter oral moisturizer she could find without any improvement.

DEFINITION
Xerostomia is a condition where the mouth is dry, usually due to a decreased or absent saliva flow.

PREVALENCE
Increases with age and probably affects approximately 30% of the population aged 65 and older.[1] Has been reported in >75% of patients at the end of life.[2]

CONSEQUENCES OF UNTREATED XEROSTOMIA
- Saliva works to hydrate, lubricate, and maintain the mucosal tissue as a barrier against microorganisms. It acts as a buffer and initiates food processing, bolus formation, and translocation. It also mediates the sense of taste.
- Decreased saliva can lead to difficulties in chewing, eating, swallowing, and talking; it also increases the risk for tooth decay, candidiasis, infections, and halitosis.[3]

LIKELY ETIOLOGIES
There are many underlying causes of dry mouth, including certain medications, cancer-related therapies, and other health conditions or illnesses (Table 47.1).

DIAGNOSIS

History
- A detailed history is likely to reveal multiple potential etiologies for dry mouth. It is important to make a detailed list of all of patient's medications and take a history of current medical problems, as well as any current or previous treatments for cancer.
- The patient will often present with complaints of oral pain, open oral lesions, dental problems, oral infection, alteration in taste, chewing or swallowing difficulties, or slurred speech. Patient may also complain that dry mouth symptoms are worse at night when saliva production is lowest.

Exam
- Dry and cracked lips—angular cheilitis
- Visible enlargement of the major salivary glands
- Swollen parotid gland
- Desiccated and sticky tongue
- Oral mucositis
- Decreased or absent saliva pooling at the floor of the mouth
- New and recurrent dental caries and enamel demineralization
- Traumatic lesions, especially in denture-wearing adults

Tests
Tests are usually not necessary unless Sjogren's syndrome is suspected.

TREATMENT OPTIONS

Nonpharmacologic
- While the evidence base for the efficacy of various treatment interventions is not strong,[4] the following strategies are recommended to help manage chronic dry mouth symptoms:
  - Address underlying causes.
  - Encourage oral hydration, e.g., frequent sips of water or sucking on pieces of ice.
  - Use humidifier during sleep.

TABLE 47.1: CAUSES OF XEROSTOMIA
(DRY MOUTH)

Categories	Conditions
Medications: 80% of the most commonly prescribed medications cause dry mouth.[1]	**Anticholinergics:** Antiemetics Antihistamines Antipsychotics Antispasmodics Antidepressants (tricyclics) Bronchodilators Diuretics **Sympatholytics:** Alpha blockers, Alpha 2 agonists Beta blockers **Opioids** **Benzodiazepines**
Cancer-related therapies	Radiation for head and neck cancers Cytotoxic chemotherapies Radioactive iodine
Systemic illness	Diabetes Renal failure HIV/AIDS Dehydration Sjogren's syndrome Scleroderma Sarcoidosis Graft vs. host disease
Oral diseases	Parotitis Sialolith (salivary calculus)

- Stimulate residual gland function, e.g., sugarless gums and candies.
- Saliva substitutes in gel and solution form.
- Apply lip lubricants or balms.
- Eat pureed or soft foods.
- Avoid alcoholic, citrus, carbonated, or caffeinated drinks.
- Avoid dry foods (moisten with broth, sauces, butter, or milk).
- Avoid acidic (e.g., with citric acid) and sugared lozenges.
- Avoid chewable vitamin C.
- Avoid overly salty foods.
- New products with enzyme systems include:
  - Potentially antimicrobial and moisturizing agents, e.g., Biotene Dry Mouth Toothpaste, Oralbalance Dry

Mouth Gel. These products have limited duration of action. Use before eating, speaking, sleeping; avoid products with surfactant sodium lauryl sulfate (SLS), as it irritates dry mucosa and inactivates enzyme systems of newer saliva.
- Antimicrobial mouthwashes (alcohol-free), e.g., chorhexidine gluconate oral rinse 0.12% bid

Pharmacologic
Pharmacologic treatments for dry mouth help to stimulate saliva production (Table 47.2).

Mrs. E's history revealed that she takes diuretics for her heart failure and opioids to control her chronic pain. She reported that attempts at alternative treatment for pain were not successful in the past. Mrs. E was started on a low dose of pilocarpine, experienced no side effects and reported complete relief of her symptoms.

PART B: ORAL MUCOSITIS

CASE
Mr. B is a 67-year-old man with laryngeal cancer s/p resection. He was admitted to the hospital five days ago for radiation therapy and chemotherapy. The palliative care team was consulted to assist with his mouth pain, which is now limiting his oral intake and ability to communicate.

DEFINITION
Mucositis refers to the painful inflammation and ulceration of the mucous membrane that lines the entire digestive tract. Oral mucositis is sometimes referred to as "stomatitis" and is often described by patients as "mouth sores."

PREVALENCE
- Oral mucositis occurs in 40% of cancer patients receiving cytotoxic chemotherapy and in about 80% of those head and neck cancer patients receiving radiation therapy.[5]
- About 75% of patients undergoing bone marrow transplantation develop symptomatic oral mucositis during treatment.[6]

LIKELY ETIOLOGIES
Oral mucositis is most frequently caused by high-dose chemotherapy agents and/or radiation therapy, as these treatments target both the healthy and cancerous cells that are dividing rapidly. Ulcerations in the mucosal layer disrupt the natural protective barrier of the mucosa and can lead to serious life-threatening infections.

TABLE 47.2: PHARMACOLOGIC TREATMENTS FOR XEROSTOMIA

Commonly Used Cholinergic Agents	Dose	Side Effects
Pilocarpine: cholinergic parasympathomimetic agent (half-life 3 hours)	5 mg PO tid; titrate to 10 mg PO tid	Increased sweating, salivation, rhinitis, urinary frequency and nausea
Cevimeline: quinuclidine derivative of acetylcholine, is a novel muscarinic receptor agonist (half-life 5 hours)	30 mg PO tid	Increased sweating, increased salivation, and nausea

RISK FACTORS

- Oral health and oral hygiene
- Reduced salivary function
- Smoking
- Alcohol
- Specific chemotherapeutic agents (e.g., Bleomycin, Cytarabine, Doxorubicin, 5 FU)
- Bone marrow transplantation
- Radiotherapy

DIAGNOSIS

History

A careful history is likely to reveal the probable causes of the mucositis. Symptoms include pain, hemorrhage, changes in taste, erythema, and swelling. Mucositis symptoms can develop two to 10 days after the start of chemo or radiation therapy and may last two to three weeks or more.[7]

Exam

- A thorough assessment of patient's oral cavity after removal of dentures (if applicable) is absolutely necessary and can often help to guide treatment. Look for ulcerative mucositis in the floor of the mouth, the lateral and bottom surfaces of the tongue, the soft palate, and the inner surfaces of the lips and cheeks.
- Mucositis usually presents on non-keratinized surfaces. For suspicious ulcerative lesions found on keratinized surfaces, culture and biopsy by an oral specialist is recommended. These lesions may be signs of infections of viral, fungal, bacterial etiology, or GVHD if patient is post-transplantation.

Assessment Scales

The mostly widely used assessment scales include:
- National Cancer Institute Common Toxicity Criteria (NCI-CTC) for bone marrow transplant, radiation therapy, or chemotherapy patients.
- World Health Organization (WHO) Oral Toxicity Scale[8]
  - Grade 1: No Changes
  - Grade 2: Soreness with erythema
  - Grade 3: Erythema, ulcers, can eat solids
  - Grade 4: Ulcers, liquid diet only
  - Grade 5: Alimentation not possible

TREATMENT OPTIONS

To date there is no strong evidence pointing to a single intervention for treating oral mucositis.[9] However, emphasis on prevention is universal, and an interdisciplinary therapeutic regimen is essential if symptoms do occur. Expert opinion and clinical practice guidelines recommend the following strategies:[7]

- Routine daily assessment using a validated assessment tool allows clinical staff to monitor oral injury over time. Additionally, assessment will provide continuity between caregivers, who will describe the affected area using similar parameters.
- Regular pain assessment is critically important, using validated, self-report pain measures.
- Standardized oral care should be implemented in order to reduce the duration and severity of mucositis.
  - Involve a dental professional in a full dental evaluation before, during, and post-treatment.
  - Maintain good oral hygiene regimen prior to and during treatment.
  - Avoid hard, spicy, or hot foods that can trigger pain.
  - Rinse frequently with saline or water with baking soda.
  - Suck on ice chips or popsicles.
- General management recommendations for oral mucositis are listed in Table 47.3.

TABLE 47.3: MANAGEMENT RECOMMENDATIONS FOR ORAL MUCOSITIS

Mouthwashes

Non-irritating agents:
There are numerous formulations of mouthwashes. Most contain at least 3 ingredients with instruction to hold in mouth for 1–2 minutes before spitting or swallowing. This process can be repeated every 4–6 hours and patient should not eat or drink for about 30 minutes after use. Formulations containing lidocaine should not be swallowed.

Some examples with sodium bicarbonate, diphenhydramine, Maalox, and viscous lidocaine 2%:
Example 1: 8.4 g of sodium bicarbonate per 1 liter of normal saline
Example 2: 8.4 g of sodium bicarbonate, 30 cc of diphenhydramine elixir in 1 liter of normal saline
Example 3: 8.4 g of sodium bicarbonate, 30 cc of diphenhydramine elixir, viscous lidocaine in 1 liter of normal saline
Example 4: 8.4 g sodium bicarbonate, viscous lidocaine/diphenhydramine 40 cc of each
Example 5: Maalox/viscous lidocaine/diphenhydramine 40 cc of each

Cleaning

Soft bristle brush — Continue as long as no uncontrolled bleeding is present; however, replace brush weekly when patient is neutropenic

Swab — An alternative to the brush that can be continued as long as tolerated and there is no uncontrolled bleeding

Floss — Can be a regular part of patient's oral care if tolerated with no uncontrolled bleeding present

Other

Artificial saliva — Every hour as needed for dry mouth (for Grade 1–5)

Petroleum-based ointment — Apply as needed to lips (for Grade 1–5)

Patient-controlled analgesia (PCA) — Preferred over continuous infusion of opioids for pain control because it involves less opioid use/hour and more effective in shortening the pain duration (for Grade 3–5)

A stepwise approach should be employed in order to utilize the appropriate treatment for the correct stage of tissue injury.

- The following interventions were *not* recommended in the clinical practice guidelines developed by the Multinational Association of Supportive Care in Cancer (MASCC) and the International Society for Oral Oncology (ISOO):[7]
  - Mouthwashes containing chlorhexidine, antimicrobial lozenges, acyclovir and its analogues, pentoxifylline, and granulocyte-macrophage-colony stimulating factor for prevention of oral mucositis
  - Sucralfate for treatment of oral mucositis following radiotherapy
  - Chlorhexidine for treatment of oral mucositis following standard-dose chemotherapy

PALLIATIVE CARE ISSUES

- Oral mucositis is a commonly encountered side effect of chemotherapy and radiotherapy treatments for head and neck cancer.
- Because mucositis is a serious dose-limiting toxicity, it can interfere with cancer treatment, causing delay or postponement that may compromise treatment regimen and lead to worsening of patient's prognosis.[5]
- The primary symptom of oral mucositis is pain that also negatively impacts nutritional intake, mouth care, and patient's quality of life.[10] Aggressive pain management, with systemic analgesics including opioids if necessary for satisfactory pain relief, is thus a key component of the treatment program.

TAKE-HOME POINTS

Xerostomia

- Although xerostomia is not life threatening, it can negatively affect patient's quality of life.
- Common etiologies for xerostomia include medications, cancer-related treatment,

systemic illness, and oral disease. There are multiple strategies and treatments that can help relieve this symptom.

Oral Mucositis

- Oral mucositis is a significant, dose-limiting, and burdensome side effect of cancer therapy.
- Prevention of mucositis, using an interdisciplinary approach to oral care, is paramount.
- Standardized oral regimens can decrease the severity and duration of mucositis.
- Regular assessment and treatment of oral pain is an essential component of symptom management.
- A stepwise approach to general management should be employed in order to utilize the appropriate treatment for the correct stage of tissue injury.

REFERENCES

1. Ship JA, Pillemer SR, Baum BJ. Xerostomia and the geriatric patient. *J Am Geriatr Soc.* Mar 2002;*50*(3):535–543.
2. Reisfield GM, Rosielle DA, Wilson GR. *Xerostomia*, 2nd Edition. Fast Facts and Concepts. December 2008; 182. http://www.eperc.mcw.edu/fastfact/ff_182.htm. Accessed December 2011.
3. Guggenheimer J, Moore PA. Xerostomia: etiology, recognition and treatment. *JADA.* Jan 2003;*134*:61–65.
4. Furness S, Worthington HV, Bryan G, Birchenough S, McMillan R. Interventions for the management of dry mouth: topical therapies. *Cochrane Database of Systematic Reviews*, 2011, Issue 12. Art. No.: CD008934. doi: 10.1002/14651858.CD008934.pub2.
5. Rodriguez-Caballero A, Torres-Lagares D, Robles-Garcia M, et al. Cancer treatment-induced oral mucositis: a critical review. *Int J.Oral Maxillofac Surg.* 2011: doi:10.1016/j.ijom.2011.10.011.
6. Bellm LA, Epstein JB, Rose-Ped A, Martin P, Fuchs HJ. Patient reports of complications of bone marrow transplantation. *Support Care Cancer.* Jan 2000;*8*(1):33–39.
7. Keefe DM, Schubert MM, Elting LS, et al. Updated clinical practice guidelines for the prevention and treatment of mucositis. *Cancer.* 2007;*109*:820–831.
8. WHO Handbook for Reporting Results of Cancer Treatment. *WHO Offset publication No. 48.* Geneva, Switzerland: World Health Organization; 1979.
9. Clarkson JE, Worthington HV, Furness S, McCabe M, Khalid T, Meyer S. Interventions for treating oral mucositis for patients with cancer receiving treatment. *Cochrane Database of Systematic Reviews.* 2010; Issue 8. Art. No.: CD001973. doi: 10.1002/14651858.CD001973.pub4.
10. Lalla RV, Sonis ST, Peterson DE. Management of oral mucositis in patients with cancer. *Dent Clin North Am.* January 2008;*52*(1):61–67.

48

Dyspepsia

CASE

Mrs. C is an 82-year-old woman with coronary artery disease, hypertension, diabetes, and early memory loss who reports frequent episodes of epigastric abdominal pain, particularly after eating. She describes the pain as a gnawing discomfort that is not alleviated with antacids. There is no associated nausea or vomiting. The pain does not radiate. Her medications include aspirin, diltiazem, lisinopril, and metformin.

DEFINITION

Dyspepsia is a broad term used by clinicians to describe symptoms that patients may have in the upper abdomen. The symptoms can include upper abdominal pain, epigastric discomfort, fullness, early satiety, bloating, or belching. There may be associated symptoms such as nausea or vomiting. The term "dyspepsia" should not be confused with "functional dyspepsia."

Functional dyspepsia is a diagnosis given to a conglomeration of gastrointestinal symptoms that persist after a negative gastrointestinal evaluation. The etiology is not known, but altered gut motility, visceral hypersensitivity, and psychological factors have been implicated.

PREVALENCE

Dyspepsia can be a symptom in 8% to 11% of patients who are referred for palliative care.

CONSEQUENCES OF UNTREATED DYSPEPSIA

Depending on the etiology, unaddressed dyspepsia can lead to an aversion to food, which may lead to weight loss, debility, and a negative impact on quality of life.

LIKELY ETIOLOGIES

- Peptic ulcer disease
- Gastritis
- GERD
- Gastroparesis
- Gallstones
- Medications
- Functional dyspepsia

Peptic ulcer disease and gastritis are more likely to occur in a patient who is also using an NSAID for pain. A patient who is on an opiate analgesic, or other medications with potent anticholinergic side effects, is more likely to have medication-induced gastroparesis.

DIAGNOSIS

History

Most medications have the potential to cause nausea in patients. NSAIDs may cause erosive disease anywhere in the gastrointestinal tract. Opioids can cause delayed gut motility. Calcium channel blockers may produce reflux-type symptoms by reducing tone in the lower esophageal sphincter as well as decreasing gut motility. A thorough history can often guide empiric therapy for a patient's dyspepsia.

- **Peptic ulcer** is often described as a gnawing or boring pain located in the epigastrum. Depending on the location of the ulcer, it may be relieved or exacerbated by meals. The patient should be questioned for any signs of recent gastrointestinal bleeding such as melena. A history of NSAID use would heighten the possibility that a patient's pain may be due to ulcers or gastritis.
- **Gastroesophageal reflux disease (GERD)** is very common among the general population. The classic symptom of reflux is epigastric burning that radiates upward into the chest, usually after meals and when patient is recumbent. In some patients, GERD may manifest as bloating or eructation after meals. Other symptoms from complications related to GERD, such as odynophagia and dysphagia related to esophagitis or esophageal ulcers, may also be present. Patients should be asked

questions about dietary and lifestyle factors that may predispose the individual to reflux. Caffeine, alcohol, tobacco, chocolates, and mints may be lead to a decrease in the lower esophageal sphincter pressure and increased reflux. In an immobile patient, remaining in a supine position for extended periods of time may lead to reflux because of the loss of gravity's aide in reducing reflux.

- **Gastroparesis:** The incidence of gastroparesis is estimated at 9.6 per 100,000 persons.[1] Gastroparesis is most common in patients with diabetes. In the palliative care patient, opioids can be a leading cause of delayed gastric emptying. A workup for gastroparesis to officially document delayed gastric emptying, however, may not be necessary or appropriate for patients with significant functional or cognitive impairment, or in patient populations where goals of care are focused on quality of life. (See Chapter 51: Gastroparesis.)
- **Biliary colic** most commonly manifests as epigastric or right upper quadrant pain. The pain may be associated with nausea and not infrequently radiates to the right scapula or shoulder. It typically occurs 30 to 60 minutes after a fatty meal, when chyme in the duodenum triggers the gallbladder to contract with subsequent, transient obstruction of a gallstone(s) at the egress of the gallbladder near the cystic duct. The pain dissipates after the stomach empties and relaxation of the gallbladder takes place, allowing the stone to "fall back down." If the stone becomes impacted, inflammation and infection can then ensue, causing cholecystitis.
- **Cholecystitis** can also occur in patients who do not have gallstones. Acalculous cholecystitis most often occurs in critically ill patients related to trauma, surgery, shock, burns, sepsis, prolonged fasting, and parenteral nutrition. It can occur one to 50 days after an inciting event. Ischemia and bile stasis have been implicated as possible cause of acalculous cholecystitis.[2]

Tests

For the elderly or seriously ill patient, the burdens and benefits of diagnostic testing should be carefully considered, taking into account prognosis, comorbidities, and goals of care (Table 48.1).

TREATMENT OPTIONS

Pharmacologic

- Treatment should be first aimed at reviewing the medications that the patient is taking. Any potentially offending medications should be discontinued, if possible. In the case of analgesics, substitution of opioids in place of NSAIDS, or use of other analgesic adjuvants should be

TABLE 48.1: DIAGNOSTIC TESTS

Procedure	Conditions	Notes
Upper GI series	GERD Esophagitis Esophageal ulcer Peptic ulcer disease	Patients must be mobile and able to move and change positions as the procedure is performed
Endoscopy	Esophagitis Esophageal ulcer Peptic ulcer disease Gastritis	The procedure requires sedation
Gastric emptying scan*	Gastroparesis	May not be necessary or appropriate for patients with significant functional or cognitive impairment
Ultrasound	Biliary colic Cholecystitis	
HIDA scan	Cholecystitis	

*Normal emptying of the stomach is usually measured by the time required for 50% emptying, which is best evaluated by the Gastric Emptying Scan. The normal T ½ is 50 to 90 minutes for men and postmenopausal women, and 50 to 100 minutes in premenopausal women.

considered. (See Chapter 29: Management of Pain in Older Adults.)

- In most patients, and probably particularly true for a palliative care patient, empiric treatment of dyspepsia with a proton pump inhibitor (PPI) should be the first line therapy. PPIs have been shown to be effective in the treatment of dyspepsia.[3] Treatment with a step-up approach using antacids, H-2 receptor antagonists, and then proton pump inhibitors has a success rate of 72%.[4]
- If therapy aimed at acid suppression fails, a trial of metoclopramide 5 mg to 10 mg prior to meals and at bedtime may be helpful if symptoms suggest delayed gastric emptying. Extended use of metoclopramide beyond 12 weeks has been associated with the development of tardive dyskinesia and Parkinsonism.[5] The risk of these potential side effects should be weighed in the context of prognosis, goals of care, and severity of symptom distress.
- Biliary colic can be mitigated by adherence to a low-fat diet and analgesics on an as needed basis.
- Episodes of cholecystitis can be treated with broad-spectrum antibiotics when they occur.

Other treatment options

- If the patient has frequent cholecystitis or chronic cholecystitis, mechanical decompression of the gallbladder may be necessary. This is usually achieved with a cholecystectomy.
- A less invasive alternative to surgery that can provide effective long-term relief for a patient who is not a candidate for surgery may be a percutaneous cholecystotomy. This procedure entails the placement of pigtail catheter into the gallbladder under fluoroscopy to achieve drainage. The procedure is usually performed under local anesthetic.[6]
- Acalculous cholecystitis can be treated with cholecystotomy or cholecystectomy.

TAKE-HOME POINTS

- Dyspepsia is a common complaint.
- Depending on the etiology, unaddressed dyspepsia can lead to an aversion to food, which may lead to weight loss, debility, and a negative impact on quality of life.
- Most cases of dyspepsia can be treated empirically, and invasive testing can be avoided.
- Treatment should be first aimed at reviewing the medications that the patient is taking. Any potentially offending medications should be discontinued, if possible.
- A less invasive alternative to surgery that can provide effective long-term relief for a patient who is not a candidate for surgery may be a percutaneous cholecystotomy.

REFERENCES

1. Jung H, Choung RS, Locke GR, et al. The incidence, prevalence, and outcomes of patients with gastroparesis in Olmstead County, Minnesota, from 1996 to 2006. *Gastro.* 2009;*136*:1225–1233.
2. Huffman JL, Schenker S. Acute acalculous cholecystitis—a review. *Clin Gastroenterol Hepatol.* Sept 9, 2009;*8*(1):15–22.
3. Delaney B, Ford AC, Forman D, et al. Initial management strategies for dyspepsia. *Cochrane Database Syst Rev.* 2005;(*4*):CD001061.
4. van Marrewijk CJ, Mujakov S, Fransen GA, et al. Effect and cost-effectiveness of step-up versus step-down treatment with antacid, H2-receptor antagonists, and proton pump inhibitors in patients with new onset dyspepsia (DIAMOND study): a primary-care-based randomized controlled study. *Lancet.* 2009;*373*:215–225.
5. Ganzini, L, Casey DE, Hoffman WF, McCall AL. The prevalence of metoclopramide-induced tardive dyskinesia and acute extrapyramidal movement disorders. *Arch Intern Med.* 1993;*153*(12): 1469–1475.
6. Teoh WM, Cade RJ, Banting SW, Mackay S, Hassen AS. Percutaneous cholecystotomy in the management of acute cholecystitis. *ANZ J Surg.* 2005;*75*:396–398.

49

Dysphagia

CASE

Mrs. S is an 83-year-old woman with hypertension, diabetes, osteoarthritis, and asthma. She presents with progressive dysphagia to solids over the past three weeks. She does not have any problems drinking liquids. The dysphagia is described as food not going down smoothly as she swallows. There is a feeling of the food getting stuck in the esophagus from time to time, but she has not had an impaction. She does not cough or regurgitate after eating. There has been a five-pound weight loss over this time. Her medications include a steroid inhaler, potassium supplements, calcium, and ibuprofen.

DEFINITION

Swallowing can be divided into two processes, the oropharyngeal phase and the esophageal phase.

- The oropharyngeal phase involves coordination of striated (voluntary) muscles to macerate the food, prepare it into a bolus, and move it into the hypopharynx, and relaxation of the upper esophageal sphincter (cricopharyngeus muscle).
- The esophageal phases involve the smooth (involuntary) muscles of the esophagus and lower esophageal sphincter. Once the bolus traverses the upper esophageal sphincter, the bolus of food is propagated through the esophagus over a 2-second span by the coordinated contractions of the esophagus.
- Swallow is completed by the transient relaxation of the lower esophageal sphincter to allow the bolus to enter the stomach.
- *Dysphagia* occurs when there is a problem with any part of the swallowing process. Dysphagia can be divided in various manners such as oropharyngeal vs. esophageal or anatomic (mechanical) vs. motility. Esophageal dysphagia can be further divided by etiology, i.e., mechanical (anatomic), or motility-related.

- The symptoms of dysphagia as reported by the patient can be quite variable. Symptoms and signs of dysphagia include:
  - Difficulty chewing hard foods such as meats
  - Difficulty initiating a swallow
  - Choking or coughing during swallowing
  - Sensation of slowed or non-passage of food through the esophagus after swallowing
  - Persistent sensation of something present in the esophagus
  - Regurgitation
  - Aspiration
  - Decreased oral intake
  - Weight loss

PREVALENCE

- Dysphagia in the geriatric population is estimated at 10% to 15%, although many patients do not report these symptoms to their health care professionals.[1,2]
- A significant decrease in esophageal motility with aging has been reported. This led to the adoption of the term "presbyesophagus" 35 years ago.[3]

CONSEQUENCES OF UNTREATED DYSPHAGIA

- Weight loss
- Loss of pleasure from eating
- Pneumonia
- Acute food impaction

LIKELY ETIOLOGIES

1. **Neurogenic dysphagia** (inability to coordinate glutition):
   - Stroke
   - Myasthenia gravis
   - Dementia and other neurodegenerative disorders
2. **Anatomic dysphagia:**
   - Hypertonic cricopharyngeus muscle
   - Diverticulum
   - Neoplasm
   - Schatzki ring

- Esophageal web
- Esophagitis:
  - Pill-induced (tetracycline, minocycline, doxycycline potassium, bisphosphonates and quinidine)
  - Reflux-induced
  - Infectious (candida, HSV, or CMV)
3. **Motility-related dysphagia**:
  - Ineffective swallow (presbyesophagus)
  - Achalasia

DIAGNOSIS

History

- A thorough history is the most valuable tool in the evaluation of a patient with dysphagia The process should begin with questions aimed at determining if the dysphagia is a problem with the oropharynx and coordinating the muscles necessary for glutition or an esophageal process, which is coordinated involuntarily.
- Further questions to determine if the dysphagia is related to solids, liquids, or both will immediately narrow the possible etiology of the dysphagia. For instance, a thorough history may determine that the problem may be due to poorly fitting dentures that prevent a patient from chewing his or her food adequately, or may arise because the patient is bed-bound and eats in a nearly supine position.
- The patient's medication list should be thoroughly reviewed to determine if any medications that can cause a pill-induced esophagitis have been prescribed.

In the case of Mrs. S, the ibuprofen and potassium can cause erosive esophagitis. The inhaled steroid that she is using can cause candida esophagitis.

Exam

- Physical examination may be helpful if the patient is discovered to have neurologic deficits that suggest a recent, perhaps otherwise silent, stroke.
- Oropharyngeal thrush in a patient who is a diabetic, immunosupressed, or on a corticosteroid (both systemic and inhaled) increases the likelihood that candida esophagitis is the cause.

Tests

- Diagnostic procedures for dysphagia are presented in Table 49.1. When deciding whether to pursue testing, the patient's comorbid conditions, prognosis, goals for care, and decision on whether or not a procedural intervention, such as an esophageal dilation, would be performed after the diagnostic test should be taken into account.
- The risk of radiographic studies and esophageal manometry is negligible.
- This estimated risk of major complications with diagnostic upper endoscopy is 0.2%. The risk of upper endoscopy with esophageal dilation is 0.5%.

TREATMENT OPTIONS

- For patients with a motility disorder of the esophagus, a soft mechanical diet can reduce symptoms. The patient should be instructed to always eat in the upright position. The patient should chew thoroughly and slowly, and should drink plenty of fluids between swallows to clear any residual food that may remain in the esophagus.
- Cessation of the offending pill may suffice to resolve symptoms in patients who have developed a pill-induced esophagitis.[5] The addition of an acid-suppressing medication, such as an H2 blocker or proton pump inhibitor, may allow faster healing.
- In patients suspected as having candida esophagitis, an empiric 10-day trial of an antifungal agent such as Diflucan is a reasonable approach, especially if the patient is immunocompromised.[6]
- Because reflux is one of the main suspected causes of presbyesophagus, empiric treatment with a proton pump inhibitor is a reasonable approach. The patient should be monitored for a response after treatment for 6 to 12 weeks. If there has been no improvement, the medication should be discontinued to avoid unnecessary polypharmacy.
- Esophageal rings and webs may be treated during by Bougie dilation after the diagnosis has been made.
- Achalasia can be treated endoscopically by Botox injections to the lower esophageal sphincter once every 3 to 22 months, with a median length of symptoms relief of 11.5 months.[7]

PALLIATIVE CARE ISSUES

- For palliative care patients who have oropharyngeal dysphagia, referral to a speech/language pathologist can often be helpful. The goals of therapy may not be the prevention

TABLE 49.1: DIAGNOSTIC PROCEDURES

Procedure	Conditions	Notes
Cine esophagram or modified barium swallow	Neurogenic causes (stroke) that impede coordination of the muscles of glutition Cricopharyngeus dysfunction	A cine or video esophagram is different than an upper GI series or esophagram. The test is often performed by a speech/swallow therapist and typically evaluates the process of glutition and the upper esophageal sphincter only.
Esophagram	Diverticulum Schatzki ring Esophageal web Neoplasm Pill-induced esophagitis Reflux-induced esophagitis Achalasia Presbyesophagus	An esophagram will be able to determine both anatomic and motility disorders of the esophagus.
Endoscopy	Diverticulum Schatzki ring Esophageal web Neoplasm Pill-induced esophagitis Reflux-induced esophagitis Infectious esophagitis	Endoscopy will not only determine anatomic causes of dysphagia, but it can also serve as a treatment intervention, e.g. a balloon or Bougie dilation, can be performed during endoscopy. The procedure usually requires sedation.
Esophageal manometry	Achalasia Presbyesophagus	Manometry is usually used as a confirmatory test, as the information it provides is limited to esophageal motility only.

of dysphagia but rather the mitigation of risk and discomfort to the patient.[4]

- Referral to a dietician can be beneficial because modification of the consistency of the food that a patient eats is sometimes sufficient to palliate patients with oropharyngeal dysphagia. Because thin liquids have a rapid oropharyngeal transit time, patients with an impaired swallow mechanism may not have time to safely swallow.
- Feeding tube placement is an option for patients who have a swallowing problem. Decisions about artificial nutrition should be based on goals of care, and with careful consideration of comorbidities, patient and family preferences and values, and prognosis.

TAKE-HOME POINTS

- Dysphagia is a common symptom in elderly patients and often is not reported to the medical team.
- A thorough history is often sufficient to make the diagnosis, or at least limit the differential diagnosis and the testing that needs to be performed.

- Many causes of dysphagia can be treated empirically.

REFERENCES

1. Lindgren S, Janzon L. Prevalence of swallowing complaints and clinical findings among 50–79 year-old men and women. *Dysphagia.* 1991;6:187–192.
2. Bloem B, Lagaay A, Van Beck W, et al. Prevalence of subjective dysphagia in community residents aged over 85. *BMJ.* 1990;31:721–722.
3. Hollis J, Castell D. Esophageal function in elderly men: a new look at presbyesophagus. *Ann Intern Med.* 1974;91:897–904.
4. Eckman S, Roe J. Speech and language therapists in palliative care: what do we have to offer? *Int J Palliat Nurs.* 2005;11(4):179–181.
5. Kikendall J. Pill esophagitis. *J Clin Gastroenterol.* 1999;28:298.
6. Mulhall B, Wong R. Infectious esophagitis. *Curr Treat Options Gastroenterol.* 2003;6(1):55–70.
7. Martinek J, Siroky M, Plottova Z, Bures J, Hep A, Spicak J. Treatment of patients with achalasia with botulinum toxin: a multicenter prospective cohort study. *Dis Esophagus.* 2003;16(3):204–209.

50

Hepatic Encephalopathy

CASE

Mrs. L is a 67-year-old with known hepatitis B cirrhosis. She is currently undergoing a liver transplant evaluation. She presents for a routine follow-up medical evaluation and has no specific complaints. Her husband, who accompanied her, says that she has not been herself for the last two weeks. He notes that she is tired during the day but has trouble sleeping at night. Last week they had to cancel their weekly bridge games because of her inability to concentrate. He wonders if she is depressed or getting Alzheimer's, and he questions if anything can be done.

DEFINITION

Hepatic encephalopathy is a reversible neuropsychological dysfunction that is associated with severe acute liver damage or advanced cirrhosis with portal hypertension. This section will focus on encephalopathy due to cirrhosis. The diagnosis also requires that all other causes of encephalopathy are ruled out.

- Encephalopathy is one of the clinical indicators of end-stage or decompensated liver disease. Other indicators of decompensated cirrhosis are ascites, hepatorenal syndrome, and variceal bleeding.
- Encephalopathy can be episodic or persistent, and it is particularly distressing to family members and caregivers. The findings, which can be subtle, include abnormalities that are picked up only on psychometric testing, reversal of sleep/wake cycles, mild personality changes, and impaired ability to concentrate. On the other hand, the encephalopathy can be so severe that the patient is comatose.
- To clarify confusing terminology, a consensus statement on the definition of hepatic encephalopathy was issued by the International Working Party at the 11th World Congress of Gastroenterology (Vienna 1998)[1] (Box 50.1)

PREVALENCE

- Due to previous inexact nomenclature, wide variety in presentation, and no simple diagnostic test, the exact prevalence of hepatic encephalopathy is unknown.
- Prevalence of cirrhosis in the United States is 5.5 million people, or 2% of the population, and end-stage liver disease is the 12th leading cause of death.[2]
- Hepatic encephalopathy is common among those with decompensated liver disease. Studies of transplant candidates found prevalence of hepatic encephalopathy as high as 40% to 78%.[3,4]

BOX 50.1 DEFINITION OF HEPATIC ENCEPALOPATHY

A multiaxial definition of hepatic encephalopathy defines both the type of hepatic abnormality and duration/characteristics of neurological manifestations.

The types of hepatic abnormality
- Encephalopathy associated with acute liver failure (Type A for acute)
- Encephalopathy associated with portal-systemic bypass without hepatocellular disease (Type B for bypass)
- Encephalopathy associated with cirrhosis and portal hypertension (Type C for cirrhosis)

CONSEQUENCES OF UNTREATED HEPATIC ENCEPHALOPATHY

Potential complications and consequences may depend on the severity of the encephalopathy:

- Poor quality of life in multiple studies even if mild[2,3]
- Inability to work or drive
- High risk of aspiration
- Poor oral intake
- Inability to adhere to medical treatments
- Inability to be cared for at home even at the end of life
- Extreme sensitivity to medications such as pain medications
- Respiratory failure due to inability to protect the airway
- Increased mortality
- High family caregiver burden

LIKELY ETIOLOGIES

Hepatic encephalopathy results from underlying liver disease with hepatocyte dysfunction and portal hypertension causing shunting of portal blood flow. The pathophysiology is not clearly understood and is likely multifold.

Risk Factors

- Ammonia production (levels do not always correlate with encephalopathy)
- Altered neurotransmitter and amino acid synthesis
- Endogenous benzodiazepines bind to g-aminobutyric acid receptors
- Swelling and impaired function of brain astrocytes, which break down ammonia[5]
- Accumulation of neurotoxic manganese in the globus pallidum[5]
- Increased nitric oxide, which may cause relative hypoperfusion of the brain[5]

Precipitating Factors

There are several conditions that may precipitate hepatic encephalopathy in patients with advanced liver disease. Many of these aggravating factors are known to elevate ammonia levels. Unfortunately, geriatric patients are more prone to some of the factors listed below, especially constipation, gastrointestinal bleeding, and infection:

- High-protein meal
- Constipation
- Hypovolemia
- Gastrointestinal bleeding
- Hypokalemia and/or metabolic alkalosis
- Hypoxia
- Transjugular intrahepatic portosystemic shunt (TIPS)
- Sedatives or tranquilizers
- Hypoglycemia
- Infection (including spontaneous bacterial peritonitis)
- Rarely, hepatoma and/or vascular occlusion (hepatic vein or portal vein thrombosis)
- Progression of underlying liver disease

DIAGNOSIS

History

- Other causes of delirium, such as drugs, substance use, withdrawal, nervous system infections, head trauma, and endocrine disorders, must be ruled out.
- If the hepatic encephalopathy is minimal to mild and persistent, it may be confused with dementia or depression.
- The diagnosis of hepatic encephalopathy should always be considered in someone who has risk factors for chronic liver disease and who presents with neuropsychiatric disturbances.

Because of the acute nature of the patient's symptoms and known history of liver cirrhosis, the patient is suspected to have hepatic encephalopathy. Upon further evaluation the patient is found to have worsening anemia and blood in her stool. GI bleeding can precipitate hepatic encephalopathy.

- The workup requires a comprehensive history, physical exam, and investigation of possible precipitating factors.

Exam

- Look for stigmata of chronic liver disease such as abdominal distention from ascites, palmer erythema, spider telengiectasias, and jaundice. (See Chapter 76: End-Stage Liver Disease.)
- Perform a thorough neurologic exam
- Evaluate for asterixis:
  - Present at grade 2 and 3 encephalopathy
  - Flapping of hands elicited by dorsiflexing at the wrists with arms outstretched
  - Not specific for hepatic encephalopathy
- Check stool for blood.

Tests

- Ammonia level:
  - Does not correlate with encephalopathy and can be elevated in conditions such as shock
  - Can be useful with other tests and findings, but not as an isolated test
- Comprehensive metabolic panel including liver enzymes
- Complete blood count
- Cultures if infection is suspected
- Diagnostic paracentesis if peritonitis suspected
- Oxygen saturation
- Abdominal ultrasound to rule out masses and portal or hepatic vein thrombosis
- Head CT
- EEG to rule out non-convulsive seizures
- Trial of lactulose

TREATMENT OPTIONS

In addition to the list of treatments below, all patients who may be candidates for liver transplantation should have an early referral to a transplant center. Advanced age is not a contraindication for transplantation.

Nonpharmacologic

- Prevent constipation.
- Avoid large protein intake at one sitting; overall protein reduction is not recommended since patients often malnourished.
- Avoid medications that may precipitate encephalopathy.
- Prevent or treat all other precipitating factors.

Pharmacologic

1. Therapies to reduce ammonia levels

Lactulose:

- Considered standard of care for encephalopathy, but never studied in well-designed prospective randomized trial
- Non-absorbed disaccharide metabolized by gut bacteria that promotes ammonium formation rather than ammonia
- Starting dose is 30 mL twice a day to four times a day, titrated to two to four soft bowel movements a day
- If patient unable to swallow, can be given as an enema

- Benefits/burdens of treatment and impact on quality of life should always be considered and discussed

Neomycin:

- Kills gut bacteria that produce ammonia
- No well-designed prospective randomized trial, although a recent Cochrane review found it more effective than lactulose[6]
- Dose is 4 to 12 grams, divided every four to six hours for no more than five or six days due to nephrotoxicity and ototoxicity.
- Mainly used for those who do not respond well to lactulose

Rifaximin:

- Stops growth of bacteria
- Dose of 400 mg taken orally three times a day was as effective as lactulose or lactilol at improving hepatic encephalopathy symptoms[7]
- Unclear if rifaximin can improve severe encephalopathy symptoms as rapidly as lactulose, and if it is cost-effective
- Used for those who respond poorly to lactulose since it is better tolerated and with less toxicity than neomycin

Other antibiotics:

- Other less studied but more easily tolerated antibiotics include vancomycin and metronidazole.

2. Treat endogenous benzodiazepines that bind to GABA receptors:
- Flumazenil is a benzodiazepine antagonist.
- Can precipitate seizures
- Short benefit duration and thus not a routine treatment

3. Treat agitation:
- If patient is agitated and there is concern about safety, can give haloperidol (0.5–1 mg) parenterally or orally, as needed.

4. Community referral for home care services and caregiver support should always be part of the treatment plan.

Mrs. L was admitted to the hospital and was started on lactulose, and her encephalopathy improved. She also had an upper endoscopy that showed a duodenal ulcer. In addition to the lactulose,

Mrs. L was treated for H. pylori with complete resolution of her encephalopathy within two weeks.

PALLIATIVE CARE ISSUES

- Patients with advanced liver disease, including those who are pursuing transplantation, should be offered palliative care to help address advance directives, goals of care, family distress, caregiver burden, and symptom management.
- Because of the cognitive dysfunction that is associated with hepatic encephalopathy, it is particularly important for a patient to designate a health care proxy as early as possible in the disease trajectory.
- Hepatic encephalopathy is associated with end-stage liver disease; therefore, all treatments should be evaluated based on a consideration of benefits and burdens given limited prognosis.

TAKE-HOME POINTS

- Hepatic encephalopathy, even if mild, can significantly impair quality of life.
- As with delirium, encephalopathy is often related to a precipitating factor; thorough evaluation of potential contributing factor(s) is therefore crucial.
- Geriatric patients with cirrhosis are more prone to some of the precipitating factors, especially constipation and polypharmacy.
- Standard treatment is lactulose, but there is limited evidence for this treatment.

REFERENCES

1. Ferenci P, Lockwood A, Mullen A, et al. Hepatic encephalopathy—definition, nomenclature, diagnosis, and quantification: Final report of the working party at the 11th World Congress of Gastroenterology, Vienna, 1998. *Hepatology.* 2002;*35*: 716.
2. Xu JQ, Kochanek KD, Murphy SL, Tejada-Vera B. Deaths: Final data for 2007. National vital statistics reports; vol 58 no 19. Hyattsville, MD: National Center for Health Statistics. 2010.
3. Arguelas MR, DeLawrence TG, McGuire BM. Influence of hepatic encephalopathy on health-related quality of life in patients with cirrhosis. *Dig Dis Sci.* 2003;*48*:1622.
4. Kalaitzakis E, Josefsson A, Bjornsson E. Type and etiology of liver cirrhosis are not related the presence of hepatic encephalopathy or health-related quality of life in a cross sectional study. *BMC Gastroenterol.* 2008;*8*:46.
5. Butterworth RF. Complications of cirrhosis. *J Hepatol.* 2000;*32*:71.
6. Als-Nielsen B, Gluud LL, Gluud C. Nonabsorbable disaccharides for hepatic encephalopathy. Cochrane Database of Systematic Reviews 2004, Issue 2. Art. No.: CD003044.
7. Bucci L, Palmieri GC. Double-blind, double-dummy comparison between treatment with rifaximin and lactulose in patients with medium to severe degree hepatic encephalopathy. *Current medical research and opinion.* 2003;*13*(2):109–118.

51

Gastroparesis

CASE

Mr. S is a 75-year-old man with poorly controlled diabetes, hypertension, and hepatitis C with hepatocellular carcinoma. He presents to your office complaining of early satiety, feeling bloated after meals, and nausea with occasional vomiting. A recent CT scan of his abdomen has shown that there is no mechanical obstruction, but he does have significant ascites. Eating is a passion of his, and he wants to know if you can give him anything to make these symptoms better.

DEFINITION

Gastroparesis is a condition of delayed emptying of the stomach due to abnormal motility of the gastric mucosa and in the absence of gastric outlet obstruction. It is most commonly associated with diabetes but can be associated with a wide range of clinical syndromes and diagnoses. Diagnosis rests on the presence of the triad of 1) early satiety and postprandial fullness, 2) nausea, and 3) vomiting.

Mr. S had this diagnostic triad and may be using the term bloating to describe postprandial fullness.

CLASSIFICATION OF SEVERITY[1]

1. Mild gastroparesis: Easily controlled. Able to maintain weight and meet nutritional needs. Patient on a regular diet or only minor modifications.
2. Compensated gastroparesis: Moderate symptom control, with need for pharmacologic agents. Can maintain nutrition with diet and lifestyle modifications. Rarely admitted to hospital.
3. Severe gastroparesis: Refractory symptoms despite maximal medical therapy. Unable to maintain nutrition needs via oral route. Frequent hospitalizations.

PREVALENCE

There have been no comprehensive studies of the prevalence of gastroparesis, particularly in terms of geriatric or palliative care populations. However, the overall prevalence of the symptom in the population at large is thought to be as high as 4%, and the majority of the cases are in women.

CONSEQUENCES OF UNTREATED GASTROPARESIS

- Anorexia
- Weight loss
- Malnutrition

LIKELY ETIOLOGIES

Causes of gastroparesis include the following:

1. Hyperglycemia/poorly controlled diabetes
2. Medications:
   - Anticholinergics and opioids
   - Tricyclic antidepressants, Ca-Channel blockers, clonidine, dopamine agonists, lithium, nicotine, progesterone-containing medications
3. Post-surgical sequelae:
   - Vagotomy and gastric resection/drainage
   - Fundoplication, esophagectomy
   - Gastric bypass surgery
   - Whipple procedure
   - Heart/lung transplant (may result in damage to vagus nerve)
4. Physiologic abnormalities of stomach:
   - Peptic ulcer
   - Gastritis (of any cause)
   - Gastric cancer
5. Ascites
6. Autonomic failure:
   - Central—CVAs, trauma, tumors, seizures
   - Peripheral—Parkinson's disease, multiple sclerosis, dysautonomias

7. Cancer:
   • Through poorly understood mechanisms, cancers that are not directly related anatomically to the stomach can cause gastroparesis, particularly unresectable upper gastrointestinal tumors.
8. Rheumatologic disease:
   • Lupus
   • Scleroderma
   • Polymyositis/dermatomyositis

Mr. S's gastroparesis most likely has multiple causes, including his poorly controlled diabetes, ascites from his liver disease, as well as opioid medications for control of his cancer-related pain, leading to constipation and slowed transit time.

OTHER DIAGNOSES RELEVANT TO GERIATRICS AND PALLIATIVE CARE

• Gastroparesis should be distinguished from gastric outlet obstruction, which can also cause delayed gastric emptying but is treated in a different manner. It should also be distinguished from more distal intestinal obstructions.
• Gastroparesis can be a cause of nausea and vomiting due to significantly decreased gastric motility.
• Physical compression of the stomach (e.g., extrinsic tumor, enlarged spleen) can result in early satiety.

DIAGNOSIS

Exam

• There are no physical exam findings that are diagnostic of gastroparesis. Signs of other disorders that can be either causative (e.g., ascites) or related (e.g., weight loss from persistent vomiting) should be noted.
• It is important to look for physical signs related to other diagnoses that may cause similar symptoms (e.g., feeling for an abdominal mass or organomegaly).

Tests

• Gastric scintigraphy (aka gastric emptying study) is the gold standard diagnostic test for gastroparesis. The patient ingests a radio-labeled solid meal and serial radiographs are taken to determine the time

it takes the stomach to empty. However, there are no generalizable standards for what the meal consists of, and varying components of the meal (i.e., quantity of liquids, fat content, indigestible fiber) can affect the time to gastric emptying.
• Other diagnostic tests that can be used to diagnose gastroparesis include ultrasound (used to visualize emptying of stomach after a liquid meal), MRI, CT scan, and isotope breath tests.
• Much less common diagnostic tests include the use of a "smart pill" (a pill that measures changes in pH, pressure, and temperature as it moves through the bowel and transmits these data transcutaneously using a wireless system) or antroduodenal manometry.
• Depending on the patient population (e.g., hospice patient near the end of life), the burdens of formalized testing may outweigh the benefits. In these cases, the triad of symptoms may be diagnostic enough so that a definitive test is not needed.

TREATMENT OPTIONS

Combining the nonpharmacologic and pharmacologic treatment modalities described below is often the most effective way to treat gastroparesis, but the degree to which elements of lifestyle and diet modification may be possible depends on the care setting and patient's clinical condition.

Nonpharmacologic

• Lifestyle modification: Eating smaller meals, allowing more time between meals for gastric emptying, walking after meals
• Diet modification: Increasing fluid intake with meals (promotes gastric emptying), minimizing fat and fiber intake, shifting caloric consumption from solids to liquids (i.e., consuming more calories in a liquid form and less in a solid form)
• Glycemic control: Hyperglycemia delays gastric emptying in the absence of neuropathy or myopathy. Prevention of wide fluctuations may be more important than maintaining tight control.
• Whenever possible, reduce or discontinue medications that may delay gastric emptying (e.g., anticholinergics, opioids).

Pharmacologic

• Pharmacologic options for gastroparesis are listed in Table 51.1. The evidence base for these medications is poor overall, and there are few head-to-head trials. As a result choice of medication and dose often consists of trial and error.

- These gastroparesis medications should not be used in gastric or bowel obstruction, as they can produce powerful contractions that can cause significant pain if a patient has a gastrointestinal obstruction.
- Because nausea and vomiting are often the most disabling aspects of gastroparesis, the medications described in table 51.1 may be beneficial because of their anti-emetic properties as well as their direct effects on the stomach. However, they may have to be combined with anti-emetic medications to reduce patients' symptoms.[3]

Other Treatments

- *Botulinim toxin* injected during endoscopy in a circumferential pattern in the pylorus may reduce spasm. Although several open-labeled studies have demonstrated the effectiveness of this treatments for pyloric spasms, randomized controlled trials have not been as convincing.
- *Direct electrical stimulation* of the gastric musculature through an implanted stimulator has been studied, but the results are mixed and this procedure is performed only at select centers. This treatment is currently approved by the Food and Drug Administration only on humanitarian grounds.
- *Gastric resection or pyloroplasty* may be needed in extreme cases, though these types of measures may not be appropriate in certain geriatric and palliative care populations.
- These more invasive treatments should be reserved for extreme cases where the benefits of the modality outweigh the

TABLE 51.1: PHARMACOLOGICAL OPTIONS[2]

Medication	Dose	Mechanism	Notes
Metoclopramide	5–20 mg every 6–8 hours	Increases gastric motility by antagonizing dopamine D2 receptor	Give 30 minutes before meals for maximum effectiveness Often the medication of first choice Also an effective anti-emetic via brainstem D2 antagonism as well as 5-HT3 receptor antagonism Because of its effect at dopamine receptors, can cause acute dystonic reactions and extrapyramidal symptoms
Domperidone	10–30 mg every 6–8 hours	Similar to metoclopramide	Not available in United States Has fewer CNS side effects than metoclopramide
Erythromycin	50–250 mg q6–q8 hours	Increases gastric motility by binding at motilin receptor	Although counterintuitive, it is more effective if given intravenously as compared to orally
Bethanacol	25 mg q6 hours	Muscarnic agonist that increases lower esophageal sphincter pressure and stimulates fundoantral contractions; does not actually induce peristalsis in stomach	Used rarely, as adjuvant to either pro-kinetic drugs or anti-emetics Multiple adverse effects, including abdominal cramping, flushing, diaphoresis, lacrimation, salivation, bronchoconstriction, urinary urgency, miosis Can have serious cardiovascular effects, including sudden hypotension and inducing atrial fibrillation in patients with hyperthyroidism
Cisapride and Tegaserod		5-HT4 receptor agonist	Both withdrawn from U.S. market due to significant cardiac risks, including sudden cardiac death (cisapride)

burdens and are in line with the patient's goals of care.

TAKE-HOME POINTS

- Gastroparesis must be distinguished from gastric outlet obstruction and other causes of nausea and vomiting.
- A workup for gastroparesis to officially document delayed gastric emptying may not be necessary or appropriate for patients with significant functional or cognitive impairment, or in patient populations where goals of care are focused on quality of life.
- When the cause of gastroparesis can be definitively determined, treatment should be directed at the underlying cause, including reducing or discontinuing medications that delay gastric emptying (when appropriate). Otherwise,

metaclopramide is often the first line of treatment.
- More invasive treatments such as the use of botulinim toxin, electrical stimulation, or surgical intervention should be reserved for extreme cases where the benefits of the modality outweigh the burdens and are in line with the patient's goals of care.

REFERENCES

1. Waseem S, Moshiree B, Draganov PV. Gastroparesis: current diagnostic challenges and management considerations. *World J Gastroenterol.* Jan 7, 2009;*15*(1):25–37.
2. Gumaste V, Baum J. Treatment of gastroparesis: an update. *Digestion.* 2008;*78*(4):173–179.
3. Mannix, K. Palliation of Nausea and Vomiting. In: Doyle D, Hanks G, Cherny NI, and Calman K, eds. *Oxford Textbook of Palliative Medicine.* New York: Oxford University Press; 2005;459–468.

52

Hiccups

CASE

Mr. E, is a 94-year-old man with history of colon cancer, which was treated with a hemicolectomy at age of 92. He had four positive lymph nodes at the time of the surgery, but he and his family decided to forgo chemotherapy due to his frailty. In two years, patient has had some weight loss and decreased energy, but otherwise minimal decline. In the last month he has started to have frequent bouts of hiccups, sometimes lasting several days and affecting the quality of his sleep. He is not sure what brings them on. He has tried many home remedies, with questionable benefit, as the hiccups would stop for a few hours or days, then recur. There seems to be no pattern that he or the family can discern. His appetite is normal, he does not have any abdominal pain, nausea, or vomiting, and his bowel habits are unchanged. He smokes six to eight cigars a week and drinks no alcohol. While initially finding the situation somewhat amusing, he has now become embarrassed, exhausted, irritable, and frustrated, mainly due to sleep deprivation.

DEFINITION

Hiccups (medical term: *singultus*) are brief, involuntary contractions of the diaphragm and intercostals muscles that result in a sharp inspiration that is abruptly interrupted by glottic closure. Depending on their duration, they can be classified as:

- Acute hiccups, hiccup bout, or non-pathologic hiccups: up to 48 hours
- Chronic hiccups:
  - Persistent: 48 hours to one month
  - Recurrent: repeated episodes of persistent hiccups
  - Intractable: last more than two months

PREVALENCE

While the lifetime prevalence of benign self-limited hiccup bouts is 100%, chronic hiccups are rare and often can be a marker of underlying disease. Because hiccups are perceived to be insignificant, their prevalence is not well documented. Chronic hiccups occur more commonly in men than in women, and estimates of prevalence in cancer patients ranges from 10% to 20%.

CONSEQUENCES OF UNTREATED HICCUPS

Hiccups can be a serious problem for elderly debilitated patients. Persistent and intractable hiccups can have significant adverse effects such as eating difficulties leading to malnutrition, dehydration, and weight loss; insomnia, which can lead to fatigue and confusion; respiratory and digestive problems; wound dehiscence in postsurgical patients, and profound social isolation and psychological distress.

LIKELY ETIOLOGIES

- Hiccups result from stimulation to the afferent limb of the phrenic or the vagus nerves, which get transmitted to a "hiccup"-mediator in the upper cervical spinal cord that interacts with nuclei in the brainstem, medullary reticular formation, and hypothalamus. The efferent limb consists mainly of the motor fibers of the phrenic nerve with accessory connections to the glottis and other respiratory muscles.
- Self-limited hiccup bouts are usually caused by gastric over-distention or excessive alcohol ingestion. But there have been more than one hundred other causes identified that may be associated with phrenic, vagus, or CNS irritation leading to chronic hiccups. The more likely etiologies in the geriatric population include:[1]
  - *CNS disorders*: trauma, vascular lesions, tumors, infection, demyelinating lesions, hydrocephalus
  - *Head and neck*: foreign bodies, tumors, cysts, goiters, vascular anomalies, neck hyperextension, injury or stimulation of recurrent laryngeal nerve (branch of phrenic nerve)

- *Ears*: foreign bodies or tumors in ear canal that stimulate the auricular branch of the vagus nerve
- *Pulmonary*: pneumonia, pleuritis, neoplasms
- *Cardiovascular*: myocardial infarction, pericarditis, aneurysms
- *Gastrointestinal*: gastric distention, GERD, esophagitis, esophageal obstruction, hiatal hernia, ulcers, gastritis, pancreatitis, cholecystitis, constipation, bowel obstruction, neoplasm
- *Infectious*: oral-pharyngeal or esophageal candida, abscesses, influenza, tuberculosis, herpes zoster
- *Metabolic*: alcoholism, uremia, electrolyte imbalances
- *Medications*: many of the medications that treat hiccups can also cause hiccups. The common offenders include steroids, methyldopa, barbiturates, cisplatin, and drugs used in general anesthesia.
- *Psychogenic*: stress, conversion disorder, malingering
- Idiopathic

On exam, Mr. E, a frail, thin, pleasant man, was lying on his bed in no acute distress. Occasional hiccups were noted, approximately once every two minutes. He was afebrile and his other vital signs were also normal. The head and neck exam was remarkable only for a soft cerumen impaction of both ears, which was removed. There were no neck or supraclavicular masses palpated. The lungs were clear bilaterally with mild decreased breath sounds at both bases. Heart sounds were regular. The abdomen had a well-healed surgical incision from the hemicolectomy and felt full and diffusely tender to deep palpation with no discrete masses. The liver edge was noted to be five cm below the costal margin and firm. Rectal exam was notable for lots of pasty brown stool in rectum without patient having the urge to evacuate. Rectal tone was a little diminished.

No labs were ordered.

Patient was given 5 mg daily of oral bisacodyl. This produced a significant increase of stool output and a transient improvement in the hiccups.

DIAGNOSIS

Chronic hiccups require a thorough evaluation with the goal of finding the underlying etiology and determining the appropriate treatment.

History

Include questions about drug and alcohol use and medications, and assess the persistence of hiccups during sleep. Perform a complete review of systems.

Exam

- Complete head and neck exam, including both ear canals (cerumen disimpaction if needed).
- Full neurological exam
- Chest and abdomen exam
- Rectal exam to rule out fecal impaction if there is a history of constipation or diarrhea

Tests

- CBC, electrolytes, and chest X-ray.
- Other tests that may be helpful if the initial workup is unrevealing include LFTs, serum calcium, CT and MRI as needed, endoscopy, brochoscopy, and EEG.

After six weeks, daily 2- to 4-hour bouts of hiccups started to recur despite optimal bowel regimen and no evidence of constipation. Despite small meals, he sometimes vomited because of the force of the diaphragmatic contractures. Mr. E's appetite decreased, his sleep suffered, and his mood became despondent. He developed fatigue and dyspnea on exertion. On physical exam, there was no evidence of constipation, but there was an increased area of diminished lung sounds at the bases, suggesting progression of pleural effusions.

TREATMENT OPTIONS

Nonpharmacologic

- Home remedies: breathing into a paper bag, swallowing sugar, drinking from the opposite side of the glass, holding breath, inducing a sneeze, being startled, etc. There are as many remedies as there have been old wives, and given the transient nature of most hiccups, all remedies "work" at some point. Most treatments do have a physiologic basis in that they interrupt the hiccup reflex arc by stimulating the vagus or phrenic nerves, interfering with normal respiration, or by increasing pCO2 levels.
- Acupuncture: efficacy is comparable to or better than prescription drug therapy.[2]
- Hypnosis.
- Behavioral techniques: distraction, small meals, fasting, vigorous exercise, though

exercise may not be an option in frail elderly patients.

Pharmacologic

- Given the lack of large randomized controlled studies, most of the treatments for hiccups are guided by literature that includes mainly case reports, anecdotal evidence, expert clinicians' experience, and small series.
- The focus of management should be in treating the underlying cause, but if none can be found, the medications in Table 52.1 may be tried.
- The following medications may also be effective and can be synergistic with the medications listed in Table 52.1:
  - Gabapentin: may be especially useful in palliative care patients with intractable symptoms,[3] as well as geriatric patients who cannot tolerate the categories of medications in the table listed above
  - Valproic acid
  - Phenytoin
  - Nifedipine
  - Sertraline
  - Amitriptyline

- Intravenous lidocaine
- Quinidine
- Ranitidine
- Simethicone
- Proton pump inhibitors

SURGICAL INTERVENTION

Surgical treatments should be a choice of last resort and are rarely indicated in the geriatric or palliative care population:

- Phrenic nerve block, transection, or electrostimulation
- Breathing pacemaker
- Vagus nerve stimulator
- Cervical epidural block
- Short-term anesthesia with or without pharyngeal stimulation

Baclofen 20 mg once daily was started and tapered up to 20 mg three times a day. This did not affect the frequency of the bouts, but it decreased their force and patient was able to sleep through the hiccups.

TAKE-HOME POINTS

- Chronic hiccups can be distressing and disabling to the geriatric patient.

TABLE 52.1: PHARMACOLOGIC TREATMENTS

Class	Examples	Benefits	Risks
Muscle relaxants	Baclofen (GABA analogue) starting with 10 mg twice daily and titrated up to 20 mg 4 times a day. This should be the first choice.	May aid in blocking the hiccup stimulus and can decrease the severity of the hiccups	Drowsiness, weakness, hypotension, nausea, constipation. Should not be discontinued drastically, and should be used cautiously in patients with renal insufficiency
Gastric motility agent	Metoclopramide starting with 10 mg three times daily. Can also be given intravenously	Acts centrally and also encourages gastric emptying	Safer than other dopamine antagonists (chlorpromazine, haloperidol), but also may be less effective
Antipsychotics	Chlorpromazine starting at 25 mg once daily and titrating up to 50 mg three or four times a day for seven to ten days. May also be given intravenously	Acts centrally in the hypothalamus by dopamine antagonism	Dystonic reactions, drowsiness, hypotension
	Haldol 2–5 mg IM, 0.5–5 mg po q 8H	May be given IM	Same as above

- Evaluation requires a complete history and physical, labs, and chest X-ray, but often a cause is not found.
- Pharmacologic treatments are guided by limited evidence, but in the absence of a clear etiology, a rational pharmacological approach in combination with an open-minded exploration of alternative therapies, such as acupuncture, makes sense for older patients and those receiving palliative care.
- Surgical interventions are rarely indicated in the geriatric or palliative care population.

REFERENCES

1. Smith HS, Busracamwongs A. Management of hiccups in the palliative care population. *Am J Hosp Palliat Care*. 2003;*20*(2):149–154.
2. Schiff E, River Y, Oliven A, et al. Acupuncture therapy for persistent hiccups. *Am J Med Sci*. 2002;*323*:166–168.
3. Tegeler ML, Baumrucker SJ. Gabapentin for intractable hiccups in palliative care. *Am J Hosp Palliat Med*. Mar 2008;*25*:52–54.

53

Nausea and Vomiting

CASE

Ms. N is an 85-year-old woman with longstanding diabetes mellitus, hypertension, and severe biventricular heart failure. She has dyspnea, moderately controlled by taking opioids and diuretics, and significant lower extremity edema. Her main complaint today is persistent nausea with occasional vomiting. She feels full all the time, but her nausea is worse after meals. She would like help controlling the nausea, as it is interfering with her quality of life and ability to function.

DEFINITIONS

Nausea is entirely subjective. It is defined either as the sensation that precedes vomiting or as the response to stimulation of the chemoreceptor trigger zone, vestibular apparatus, gastrointestinal lining, or cerebral cortex. Patients may report feeling "queasy" or "sick to the stomach."[1]

Vomiting is a specific neuromuscular response, involving the rapid, forceful expulsion of gastric contents in a retrograde manner from the stomach up to and out of the mouth. Vomiting is associated with contraction of the abdominal and chest wall musculature.[1]

PREVALENCE

- While most people have experienced transient nausea and vomiting, frequent episodes of nausea are relatively uncommon in the general population, occurring more than once per month in only 8% of people.[2]
- Vomiting is even less common, with only 2% of people having more than one monthly episode.[2]
- At the end of life, nausea occurs in 60% to 70% of cancer patients and up to 70% of patients with a variety of diagnoses.[3,4] Vomiting is less common in the final weeks of life, with about 30% of patients affected.[5]

CONSEQUENCES OF UNTREATED NAUSEA AND VOMITING

- Distress
- Decreased appetite and intake
- Weight loss
- Dehydration
- Electrolyte imbalances
- Mallory-Weiss tears (bleeding mucosal lacerations of the distal esophagus and proximal stomach)[6]
- Boerhaave's syndrome (rupture of the esophagus)[1]

LIKELY ETIOLOGIES

Vomiting is the result of vomiting center input (via vagal nerve) from one of the four afferent sites (Figure 53.1):

1. Chemoreceptor trigger zone (dopamine and serotonin receptors):
   - Drugs (opioids, chemotherapy agents, digoxin)
   - Metabolic disorders (uremia, hypercalcemia)
   - Toxins (bacterial, tumor-related, radiotherapy)
2. Vestibular apparatus (cholinergic, histamine receptors):
   - Toxic drug effects (non-steroidal anti-inflammatory drugs, opioids)
   - Meniere's, motion sickness, labyrinthitis, benign positional vertigo
   - Tumors: acoustic neuroma, brain tumor, cranial metastases
3. Direct gastrointestinal irritation (serotonin, histamine receptors):
   - Gastric/intestinal distention (gastroparesis, stasis, constipation, obstruction)
   - Gastric irritation/mucosal irritation (drugs, blood, alcohol, gastro-esophageal reflux disease)
   - Liver (inflammation, capsular stretch, biliary obstruction)

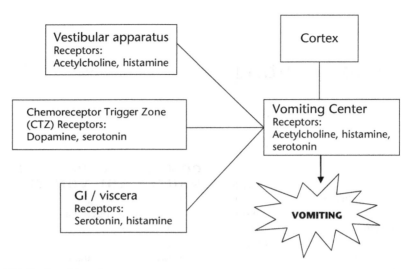

FIGURE 53.1: Pathophysiology of vomiting.

4. Cortical (histamine, serotonin, cholinergic receptors):
   - Pain, fear, emotional factors, anxiety (anticipatory nausea and vomiting)
   - Increased intracranial pressure, meningitis, CNS malignancy

DIAGNOSIS

The workup requires a comprehensive history, physical exam, and investigation of possible etiologies. Choice of treatment should be based on the pathophysiology and the specific neurotransmitter receptors involved.

History

- Identify contributing medications and eliminate them if possible.
- Clarify duration, frequency, severity, timing:
  - Acute: drug-related, viral, pancreatitis, cholycystitis
  - Insidious: gastroparesis, metabolic disorder, GERD
- Timing:
  - Upon awakening: increased intracranial pressure, uremia
  - Post-prandial: gastroparesis
- Associated symptoms: pain, headache, early satiety

Exam

- Evidence of dehydration: hypotension, orthostasis, tachycardia, weight loss
- Abdominal exam:

- Inspection: distension, visible peristalsis
- Auscultation: succussion splash (gastroparesis or gastric outlet obstruction), high-pitched bowel sounds (obstruction), absent bowel sounds (ileus)
- Percussion/palpation: masses, hepatomegaly
- Rectal exam: rule out impaction, look for blood in stool
- Evidence of other systemic diseases

Tests

Order tests based on the results of the history and exam. Goal is to assist in identifying the cause and/or evaluate for consequences such as electrolyte imbalance, dehydration, alkalosis, or malnutrition, and signs of organ insufficiency:

- CBC
- BMP
- Drug levels for patients taking digoxin, theophylline
- Liver enzymes
- Chemistry panel

Imaging

Imaging may not be necessary, but if consistent with appropriate and achievable goals of care, imaging is helpful especially when the etiology is elusive.

- Abdominal X-ray: May indicate obstruction, pseudo-obstruction

- Upper GI barium study +/- small bowel follow-through: Can reveal obstruction, mucosal lesion
- Abdominal CT scan: Detect and diagnose obstruction and evaluate other organs
- Gastric emptying scan: Quantifies rate of transit of solids and liquids
- Esophogastroduodenoscopy: Allows for mucosal exam and intervention (i.e., stenting for intrinsic or extrinsic obstructions)

TREATMENT OPTIONS

Etiology of nausea and vomiting is often multifactorial (i.e., opioids, liver capsular stretch, uremia, and constipation). It is important to address as many etiologies as possible.

NONPHARMACOLOGIC

- Avoid strong smells or other triggers.
- Eat small meals.
- Utilize relaxation and breathing techniques to reduce stress.
- Consider acupuncture stimulation of the P6 point above the wrist. (Numerous studies report benefit of acupuncture for post-op and chemo-induced nausea and vomiting, with decreased nausea and decreased vomiting frequency.)[7,8]

PHARMACOLOGIC

Pharmacologic management is outlined in Table 53.1.[9]

TABLE 53.1: PHARMACOLOGIC MANAGEMENT OF NAUSEA AND VOMITING[9]

Drug	Neurotransmitters/ Mechanism	Side Effects/Issues	Dosing
Antipsychotic; dopamine antagonist	D2 antagonist	Extrapyramidal symptoms (EPS), sedation	Haloperidol: 0.5 mg–5 mg/dose Q8h (SC/IV = ½ PO)
Antipsychotics	H1 antagonist, ACH antagonist, lessor D2 antagonist	EPS	Chlorpromazine: 0.5 mg–1 mg/kg Q8h (IV = PO)
Promotility agent; dopamine antagonist	D2 antagonist, 5HT4 agonist at gut	Increases GI motility Good for gastroparesis, bad for total mechanical obstruction	Metoclopramide: 5–15 mg before meals and bedtime (IV/SC = PO)
Antivertigo/ Antiemetic	ACH-M1 antagonists H1 antagonists	Anticholinergic side effects, likely bad choices in elderly, delirious, or cognitively impaired patients	Scopolamine: 0.5 mg transdermal PATCH Q3d Meclizine: 25 mg TID
Serotonin receptor antagonist	5HT3 antagonist	Costly	Granisetron: 1 mg q12h Ondansetron: 0.15 mg/kg/dose Q6h (max. 8 mg/d)
Steroids	Capillary permeability Intracranial pressure Edema, capsular stretch	Hypertension, gastritis, osteoporosis, myopathy, mood swings, hyperglycemia, immunosuppression, delirium	Dexamethasone: 6–1 0mg load then 2–4 mg bid or qid for maintenance Prednisone: 1.5 mg dexamethasone = 10 mg prednisone
Antihistamine	H1 antagonist	Sedation Can cause confusion in older adults	Diphenhydramine: 1 mg/kg/dose PO q4h (max: 100 mg/dose) Hydroxyzine: 0.5–1.0 mg/kg/dose Q4h (max: 600 mg/day)
Somatostatin analogue		Costly	Octreotide: 50–100 micrograms subQ TID, can increase to 900 mcg per day[10]

PALLIATIVE CARE ISSUES

Chemoreceptor trigger zone is often involved in nausea at the end of life; therefore, a dopamine or serotonin antagonist can be very helpful.

TAKE-HOME POINTS

- Determine the etiologies of nausea and vomiting if possible.
- Correct reversible causes, remove offending drugs if possible, and rotate opiates.
- Treat the symptom if the etiology cannot be determined.

REFERENCES

1. Quigley EMM, Hasler WL, Parkman HP. AGA Technical review on nausea and vomiting. *Gastroenterology.* 2001;*120*:263–286.
2. Spiller RC. ABC of the upper gastrointestinal tract: anorexia, nausea, vomiting, and pain. *BMJ.* 2001;*323*:1354–1357.
3. Fainsinger R, Miller MJ, Bruera E, Hanson J, Maceachern T. Symptom control during the last week of life on a palliative care unit. *J Palliat Care.* 1991;*7*(1):5–11.
4. Reuben DB, Mor V. Nausea and vomiting in terminal cancer patients. *Arch Intern Med.* 1986;*146*(10):2021–2023.
5. Wood GJ, Shega JW, Lynch B, Von Roenn J. Management of intractable nausea and vomiting in patients at the end of life. *JAMA.* 2007;*298*(10):1196–1207.
6. Mallory GK, Weiss S. Hemorrhages from lacerations of the cardiac orifice of the stomach due to vomiting. *Am J Med Sci.* 1929;*178*:506.
7. Ezzo J, Vickers A, Richardson MA, et al. Acupuncture-point stimulation for chemotherapy-induced nausea and vomiting. *Journal of Clinical Oncology.* 2005;*23*(28): 7188–7198.
8. Streitberger K, Ezzo J, Schneider A. Acupuncture for nausea and vomiting: an update of clinical and experimental studies. *Auton Neurosci.* 2006;*129*(1-2):107–117.
9. Policzer JS, Sobel J. Management of selected non-pain symptoms of life-limiting illness. Hospice/Palliative Care Training for Physicians: UNIPAC. Vol 4. 3rd ed. Glenview, IL: American Academy of Hospice and Palliative Medicine; 2007.

54

Urinary Retention

CASE
Mr. C is an 82-year-old male with a history of diabetes, hypertension, constipation, and osteoarthritis. He takes insulin, hydrochlorothiazide, milk of magnesia as needed for constipation, and Tylenol with codeine as needed for pain. During a routine office visit, he mentions that he occasionally feels like he has to force his stream of urine out. He does not feel like his bladder is emptied after urination.

DEFINITION
Urinary retention (UR) is the inability to empty the bladder by voiding urine voluntarily. UR can be an acute event that presents with abdominal or pelvic discomfort and a sudden loss of the ability to urinate. UR may also be chronic, characterized by an intermittent or continuous inability to empty the bladder, with varying degrees of retention.

PREVALENCE
Prevalence of UR varies according to care setting, sex, and age of patient, and whether retention is acute or chronic. In the outpatient setting, the incidence of acute retention in men ranges from 4.5 to 6.8 per 1,000 men per year, and the rate increases with age.[1] The prevalence in women is not well studied.

CONSEQUENCES OF UNTREATED URINARY RETENTION
- Acute onset UR is common in geriatrics and palliative care patients and presents with abdominal pain, generalized discomfort, and delirium.
- Chronic urine retention is often asymptomatic but becomes clinically significant when it results in distressing voiding dysfunctions, or when it leads to serious complications, including:
  - Urinary stasis in the bladder can cause recurrent urinary tract infections.
  - Overflow incontinence occurs when the bladder volume reaches its capacity to store urine, resulting in leakage.
- Chronic retention can progress to permanent retention. As the detrusor muscle remains stretched, the muscle wall is eventually replaced by connective tissue, becomes fibrotic, loses its tone and ability to contract appropriately, then weakens. This complication is commonly seen in elderly males with longstanding untreated benign prostatic hypertrophy (BPH). If the enlarged prostate is treated, the patient may still experience urine retention due to a weak detrusor muscle.
- Hydronephrosis is often a consequence of prolonged and severe urine retention. Untreated hydronephrosis can lead to renal failure.

LIKELY ETIOLOGIES
Urinary retention is caused by bladder outflow obstruction or impairment of the bladder detrusor muscle (i.e., the bladder does not contract appropriately).

1. **Outflow obstruction** prevents urine from passing. Factors may be intrinsic (inside the bladder or urethra) or extrinsic (outside the bladder or urethra).
   - Benign prostatic hypertrophy (BPH) is the most common obstructive cause.
   - For patients with serious illness, outflow obstruction may be caused by tumors of the urethra, bladder or prostate, or gynecological surgeries or malignancies.
   - Other causes include:
     - Urethral strictures (s/p urethral instrumentation, perineal trauma, urethritis, idiopathic)
     - Bladder stones
     - Prolapse of pelvic organs in women (uterocele, rectocele, cystocele)
     - Urethral polyps
     - Fecal impaction
     - Infection-prostatitis (the most common infectious cause), cystitis

- Trauma-pelvic injuries, penile injuries, traumatic pelvic instrumentation

2. **Impairment of the detrusor muscle** prevents the evacuation of stored urine from the bladder. Causes include:
   - Neurologic: Conditions involving upper motor neurons, lower motor neurons, or peripheral nerves that cause impaired sensory and/or motor innervation of the bladder or urethral sphincter. These include diseases or conditions that affect the brain, spinal cord, and/or peripheral or autonomic nerves, including stroke, dementia, Parkinson's disease, tumors, normal pressure hydrocephalus, spinal cord injuries, herniated discs, and peripheral neuropathy.
   - Long-standing chronic obstruction (See "Complications" below.)
   - Detrusor hyperactivity with incomplete contractions (DHIC): a common and often unrecognized problem in very elderly patients. Patient experiences urge symptoms, but the detrusor muscle fails to contract adequately to release urine. (See Chapter 55: Urinary Incontinence.) Diagnosed by urodynamic testing.
   - Pharmacologic: Anticholinergic medications inhibit detrusor muscle contractions and sympathomimetics increase smooth muscle tone around the bladder neck, causing urinary retention. These include antihistamines (diphenhydramine), muscle relaxants (baclofen), antipsychotics (haloperidol), antidepressants (amitripytiline), anticholinergics (oxybutinin, scopolamine), antiparkinsonian agents (levodopa), sympathomimetics (psudoephedrine), opioids, and many others.

DIAGNOSIS

History

- Symptoms of urinary incontinence: decreased stream, dribbling, and hesitancy
- Past history of urine retention
- Urologic or gynecologic problems, surgeries, radiation
- Pelvic trauma
- Lower back pain
- Neurologic symptoms in lower extremities

- Other symptoms that suggest infection-frequency, dysuria, hematuria
- Bowel habits, especially constipation
- Review all medications—both prescription and over-the-counter

Exam

- Lower abdominal: assess for distended bladder, tenderness.
- Gynecological, supine and standing: assess for prolapsed pelvic organs.
- Rectal: assess for masses, fecal impaction, perineal sensation, rectal sphincter tone, prostate size.
- Focused neurologic examination: strength, sensation, deep tendon reflexes, muscle tone

Tests

- Diagnostic testing should be guided by the findings of the history and physical exam. Prognosis and achievable goals of care, as determined in discussions between patient, family, and medical team should also be taken into account.
- In the palliative care population, the benefit of imaging and other diagnostic procedures must be considered in the context of prognosis, comorbidities, testing burden, patient/family preferences, and achievable goals of care.
- Testing options include:
  - Post-void residual evaluation: The patient urinates to empty the bladder as much as possible. The amount of urine left in the bladder is called the "post-void residual." Less than 100 cc is considered normal. Greater than 200 cc is indicative of retention. The clinician can check the post-void residual with a catheter, with ultrasound, or via a bladder scanner.
  - Urinalysis and urine culture.
  - Renal function: do complete blood count if systemic infection or hydronephrosis suspected.
  - If neurological etiology is suspected, radiological imaging of pelvis or spine may be indicated.
  - Urodynamic testing also may facilitate management strategies.

TREATMENT OPTIONS

Treatment options for urinary retention are determined by the underlying etiology.

1. **Acute UR:**
   - Should be managed by immediate and complete bladder decompression

by catheter. Historically, partial and slow decompression via draining and clamping of the catheter was recommended to reduce the complications of hematuria, hypotension, and post-obstructive diuresis. Evidence no longer supports the need for this practice, and rapid decompression can be safely performed, with close monitoring of elderly patients for these complications.

- The optimal length of time to leave the catheter in place has not been determined. A voiding trial without a catheter can be performed after two to three days. Men have greater chance of voiding freely when the catheter is removed if they are treated with an alpha blocking agent for three days starting at the time of catheter insertion.[2,3]

2. **Chronic UR:**
   - Intermittent catheterization is the management strategy of choice for patients with chronic UR. Intermittent catheterization poses the least risk of complications such as renal failure, upper urinary tract deterioration, and urospesis.
   - Patients with the cognitive and functional ability, manual dexterity, and positive motivation can successfully self-catheterize. In the community setting, intermittent catheterization can be safely performed under clean circumstances.
   - The use of indwelling catheters should be avoided because of associated complications such as infection, bladder stones, and cancer. Indwelling urethral catheters can also cause periurethral abscesses or bladder and urethral erosions.[4]
   - Indwelling catheter may be recommended if the patient or caregiver is not able to perform intermittent catheterization due to dementia, poor functional status, or difficulty passing a catheter.

NONPHARMACOLOGIC

- For medication-induced UR, adjust or eliminate those medications that are suspected to cause or exacerbate symptoms, e.g., anticholinergic, sympathomimetic agents in an elderly male with known prostatic hypertrophy.
- Prevent/treat constipation and fecal impaction that can cause or exacerbate retention.

PHARMACOLOGIC

- Urinary tract infection or prostatitis should be aggressively treated.
- Alpha 1 (terazosin, doxazosin) or alpha 1a-(alfuzosin, silodosin, tamsulosin) receptor antagonists relax the smooth muscle of the internal urethral sphincter at the bladder neck and prostatic capsule. For men with BPH, these medications have been shown to increase the chance of voiding successfully after initial treatment with catheter for acute UR.
- Nonspecific alpha blockers cause orthostatic hypotension and reactive tachycardia. They should be given at a low dose and tapered up as the blood pressure will tolerate. The newer alpha 1a-blockers work specifically at the urethral sphincter, have very few side effects, and do not need to be tapered up to an optimal dose.
- 5-alpha-reductase inhibitors (e.g., finasteride, dutasteride) selectively block the conversation of testosterone to 5-alpha-dihydrotestosterone, thereby decreasing the size of the prostate. These medications are not indicated in the treatment of acute retention, as their mechanism of action is slower.
- Combination therapy with both 5-alpha-reductase-inhibitors and alpha blockers is the most effective treatment in reducing acute urinary retention in a male with a urethral outlet obstruction due to benign prostatic hypertrophy.[5]

SETTING CONSIDERATIONS

Hospital

- Urinary incontinence is NOT an indication for placing a bladder catheter.
- Acute retention is common in the acute care setting. Multifactorial causes include medications, fecal impaction, and immobility.
- Catheterization should be done under sterile conditions to prevent/delay introduction of bacteria into the bladder.
- For patients with chronic indwelling catheters, prevalence of asymptomatic bacteriuria is 100%. Patients with

short-term catheters develop bacteriuria at a rate of 2% to 7% per day.[6]

Home

- Several factors, including patient characteristics, prognosis, functional status, and patient and family preference, will determine whether intermittent or indwelling catheters should be employed.
- Indications for catheterization for more than 14 days include:[7]
  - UR that cannot be treated medically or surgically, and when alternate therapy is not feasible
  - UR that cannot be managed with intermittent catheterization
  - Urine loss that leads to contamination of stage 3 or 4 pressure ulcers, and impeding healing despite appropriate nursing care
  - Terminal illness or severe impairment that makes positioning for urination uncomfortable or painful
- Catheterization at home can be done under clean circumstances. Sterile conditions are not required.

Hospice

- Hospice patients are at high risk of urine retention due to medications such as opioids, anticholinergics, and antipsychotics, as well as fecal impaction and immobility.
- When patient comfort is the primary goal, indwelling catheterization may be considered to reduce pain and discomfort associated with frequent turning and repositioning for incontinence care and skin integrity.

PALLIATIVE CARE ISSUES

Urologic considerations for patients with chronic, progressive health care conditions include:[8]

- Urinary system dysfunction in the context of serious illness may be caused by the disease process, or may be an indirect adverse effect of medical interventions or medications.
- Weakness and debility associated with advanced disease will require special considerations for the management of urologic function.

- Urinary system dysfunction may be very distressing and can significantly affect quality of life for patients and caregivers.
- Despite the lack of evidence-based strategies available to address urological issues at the end of life, seriously ill patients should receive appropriate management for urologic symptoms based on expert consensus or accepted practice guidelines.
- Intermittent catheterization should be the first choice of treatment for UR whenever feasible. For palliative care patients with advanced prostate or other pelvic cancer, an indwelling catheter may sometimes be indicated to maintain urinary patency. The choice of intermittent or indwelling catheterization should be based on prognosis, symptom burden, patient/family preferences and goals for care.

Mr. C's physical exam reveals a distended bladder and a smooth, enlarged prostate. A post-void residual (PVR) measurement is performed in office with bladder scanner and detects 350 cc urine, which is drained with a straight catheter. The diagnosis is prostatic enlargement with urinary retention. Tamsulosin 0.4mg daily and finasteride 5.0 mg daily are prescribed. Mr. C also received counseling on maintaining good bowel movements and avoiding certain medications such as diphenydramine and pseudoephedrine. One month later, he returns for a follow-up visit. PVR is 80 cc urine. His symptoms have resolved, and he is grateful for the care he has received.

TAKE-HOME POINTS

- Acute urinary retention is a medical emergency requiring immediate decompression.
- Chronic urinary retention may present with no symptoms or atypical symptoms.
- Most common causes of urinary retention include obstruction, infection, pharmacologic, neurological impairment, trauma, and postsurgical complication.
- Urinary system dysfunction in the context of serious illness may be caused by the disease process, or may be an indirect adverse effect of medical interventions or medications.
- Always review the patient's medications as a cause or a contributing factor in urine retention.

- For patients with chronic UR, the preferred treatment is intermittent rather than indwelling catheterization.

REFERENCES

1. Meigs JB et al. Incidence rates and risk factors for acute urinary retention: the health professionals follow up study. *J Urol.* 1999;*162*(2):481–487.
2. McNeill SA, Hargreave TB, et al. Alfuzosin once daily facilitates return to voiding in patients in acute urinary retention. *J Urol.* 2004;*171*:2316–2320.
3. Lucas MG, Stephenson TP, Nargund V. Tamsulosin in the management of patients in acute urinary retention from benign prostatic hyperplasia. *BJU Int.* 2005;*95*(3):354–357.
4. Newman D. The indwelling urinary catheter: principles for best practice. *J Wound Ostomy Continence Nurs.* 2007;*34*(6):655–661.
5. McConnell JD, Roehrborn CG, Bautista OM, et al. The long-term effect of doxazosin, finasteride, and combination therapy on the clinical progression of benign prostatic hyperplasia. *N Engl J Med.* 2003;*349*(25):2387–2398.
6. Nicolle LE et al. Infectious Diseases Society of America guidelines for the diagnosis and treatment of asymptomatic bacteriuria in adults. *Clin Infect Dis.* 2005;*40*(5):643–654.
7. Cochran S. Care of the indwelling urinary catheter: is it evidence based? *J Wound Ostomy Continence Nurs.* 2007;*34*(3):282–288.
8. Baker B, Ward-Smith P. Urinary incontinence nursing considerations at the end of life. *Urol Nurs.* 2003;*31*(3):169–172.

55

Urinary Incontinence

CASE

Mrs. R is a 78-year-old woman with hypertension, osteoarthritis, diabetes mellitus, and gait instability, now diagnosed with metastatic breast cancer. During a regular office visit, she complains of having to urinate frequently, so much that it disrupts her daily activities and social life. She wears pads due to occasional leakages of urine when she cannot get to the bathroom in time. She was looking forward to a trip with her local social club on a cruise to the Caribbean, but she has decided against the trip because of her frequent urination. She is afraid of "wetting herself" and having to let her cabin-mate see her pads in the garbage. She admits to embarrassment and low self-esteem, and also describes feeling "blue" because of impact of this condition on her quality of life.

DEFINITION

- Normal urination involves a complex interaction of pathways connecting the cerebral cortex, spinal cord, bladder, and urethra. The main receptors involved are:
  1. Cholinergic (muscarinic): innervate the bladder wall
  2. Sympathetic (alpha 1-a): innervate the internal urethral sphincter
- Urinary continence requires intact lower urinary tract function, cognitive and functional ability to recognize signals to void and use a toilet, the motivation to maintain continence, and an environment that facilitates the process.
- *Urinary incontinence* (UI) is defined as the involuntary loss of urine. It can present as a problem ranging from occasional leakage to complete inability to hold any urine. UI may be transient (acute) or chronic. Types of chronic UI include stress, urge, mixed, overflow, and functional. Patients often present with more than one type.

PREVALENCE

- Prevalence reports vary depending on how the condition is defined and the population studied. Underreporting by patients and lack of recognition by physicians are common.
- UI affects approximately 15% to 30% of elderly persons living in the community, 35% of elderly in the acute-care hospital setting, and at least 50% of nursing home residents.[1,2]

CONSEQUENCES OF UNTREATED URINARY INCONTINENCE

Untreated UI can lead to the following conditions:

- Depression
- Decreased socialization, activities in public
- Caregiver stress
- Potential for institutional placement
- Pressure ulcers
- Skin rashes
- Possible falls
- Financial burden to patient, caregiver, facility

PREDISPOSING FACTORS

Incontinence is not a normal part of aging, but age-related changes occurring in the genitourinary tract are known to be predisposing factors. These changes include:

- Decreased maximum capacity of the bladder to store urine
- Decreased bladder contractility
- Increased post-void residual of the bladder
- Increased involuntary contractions of the bladder
- Increased excretion of urine in the evening and nighttime
- Decreased estrogen levels in women after menopause
- Increased prostate size
- Shortened length of the urethra in women

LIKELY ETIOLOGIES

- There are numerous causes of urinary incontinence in older persons. Acute incontinence is characterized by the sudden onset of potentially reversible causes represented by the mnemonic acronym D-I-A-P-P-E-R-S.[3] (Box 55.1).
- Chronic incontinence is often multifactorial in origin, with overlapping categories/types (Table 55.1).

URINARY INCONTINENCE IN PALLIATIVE CARE POPULATION

- In the palliative care population, urinary incontinence is often due to factors unrelated to the urinary tract itself. These include functional decline, weakness, fatigue, restraints such as bed rails, therapeutic interventions, medication side effects, or progression of disease.
- Common causes of UI also include malignancies of the genito-urinary and gynecological systems: cancers of the cervix, bladder, and rectum. UI can also occur as a side effect of treatment for these malignancies, i.e., radiotherapy, surgery, or a chemotherapy regimen.
- Other diseases, such as Parkinson's, dementia, and HIV/AIDS, can progress to a stage of weakness and debility that requires special consideration for management of urologic function.[4]
- The diagnostic recommendations discussed below are applicable to the general geriatric patient population. Palliative care patients should also be routinely assessed for UI. However, if no readily reversible cause is identified, the decision to continue the workup should take into consideration prognosis, patient and family goals of care, and the burden of the proposed diagnostic procedures.

DIAGNOSIS

- Because urinary incontinence is generally underreported by patients, it is important to always inquire about urinary symptoms. UI may have a reversible cause, and therefore a comprehensive medical and environmental evaluation is always indicated. Treatment options will also be guided by type of incontinence.[5]
- Explore meaning and impact of UI to patient, such as embarrassment, loss of control, and the feeling of being a burden. Assess emotional/psychological impact; screen for depression in both patient and caregiver.[6,7]

History

- Obtain past medical history, surgical history (urological or gynecological),

---

BOX 55.1   REVERSIBLE CAUSES OF URINARY INCONTINENCE (D-I-A-P-P-E-R-S)

Delirium—confusional state

Infection—may present as incontinence (new symptoms or worsening of chronic symptoms) without other signs or symptoms of dysuria, hematuria

Atrophic vaginitis—common symptom in post-menopausal women. Can cause urgency, dysuria, mimics a urinary tract infection

Psychological—depression

Pharmaceuticals—extensive list of both prescription and over-the-counter; caused by different mechanisms; common categories are diuretics, anticholinergic agents (e.g., antihistamines, antipsychotics, tricyclic antidepressants), alpha receptor antagonists (e.g., doxazosin), alpha receptor agonists (e.g., pseudoephedrine), opioid analgesics

Excess output—congestive heart failure, hypergycemia

Restricted mobility

Stool impaction—can cause urethral obstruction resulting in overflow (e.g., dribbling symptoms)

TABLE 55.1: CHRONIC INCONTINENCE

Type	Risks	Pathophysiology	Symptoms
Urge, detrusor overactivity (DO) Detrusor hyperactivity with incomplete contractions (DHIC)	Age, CNS diseases (dementia, strokes, Parkinson's), bladder-infection, inflammation, stones, early BPH Older, female	"Uninhibited" bladder contractions Caused by aberrant afferent/efferent sensory nerve pathways regulating bladder contractions Patients have the above problem, but the bladder cannot appropriately contract for emptying.	Frequent urge to urinate at any time during the day and night hours Amount of urine leaked varies depending on the volume of urine in the bladder at the time. Same as above; diagnosis made by urodynamics as symptoms are similar to DO
Stress	Age, multiparity, obesity, drugs (diuretic, alpha antagonist)	Intraabdominal pressure exceeds urethral sphincter pressure	Loss of urine with any maneuver that causes a valsalva effect, e.g., cough, laugh, sneeze, standing up
Mixed—urge and stress		Unknown	Symptoms of both disorders exist
Overflow: 2 different mechanisms: (1) urethral outflow obstruction (2) bladder storage and emptying	Age, male, drugs (alpha agonists) Neuropathy (diabetes), drugs (anticholinergics)	Urethral outflow obstruction, e.g., BPH Incomplete detrusor contractions e.g., Neurogenic bladder	Patient has to stand and force out stream of urine Splaying of stream Patient may not realize overflow exists, as "incomplete emptying" urination may occur as "overflow" of urine out of bladder
Functional	Age, ambulation problem, physical disability	Often seen in elderly patients who have underlying age-related changes and/or minimal pathophysiology but cannot get to the toilet in time	Patient loses urine on the way to the toilet

medications (prescribed and over-the-counter), any other treatments attempted for this problem, or history of bowel problems. Identify any acute or transient causes of incontinence as listed above.

- Mainstay of evaluation is a voiding diary for 48 to 72 hours. Patient or caregiver keeps track of time/volume of normal voids, time/volume of incontinence episodes, any associated symptoms, e.g., urge, time of intake of medications and fluids.
- The diagnosis of urge incontinence can often be made with a simple question: "Do you experience such a strong and sudden urge to urinate that you leak before reaching the toilet?"
- Diagnosis of stress incontinence can also be reliably made by asking about leakage with stress maneuvers (coughing, laughing, bending over, running, changing position).
- The diagnosis of overflow incontinence varies according to the underlying etiology. Patients with chronic retention may not have any complaints or symptoms. Others, especially men with BPH, will complain of difficulty getting urine stream to begin, post-void dribbling, or feeling of incomplete emptying.

- When considering the possibility of functional incontinence, assessment should include the patient's physical and cognitive functional status, home environment, and caregiver support system.

Exam

- Cardiovascular/pulmonary: assess volume status
- Abdomen: masses, tenderness, bladder distension
- Extremities: joint mobility, venous insufficiency, edema
- Gynecological: atrophy of vaginal mucosa, pelvic muscle laxity
- Rectal: masses, fecal impaction, prostatic enlargement
- Neurological: assess mental status, signs of Parkinsonism, cerebrovascular accidents, neuropathies, spinal cord disease, or cord compression.

Tests

- Laboratory tests include urinalysis, urine culture, urea nitrogen, creatinine, glucose, calcium
- Stress test: The patient should stand in the exam room with a full bladder and cough as hard as she/he can. If there is leakage of urine, the diagnosis of stress incontinence can be made. This test loses sensitivity if the bladder is not full.
- Post-void residual: Less than 100 cc is considered normal. Greater than 100 cc indicates retention. (See Chapter 54: Urinary Retention.) Post-void residual can be obtained with a catheter, by means of a bladder scanner, or via ultrasound.

TREATMENT OPTIONS

- Treatment of UI should focus on eliminating or mitigating any underlying causes, identifying treatment strategies, managing the condition, enhancing self-esteem, and maximizing quality of life. Reassure patients and families that there are many alternatives to "adult diapers," which should be a strategy of last resort.
- The degree of symptom burden and inconvenience for the patient and caregiver will guide treatment options. Behavioral interventions require a motivated patient, and many medications have side effects that may outweigh the need for or benefit of management.[3]
- In older patients, various therapies, most notably bladder training and pelvic muscle exercise (Kegels), are effective for the different types of urinary incontinence (Table 55.2).[8]

TABLE 55.2: TREATMENT OF URINARY INCONTINENCE BY TYPE

Urge Urinary Incontinence (Detrusor overactivity)	
Treatment Strategy	Treatment Options
Behavioral therapy: exercises focusing on delaying voiding, suppressing premature urges, and increasing bladder capacity. Effectiveness depends on the patient's cognitive status and motivation.	*Bladder training*—If the patient is cognitively intact and motivated, this method focuses on suppressing abnormal urges, scheduling, and gradually extending the voiding intervals.
	Prompted voiding—Patient is asked if he or she needs to urinate on a regular timed basis and brought to the toilet. Positive feedback is provided when patient uses the toilet and remains dry.
	(*For bladder training and prompted voiding, timing is determined by the patient's initial response. These methods may take weeks to months to have an effect.*)
	Scheduled toileting—Preferred method for cognitively impaired patients who cannot follow commands as needed for other types of behavioral training. Caregiver toilets the patient on a regular schedule—every two hours while awake is recommended.
	Adjusting the timing and amount of fluid intake

(continued)

TABLE 55.2: (CONTINUED)

Treatment Strategy	Treatment Options
Pharmacologic treatment—can be used in conjunction with behavioral training	*Anti-cholinergic medications* suppress abnormal/premature contractions of the bladder by blocking the muscarinic receptors on the detrusor muscle wall. (*Note: Use caution in older adults due to negative impact on cognitive performance, constipation, dry mouth, and orthostatic hypotension[9]*)
	Short acting: oxybutynin (immediate release)—not recommended due to its side effect profile, which includes dry mouth and constipation
	Long acting: Provide an advantage over the short-acting oxybutynin, as they have fewer anticholinergic side effects and can be tolerated for short-term treatment at low doses Oxybutynin (extended release—oral; transdermal patch) Tolterodine (Detrol), darifenacin (Enablex), trospium (Sanctura), solifenacin (Vesicare) (*Note: Some patients may have a skin reaction at the transdermal patch site. There is also some concern over the CNS and ophthalmologic side effects of these medications.*)
	Tricyclic antidepressants, e.g. imipramine Have both alpha agonist (weakly inhibits the reuptake of norepinephrine) and anticholinergic properties for patients with both urge and stress incontinence. Not FDA approved for urinary incontinence, but some studies have demonstrated effectiveness. Adverse effects include orthostatic hypotension, constipation, dry mouth, and confusion in older patients.
Botulism toxin	May relieve symptoms that do not respond to anti-cholinergic or behavioral therapy Injected into the detrusor muscle or by instillation into the bladder Can cause post-treatment urinary retention
Electrical stimulation therapy	Treatment option for more severe cases of urge incontinence that have not responded to conservative management with behavioral, physical therapy, or pharmacological strategies The pudendal nerves are electrically stimulated and modulate neural reflexes that control bladder and pelvic floor muscles[10]

Stress Urinary Incontinence	
Treatment Strategy	Treatment Options
Behavioral	Kegel exercise: Patients are instructed to tighten their pelvic floor muscles while relaxing their abdominal, thigh, and gluteal muscles, gradually increasing the number and duration of contractions Recommend at least 30 contractions during the day, holding each contraction for 10 seconds at a time
Pharmacologic	Alpha adrenergic agonists stimulate the alpha receptors on the internal urethral sphincter to contract. Examples include pseudoephedrine and phenylephrine. *These medications are not recommended due to their side effect profile, including tachycardia and restlessness.*
	Hormone replacement therapy is no longer recommended, as it may worsen incontinence symptoms.
	Duloxetine (FDA-approved as an antidepressant): A serotonin and norepinephrine reuptake inhibitor; has been shown to provide significant subjective improvements in quality of life and perception of incontinence; not FDA-approved for the treatment of stress incontinence

(continued)

TABLE 55.2: (CONTINUED)

Treatment Strategy	Treatment Options
Injection of bulking agents into the bladder neck	Examples include collagen, autologous fibroblasts/myoblasts. These can reduce incontinence episodes but often must be repeated
Pessaries	Provide bladder neck support for prolapsed uterus or bladder and can improve continence in women These devices have been helpful in place of or in conjunction with other treatment modalities.
Surgery	Several types of surgeries are available. Retropubic colposuspension and pubovaginal sling are considered most effective. While surgery may be considered when other treatment options have failed, success rates vary and relevant studies are mostly nonrandomized and uncontrolled. Surgery is not likely to be appropriate in the palliative care population.

Overflow Urinary Incontinence

Treatment Strategy	Treatment Options
Nonpharmacologic	Review medications and eliminate any that may be contributing factor, e.g., anticholinergic or alpha-adrenergic medications Treat constipation and fecal impaction
Pharmacologic	*Outflow obstruction*: Alpha receptor antagonists: Older medications (doxazosin) are nonspecific alpha receptor blockers with major side effect of orthostatic hypotension. Newer medications are specific to alpha 1 (terazosin, prazosin) and alpha 1a (tamsulosin, alfuzosin, silodosin) receptors that innervate the urethral sphincter and have much less orthostasis side effect. *Underactive detrusor*: Cholinergic agents such as bethanochol are used, but based on randomized, placebo-controlled studies, do not appear to improve outcomes.

Catheterization	Employed when a patient's urinary retention has not resolved after both nonpharmacologic and pharmacologic treatments have been sufficiently explored
	Intermittent catheterization is the preferred choice, with training for either the patient with good cognition and manual dexterity, or an available and willing caregiver. Carries less risk of infection, bladder stones, and other complications than a chronic indwelling catheter.
	Catheterization at home does not require sterile technique as in a health care facility
	Indwelling bladder catheter is placed if the patient or caregiver cannot perform intermittent catheterization. Indications include:
	  Bladder outlet obstruction that cannot be managed using other methods
	  Non-healing stage III or IV skin ulcers that are exposed to urine
	  For older or seriously ill adults who would suffer pain and discomfort from routine incontinence care, or when pain and
	  immobility restricts toileting[11] (See Chapter 54: Urinary Retention)

Functional Incontinence

Treatment Strategy	Treatment Options
Identify and address environmental barriers to safe and timely toileting	Provide pain relief Provide appropriate assistive devices and/or a bedside commode Conduct a home safety evaluation

PALLIATIVE CARE ISSUES[12]

- Urinary incontinence is not a normal part of aging, but it is a common symptom for older patients due to therapeutic interventions, functional decline, and disease progression.
- Urinary incontinence is very distressing and can take a major toll on patients and caregivers alike. Assessment and symptomatic management in the context of advanced illness will provide dignity and improve quality of life, and should therefore be an important component of the plan of care.
- If assessment does not point to a clearly reversible cause of UI, the benefit of further workup should be weighed against the goals for care and the burden of proposed evaluation and intervention.
- Weakness and debility associated with advanced disease will require special considerations for the management of functional UI. Effective strategies include providing adaptive equipment and assistive devices for impaired mobility, scheduling voids, assistance with transfers, and use of a bedside commode.
- For palliative care patients, an indwelling catheter may be indicated to facilitate skin care or to reduce the pain or discomfort of movement and frequent perineal care. The decision for indwelling catheterization should be based on prognosis, symptom burden, patient/family preferences, and goals for care.

Mrs. R was diagnosed as having a combination of urge and stress incontinence. She was advised about how to perform Kegel and "bladder training" exercises over the next four weeks. In addition, her diabetes was brought under better control and she was instructed to take around-the-clock Tylenol for her osteoarthritis pain. The combination of these recommendations decreased the number of her incontinent episodes during the day and night. She was able to enjoy the cruise with her friends.

TAKE-HOME POINTS

- Remember to inquire about urinary symptoms, as patients frequently do not report them.
- Evaluate patient for any treatable causes of new or worsening urinary incontinence.

- Review the patient's medications, both prescription and non-prescription, for a cause of incontinence.
- Urinary incontinence is very distressing and can take a toll on patients and caregivers alike. Treatment choices and management strategies should be based on patient preferences and goals of care, with focus on enhancing self-esteem and maximizing quality of life.
- Nonpharmacologic treatment options should always be employed first.
- Assessment and symptomatic management in the context of advanced illness will provide dignity and improve quality of life, and should therefore be an important component of the plan of care.
- If no readily reversible cause of UI is identified for a palliative care patient, the decision to continue the workup should take into consideration prognosis, patient and family goals of care, and the burden of the proposed diagnostic procedures.

REFERENCES

1. Fanti A, Newman DK, Colling J, et al. *Urinary incontinence in adults: acute and chronic management 1996; Agency for Healthcare and Policy Research (AHRQ)*, Publication No. 92-0047: Rockville, MD.
2. Sier H, Ouslander J, Orzeck S. Urinary incontinence among geriatric patients in an acute-care hospital. *JAMA*. 1987;*257*(13):1767–1771.
3. Guzzo TJ, Drach GW. Major urologic problems in geriatrics. *Med Clin N Am*. 2011;*95*:253–264.
4. Baker B, Ward-Smith P. Urinary incontinence nursing considerations at the end of life. *Urol Nurs*. 2003;*31*(3):169–172.
5. Holroyd-Leduc JM et al. What type of urinary incontinence does this woman have? *JAMA*. Mar 26, 2008;*299*(12):1446–1456.
6. Melville JL, Delaney K, Newton K, Katon W. Incontinence severity and major depression in incontinent women. *Obstet Gynecol*. 2005;*106*(3): 585–592.
7. Cassells C, Watt E. The impact of incontinence on older spousal caregivers. *Obstet Gynecol*. 2003;*42*(6):607–616.
8. Shamliyan TA et al. Systematic review: randomized controlled trials of non-surgical treatments for urinary incontinence in women. *Ann Intern Med*. 2008;*148*:459–473.

9. Campbell N, Boustani M, Limbil T, et al. The cognitive impact of anticholinergics: a clinical review. *Clin IntervAging*. 2009;4:225–233.

10. Brazzelli M, Murray A, Fraser C. Efficacy and safety of sacral nerve stimulation for urinary urge incontinence: a systematic review. *J Urol*. 2006;*175*:835–841.

11. Cochran S. Care of the indwelling urinary catheter: is it evidence based? *J Wound Ostomy Continence Nurs*. 2007;*34*(3):282–288.

12. Kapo J, Morrison LJ, Liao S. Palliative care for the older adult. *J Palliat Med*. 2007;*10*:185–209.

56
Bleeding

CASE
Mrs. M is a 78-year-old female with a history of osteoarthritis, hypertension, and adult onset diabetes. She presents to her geriatrician with complaints of fatigue, weakness, occasional palpitations, and vague abdominal discomfort.

DEFINITION
Bleeding is the loss of blood or blood escaping from the circulatory system. Associated symptoms depend on the duration and rate of bleeding.

PREVALENCE
Bleeding is a common problem, especially in the elderly population. Risk of bleeding increases significantly with patient age.

CONSEQUENCES OF UNTREATED BLEEDING
Progressive blood loss with anemia can result in:

- Weakness, fatigue
- Palpitations and cardiac complications (myocardial ischemia/infarction)
- Dizziness and syncope
- Hypotension and hypovolemia with cardiovascular collapse in severe situations

LIKELY ETIOLOGIES
Many factors can lead to blood loss. In older adults, the most common causes include disease-associated bleeding, disorders of coagulation, and thrombocytopenia.

1. Disease-associated bleeding
   - Upper GI (more common): Ulcers +/- NSAIDs or aspirin, esophagitis, duodenitis, Mallory-Weiss lesions, gastric cancer
   - Lower GI: Diverticular bleeding (strongly associated with aspirin), colitis, angiodysplasia, colon cancer
   - Other disease related causes include: gynecological (uterine cancer), GU (bladder cancer or infection)

2. Coagulopathy/Bleeding Disorders
   - Due to anticoagulant treatment (warfarin, heparin), or antiplatelet treatment (aspirin, ticlopidine, clopidogrel, and NSAIDs)
   - Vitamin K deficiency due to:
     - Antibiotic treatment
     - Poor diet
     - Vitamin K is necessary for synthesis of factors II, VII, IX and X.
   - Liver disease:
     - Clotting factors synthesized in the liver
     - With reduced factor synthesis → reduced factors and prolonged PT/PTT
   - Kidney disease:
     - Acquired platelet defect in renal failure and in poorly dialyzed patients
   - Acquired hemophilia:
     - Rare disorder (1.3 to 1.5 cases/ million people).
     - Acquired factor VIIII inhibitor (acquired hemophilia A) is most common.[1]
     - More often in older patients; median age at diagnosis 64 years old.
     - Associated with: Lupus, rheumatoid arthritis, malignancy lymphoproliferative disease, drug reactions, idiopathic (50% of cases).
     - Suspect with severe bleeding, often in the postoperative setting.
     - Disseminated Intravascular Coagulation (DIC):[2] Consumption of clotting factors leading to both bleeding and clotting; occurs in 1% of hospital admissions;always results from an underlying condition (sepsis, trauma, malignancy).

3. Thrombocytopenia
   - Due to medication (most often antibiotics)
   - Splenomegaly and portal hypertension in liver disease

- DIC
- Hematologic disorders: Immune thrombocytopenia purpura, myelodysplastic syndrome, leukemia, or other malignancy with bone marrow involvement

DIAGNOSIS

History

When taking a history, inquire about the following:

- Nosebleeds
- Bleeding from the mouth or gums, especially when brushing teeth
- Bruising
- Bleeding with cuts, abrasions, immunizations, or other injections
- Gastrointestinal or genitourinary bleeding
- Hemarthroses (bleeding into the joints)
- Delayed wound healing
- Use of prescription, nonprescription, and herbal medications
- Comorbid medical conditions, including liver disease, collagen and vascular disorders, underlying malignancies

Exam

Examine for evidence of bleeding:

- Stool test for guaiac
- Skin and soft tissue bleeding
- Petechiae—small capillary hemorrhages; asymptomatic; not palpable; found on extremities (with increased venous pressure)
- Ecchymoses—purple and superficial
- Mucocutaneous bleeding-epistaxis; evidence of gum and mouth bleeding
- Hemarthrosis-bleeding into joints seen in hemophilia

Tests

- CBC including platelet count
- Coagulation panel including PT, PTT, fibrinogen
- Chemistry including creatinine and LFTs
- Further coagulation studies as indicated:
  - Bleeding time
  - Clotting factor levels
  - Platelet aggregation assays
- Evaluation for GI bleeding:
  - Upper/lower endoscopy
  - If non-diagnostic, further evaluation with capsule endoscopy or small bowel series indicated

- CT scan of the abdomen/pelvis
- Evaluation for GU bleeding:
  - Urinalysis with microscopic evaluation
  - Cystoscopy
  - CT scan of the abdomen/pelvis
- Evaluation for GYN bleeding:
  - GYN examination
  - Pelvic ultrasound/CT scan of the abdomen/pelvis

On exam, Mrs. M is found to be tachycardic, pale, and with moderate mid-epigastric tenderness. Stool is black and guaiac positive. Hemoglobin is 7g/dL. On further questioning, Mrs. M reports significant increase in her arthritis-related joint pain for the past three months and use of aspirin and ibuprofen.

TREATMENT OPTIONS

Nonpharmacologic

Blood product support for symptomatic anemia and bleeding:

- Red blood cells
- Platelets
- Fresh frozen plasma
- Cryoprecipitate

For GI bleeding:

- Endoscopic interventions with EGD/colonoscopy to treat bleeding source:
  - Cautery, injection, polypectomy
  - Surgical intervention as indicated (e.g. resection of colonic malignancy)

Pharmacologic

- Cessation of contributing medications: Aspirin, NSAIDs, anticoagulants (warfarin and heparin)
- Treatment of ulcer disease:[3] Proton pump inhibitor and H-2 blockers
- Reversal of anticoagulant effect:
  - Vitamin K administration (PO or SC) to reverse warfarin effect
  - Protamine sulfate to reverse heparin
- Bleeding in renal failure:
  - Optimize dialysis in end-stage renal failure
  - DDAVP to improve platelet function

The patient is admitted for further evaluation, and an upper endoscopy demonstrates a large duodenal ulcer with stigmata of recent bleeding. The ulcer is cauterized with no further bleeding, and Mrs. M receives 2 units of packed red blood cells for her symptomatic anemia. The patient is advised to avoid NSAIDs and aspirin.

PALLIATIVE CARE ISSUES

- Approach to treatment of bleeding should take into consideration underlying disease states, prognosis, cognition, patient preferences, goals of care, and function.
- GI bleeding in the elderly is usually not associated with mortality and can be managed medically.
- Acute treatment is intended to hemodynamically stabilize the patient and allow time for evaluation.
- Should a malignancy be diagnosed, the approach and level of intervention should be dictated by patient preference, patient performance status, and achievable goals of care.
- In the setting of terminal illness, aggressive treatments and transfusion support may not be indicated. Transfusion for a short period of time may be an option, however, to allow patient and family to settle legal, financial, and business affairs, and to mentally, emotionally, and spiritually prepare for the end of life.
- When it is a patient's wish to die at home, and if there is a possibility of uncontrollable bleeding at the end of life, caregiver education, reassurance, and support should be provided in advance. (See Chapter 15: Dying at Home.)

TAKE-HOME POINTS

- Bleeding is very common in geriatric populations, particularly with chronic conditions requiring multiple medications.
- The cause of bleeding can usually be identified through a careful history and exam.
- Contributing medications should be withdrawn (aspirin, ticlopidine, clopidogrel, and NSAIDs).
- A treatment plan based on prognosis and aligned with achievable goals of care should be developed to prevent or reverse underlying cause.

REFERENCES

1. Franchini M, Lippi G. Acquired factor VIII inhibitors. *Blood*. Jul 15, 2008;*112*(2):250–255. Epub 2008 May 7.
2. Kitchens CS. Thrombocytopenia and thrombosis in disseminated intravascular coagulation (DIC). *Hematology Am Soc Hematol Educ Program*. 2009;*1*: 240–246.
3. Pilotto A, Franceschi M, Maggi S, Addante F, Sancarlo D. Optimal management of peptic ulcer disease in the elderly. *Drugs Aging*. Jul 1, 2010;*27*(7): 545–558.

57

Thrombosis

CASE

Mr. J is a 73-year-old male with a history of hypertension, hypercholesterolemia, and recent left knee replacement who presented to his geriatrician with a two-week complaint of a swollen and tender distal left calf.

DEFINITION

Thrombosis is the formation of a thrombus (clot) in a vein or artery. Arterial clots are associated with myocardial infarction, cerebrovascular accidents, and peripheral vascular disease. Venous clots are most commonly seen in deep venous thromboses of the lower extremities and in the pulmonary vasculature, but they can also occur in the upper extremities (10%), often associated with an indwelling catheter.

Thromboses of the vena cava/pelvic veins and unusual locations (mesenteric veins and dural sinus) are less common.

This section will focus on venous thromboembolic disease.

INCIDENCE

- Deep vein thrombosis (DVT) has a dramatic increase in annual incidence by age:
  - 40–49 years old: 100 cases per 100,000 persons/year
  - 70–79 years old: 700 per 100,000 persons/year
- Pulmonary embolism (PE)[1] also increases with age and is a common cause of death in people ≥70 years old. Often found during autopsies as a cause of death
  - 40–49 years old: 20 per 100,000 persons/year
  - 70–79 years old: 300 per 100,000 persons/year

CONSEQUENCES OF UNTREATED THROMBOSIS

- Untreated DVT can result in lymphedema, post-phlebitic changes, pain, functional impairment, and migration of clot to lungs → PE.
- Untreated PE can result in respiratory insufficiency, respiratory failure, pulmonary hypertension, heart failure, cardiac arrhythmia, and death.

LIKELY ETIOLOGIES[2]

- The risk of DVT/PE is increased in geriatric population due to multiple comorbidities.
- **Acquired risk factors** in older patients include:
  - Immobility due to illness or recent surgery (orthopedic, pelvic, neurosurgery, major vascular, and cancer)
  - Cancer
  - Recent indwelling catheter placement (a risk for upper extremity DVT)
  - Myeloproliferative disorder (especially polycythemia vera and essential thrombocytosis)
  - Nephrotic syndrome
  - Antiphospholipid syndrome
  - Prior thrombotic event
- **Inherited risk factors** are not often suspected in older adults, but evaluation should be considered in the event of two or more thrombotic episodes without a risk factor, or with an unusual site of thrombosis (mesenteric veins or dural sinus).
- Inherited prothrombotic factors include factor V Leiden mutation, prothrombin gene mutation, homocysteine level, protein C or S deficiency, and antithrombin activity.

DIFFERENTIAL DIAGNOSIS

Differential diagnoses relevant to geriatrics and palliative care include:

For DVT:
- Superficial thrombophlebitis: benign course; treat symptoms with

warm compresses, analgesics, and anti-inflammatory meds

- Superficial vein thrombosis: tender and palpable superficial veins; less severe than DVT; may progress to DVT/PE
- Extremity injuries
- Cellulitis or other extremity infections
- Lymphangitis
- Venous insufficiency (especially with a history of DVT)

For PE:

- Pneumonia
- CHF
- COPD exacerbation
- Myocardial infarction
- Pericarditis

DIAGNOSIS

Clinicians should maintain a high index of suspicion to diagnose DVT/PE. Use clinical pre-test probability and D-dimer to choose which patients require further evaluation with imaging studies.

Exam

Patients with suspected DVT:

- Tender, warm, erythematous, edematous, or asymmetric extremity
- Palpable cord (thrombosed vein)
- Superficial venous dilation

Patients with suspected PE:

- Patients report sudden onset or worsening dyspnea, orthopnea, pleuritic chest pain, cough, wheezing, or hemoptysis with no alternate explanation.
- Abnormal vital signs: Tachycardia; tachypnea, hypoxia, hypotension and shock in severe cases
- Abnormal pulmonary exam: Rales; decreased breath sounds
- Distension of jugular veins

Tests

For suspected DVT:

- Assess patient pretest probability with a tool such as the Wells score:
  - Incorporates risk factors and clinical signs and assigns a score resulting in low, moderate, or intermediate probability for DVT[3]

- Low pretest probability → median negative predictive value to rule out DVT of 96% (range 87–100)
- Low pretest probability and negative D-dimer → median negative predictive value to rule out DVT → 99% (range 96–100)
- High pretest probability → positive predictive value <75%; need to evaluate with doppler for DVT
- Doppler (compression) ultrasound is the most common study ordered:
  - Noninvasive; for proximal lower extremity DVT, sensitivity is 94% and specificity 100%
  - If initial Doppler is negative and suspicion is high, repeat doppler within five to seven days
- Venography is the gold standard exam; invasive study that is used when Doppler studies are equivocal or not able to be done.

For suspected PE:

- Assess pretest probability with a tool such as the Wells score:
  - Incorporates risk factors and clinical signs and assigns a score resulting in low, moderate, or intermediate probability for PE[4]
  - Low pretest probability and negative D-dimer → rule out PE
  - Patient with positive D-dimer and likely/ unlikely to have PE; should be further evaluated with CT angiogram
- V/Q scan: Widely used but has low specificity
  - High probability scan is diagnostic of PE, but seen only in 20% to 40% of patients; if there is less than high probability, may need further imaging for evaluation
  - If a V/Q scan is performed:
    - Low probability V/Q + low clinical probability → r/o PE
    - Normal V/Q + low/intermediate/high clinical probability → r/o PE
    - High probability V/Q + high clinical probability → confirms PE
- CT angiogram with intravenous contrast:
  - Used more frequently to diagnose PE
  - Cannot be used for a patient with renal insufficiency
  - Risk of renal injury
  - Radiation exposure

- Pulmonary angiogram is the gold standard:
  - Expensive and invasive
  - Risk of renal injury
  - Radiation exposure

Additional studies which may be helpful include:

- Echocardiogram
- EKG

Labs

1. Baseline panel:
   - CBC
   - PT/INR/PTT
   - D-dimer:
     - Demonstrates fibrinolysis of cross-linked fibrin
     - Negative test has a high negative predictive value for DVT/PE if used in patients with low or moderate pretest probability
     - Positive test not helpful in establishing a diagnosis
2. When inherited hypercoagulable state is suspected, evaluate with hypercoagulable panel, including:
   - Factor V Leiden mutation, prothrombin gene mutation, homocysteine level, protein C/S levels, antithrombin activity
   - Most often in patients < 50 years old
3. If acquired hypercoagulable state is suspected, evaluate for:
   - Antiphospholipid antibodies (lupus anticoagulant and anti-cardiolipin antibodies)
   - Cancer
   - Myeloproliferative disorder (CML, myelofibrosis, polycythemia vera, essential thrombocytosis)
   - Nephrotic syndrome

On examination, the patient had an asymmetrical and enlarged left distal lower extremity. Lower extremity pulses were within normal limits, and there was no evidence of infection. Mr. J was referred for a Doppler ultrasound examination, which demonstrated a deep venous thrombosis in the proximal femoral vein.

TREATMENT OPTIONS[5]

Treatment should be initiated when a diagnosis of DVT/PE is suspected or confirmed. An untreated DVT can progress to PE in up to 50% of patients.

Nonpharmacologic

- If a patient has a DVT and is at risk for proximal DVT or PE but is NOT a candidate for anticoagulation, then placement of an inferior vena cava (IVC) filter can be considered.
- A filter can also be placed if a patient has recurrent VTE even with adequate anticoagulation. The IVC filter can be temporary (removable) or permanent.
- Complications of IVC filters include local complications related to the insertion process, DVT at the site of insertion, and filter migration.

Pharmacologic[6]

Anticoagulation is the most common pharmacologic treatment for patients with DVT/PE.

Rationale for anticoagulation:

- Prevents thrombus extension or recurrence and reduces risk of death due to fatal PE.
- Reduces risk of postphlebitic syndrome in patients with DVT, venous insufficiency.
- Reduces risk of pulmonary hypertension due to chronic PE.

Approach to anticoagulant treatment:

- Treatment plan should be consistent with established goals of care.
- Anticoagulant choices include unfractionated heparin, low molecular weight heparin, fondaparinux, and warfarin (an oral vitamin K antagonist).
- If patient is appropriate candidate, and treatment is aligned with goals of care, begin with a five-day course of selected anticoagulant agent. Use the anticoagulant concurrently with warfarin at a therapeutic dose to achieve an INR 2–3 for at least 24 hours.
- After approximately five days, the heparin, low molecular weight heparin or fondaparinux should be discontinued while the warfarin is continued for at least three months.
- Elderly patients are more sensitive to warfarin: use an initial daily dose of less than 5 mg/day. Use an even lower dose in patients with heart failure, liver disease, if at high risk for bleeding, debilitated or with poor nutrition.

Selecting the appropriate anticoagulant agent:

- Choice of which anticoagulant to use should be guided by functional/cognitive status, prognosis, benefit-burden analysis, cost considerations, ability of patient/family to administer and monitor, insurance coverage, and goals of care. Clinicians should also consider the following issues when selecting an anticoagulant agent:
  - *Low molecular weight heparin* is best for most patients
    - Anti-Xa levels should be checked only in special circumstances (renal insufficiency, morbid obesity, low body weight).
    - Can be used with mild to moderate renal insufficiency (creatinine clearance 30–80 mL/min).
  - *Unfractionated heparin (IV):*
    - Increased risk for bleeding
    - Hypotension due to PE
    - Obesity or anasarca (concern for SC absorption)
    - Possible thrombolysis
    - Monitor by using aPTT
  - *Fondaparinux*
    - A synthetic anticoagulant that catalyzes factor Xa inactivation by antithrombin
    - Contraindicated in patients with creatinine clearance <30 mL/min
    - Use with caution in patients with mild to moderate renal insufficiency (30 to 80 mL/min)
  - *Warfarin*
    - For long term use
    - Disadavantage is the need for INR monitoring; blood draws to verify therapeutic levels

Duration of treatment:

Duration of anticoagulant treatment is based on the risk of recurrent DVT/PE:

- Proximal DVT or PE in a patient with reversible (e.g., following surgery, trauma, immobilization) risk factors → 3 months
- Patients with non-reversible risk factors (malignancy and inherited thrombophilias) → lifelong
- Patient with idiopathic DVT → often requires prolonged treatment based on risk of recurrence vs. risk of bleeding

- Patients with recurrent DVT/PE (≥2 episodes) → indefinite warfarin

Pulmonary examination was normal and a pulmonary embolism was not suspected. The patient was treated with anticoagulants for three months.

PALLIATIVE CARE ISSUES

- Performing a risk-benefit ratio assessment of anticoagulation is essential given comorbid conditions in older adult and geriatric population.
- Considerations in older adults include:
  - Increased risk for bleeding, especially with concurrent aspirin, clopidogrel or NSAID therapy
  - Risk of recurrent falls especially if the patient has an unstable gait or peripheral neuropathy
  - Cognitive impairment
  - Drug-drug interactions (especially with warfarin)
  - Prior history of cerebral hemorrhage, GI bleeding, or hypertension
  - If on warfarin, consider the patient's ability to access warfarin clinic for INR monitoring.

TAKE-HOME POINTS

- Older adults have a significantly increased risk of DVT and PE compared to younger populations.
- Multiple comorbidities including malignancy and immobility contribute to the increased risk.
- Clinicians should have a high index of suspicion in diagnosing DVT and PE.
- The most common studies used are Doppler ultrasound for DVT and either V/Q scan or CT angiogram for PE.
- Carefully weigh risks and benefits of diagnostic evaluation and anticoagulation therapy in the context of goals of care, prognosis, and functional/cognitive capacity.
- Consider a reduced dose of warfarin in older adults given increased risk for bleeding complications.

REFERENCES

1. Stein PD, Matta F. Acute pulmonary embolism. *Curr Probl Cardiol.* Jul 2010;35(7):314–376.
2. Engbers MJ, van Hylckama Vieg A, Rosendaal FR. Venous thrombosis in the elderly: incidence, risk

factors and risk groups. *J Thromb Haemost*. Oct 2010;8(10):2105–2112.

3. Wells PS, Anderson DR, Rodger M, et al. Evaluation of D-dimer in the diagnosis of suspected deep-vein thrombosis. *N Engl J Med*. 2003;*349*:1227.

4. van Belle A, Buller HR, Huisman MV, et al. Effectiveness of managing suspected pulmonary embolism using an algorithm combining clinical probability, d-dimer testing and computed tomography. *JAMA*. 2006;*295*:172.

5. Spyropoulous AC, Merli G. Management of venous thromboembolism in the elderly. *Drugs Aging*. 2006;*23*(8):651–671.

6. Robert-Ebadi H, Le Gal G, Righini M. Use of anticoagulants in elderly patients: practical recommendations. *Clin Interv Aging*. 2009;*4*:165–177. Epub 2009 May 14.

58

Lymphedema

CASE

Ms. G is a 69-year-old female who has been in and out of the hospital suffering from graft vs. host disease after a bone marrow transplant a few months ago. She is on an ever-changing list of medications. For several years, she has had intermittent swelling in both lower extremities, especially the feet and ankles. The condition has recently gotten worse. The swelling now affects her mobility and balance, causing discomfort, exacerbating the neuropathy in her feet, prohibiting her from wearing any of the shoes in her closet, and now is contributing to significant functional impairment and emotional distress.

DEFINITION

Lymphedema (aka lymphostatic edema) is an abnormal accumulation of protein-rich fluid in the interstitial spaces, resulting in the swelling of an extremity or body part.

PREVALENCE

Considering all causes, one out of every 40 people in the world may be affected by lymphedema.[1] The leading cause of lymphedema worldwide is lymphatic filariasis, which affects 750 million people.[2] Other types of secondary lymphedema affect another 140 million to 250 million worldwide.[3]

LIKELY ETIOLOGIES

Lymphedema is usually classified as primary (hereditary) or secondary (acquired).

1. **Primary lymphedema**
   - Causes: dysplasia of the lymphatic structures; can be hereditary or congenital
   - Usually affects the lower extremities but can also affect other parts of the body
   - The condition typically starts distally and migrates proximally
2. **Secondary lymphedema**
   - Causes:
     - Iatrogenic
     - Trauma

- Obesity
- Infection or inflammation
- Filariasis (common in tropical and subtropical regions)
- The condition typically, but not always, starts proximally and migrates distally.
- Secondary lymphedema in the United States and the other Western industrialized nations is frequently the result of cancer treatments such as lymph node dissection and/or radiation therapy. Approximately one-third of breast cancer patients will develop lymphedema of the upper extremity, depending on the type of surgery, radiation, age, and weight of the patient.[2]

CONSEQUENCES OF UNTREATED LYMPHEDEMA

- Cellulitis is the major complication of lymphedema.
- Loss of mobility, discomfort, joint problems, muscle weakness from lack of use, eventually leading to disability and possibly disfigurement.
- Skin breakdown, such as papillomatosis, hemosiderin, hyperkeratosis, fungal infections, lymphorrhea.
- Psychosocial issues: depression, social isolation, anxiety, fear, and anger.
- In rare cases, angiosarcoma (Stewart-Treves syndrome).

CLASSIFICATION

A classification scheme is used to describe the severity of lymphedema.

- **Stage 0:** Latency
  - Can be asymptomatic
  - A sense of fatigue in the limb
  - A sense of heaviness in the limb

- **Stage 1:** Reversible
  - The limb swells during the day, reduces on elevation.
  - Pitting upon pressure
  - No fibrosis
- **Stage 2:** Spontaneously irreversible
  - The limb swells during the day, no longer reduces on elevation.
  - Minimal pitting
  - Clinical fibrosis
- **Stage 3:** Elephantiasis
  - Tissue fibrosis
  - No pitting
  - Skin changes: hyperkeratosis, papillomatosis, lymphorrhea, fungal infections
  - Decreased mobility, disability
  - Increased risk of cellulitis

DIAGNOSIS

History

Detailed history should focus on:

- Past surgeries: Determine if lymph nodes were removed; if so, identify location, number removed, and number positive for cancer; also if other cancer treatments such as radiation therapy or chemotherapy were offered.
- Personal and family cancer history
- Personal history of thyroid, vascular, cardiac, pulmonary or renal disease
- Any acute or chronic infections
- Duration, presentation, location of symptoms, and previous interventions
- Careful review of all medications
- Assessment of patient's social environment including work situation, recreational activities.

Exam

Inspection and palpation of the affected areas with focus on:

- Skin and nail changes, including scars, appearance of the skin or nail, temperature, and symmetry (on both extremities)
- Signs of infection
- Evaluation of ulcers
- Documentation of edema stage as well as whether or not it is pitting
- Evaluation of how lymphedema impairs or limits ADLs and IADLs

Tests

- The physical exam together with the history should provide information as to whether DVT, tumor obstruction of lymphatic pathways, and tumor recurrence should be further evaluated.
- Further workup may not be necessary or appropriate for patients with significant functional or cognitive impairment, or in patient populations where goals of care are focused on quality of life.
- If the results of testing will have a clinical impact on treatment decisions, consider:
  - Indirect lymphoscintigraphic function test, lymphangiography, fluorescent microlymphography, MRI, CT, or ultrasound
  - Bioelectrical Impedance Analysis: a quick, noninvasive technique that uses electrodes to measure the difference in the amount of fluid between the affected and unaffected limb. Can be used preoperatively to establish a normal baseline and then periodically after surgery to monitor changes in fluid from that baseline, thereby detecting the onset of lymphedema before symptoms or visual awareness occurs.

TREATMENT OPTIONS

Nonpharmacologic

Lymphedema is a chronic, generally incurable condition that requires lifelong care and attention, as well as continuing psychosocial support. The commitment and participation of the patient is essential to an improved outcome.[4]

- Conservative therapeutic approach includes:
  - **Stage 0:** A compression garment is recommended as a prophylactic measure to be worn when traveling on airplanes, or at other times when the patient feels the need, such as in strenuous exercising. (For arm edema, it is recommended that the patient have both a sleeve and a glove.) The patient is made aware of the standard guidelines for prevention.
  - **Stage 1:** A compression garment may be all that is needed.
  - **Stages 2 and 3:** To date, success in lymphedema treatment is attributed primarily to Combined Decongestive Therapy.[2,3,5]

- Combined Decongestive Therapy (CDT) is a two-phase program consisting of multilayered bandaging during an intensive phase and the wearing of compression garments during the maintenance phase (Table 58.1). The goals of CDT include:
  - Reduction of swelling, fibrosis, and risk of infection
  - Maintaining health of the skin

- Resolving long-standing wounds
- Increasing mobility
- Enhancing qualify of life and improving patient self-image
- The following may be used as adjunct therapies during the maintenance phase of CDT.
  1. **Intermittent pneumatic compression**: Pneumatic compression

---

TABLE 58.1: COMBINED DECONGESTIVE THERAPY[4]

CDT Phase I—Intensive Phase

The standard duration of this phase is approximately 10–20 days. The patient remains bandaged for approximately 22 hours each day during this period.

Skin care	The skin must be kept clean and well hydrated to avoid infection. Skin should be moisturized with an unscented, low pH moisturizer on a daily basis.
Manual Lymph Drainage (MLD)[a]	A specific manual technique using gentle, rhythmic strokes that stretch the skin, thereby working on the superficial lymphatics, enhancing lymph flow from an area of congestion to an area of more viable lymphatics
Compression Bandaging	Limb is wrapped in several layers of different types of bandages ranging from foam to short stretch bandages
Moderate Exercises	Gentle exercises of the limb geared toward further mobilizing fluid while the patient is in the bandages

CDT Phase II—Maintenance

Patient compliance is necessary to successfully maintain the reduction results of CDT.

Skin Care	Attention paid to keeping the delicate, often fragile skin of the palliative/geriatric patient clean and well hydrated is important for the prevention of infection and for maintaining the integrity of the skin.
Medical Grade Compression Garments	Compression is the most important part of maintenance. Needed by some patients 24/7 in order to maintain the reduction achieved in CDT Compression garments can be difficult for the patient to put on and remove. A caregiver may be needed to assume this task. When choosing garments, consideration should be given to these limitations, as well as to the fragility of the skin and the patient's ability to tolerate wearing the garment. For arm lymphedema, patients should be given a sleeve and a glove to prevent swelling of the hand.
Self-Bandaging	Patients are often instructed how to bandage themselves at night, but many lack the capacity to do so. This task often falls to a caregiver, who may find it physically taxing and an additional stressful burden. In addition, incorrectly applied bandages could cause further compromise the affected limb. An alternative to self-bandaging is to wear non-pneumatic compression garments, which are designed specifically to be worn at night. Many types are comfortable, with Velcro straps making them adjustable to accommodate fluctuations in limb girth, and easy to put on.
Manual Lymph Drainage	Patients are often taught to do self-MLD. A caregiver may also want to learn to perform the procedure. If possible, periodic MLD treatments by a trained therapist would be beneficial. Helps to enhance lymphatic flow; gentle touch of MLD works on the ANS, inducing the relaxation response
Remedial Exercises	If the patient is unable to perform simple exercises, a caregiver can perform passive exercise, depending on patient tolerance.

[a] MLD should not be confused with massage therapy, which is contraindicated for the lymphedema patient. Even effleurage (a light massage stroke) is considered too heavy.

devices use a plastic sleeve or stocking that is inflated intermittently and applies sequential pressures over the affected limb. After compression is achieved, an elastic knit sleeve is applied to maintain edema reduction. Considerations include:

- Although Medicare and other insurance companies reimburse for the compression pumps, there are numerous conflicting conclusions regarding its efficacy.
- Should never be used in place of CDT in Phase I or compression garments in Phase II.
- If used improperly, complications can arise to the areas adjacent to the pump sleeve.
- Not all patients are candidates for this modality.

2. **Exercise**: Although originally discouraged for lymphedema patients, the evidence supporting the safety and benefits of exercise has been growing. In a study of breast cancer survivors with lymphedema, gradually progressive weight lifting had no significant effect on limb swelling, and there was a decrease in exacerbations of lymphedema, reduced symptoms, and increased strength.[6] A properly fitting compression garment should always be worn during exercise.

Mrs. G was referred for MLD treatments to address the swelling in both of her legs, but it was quickly determined that she would benefit from CDT. She received 5 days of intensive treatment, after which she was measured for custom-made medical grade compression garments. CDT resulted in a significant reduction of the circumference of both legs, which returned her columnar, edematous limbs to their normal contour.

Pharmacologic

- Diuretics are not recommended as a stand-alone treatment for lymphedema. When diuretics are discontinued, the tissues will frequently fill back up quickly, often more than prior to the diuretic use. Diuretics may become necessary, however, in malignant lymphedema, or in the context of comorbidities such as CHF, or kidney or liver disease.
- Benzopyrones (Venalot, Paroven, coumarin), are not recommended for the treatment of lymphedema because they can take months to have an effect and have also been proven to cause liver toxicity.

Surgical Interventions

- Surgical approaches for lymphedema are not curative and should be reserved for those cases where conservative treatment with CDT has clearly been unsuccessful.
- The goals of surgical interventions are to reduce of the volume of affected areas, to improve function, and to prevent or mitigate complications of the condition. Surgical procedures include microsurgery (lymphovenous anastomoses or LVA), liposuction, debulking (in cases of obesity), and lymph node transplantation (often done during reconstruction). Compression garments must still be worn afterward to control the condition.
- Surgery should be considered only when the potential benefits clearly outweigh the burdens and are aligned with the patient's goals of care.

THERAPIST QUALIFICATIONS

- Lymphedema treatment should be performed only by a certified lymphedema therapist. The following professionals are eligible for such training: physical therapists, occupational therapists, nurses, licensed massage therapists, physical therapist assistants, and occupational therapist assistants.
- Sources for referrals are www.lymphedemapeople.com, National Lymphedema Network (www.lymphnet.org), www.klosetraining.com, www.vodderschool.com, and www.acols.com.

INSURANCE REIMBURSEMENT

- Lymphedema can be an expensive condition to treat. Daytime compression garments are quite costly and need to be replaced approximately every six months. Intensive treatment is time consuming and labor intensive.
- Medicare currently does not reimburse for compression garments or bandaging supplies; nor does Medicare reimburse for lymphedema treatment performed by those nurses or licensed massage therapists, who are also qualified certified lymphedema therapists (CLT).
- Medicare does reimburse for clinical services performed by occupational therapists, physical therapists, occupational

therapist assistants, and physical therapist assistants, even if they are not certified in the treatment of lymphedema.

- The Women's Health and Cancer Rights Act of 1998 indicates that if an insured's coverage consists of payment for a mastectomy, then that patient must also be covered for "Prostheses and physical complications of all stages of mastectomy, including lymphedema."
- Some private insurance plans have restrictions on lymphedema treatment, bandaging supplies, and the types of compression garments that qualify for reimbursement.

PALLIATIVE CARE ISSUES

- Lymphedema is an underdiagnosed condition and is often dismissed as an inconsequential condition of patients with long-term serious illnesses.
- Clinicians should be aware of the signs, symptoms, and causes of lymphedema. Early diagnosis and treatment increases the manageability of lymphedema. If left untreated, the condition will progress, causing disfigurement, long-term disability, severe reduction in quality of life, a loss of independence, increased caregiver burden, and frequent hospitalizations due to infections.
- Lymphedema is a chronic, progressive condition that requires lifelong maintenance treatment. Effective management of lymphedema requires a comprehensive care model that addresses the patient's fears and concerns, arranges for appropriate referrals, and takes into consideration the patient's prognosis, goals for care, functional status, and cognitive abilities.

Mrs. G's improvement had a major impact on her physical and emotional state. Her neuropathy was less bothersome, and she was able to ambulate more easily, as well as wear normal shoes. While she does not like wearing the compression garments, she realizes the importance of maintaining her lymphedema reduction and has been compliant in her maintenance. She wears them most days but occasionally takes a day or two off with little compromise. She gets periodic MLD treatments as well.

TAKE-HOME POINTS

- Lymphedema is a chronic, progressive condition that requires lifelong maintenance treatment.
- Clinicians should be informed regarding the signs, symptoms, and causes of lymphedema, as early diagnosis and treatment is key to effective management.
- The lynchpin of treatment is Combined Decongestive Therapy (CDT), which must be provided by a certified lymphedema therapist (CLT).
- Compression is essential for the management of lymphedema. The wrong garment can be worse than no garment. Therefore, a patient should be given the garment that is *needed* by that patient, not just a garment that will be reimbursed for by the patient's insurance provider.

REFERENCES

1. Slavin SA, Schook CC, Greene AK. Lymphedema management. In Davis M, Feyer P, Ortner P, Zimmerman C (Eds). *Supportive Oncology* (p. 211–220); Philadelphia: Elsevier Inc; Philadelphia. 2011.
2. Koul R, Dufan T, Russell C, et al. Efficacy of Complete Decongestive Therapy and manual lymphatic drainage on treatment-related lymphedema in breast cancer. *Int J Radiat Oncol Biol Phys.* 2007;67(3):841–846.
3. Lee BB, Andrade M, Bergan J, et al. Diagnosis and treatment of primary lymphedema. Consensus document of the International Union of Phebology. *Int Angiol.* 2010;29(5):454–470.
4. International Society of Lymphology Executive Committee. The diagnosis and treatment of peripheral lymphedema. *Lymphology.* 2003;36:84–91.
5. Cheifetz O, Haley L. Management of secondary lymphedema related to breast cancer. *Can Fam Physician.* 2010;56:1277–1284.
6. Schmitz KH, Ahmed RL, Troxel A, et al. Weight-lifting in women with breast-cancer-related lymphedema. *N Engl J Med.* 2009;361:664–673.

59

Pressure Ulcers

CASE

Mrs. P is an 85-year-old woman with dementia and hypertension who develops a pressure ulcer while hospitalized with pneumonia and delirium. She is now home, and a home health nurse is visiting her for wound care. Her daughter seeks your advice because it is two weeks post hospital discharge, and the wound has not healed.

DEFINITION

A *pressure ulcer* is a localized injury to the skin and/or underlying tissue, usually over a bony prominence, as a result of pressure, or pressure in combination with shear and/or friction. Most common locations of pressure ulcers include:

- Sacrum
- Heels
- Ischium
- Trochanter

PREVALENCE

The prevalence of pressure ulcers is 0.4% to 38% in acute care populations, 0% to 17% in patients cared for at home,[1] 14% to 28% of hospice patients, and 2% to 28% of nursing home patients.[2]

CONSEQUENCES OF UNTREATED PRESSURE ULCERS

- Pain
- Infection (osteomylitis, cellulitis, sepsis)
- Undermining
- Tunneling (leading to a fistula)

DIFFERENTIAL DIAGNOSIS

- Arterial ulcers: often occur on lateral lower leg or toes, are very painful, with demarcated borders
- Venous ulcers: often occur on medial lower leg, are very painful, with irregular borders
- Diabetic neuropathic ulcers: on feet, toes, heels, often with callus

LIKELY ETIOLOGIES

1. *Pressure* is the most direct cause of ulcers.
   - Pressure leads to decreased blood flow and tissue anoxia, which then leads to increased capillary permeability and edema and eventually cell death.
   - Process starts at the epidermis, thus when visualized at dermis, a larger epidermal area is affected.
   - Low pressure over prolonged period is more damaging than high pressure for a short time.
2. *Shear* occurs when parallel surfaces move at different rates (for example, when a patient is sitting in bed and the bones and tissue slide down but the skin sticks to the sheet and kinks the blood vessels).
3. *Friction* occurs when two surfaces move across each other (for example, when patient is dragged across sheets), which removes outer skin.
4. *Moisture* causes maceration of skin leading to breakdown.
   - Fecal incontinence is more damaging than urinary incontinence.
   - Dry skin leads to cracks and the outer layer can flake off, allowing for underlying dermis exposure.

RISK FACTORS

- Immobility (post surgical, spinal cord injury)
- Sensory loss and decreased position changes
- Obesity
- Contractures, fractures, musculoskeletal disorders
- Age (because of weight loss, decreased skin elasticity)
- Poor nutritional status
- Diabetes
- CVA/Altered mental status (dementia)
- Incontinence (fecal, urine)
- Peripheral vascular disease
- History of pressure ulcer

RISK ASSESSMENT

- Although there are no specific frequency recommendations, risk assessment should be performed on a regular basis, including after a hospitalization or in the event of any changes in status. Assessment scales include:
  - **Braden Scale**: Assesses five areas: sensory perception, moisture, activity, mobility, nutrition, friction, and shear. Rates each area as completely limited, very limited, slightly limited, or no impairment. When Braden Scale score is 16 or less, implement Pressure Ulcer Prevention Protocols (http://www.bradenscale.com).
  - **Norton Scale**: Uses five criteria to assess patients' risk for pressure ulcers: physical condition, mental condition, activity, mobility, and incontinence. Scores of 14 or less indicate liability for ulcers; scores of <12 indicate very high risk (http://www.rd411.com/wrc/pdf/w0513_norton_presure_sore_risk_assessment_scale_scoring_system.pdf).

REVERSE STAGING

- The National Pressure Ulcer Advisory Panel (NPUAP) has taken the position that once an ulcer has reached an advanced stage, it should not be down-staged as it heals.
- Based on this conclusion, the Centers for Medicare and Medicaid Services (CMS) revised the Minimum Data Set (MDS) guidelines for pressure ulcer risk assessment and staging, which now state that applying the pressure ulcer staging system in reverse order is erroneous and can lead to inappropriate wound care and reimbursement (www.cms.hhs.gov/NursingHomeQualityInits/01_Overview.asp#TopOfPage).

PREVENTION

1. Use moisturizing/barrier cream:
   - Prevents cracks in the skin
   - Creates a barrier so stool and urine do not touch skin
   - Reduces friction
2. Reduce pressure, sheer, and friction:
   - Turning and regular positioning
   - See pressure reducing mattresses below (group I).
   - Sheer reduction: maintain head of bed at or below 30 degrees to prevent shear-related injury.
   - Pillow bridging to free float heels
3. Monitor nutrition:
   - Provide nutritional supplement if indicated and consistent with prognosis and goals of care.
   - Maintain hydration.
4. Manage moisture due to:
   - Fecal and urinary incontinence
   - Perspiration

DIAGNOSIS

History

A detailed history should seek to identify risk factors and predisposing factors since they are critically important in preventing the development of ulcers.

Exam

- The examination requires a careful probing and measurement of the wounds. A thorough exam will help differentiate pressure ulcers from venous ulcers, arterial ulcers, and diabetic neuropathic ulcers.
- An accurate use of terminology is essential to allow the physician and nurse doing the wound care to create appropriate plans of care (see Table 59.1).

Tests

Wound cultures at the bedside are not helpful. Wounds are often colonized with bacteria, but not infected. If cellulitis and osteomyelitis are suspected, systemic antibiotics are indicated. Topical antibiotics are not effective.

TREATMENT OPTIONS

1. Pain management
   - Dressing removal and cleansing of the wounds are the most painful aspects of wound care, are very distressing to patients, and are rarely managed with preemptive analgesia.
   - Wound care and treatment involves turning and repositioning, often a source of great pain to the patient. Strategies to mitigate pain include:
     - Involve the patient; determine if the patient can remove his or her own dressings.
     - Premedicate with oral medications 30 minutes before wound care.

TABLE 59.1: ASSESSMENT OF PRESSURE ULCERS

Assessment	Description
Stage[1]	**Stage I: Non-blanchable redness of intact skin;** usually over bony prominence; discoloration of skin, warmth, edema, hardenss, pain may also be present **Stage II: Partial-thickness skin loss or intact/open blister** involving epidermis, dermis or both **Stage III: Full-thickness skin loss (fat visible)** involving damage or necrosis of subcutaneous tissue that may extend to fascia; bone, tendon, muscle not exposed **Stage IV: Full-thickness skin loss (muscle/bone visible)** with extensive destruction, tissue necrosis, or damage to muscle, bone or support structures Unstageable/Unclassified: **Full thickness skin or tissue loss**—depth unknown; depth of ulcer completely obscured by slough and/or eschar; staging can be determined after slough/eschar removed Suspected Deep Tissue Injury: **Depth unknown:** Purple/maroon localized area of intact skin or blood-filled blister due to damage of underlying dolft tissue from pressure and/or shear
Location	Sacrum, heels, trochanter, ischium
Size	Area, depth, probe for sinus tracts, tunneling, or undermining
Drainage	Amount, purulence, and odor. Types of drainage: serosanguinous, serous and purulent
Necrosis	Beige, gray, brown material often with high exudates, slough, or eschar
Granulation	Identify as wound healing, pink/red epithelializing tissue
Fibrin	Yellow tissue, healthy
Eschar	Thick brown devitalized tissue, unstageable as cannot probe depth of wound
Cellulitis or abscess	Redness and warmth around wound, fluctuance

- Use around-the-clock medications for continuous wound pain.
- EMLA cream (Eutectic Mixture of Local Anesthetics), a combination of lidocaine and prilocaine, has been shown to provide pain relief during dressing changes and is generally well tolerated (some burning and slight local redness). It should be applied directly on the wound and covered with plastic wrap for 20 minutes. If not effective, increase pretreatment to 45 minutes to 60 minutes prior to dressing change. Generally 5% EMLA cream is used; apply 1 g (1 mL) of cream per 10 cm² of ulcer area up to a maximum of 10 g.[3]
- Applying lidocaine gel to the wound bed prior to irrigation is a frequently used strategy, but the evidence for this approach is less robust. Lidocaine gel may be mixed with a zinc cream. Apply up to a maximum of 10 g of lidocaine.[2]

2. Psychosocial needs
   - Assess for poor self-image, isolation from family, and lack of privacy due to wound care routines.
   - Make referrals for counseling when appropriate.
3. Pressure reduction (all stages)
   - Turning regularly or other position changes if possible
   - Pillow bridges, heal boots
4. Assess and treat infection
   - Cellulitis, osteomylitis
5. Nutritional support[3]
   - Evidence for giving vitamin C is limited, but if patient is deficient then add short-term daily supplementation (50 mg to 100 mg).
   - Protein supplementation does seem to help wound healing,[4] but evidence is limited.
   - Recommendations include protein 1.25 to 1.5 g/kg/day and minimum of 30 to 35 kcal per kg body weight per day unless contraindicated, as in renal failure.[5]

SUPPORT SURFACES

- A variety of pressure-relieving surfaces (beds, mattresses, mattress overlays, cushions) are routinely used for pressure ulcer prevention. Although evidence is limited, mattress overlays on operating tables may decrease the incidence of postoperative pressure ulcers. Higher specification foam mattresses and specialized sheepskin overlays also reduce pressure ulcer incidence, compared with the standard hospital mattress. Study results are mixed comparing dynamic versus static surfaces for prevention of pressure ulcers.[1]

- Reimbursement for these support surfaces, based on use for prevention (group I) or for treatment (group I, II, III), is available from Medicare. Specific Medicare criteria are described in Table 59.2.

WOUND CLEANSING OR IRRIGATION

1. For all stage wounds:
   - Clean granular wounds: shower, bulb syringe, piston syringe.
   - Chronic wounds and necrotic, infected, tunneling, or undermining wounds require pressurized irrigation with normal saline. Attach canyon tunneling device or use splash guards as needed.
   - Drinkable tap water can be used when a patient does cleansing in a shower.
2. For stage I, II wounds:
   - *Moisturizing*: Clean area with normal saline and gauze; apply barrier cream twice a day and after soiling.
   - *Debridement*: Selection of debridement method should be based on patient's condition, goals of care, ulcer status, care setting, and professional accessibility and capability (Table 59.3).[6] Do not debride eschar on heel unless septic, especially if there is suspected decreased blood supply to foot.

WOUND DRESSINGS

The goal of wound dressing is to maintain a moist wound surface surrounded by dry skin.[5] See Table 59.4 for a description of different types of wound dressings.

TABLE 59.2: SUPPORT SURFACES AND MEDICARE CRITERIA FOR COVERAGE

Category	Group I	Group II	Group III
Examples	1) 4–6 inch foam 2) Air (powered or non-powered, < 5 inches) 3) Gel 4) Water 5) Alternating pressure overlay	Low air loss bed Alternating pressure mattress	Air fluidized therapy (specialty bed)
Materials	# 1–4 above non-powered, 5 is powered	Powered, has air sacs containing warm air	Powered, contains silicone-coated beads that liquefy when air is pumped through them
Medicare criteria for coverage	*Criteria:* Complete immobility OR Limited mobility PLUS ONE RISK FACTOR: Impaired nutrition Incontinence Altered sensory perception Compromised circulation	*Criteria:* MULTIPLE stage 2 ulcers on pelvis or trunk, and a group I support surface has been used for 1 month, and the ulcers have worsened or remained the same OR Large or multiple stage 3 or 4 ulcers on trunk or pelvis OR Flap or graft surgery within 60 days and was on group 2 or 3 in hospital prior to discharge	*Criteria:* All of the following: Stage 3 or 4 ulcer Bed- or chair-bound (Without bed, patient would be institutionalized) Order written by MD based on a comprehensive assessment and evaluation Group 2 surface and comprehensive therapy tried for > 1 month with worsening or no improvement Trained adult caregiver Physician directs monthly No pulmonary disease[1]

TABLE 59.3: DEBRIDEMENT METHODS

Type of Debridement[6]	Description	Advantages/Disadvantages
Mechanical (not recommended)	Wet to dry dressings or other physical force	May remove healthy tissue, possibly painful, DO NOT USE
Sharp	Scalpel or scissors to remove large amounts of tissue	Quick, pain control needed, requires good vascular supply to wound
Biosurgery	Larvae to digest devitalized tissue	Quick, effective, often used in other countries, patient/family emotional response
Enzymatic[a]	Topical debriding agent to dissolve devitalized tissue	Takes 3–7 days, healthy tissue can get debrided
Autolytic	Use of synthetic dressings to allow self-digestion by natural ulcer fluids	Takes longer
Hypergels	20% hypertonic saline gauze—absorbs and debrides20% hypergel—placed on dry eschar to soften	Does not require prescription

Note. Table adapted from Cobbs EL, Duthie EH, Murphy JB, eds. *Geriatrics Review Syllabus: A Core Curriculum in Geriatric Medicine.* 5th ed. Malden, MA: Blackwell Publishing for the American Geriatrics Society; 2002: 207.
[a] All papain-urea enzymatic debriding agents were taken off the market in 11/08 after several anaphylactic reactions were documented. Currently the only enzymatic agent available is collagenase.

ODOR CONTROL

- Foul odor emanating from a wound can lead to social isolation, depression, diminished quality of life for the patient, and distress for caregivers, family members, and professionals.
- The goals of treatment include reducing or eliminating odor, absorbing exudates,

controlling pain, and managing infection. (See Chapter 61: Malodorous Wounds.)

NON-HEALING WOUNDS

Despite careful monitoring and appropriate and meticulous treatment using the options described above, some wounds do not heal. Considerations in the event of wounds that do not heal include:

TABLE 59.4: WOUND DRESSINGS[5]

Dressing	Indication	Contraindication	Example	Other Comments
Transparent film	Stage I, II Protection from friction Superficial wound	Drainage	Tegaderm Op-Site	Change q 2–4 days depending on drainage
Hydrocolloid	Stage II, III Low drainage Autolytic debridement	Infections Packing Wounds with increased drainage	DuoDerm Comfeel Nu-derm	Change q 3–5 days
Hydrogel	Stage II, III, IV shallow minimally draining granulating wounds	Maceration Excessive exudates	SoloSite gel Restore gel	Apply on gauze Change 1 time/day
Alginate or Hydrofiber	Stage III, IV for moderately/heavily draining wounds	Dry wound	AlgiSite Seasorb	Apply within wound boarders Change 1 x per day
Foam	Stage II, III can be a surface foam or applied in wound as a packing	Dry wound	Allevyn foam Curafoam	Change 1 time/day

Note. Adapted from: Ruben DB, Herr KA, Pacala JT, et al. *Geriatrics At Your Fingertips*, 12th Edition. New York: The American Geriatrics Society; 2010: 236.

- All pressure ulcers are colonized with aerobic and anaerobic bacteria; wound irrigation/cleansing is the most important aspect of minimizing bacterial colonization. Wound cultures are almost never helpful, but if done, perform after irrigation/cleansing. Systemic antibiotics are indicated for cellulitis and osteomylitis.
- Trial of silver dressing works best in slow healing wounds with excessive drainage after two weeks of usual treatment. Apply silver sulfadiazine or mupirocin ointment in wound. (All the dressings in Table 59.4 are impregnated with silver, i.e., silver alginate, silver hydrogel.)
- Adjunctive therapies include negative pressure wound therapy (NPWT), also known as vacuum-assisted wound closure. Advantages include fewer dressing changes and accelerated wound healing. Disadvantages include cost and need for patient to carry the portable pump. NPWT is contraindicated for patients with fragile skin due to age or chronic corticosteroid use.
- Surgical option for wound closure: Most pressure ulcers can be effectively managed using basic wound care practices and dressings. For patients who may benefit from rapid wound closure, and if appropriate in context of prognosis, functional status, and goals for care, surgical procedures are available (e.g., skin grafts, skin flaps).

TAKE-HOME POINTS

- Assessment and reduction of risk is the most important aspect of pressure ulcer prevention.

- Patient preferences and concerns should be identified and taken into consideration when planning treatment of wounds.
- Once pressure ulcers do develop, local wound care and pressure relief are the most important strategies.
- Wound care is often a source of significant pain to the patient. Appropriate pain control must be instituted to manage discomfort during repositioning, wound cleansing and dressing.

REFERENCES

1. Reddy M, Gill S, et al. Preventing pressure ulcers: a systematic review. *JAMA.* 2006;*296*:974.
2. Alvarez OM, Kalinski C, et al. Incorporating wound healing strategies to improve palliation (symptom management) in patients with chronic wounds. *J Palliat Med.* 2007;*10*(5):1161–1189.
3. Evans E, Gray M. Do topical analgesics reduce pain associated with wound dressing changes or debridement of chronic wounds? *J Wound Ostomy Continence Nurs.* 2005;*32*(5):287.
4. Reddy M, Gill S, et al. Treatment of pressure ulcers: a systematic review. *JAMA.* 2008;*300*:2647.
5. Ruben D, Herr K, et al. *Geriatrics at your Fingertips: 2010*, 12th edition. New York: The American Geriatrics Society; 2010.
6. Bergstrom N, Bennett MA, Carlson CE, et al. Pressure Ulcer Treatment. Clinical Practice Guideline. Quick Reference Guide for Clinicians, No. 15. Rockville, MD: U.S. Department of Health and Human Services, Public Health Service, Agency for Health Care Policy and Research. AHCPR Pub. No. 95-0653. Dec. 1994.

60

Pruritus

CASE

Mrs. H is a 73-year-old female with history of hepatitis B cirrhosis who presents with new liver masses. She was started on morphine five days ago for worsening right upper quadrant pain. There is a one-year history of lower extremity itching that has become generalized in the last month and worsened in the last week. The patient is jaundiced. Skin exam is positive for xerosis, a tender right upper quadrant pain, and myoclonus.

DEFINITION

Pruritus is the unpleasant sensation that provokes desire to scratch. Scratching on or near affected skin area diminishes or arrests the itch sensation. Pruritis can be acute and self-limited or chronic and persistent (including intractable pruritus). It may be localized (defined skin regions) or generalized pruritus (large body surface areas).

PREVALENCE

Pruritis is the most common symptom of skin disease in the elderly.

CONSEQUENCES OF UNTREATED PRURITUS

- Diminished quality of life including insomnia, anxiety, depression.
- Secondary effects of repeated scratching include excoriation, lichenification, impetigo, prurigo nodularis.[1]

CLASSIFICATION

Pruritis can be divided into two general categories: dermatological (originates in the skin) and nondermatological (originating outside the skin). See Table 60.1 for a pathophysicology-based classification of pruritis.

DIAGNOSIS

History

In the absence of a primary skin condition, look for systemic/neurogenic/neuropathic causes. Review allergy history and all medications, especially recently introduced drugs.

Exam

Complete skin exam including scalp, nails, and mucous membranes; look for signs of liver/renal disease/cancer/thyroid dysfunction.

Tests (based on categorization into dermatological, non-dermatological pruritus or both):

- Hepatic, renal, thyroid panel
- Peripheral eosinophil count
- Parasite workup
- Blood smear
- Cancer screening

Mrs. H's lab tests revealed a total/direct bilirubin 24/17, alkaline phosphatase 800 and serum creatinine of 8 (baseline 1.2 six weeks ago). An ultrasound confirms biliary obstruction and two new liver masses. The diagnosis is initial localized dermatological pruritus secondary to xerosis with superimposed generalized non-dermatological systemic/neurogenic pruritus in the setting of cholestasis, opioids, and uremia.

TREATMENT OPTIONS

There are no generally accepted universal therapies; medications may need to be used in combination.

Nonpharmacologic

- Investigate possible pet, pollen, food, linen/clothing (wool) allergies.
- Use non-alcohol, fragrance-free skin products; review ingredients for possible allergenic content.
- Limit bathing and use lukewarm (not hot) water, which increases hydration; use mild soap or substitute; take oatmeal (Aveeno) baths; pat (do not rub) skin dry with soft towel.
- Wear loose clothing, keep surroundings cool; use humidifier during winter.

TABLE 60.1: PATHOPHYSIOLOGY-BASED CLASSIFICATION[2-5]

Dermatological (pruritogenic) pruritus: originates in the skin
  Xerosis (dry skin; most common in the elderly and falls in category of "senile itch")
  Atopic dermatitis/eczema, psoriasis, infestations (scabies)
  Fungal (tinea/candida)
  Autoimmune diseases (bullous pemphigoid, pemphigus, drug-related hypersensitivity vasculitis, erythema multiforme, toxic epidermal necrolysis)
  Mycosis fungoides

Non-dermatological pruritus: originates outside the skin
  Systemic: (organ-based, metabolic, cancer, infections; overlaps with neurogenic mechanisms):
    Lymphoma (Hodgkin's, T-cell lymphoma)
    Leukemia, macroglobulinemia
    Endocrine abnormalities (hyper/hypothyroid; diabetes)
    Liver (cholestasis/hepatitis)
    Uremia
    HIV
    Polycythemia vera
    Adverse drug reactions (aspirin, opioids, amphetamines)
    Dermatographism

  Neurogenic: central neurological dysfunction in absence of primary nerve or skin damage; often associated with central/spinal opioid receptor stimulation
    Exogenously administered opioids and their metabolites
    Endogenous opioid peptides which accumulate in renal failure and cholestasis

  Neuropathic: primary neurological disorder without primary skin involvement associated with sensory "neuropathic" components (alloknesis and hyperknesis)
    Peripheral:
      Post-herpetic neuralgia
      HIV and chemotherapy-induced polyneuropathies
      Brachio-radial pruritus due to cervical spine disease related nerve root injury
      Ano-genital pruritus due to lumbo-sacral radiculopathy
      Nerve entrapment
      Tumor
    Central:
      Stroke
      Abscess tumor, where it can be unilateral
      Multiple sclerosis, where it is characteristically sudden and lasts only seconds or minutes; treated with neuropathic adjuvants

  Psychogenic:
    Depresson
    Anxiety
    Schizophrenia associated-parasitophobia

  Mixed or multifactorial: more common in geriatric patients with serious chronic illness or at end-of-life

- Avoid scratching; maintain short nails; wear cotton gloves during sleep.
- Reduce stress and address anxiety and depressive states.

Pharmacologic[6]
- The rules of geriatric drug dosing apply with attention to age-related pharmacological changes, including increased volume of distribution for fat-soluble drugs and decreased hepatic metabolism and renal excretion leading to increased half-lives.
- Be alert for adverse drug effects such as lethargy, delirium, bowel and bladder dysfunction, and falls. Lower starting doses and extended dosing intervals are appropriate.

- Emollients (skin softeners that also moisturize by slowing water loss and increasing skin water content) should be applied immediately after bathing and twice a day. Products include Aquaphor, Eucerin, Cera-Ve, Lachydrin, urea-based and emollients with anesthetic components from added menthol (1%–2%), camphor, and phenol (0.5%–1%).
- Topical anesthetics for localized itch areas (small amounts and limited time trial): benzocaine, tetracaine, lidocaine, and prilocaine (both found in EMLA cream), doxepin 5% cream, capsaicin 0.025/0.075%; pramoxine 1%.
- Topical steroids should be used when an inflammatory skin condition exists.

Setting Specific Medications[6,7]

1. **Pruritogenic (histaminic) pruritus**
   - Hydroxyzine 25–50 mg q8h
   - Doxepin 10–25 mg qhs
2. **Uremic pruritus**[8,9] Incidence and severity not correlated with age, type of renal disease, or dialysis adequacy.
   - Gamma linolenic acid 2.2% (primrose oil) cream bid
   - Gabapentin 100–300 mg q post dialysis
   - UVB phototherapy x 6 weeks
   - Naltrexone 25–75 mg daily if severe itching (Avoid opioid antagonists in patients receiving opioids.) Also consider the following:
     - Thalidomide 50–100 mg daily
     - Ondansetron 4–8 mg q8h
     - Cholestyramine 4–16 gm daily
     - Nalfurafine 5 microgram IV q post dialysis x 2–4 weeks
     - Butorphanol 1–4 mg daily intranasally
     - Short-term therapy of localized pruritus: tacrolimus 0.03% bid
3. **Neuropathic pruritis**
   - Gabapentin (reduces substance P and glutamate release) 300–1200 mg qd (adjust with renal disease)
   - Local therapy:
     - Capsaicin cream 0.025%, 0.075% apply 3–4 times/day for 14–28 days
     - Menthol-based skin products
4. **Psychological pruritis**
   - Selective serotonin reuptake inhibtors (SSRIs), e.g., paroxetine, fluvoxamine

- Refer for assessment and possible cognitive behavioral therapy (CBT) intervention
5. **Cholestatic pruritus**[10,11]
   - Mechanisms: bile salt effect given response to cholestyramine and stenting; biliary obstruction that may cause elevated endogenous opioid peptides via increased hepatic synthesis
   - Naloxone and Naltrexone relieve itch; H1 blockers do not.
   - Treatment options include:
     - Cholestyramine (4–16 gms/day)
     - Phototherapy
     - Naloxone 0.4 mg bolus then 0.2 micrograms/kg/min infusion
     - Naltrexone 25–50 mg/day
     - Rifampicin 300–600 mg/day (PO)
     - Ursodeoxycholic acid 10–15 mg/kg/day
     - Serotonin reuptake inhibitors (e.g., sertraline 75–100 mg/d)
     - Endoscopic or percutaneous biliary tree decompression should be strongly considered in biliary obstruction
6. **HIV**[1]
   - Idiopathic HIV pruritus is a diagnosis of exclusion. Management should be directed at the underlying condition.
   - Consider phototherapy for some HIV-associated dermatoses and idiopathic pruritus.
   - By reconstituting immune system, HAART improves some skin diseases, but temporarily worsens others. Unless there is strong concern for drug allergy, HAART does not need to be stopped.
7. **Severe (intractable) pruritus:**[10] Possible association with circadian rhythms and tendency to be worse at night. Treatment options:
   - Doxepin 10–30 mg qhs; H1 and H2 blocker properties, sedating, antidepressant. Use caution in geriatric population.
   - Paroxetine 20–40 mg daily; especially in malignant disease; down-regulation of serotonin type 3 receptor; effect within 24-48 hours
   - Mirtazapine 15–30 mg qhs; H1 blocking effect; may last 4–6 weeks
   - Propofol 10–15 mg IV bolus, then 1 mg/kg/hr IV

- Flourinated steroids topical; systemic corticosteroids

8. **Opioid-induced pruritus**
   - Major effect probably secondary to central opioid receptor activation, possibly peripheral; may also be related to nonimmune release of histamine by certain opioids (morphine).
   - Occurs in up to 10% of patients who are given opioids. Most often associated with intraspinal and intravenous injection, morphine, and in opioid-naive patients.
   - Itching occurs, especially around face. Treatment options include:
     - Rotate opioid; fentanyl is less pruritogenic.
     - Consider treating with k-opioid receptor agonist (butorphanol).

Initial steps in Mrs. H's treatment included discontinuing morphine because of acute renal failure, and rotating to fentanyl. Cholestyramine was started, and also butorphanol (at 50% usual dose and Q6H). Aggressive skin care with emollients was instituted. After a discussion with Mr. H to review her goals of care and treatment preferences, she was referred for evaluation for biliary stent or percutaneous T-tube drainage.

PALLIATIVE CARE ISSUES

- Pruritus is a very common symptom in the geriatric palliative care patient population. While some patients respond well to treatment, management can be challenging. In severe cases, pruritis can be incapacitating.
- Scratching associated with pruritis can lead to skin excoriation, infection, and scarring. Itching is not usually considered a 'pain state," but the discomfort it causes can be just as distressing, frequently causing agitation, alteration of mood, and sleep disorders.
- Pruritus is perceived as very bothersome to patients, and has a negative impact on several domains of quality of life, including physical well-being, psychological health, social interactions, and family relationships.[12]
- Some of the pharmacological treatment options for pruritus may cause sedation or drowsiness, especially in older or seriously ill patients.
- Because stress can aggravate chronic itching, patients should receive psychological support and education on behavioral interventions that may help reduce their symptom burden. Complementary and alternative approaches such as acupuncture, meditation and yoga may also help to mitigate stress levels. (See Chapter 17: Complementary and Alternative Medicine.)

TAKE-HOME POINTS

- Proper classification of pruritis into dermatological or nondermatological categories will facilitate diagnosis and treatment.
- In seriously ill geriatric patients, look for multiple causes. If underlying cause is not reversible, priority should be given to symptom relief and establishing achievable goals of care.
- General nonpharmacological and pharmacological measures are the mainstay of treatment.
- In each setting, therapy should be individualized.

REFERENCES

1. Singh F, Rudikoff D. HIV-associated pruritus: etiology and management. *Am J Clin Dermatol.* 2003;*4*(3):177–188.
2. Binder A., Koroschetz J, Baron R. Disease mechanisms in neuropathic itch. *Nat Clin Pract Neurol.* 2008;*4*(6):329–337.
3. Paus R, et al. Frontiers in pruritus research: scratching the brain for more effective itch therapy. *J Clin Invest.* 2006;*116*(5):1174–1186.
4. Twycross R, et al. Itch: scratching more than the surface. *QJM.* 2003;*96*(1):7–26.
5. Yosipovitch G, Greaves MW, Schmelz M. Itch. *Lancet.* 2003;*361*(9358):690–694.
6. Roberts WE. Dermatologic problems of older women. *Dermatol Clin.* 2006;*24*(2):271–280, viii.
7. Summney BT. Pruritus (2009). In Walsh TD, Caraceni AT, Fainsinger R, et al. (Eds) *Palliative Medicine.* Philadelphia: W.B.Saunders Elsevier; 910–913.
8. Manent L, Tansinda P, Vaglio A. Uraemic pruritus: clinical characteristics, pathophysiology and treatment. *Drugs.* 2009;*69*(3):251–263.
9. Keithi-Reddy SR, et al. Uremic pruritus. *Kidney Int.* 2007;*72*(3):373–377.
10. Greaves MW. Itch in systemic disease: therapeutic options. *Dermatol Ther.* 2005;*18*(4):323–327.
11. Kremer AE, et al. Pathogenesis and treatment of pruritis in cholestasis. *Drugs.* 2008;*68*(15): 2163–2182.
12. Chen SC. Pruritis. *Dermatol Clin.* 2012;*30*: 309–321.

61

Malodorous Wounds

CASE
Mrs. J is a 78-year-old woman who has had a recent fall with a hip fracture. During her hospitalization and rehabilitation she developed pressure ulcers. She is currently ready to be discharged with continued home nursing for her wounds. She reluctantly divulges that she is embarrassed by the smell of her wounds and that she does not want to go home because of the odor. Her family has been bringing in room deodorizers and potpourri, but family members are generally reluctant to visit Mrs. J because of the smell. She asks if there is anything that can be done.

DEFINITION
A *malodorous wound* is one that has a foul odor. Types of malodorous wounds include:

- Arterial ulcers: often lateral lower leg or toes, very painful with demarcated borders.
- Venous ulcers: often medial lower leg, painful with irregular borders.
- Diabetic neuropathic ulcers; feet, toes, heels, often with callus.
- Pressure ulcers: can be at any pressure point or caused by friction or shear (See Chapter 59: Pressure Ulcers.)
- Fungating wounds: cancerous or malignant wounds (primary or metastatic lesions).

LIKELY ETIOLOGIES
- Necrotic tissue and bacteria within the wound are the causes of the odor. Anaerobic organisms, primarily bacteriodes, cause the bad odor by releasing the compounds putrescine, cadaverine, unstable sulphur compounds, and short-chain fatty acids. These odors are pungent or rotten-smelling.
- Aerobic organisms such as pseudomonas and klebsiella also produce a malodorous odor, which has been described as more fruity and ripe smelling.[1]
- Poor wound care practices can also be a potential cause of malodorous wounds.

- Primary cancers of the skin that can fungate include squamous cell, basal cell, and melanomas.[2] Other cancers that can metastasize to the skin and fungate include breast (30%), nasal sinuses (20%), larynx (16%), and oral cavity (12%). In women, the most common cancers that metastasize to the skin are breast (69%), colon (9%), melanoma (5%), ovary (4%), and lung (4%). In men, they are lung (24%), colon (19%), and oral cavity (12%).[3]

CONSEQUENCES OF UNTREATED WOUND ODOR
- Social isolation
- Depression
- Shame
- Embarrassment
- Diminished quality of life
- Distress to caregivers, both family members and professionals

DIAGNOSIS
Wound evaluation should include identification of the type of wound (See Chapter 59: Pressure Ulcers). All wounds should be assessed for the presence of a foul odor.

TREATMENT OPTIONS
The goals of treatment for wound odor include:

- Reducing or eliminating odor, absorb and contain exudates
- Controlling pain and manage infection when medically feasible and consistent with goals of care
- Improving quality of life[4]

Recommended treatment options:

1. **General wound care**
   - Assess for pain, premedicate prior to local wound care.
   - Cleansing/irrigation of wound (See Chapter 59: Pressure Ulcers.)

- Change dressings more frequently to control odor.
- Absorb exudates with foam or alginate dressings.

2. **Debridement**: When clinically indicated and medically appropriate, necrotic tissue should be removed (debridement). Extra care must be taken in fungating wounds as they tend to bleed.

3. **Topical control of odor**
   - Metronidazole gel (0.75%) (off-label use) applied into wound daily is effective against both anaerobic and aerobic organisms. This decreases wound odor (in 3–7 days),[5,6] decreases drainage, improves wound appearance, and can sometimes decrease pain. The gel formulation can cause stinging or burning sensation, as it contains alcohol; should this occur, switch to the cream (1%).[7] The wound should be covered with appropriate secondary dressing such as foam or alginate.
   - Hydrogel: There have been two small randomized controlled trials of metronidazole that have shown a decrease in odor.[8,9]
   - Crushed metronidazole tablet (250 mg or 500 mg). Apply and then cover with a petroleum-impregnated dressing.[10] (This is off-label use.)
   - Systemic antibiotics: If there is evidence of clinical infection and if consistent with the goals of care.
   - Impregnated charcoal dressings as a primary or secondary dressing. The malodorous microorganisms, bacteria, and small gas molecules are chemically attracted to the activated charcoal and then securely attach via adsorption.[11]
   - Broad spectrum topical antibiotic ointments including silver products.

4. **Alternative topical treatments**: Treatments discussed in the literature, but not supported with robust evidence, include:
   - Yogurt or buttermilk: Mechanism is unclear but possibly due to low pH of lactobacillus inhibits growth of bacteria.[12]
   - Sugar: Inhibits bacteria growth through its antimicrobial properties and absorbing fluid and starving bacteria of fluid. May cause a burning sensation initially.[12]

- Honey: Similar antimicrobial properties as sugar. Some honeys cause slow release of hydrogen peroxide, which also has antimicrobial properties. May cause a burning sensation.[12] Medical grade honey is mostly from the manuka type and has been irradiated to prevent botulism. This is prepared into gels or sheets combined with an alginate. Several products are FDA-approved.[13]
- Dakins solution: A controversial strategy is the use of cleansing with disinfectant solutions such as Dakins (0.025–0.005% sodium hypochlorite). This treatment is very toxic to granulation tissue and surrounding tissue must be protected carefully. The Wound, Ostomy and Continence Nursing organization does not recommend the use of a dilute Dakin's solution for the management of acute and chronic wounds. It is nevertheless widely considered to be an appropriate treatment option for select wounds in which the patient's condition and tolerance of treatment are considered. The clinician should also consider dilution strength, frequency of dressing change, and duration of treatment when using Dakin's solution for the management of an acute or chronic wound.[14]

5. **Environmental control of odor**: These methods decrease the odor from short chain fatty acids but not from putrescine and cadaverine compounds; they are therefore rarely completely effective. (Note: Proper disposal of old wound dressings is important.)
   - Aromatherapy
   - Room deodorizers
   - Potpourri
   - Cat litter
   - Vinegar

The nursing team begins more frequent wound irrigation, including premedication for any wound pain. Charcoal dressings are used for the odor. After two weeks, the wound smells better when covered, but it still has excessive exudates and a foul odor when wound dressing is removed.

The dressing is changed to an alginate to better absorb the exudates, and some necrotic material is debrided chemically. The exudates decrease, but the wound odor continues. Topical metronizadole gel is applied to the wound daily with a foam dressing. The wound maintains a moist environment without exudates, and the patient and daughter note a decrease in odor in two days, with almost complete resolution in one week. The metronizadole gel is continued for an additional five days. The patient returns to her daughter's house, where she continues to receive regularly scheduled wound care visits by a home care nurse.

TAKE-HOME POINTS

- Necrotic tissue and bacteria cause wound odor.
- Foul odor emanating from a wound can lead to social isolation, depression, and diminished quality of life for the patient, and distress for caregivers, family members, and professionals.
- The goals of treatment include reducing or eliminating odor, absorbing exudates, controlling pain, managing infection, and improving quality of life.
- Treatment options include debridement to remove necrotic tissue, topical odor control (metronidazole gel, antibiotic cream, charcoal impregnated dressings), and systemic antibiotics where clinically indicated and if consistent with the goals of care.

REFERENCES

1. Fleck CA. Fighting odor in wounds. *Adv Skin Wound Care*. 2006;*19*(5):242–244.
2. Dowsett C. Malignant fungating wounds: Assessment and management. *Br J Community Nurs*. 2002;*7*(8):394–400.
3. Helm T. Dermatologic Manifestations of Metastatic Carcinoma of the Skin. *Medscape*, 2010. http:// emedicine.medscape.com/article/1101058. Accessed June 2013.
4. Langemo D, Anderson J, Hanson D, et al. Managing fungating wounds. *Adv Skin Wound Care*. 2007;*20*(6):312–314.
5. Bale S, Tebble N, Price P. A topical metronidazole gel used to treat malodorous wounds. *Br J Nurs*. 2004;*13*(11):S4–S11.
6. Kalinski C, et al. Effectiveness of a topical formulation containing metronidazole for wound odor and exudate control. *Wounds*. 2005;*17*(4):84–90.
7. Alvarez O, et al. Incorporating wound healing strategies to improve palliation (symptom management) in patients with chronic wounds. *J Palliat Med*. 2007;*10*(5):1161–1189.
8. Ashford R, Plant G, Maher J, et al. Double-blind trial of metronidazole in malodorous ulcerating tumors. *Lancet*. 1984;*323*(8388):1232–1233.
9. Bower M, Stein R, Evans T, et al. A double-blind study of the efficacy of metronidazole gel in the treatment of malodorous fungating tumor. *Eur J Cancer*. 1992;*28A*:888–889.
10. Bauer C, Gerlach M, Doughty D. Care of metastatic skin lesions. *J Wound Ostomy Continence Nurs*. 2000;*27*:247–251.
11. Lee G, Anand S, Rajendran S. Efficacy of commercial dressings in managing malodorous wounds. *Br J Nurs*. 2007;*16*(6):S14–S20.
12. Wilson V. Assessment and management of fungating wounds: A review. *Br J Community Nurs*. 2005;*10*(5):S28–S34.
13. Lee D, Sino S, Khachemoune A. Honey and wound healing: an overview. *Am J Clin Dermatol*. 2011; *12*(3):181–190.
14. Cornwell P, Arnold-Long M, Barss S, Varnado M. The use of Dakin's solution in chronic wounds: a clinical perspective case series. *J Wound Ostomy Continence Nurs*. 2010;*37*(1):94–104.

SECTION V

Diseases and Syndromes

62

Frailty

CASE

Mrs. K is a 92-year-old woman with long-standing bronchiectasis. Over the last few years she has had increasing complaints of fatigue and in the last three months has experienced two hospitalizations related to pneumonia and hyponatremia. During her most recent hospitalization, she was diagnosed with heart failure related to aortic regurgitation. Since these hospital admissions, it has become increasingly difficult for her to make her outpatient doctor appointments. She has lost 20 lbs in the last year. Although she remains independent in her activities of daily living, she finds it exhausting to keep up with her apartment and has hired a helper for some tasks during the week. She reluctantly admits to a fall one week prior when she felt weak on the way to the bathroom, but minimizes the event and denies injury. She admits to a depressed mood and has anxiety over what her future holds.

DEFINITION

Frailty is a physiologic syndrome of aging that is associated with a high risk for adverse outcomes. While definitions vary, most include the following symptoms:

- Weakness
- Fatigue
- Weight loss, loss of muscle mass (sarcopenia)
- Slowed performance
- Low activity
- Possibly: cognitive compromise or depression

PREVALENCE

Because definitions vary, prevalence is difficult to measure. However, in community-dwelling older adults, estimates of the prevalence of frailty ranges from 6% to 25% of those >65 and up to 36% of those aged 85 years and older.[1] The prevalence of frailty increases with age, multi-morbidity, and illness severity.

LIKELY ETIOLOGIES

Frailty is not the outcome of a single etiology but rather reflects a cycle of physiologic decline marked by sarcopenia, immune dysfunction, neuroendocrine dysregulation, and molecular mechanisms (Figure 62.1). This decline can be age-related and/or impacted by disease.[2]

DIAGNOSIS

History and Exam

A comprehensive history and exam should include screens for weight loss, weakness, fatigue, pain, cognition, depression, and falls (Table 62.1). Additionally, clinicians should assess how many of these factors may be impacting activities of daily living (ADLs) and also identify any underlying conditions that may be exacerbating symptoms.

Tests

There are no specific tests for frailty, and frailty remains a clinical diagnosis based on history and physical exam.

TREATMENT OPTIONS

Treatment should focus on symptom management and psychosocial support. Table 62.2 summarizes management recommendations for common symptoms related to frailty.

PALLIATIVE CARE ISSUES

- When frailty is associated with advanced illness, symptoms will likely progress as the disease progresses. However, timely recognition of frailty is important, since it may help uncover treatable underlying conditions such as medication interactions, depression, or infection.[5]
- Frailty itself is predictive of adverse outcomes, including further functional decline, falls, recurrent hospitalizations, and death. As with many chronic diseases

TABLE 62.1: ASSESSMENT OF FRAILTY[3]

Frailty Characteristic	Assessment
Unintentional weight loss (> 10 pounds in the last year)	"In the last year, have you lost more than 10 pounds unintentionally (i.e., not due to dieting or exercise)?"
Weakness/loss of strength (lowest 20% by gender/body mass index)	*Women* ≤ 17 kg for BMI ≤ 23 ≤ 17.3 kg for BMI ≤ 23.1–26 ≤ 18 kg for BMI ≤ 26.1–29 ≤ 21kg for BMI ≤ *Men* ≤ 29 kg for BMI ≤ 24 ≤ 30 kg for BMI 24.1–26 ≤ 30 kg for BMI 26.1–28 ≤ 32 kg for BMI > 28
Fatigue	Self-report of feeling that everything done in the last week "was an effort," or "inability to get going" in the last week
Slowness	Observed walking for 15 feet at usual pace: *Women* Time ≥ 7 sec for height ≤ 159 cm Time ≥ 6 sec for height >159 cm *Men* Time ≥ 7 sec for height ≤ 173 cm Time ≥ 6 sec for height > 173 cm
Low physical activity	Minnesota Leisure Time activity questionnaire (short version) Women: energy < 270 kcal on activity scale (18 items) Men: energy < 383 kcal on activity scale (18 items)

TABLE 62.2: FRAILTY MANAGEMENT RECOMMENDATIONS[4]

Symptom	Management Recommendations	Specific Interventions for Mrs. K
Weight loss	Liberalize diet restrictions Recommend frequent, small meals Consider nutritional drinks Address oral care, denture problems Inquire about access to food (See Chapter 42: Anorexia and Cachexia)	*Family meeting to explain the weight loss as a reflection of her progressive disease* *Addition of oral nutritional supplement, as tolerated* *Foods of choice are encouraged. Mrs. K had previously been quite dedicated to a "healthy diet" and now allows herself chocolate daily.*
Weakness/Slowness	Recommend strength training Recommend tai chi if available Consider referral for rehab evaluation or physical therapy	*Physical therapy was initiated due to falls, but had added benefit in supporting energy conservation techniques such as implementing bedside commode.* *Use of wheelchair encouraged for transport so Mrs. K could then walk to the table at a restaurant or stand for a bit to socialize with friends, maximizing meaningful relational interactions*

(continued)

TABLE 62.2: (CONTINUED)

Symptom	Management Recommendations	Specific Interventions for Mrs. K
Fatigue	Educate re: energy conservation Treat underlying conditions (heart failure, anemia, insomnia, etc.) Review and eliminate medications that cause fatigue Increase physical activity (See Chapter 30: Fatigue)	*A review of Mrs. K's prescriptions does not identify any medications known for sedation.* *Physical therapy sessions will increase physical activity; teach energy conservations.*
Depression	Prescribe selective serotonin reuptake inhibitors (SSRIs) Explore patient's concerns Offer information about support groups Consider cognitive behavioral therapy Schedule more frequent follow-up appointments (See Chapter 64: Depression)	*Mrs. K was unable to tolerate multiple classes of antidepressants due to side effects and/or hyponatremia.* *Initiated home visit cognitive behavioral therapy for depression and anxiety* *Although benzodiazepines are not first-line agents for anxiety treatment in older adults, low-dose lorazepam 0.5mg, ½ tab every 8 hours was effective in easing her anxiety symptoms.*
Falls	Review and eliminate medications that may contribute to falls Educate re: home safety; order home safety assessment Recommend strength and balls exercises Consider physical therapy referral (See Chapter 63: Falls)	*Refer to physical therapy for balance, strengthening, and education on safe transfers* *Educate family and patient about environment optimization, i.e., removal of throw rugs, addition of grab bars to her bathroom.*
Pain	Prescribe an analgesic on a standing or regular basis, with doses as needed for pain not controlled by standing order Prescribe a laxative for patients receiving opioids (See Chapter 29: Management of Pain in Older Adults)	*Mrs. K does not have pain.*

and syndromes, prognostication can be challenging because death is often caused by unpredictable infections and other complications.

- The National Hospice and Palliative Care Organization has published guidelines for determining prognosis for non-cancer diseases that can be applied to frail older adults. Guideline criteria include:
  - Multiple emergency department visits or inpatient hospitalizations over the prior six months
  - A recent decline in functional status
  - Unintentional, progressive weight loss of more than 10% over the prior six months

TAKE-HOME POINTS

- Frailty is a well-recognized clinical syndrome that is predictive of adverse geriatric outcomes.
- Recognition of frailty and targeted interventions may benefit patients by preventing frailty or by preventing the adverse outcomes of frailty.
- Prognostication for frailty can be challenging because death is often caused by unpredictable infections and other complications. National Hospice and Palliative Care Organization guidelines for determining prognosis for non-cancer

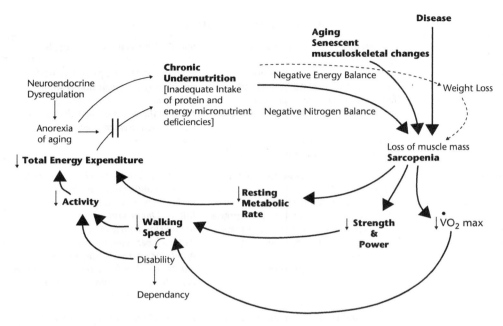

FIGURE 62.1: Cycle of frailty.

diseases can be applied to frail older adults. They include:

- Multiple emergency department visits or inpatient hospitalizations over the prior six months
- A recent decline in functional status
- Unintentional, progressive weight loss of more than 10% over the prior six months

REFERENCES

1. Rockwood K, Howlet SE, MacKnight C, et al. Prevalence, attributes, and outcomes of fitness and frailty in community-dwelling older adults: report from the Canadian Study of Health and Aging. *J Gerontol A Biol Sci Med Sci.* 2004;59:1310–1317.

2. Fried LP, Walston J. Frailty and failure to thrive. In: Hazzard WR, Blass JP, Ettinger WH Jr, Halter JB, Ouslander J, eds. *Principles of Geriatric Medicine and Gerontology* 4th ed. New York NY: McGraw Hill; 1998;1387–1402.

3. Fried LP, Tangen CM, Walston J, Newman AB, et al. Frailty in older adults; evidence for a phenotype. *J Gerontol.* 2001;56(3):M146–156A.

4. Boockvar KS, Meier DM. Palliative care for frail older adults: "There are things I can't do anymore that I wish I could…" *JAMA.* 2006;296(18): 2245–2253.

5. Walston J, Fried L. *Frailty and Its Implications for Care.* in Meier DE and Morrison RS (Eds). Geriatric Palliative Care. Oxford University Press; New York, NY. 2003; pp. 93–109.

63

Falls

CASE

Mrs. C is an 81-year-old female with hypertension, osteoarthritis, and depression who comes in for an evaluation after a recent fall. She reports rushing to answer the phone and tripping in her kitchen. She denies any chest pain, palpitations, loss of consciousness, head trauma, or other injury. She acknowledges she was wearing her reading glasses at the time, and because she was in a hurry, she was not using her cane. This is the second fall she has had this year, and she'd like advice on how she can prevent future falls. She has become reluctant to go out on her own because she is afraid of falling.

DEFINITION

A fall is defined as unintentionally coming to rest on the ground or other lower level not due to overwhelming intrinsic or environmental cause and without loss of consciousness.

PREVALENCE

- Approximately 30% of community-dwelling adults over the age of 65, and 50% of those in long-term care will fall every year.[1]
- A third of these falls result in injury and 5% to 10% result in serious injury such as lacerations, fractures, or head trauma.[1] These injuries, in turn, can cause pain, functional impairment, disability, and even death.
- Unintentional injury is the fifth leading cause of death in the elderly.[2] Falls or fear of them can lead to withdrawal, deconditioning, social isolation, depression, and loss of independence.
- Falls are a leading cause of nursing home placement.[1]

LIKELY ETIOLOGIES

- Rates of falling and injury increase with age, as older adults are more susceptible due to multiple medical problems and age-related physiologic decline.
- Older adults accumulate impairments in multiple domains that predispose them to falling when exposed to precipitating challenges, such as acute illness or tripping hazards (Figure 63.1).

Most Common Risk Factors[2]

More than 25 risk factors for falling have been identified in over 80 studies, and the risk of falling increases with increasing number of risk factors.[1]

- Muscles weakness
- History of falls
- Gait impairment
- Balance problems
- Poor vision
- Arthritis
- Depression
- Cognitive impairment at age > 80
- ADL dependency
- Polypharmacy
- Environmental hazards
  - Clutter obstructing walking paths
  - Electric cords
  - Slippery throw rugs and loose carpets
  - Poor lighting
  - Lack of nonslip bathmats or grab bars
  - Unsafe footwear
  - Climbing or descending stairs

High-Risk Medications for Falls[1]

Polypharmacy, defined as the use of four or more medications simultaneously and common among older adults, is a risk factor for falling. The following specific medications are also associated with increased fall risk:

- Anticonvulsants
- Benzodiazepines
- Class IA antiarrhythmics
- Neuroleptics
- Serotonin reuptake inhibitors
- Tricyclic antidepressants

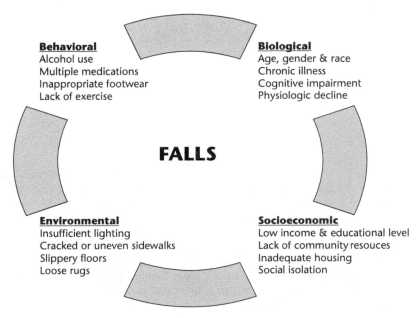

Behavioral
Alcohol use
Multiple medications
Inappropriate footwear
Lack of exercise

Biological
Age, gender & race
Chronic illness
Cognitive impairment
Physiologic decline

FALLS

Environmental
Insufficient lighting
Cracked or uneven sidewalks
Slippery floors
Loose rugs

Socioeconomic
Low income & educational level
Lack of community resouces
Inadequate housing
Social isolation

FIGURE 63.1: Fall risk factors.

FALLS AND PALLIATIVE CARE PATIENTS

In addition to polypharmacy and the use of high-risk medications, delirium was identified as a significant factor in falls of cancer patients hospitalized for palliative care.[3]

Mrs. C had several risk factors for falling:

- *History of arthritis and depression*
- *Wasn't using assistive device and was wearing reading glasses at time of fall*
- *Possible tripping hazards in the home*
- *Fear of falling and restriction of activity that further increases risk of falling*

DIAGNOSIS

Fall History

- Circumstances and associated symptoms
- Chronic conditions
- Medications
- Functional status and mobility
- Substance use

Exam

- Orthostatic vital signs
- Visual acuity testing
- Musculoskeletal and neurologic exam
- Gait and balance assessment
- Cognitive evaluation

Tests

Recommended routine tests include:

- EKG
- Complete blood count
- Chemistry panel
- TSH
- Vitamin B12 level
- Vitamin D level
- Drug levels (such as digoxin, or INR if on anticoagulation)

If indicated by individual fall history may include:

- Imaging studies (X-rays, head CT, etc.)
- Cardiac testing for arrhythmia
- EEG or vestibular testing

EXPECTED DISEASE COURSE

- Half of those individuals who fall will do so repeatedly, so prevention is crucial. Risk factors such as age, sex, cognitive impairment, and certain medical conditions are intrinsic and cannot be changed.
- Other risk factors, such as poor balance, impaired gait or muscle strength, depression, orthostasis, vision impairment, or polypharmacy can potentially be modified.[1]

TREATMENT OPTIONS

- Interventions that are effective in preventing falls in community-dwelling older adults:
  - Professionally supervised balance and gait training, and/or vestibular rehabilitation
  - Tai chi group exercise
  - Dose reduction/withdrawal of high-risk medications
  - Home hazard modifications in patients with history of falls
  - Cardiac pacing in appropriate patients

- The most consistently effective approach is a multifactorial assessment with targeted interventions including medication review and reduction; strength, balance, and gait training; management of postural hypotension, and environmental modifications.[1] (Table 63.1)

SETTING CONSIDERATIONS

- In contrast to the evidence pointing to successful management of fall risk in the community, interventions to prevent falls have not consistently been proven

TABLE 63.1: THERAPEUTIC APPROACH TO FALL PREVENTION

Risk Factor	Provider Intervention	Patient Education
Polypharmacy (4 or more medications)	Review and reduce medications at every visit Avoid high-risk medications Prescribe nonpharmacological treatments, like exercise, whenever possible	Keep an updated medication list and bring it to every visit with all health care providers Buy all medications at one pharmacy and do not take over-the-counter medications without asking your physician Inquire about side effects or interactions with medications you are already taking
Gait instability	Physical therapy for strength, balance, and gait training Recommend tai chi Prescribe an assistive device (such as cane or walker) and review patient's use of it	Stand upright, take full steps Use caution on stairs and uneven ground Correctly use walking aid such as a cane or walker Keep hands free to use railings Consider an emergency call device to use in the case of a fall
Postural hypotension	Check orthostatic vital signs *Geriatric tip:* BP is a more sensitive indicator of orthostasis than HR in older adults Reduce medications that may contribute Liberalize salt in patient's diet	Drink sufficient water every day Get up from sitting slowly Clench your fists and pump your ankles 10 times before standing to help raise your blood pressure a little before you get up
Vision impairment	Ask about vision problems, such as difficulty driving, watching TV, or reading due to poor vision Test visual acuity and consider ophthalmology referral	Have yearly vision checkups Keep eyeglasses clean and never walk while wearing reading glasses Allow time for eyes to adjust to changing levels of light Ensure adequate lighting throughout the home
Environmental hazards	Do home visit or refer to visiting nurse to assess home safety Give patient or caregiver checklist to assess home hazards (available from www.stopfalls.org or www.homesafetycouncil.org)	Use nightlights Install grab bars and bathmats Remove slippery throw rugs Wear appropriate footwear that covers entire foot and has thin sole with low heel

effective in long-term care and acute-care settings.[4]

- However, given the many elements that contribute to falls in older adults, a multifactorial assessment with targeted interventions as outlined above is still the recommended approach to patients in these settings.

Mrs. C's orthostatics are checked to see if her antihypertensive medications need to be decreased. A medication review is conducted for possible reduction of any that are unecessary, particularly psychotropics. She receives a referral for PT and information about how to join a local tai chi class for seniors, not only for a socializing opportunity but also to improve balance. Mrs. C is also given an individualized home safety checklist that addresses the tripping hazards in her home.

TAKE-HOME POINTS

- Clinicians should ask all older adults about any falls in the past year.
- Assess for five modifiable risk factors: polypharmacy, vision impairment, orthostasis, gait and balance instability, and environmental hazards.
- Consider withdrawal or dose reduction of high-risk medications.

- For palliative care patients, prevention and management of delirium is important.
- Patients and caregivers should receive education on strategies to prevent falls.

REFERENCES

1. Tinetti ME. Preventing falls in elderly persons. *N Engl J Med.* Jan 2003;*348*(1):42–49.
2. American Geriatrics Society, British Geriatrics Society, and American Academy of Orthopedic Surgeons Panel on Falls Prevention. Guideline for the prevention of falls in older persons. *J Am Geriatr Soc.* 2001;*49*:664–672.
3. Pautex S, Hermann FR, Zulian GB. Factors associated with falls in patients with cancer hospitalized for palliative care. *J Palliat Med.* July/August 2008;*11*(6):878–884.
4. Coussement J, De Paepe L, Schwendimann R, Denhaerynck K, Dejaeger E, Milisen K. Interventions for preventing falls in acute- and chronic-care hospitals: A systematic review and meta-analysis. *J Am Geriatr Soc.* Jan 2008;*56*(1): 29–36.

64

Depression

CASE

Mrs. B is an 80-year-old with a history of coronary artery disease, hypertension, anemia, and advanced heart failure (EF 15%) who is admitted to hospital with dehydration and is found to have weight loss of eight pounds over past two months. She had two recent hospital admissions for worsening dyspnea at rest. Patient reports loss of appetite, lack of energy, and loss of interest in going to her senior center and playing bingo, which she has enjoyed in the past. The visiting nurse alerts you that recently Mrs. B has reported being distressed by her progressive dependence.

On her follow-up visit, Mrs. B appears sad. She denies suicidal ideation and says she does not have a fear of death. Her goals of care include a preference for comfort care. She has repeatedly declined any invasive treatment including AICD placement. Patient has no history of depression or anxiety.

DEFINITION

Depression is a psychiatric syndrome of dysphoric mood and associated symptoms (Table 64.1), present for a significant period of time. Depression is a real and serious illness. Older adults with advanced diseases are particularly vulnerable to depression.

PREVALENCE

- Depression in older adults ranges from 5% to 10%. Prevalence of depression with advanced and life-threatening conditions is up to 75%.[1]
- In a study of older adults with serious illness (CHF and cancer) who visited the emergency department, over 50% of patients met criteria for intervention for anxiety and depression.[2]
- Although there are many studies on depression in cancer patients, there are relatively limited published data on depression in elderly patients with other serious illnesses. Information in this chapter has therefore been extrapolated

from existing data on patients with cancer and depression in older adults without serious illness, as well as expert opinion.

CONSEQUENCES OF UNTREATED DEPRESSION

Untreated depression in older adults augments disability and has a negative impact on quality of life. Depression in late life is also associated with medical morbidity and mortality.[3] Depression is often unrecognized and untreated due to:

- Patient reluctance to report the symptoms of depression
- Difficult distinction between depression symptoms and "appropriate sadness" or normal grief
- Difficulty differentiating vegetative symptoms of depression from underlying medical disease (anorexia, weight loss, lack of energy, sleep disturbance, etc.)

TABLE 64.1: DSM-IV CRITERIA FOR MAJOR DEPRESSION

Five or more of the following symptoms with at least one symptom being either depressed mood or anhedonia:
Persistent low or depressed mood
Anhedonia
Significant weight loss or gain
Insomnia or hypersomnia
Psychomotor agitation or retardation
Fatigue or loss of energy nearly every day
Feelings or loss of energy nearly every day
Diminished ability to think or concentrate or indecisiveness nearly every day
Recurrent thought of death (not just fear of dying, recurrent suicidal ideation)

Adapted from Major Depressive Episode. In: *Diagnostic and Statistical Manual of Mental Disorders, Fourth Edition*. Washington, DC: American Psychiatric Association, pp. 349–356.

- Believing depression is a normal reaction to advanced illness
- Concerns about the cost of treatment, interactions, and medication side effects
- Initiating treatment late in the process of illness when there is insufficient time for therapeutic benefit

RISK FACTORS

- In a systemic review and meta-analysis, significant risk factors for depression in community-dwelling elderly included bereavement, sleep disturbance, disability, prior depression, and female gender.[4]
- In palliative care patients, prominent risk factors included terminal diagnosis, comorbidities, physical disability, and poor pain management (Table 64.2).[5]

TABLE 64.2: RISK FACTORS FOR DEPRESSION IN PALLIATIVE CARE PATIENTS[5]

Having a terminal diagnosis

Certain types of cancer: pancreatic cancer, brain tumors

Comorbidities: hypothyroidism, coronary artery disease, macular degeneration, diabetes mellitus, Alzheimer's disease, Parkinson's disease, multiple sclerosis, stroke, Huntington's disease

Physical disability

Poor pain and symptom control

Metabolic abnormalities: hypercalcemia, tumor-generated toxins, uremia, abnormal liver function

Medications: amphotericin, centrally acting antihypertensive agents, H2-blockers, metoclopramide, cytotoxic drugs, corticosteroids, interferon, interleukin

Radiation therapy

Malnutrition

Cognitive loss

Previous personal history of depression

Family history of depression

Age of the patient, more common in younger patients

Request to withhold or withdraw treatment

Requests for assisted suicide

Substance abuse

Poor social support

Lack of close confiding relationships

Financial strain

DEPRESSION AND RISK OF SUICIDE IN PATIENTS WITH SERIOUS ILLNESS

- Although there is an increased risk for suicidal ideations in patients with cancer associated with poor performance status, advanced stages, and depression, the most significant risk factors are older age and severe depression.[6]
- Although some studies associated pain with increased suicidality in patients with cancer,[7,8] several other studies failed to show any significant associations in cancer patients receiving palliative care.[9,10] However, pain is known to be significantly associated with declining physical functioning, and therefore could contribute to suicidal ideation even if direct association is not shown.[11]

DIAGNOSIS

- Because depression is very common and unrecognized in the elderly with advanced and serious illness, it is important to screen for depression in this group of patients.
- Depression should be distinguished from grief, which is the universal emotional response to the loss or absence of someone or something previously present and valued. See Table 64.3 for a comparison of grief vs. depression in patients at the end of life.[12]

History

A thorough history should be elicited, paying particular attention to risk factors such as life stressors, previous episodes of depression, family history of depression or suicide, substance abuse, and social supports.

Screening

- Depression is common and often unrecognized in the elderly. It is very challenging to differentiate symptoms of depression from normal reaction to life-threatening conditions; therefore, it is important to screen the older adults with serious illness for depression (Table 64.3).
- Useful assessment tools include the Patient Health Questionnaire (PHQ9, http://www.integration.samhsa.gov/images/res/PHQ%20-%20Questions.pdf), the Geriatric Depression Scale (http://www.stanford.edu/~yesavage/GDS.html), and a single-item question: "Are you depressed?"

TABLE 64.3: GRIEF VS. DEPRESSION IN TERMINALLY ILL PATIENTS[12]

Dimension	Grief	Depression
Symptoms	Sleep and appetite disturbance, change in behavior patterns, agitation, impaired concentration, social withdrawal	Symptoms are similar, but in addition there are feelings of worthlessness, guilt, hopelessness, and thoughts of suicide
Prevalence	Almost all terminally ill patients experience grief.	Major depression occurs in 1%–53% of terminally ill patients
Intensity	Feelings and emotions result from a particular loss Patients can usually cope with this level of distress on their own.	Patients experience feelings and behaviors that meet criteria for a major psychiatric disorder. Medical or psychiatric intervention is usually necessary
Duration	Episodic Feelings advance and recede in waves	Constant and unremitting
Thinking about death	May report passive wishes for a hastened death	Persistent and intense suicidal ideation
Hope for the future	Patients have capacity for pleasure; able to look forward to the future	No enjoyment in life; no ability to see future in positive terms

Applying Diagnostic Criteria to Geriatric Palliative Care Patients

- It is difficult to differentiate the physical symptoms of depression (weight change, fatigue, and loss of energy) from underlying medical conditions in older patients with serious illness.[13]
- Assessment may be further complicated by conditions such as delirium, cognitive impairment, and dementia in older adults.
- Clinicians are therefore advised to focus their attention on the cognitive symptoms of worthlessness, hopelessness, excessive guilt, and thoughts of self-harm.[14]
- Endicott proposes the following "substitutions" for DSM-IV depression criteria in cancer patients that may also be generalizable to other patients with serious illness:[15,16]
  - Tearfulness or depressed appearance
  - Brooding, self-pity, pessimism
  - Social withdrawal
  - Lack of reactivity, cannot be cheered up

Tests

Workup should focus on ruling out reversible medical problems that can present with depression as a symptom. Test for electrolytes, calcium, and thyroid function.

TREATMENT OPTIONS

- In patients with serious illness, pharmacologic and nonpharmacologic interventions should be employed simultaneously.
- Intervention trials should be at least 3 weeks in duration to allow effectiveness to be determined. In the event of acute suicidal ideation, inpatient treatment and psychiatry consultation is indicated for close monitoring of medications, which should be titrated up to the effective dose quickly and evaluated more rapidly. ECT may also be considered.
- Even in patients with limited prognosis, treatment of depression can improve quality of life and should be addressed. For patients with life expectancy < 6 weeks, consider psychostimulants like methylphenidate and modafinil for faster onset of action.
- Appropriate referral to community mental health or home health services, or to hospice as indicated, will ensure ongoing monitoring and support.

Nonpharmacologic Treatment
Psychotherapy

- There are limited controlled trials of psychotherapy in older patients with serious medical illness. Some clinical reports suggest that pharmacological treatment is likely to be more effective in treatment of depression in older adults with serious medical illness when offered concurrently with supportive psychotherapy, especially therapeutic modalities that promote adaptive coping.[17]

- Psychological treatment is the preferred modality for patients who are unable to tolerate pharmacologic treatment. The two most common methods evaluated in clinical studies or described by pilot reports are Problem solving therapy and Reminiscence therapy. Other methods used with seriously ill patients include Dignity psychotherapy and Meaning-centered group psychotherapy.

  - *Problem solving therapy (PST)*: a structured time-limited treatment that focuses on building effective coping skills by helping the patient set achievable goals to solve practical and social problems. Patients with life expectancy of months to a year are potentially appropriate candidates for this intervention.
  - *Reminiscence therapy*: based on facilitated recollection and sharing of past experiences to enhance well-being and interpersonal functioning.
  - *Dignity psychotherapy*: shown to enhance sense of meaning, purpose, and well-being at the end of life by leaving a written legacy behind for loved ones.[18]
  - *Meaning-centered group psychotherapy*: helps patients with serious illness develop and/or maintain a sense of meaning and purpose in life. It is an eight-week intervention and involves life story telling, psycho-education and experiential exercises.

- Both reminiscence and dignity psychotherapy are appropriate for patients with serious medical illness and can be used in patients with life expectancy of days-to-week, and weeks-to-month. Meaning-centered group psychotherapy can be used in patients with life expectancy of months-to-year.
- These treatments are offered by psychotherapists or psychologists; other clinicians on the palliative care team (LSW, NP, and RN) can also be trained to offer these methods to patients when appropriate.

Electroconvulsive Therapy (ECT)

- ECT is a safe and effective treatment for older adults with depression that is refractory to other treatment modalities; data available on efficacy is limited, mainly in case reports[19,20]
- ECT is a treatment of choice for older adults who are unable to tolerate oral treatment or have psychotic features. ECT should also be considered in the event of comorbid severe mood disorder, significant disability associated with depression, or poor or no response to trial of treatment
- Although there is no absolute contraindication for ECT, the following specific conditions may be associated with substantially increased risk and should be carefully weighed when considering ECT treatment:[21,22]
  1. Cardiovascular/CNS:
     - Unstable or severe cardiovascular conditions such as recent myocardial infarction, poorly compensated congestive heart failure, and severe valvular cardiac disease
     - Aneurysm or vascular malformation that might be susceptible to rupture with increased blood pressure
     - Increased intracranial pressure, as may occur with some brain tumors or other space-occupying cerebral lesions including subdural hematoma, intracranial arachnoid cysts, or normal-pressure hydrocephalus
     - Recent cerebral infarction
  2. Pulmonary conditions such as severe chronic obstructive pulmonary disease, asthma, or pneumonia
  3. Metabolic abnormality (hypo- or hyperkalemia)
  4. Anesthetic risk rated as ASA level 4 or 5.
     - Although there is an increased risk of complications with ECT in older adults due to comorbid medical and neurological conditions, a recent study comparing frequency of side effects with ECT compared to pharmacotherapy showed that ECT resulted in fewer side effects (particularly cardiovascular and gastrointestinal) and greater efficacy than pharmacological management.[23] This study emphasizes that ECT might be a safer and perhaps the most effective form of treatment and should be considered in carefully selected older adults.

Pharmacologic Treatment

- For moderate to severe late-life depression, psychotherapy should be supplemented with pharmacotherapy (Table 64.4).
- In older adults, initial dosing should be reduced due to potential for side effects and decreased drug clearance; medications may not show efficacy for four to six weeks.
- Older patients may be hesitant to take medication to treat their depression.

During the exam, Mrs. B appears withdrawn and lacks her usual humor. She scores 16 in PHQ9 questionnaire. You explain that her depression is very likely causing her recent symptoms, and you both agree to start her on sertraline 25 mg and mirtazapine 7.5 mg at night to help with her sleep and appetite. You also make a referral to a psychotherapist. She will return for a follow-up appointment in three weeks.

MANAGEMENT OF DEPRESSION AS A CHRONIC DISEASE

- Depression is a relapsing illness; treatment should be continued if well tolerated.
- Comorbidities require the clinician to consider medication side effects and interactions including nausea, vomiting, and loss of appetite.
- Antidepressants are available only in the oral form, limiting access for some patients. If patient is unable to take oral medication, nonpharmacological treatment and perhaps ECT should be considered.
- Depression is a burden for family members who are already stressed by the demands of caregiving for loved ones with serious medical illness. Clinicians should inquire about family members' medical and emotional health. Clinicians should also educate family members about the effects of depression and the role of its treatment for the patient's general well-being.

At a follow-up appointment, Mrs. B reports some improvement in her appetite, sleep, and energy level, although she continues to lack the motivation to return to her senior center and resume her favorite activities. She has been receiving weekly psychotherapy. After confirming that she does not have hyponatremia, you decide to increase her sertraline to 50 mg daily, and to continue with mirtazapine at 7.5 mg at night.

WHEN TO REFER TO PSYCHIATRY[24]

- Clinician is uncertain about diagnosis and treatment of depression
- For patients with poor response to initial treatment trial
- Complex presentation, e.g., psychotic depression
- Patient is suicidal
- Patient is requesting a hastened death
- If clinician is considering ECT as a treatment option

WHEN TO CONSIDER HOSPITALIZATION

If patient is actively suicidal, has life-threatening weight loss, or in the event of limited oral intake or dehydration, consider hospitalization for assessment and determination of an appropriate intervention.

PALLIATIVE CARE COMANAGEMENT

In an RCT of lung cancer patients, palliative care comanagement (offered at the same time as primary oncology care) was shown to markedly reduce depression through a combination of pharmacotherapy and intensive psychological support.[25]

TAKE-HOME POINTS

- Depression is common among older adults with serious illness.
- Depression in older adults with serious illness is often unrecognized because of difficulty in differentiating symptoms of illness from depression.
- Remain hypervigilant in diagnosing and treating depression in older patients with serious illness. Treatment of depression is likely to improve patients' quality of life.
- When treating depression in older adults with serious medical illness (especially patients with life expectancy of days-to-week, or weeks-to-month), consider psychostimulants because of rapid onset of action, decreased sedation from opioids, and tolerable side-effect profile.
- Consider ECT if patient is not responding to above treatment within three to six weeks of optimal treatment, or has life-threatening weight loss, limited oral intake, or dehydration.

TABLE 64.4: PHARMACOLOGIC TREATMENT

A. For Patients with Prognosis of Months to Years:

Class of Drug	Medication	Half-life(hrs)	Dosage (mg/day)	Most Common Side Effects	Precautions	Most Useful
Tricyclic antidepressant	Desipramine	14.3–24.7	10–100	Anticholinergic side effects	Anticholinergic side effects	In patients with seizure Sedation is desirable
	Nortriptyline	15–39	10–100	Anticholinergic side effects	Anticholinergic side effects	In patients with seizure Sedation is not desirable
SSRIs	Citalopram	33–37	20–40	Hyponatremia, headache, nausea, dizziness	Dose adjustment in patient with severe renal impairment	
	Escitalopram	22–32	10–20	Hyponatremia, headache, nausea		If anxiety and depression coexist
	Fluoxetine	4–6 days	10–60	Hyponatremia, loss of appetite, nausea	Multiple drug-drug interaction due to extensive P450 CYP2D6 metabolisim Risk of withdrawal if abruptly stopped	
	Paroxetine	15–22	25–75	Diaphoresis, loss of appetite, nausea, hyponatremia	Multiple drug-drug interaction due to extensive P450 CYP2D6 metabolisim Risk of withdrawal if abruptly stopped	
	Sertraline	22–32	25–200	Hyponatremia	Lower dose in liver impairment	
SNRIs	Duloxetine	11–16	30–90	Diaphoresis, nausea, diarrhea, dizziness	Do not use in patients with hepatic failure Adjust dose in patients with renal impairment	If anxiety and depression coexist Also in patients with neuropathic pain

	Drug	Half-life	Dose (mg)	Adverse effects	Dose adjustment	Comments
Others	Venlafaxine	3–7	37.5–375	Hypertension (much less with extended-release form) dizziness, nausea	Dose adjustment in patient with liver and renal impairment Risk of withdrawal if abruptly stopped	If anxiety and depression coexist
	Bupropion	12–30	100–450	Headache, insomnia	Reduce dose and frequency in patients with hepatic and renal failure	It inhibits weakly the neuronal uptake of dopamine, therefore preferred in treatment of depression in patients with Parkinson's disease
	Mirtazapine[a]	25–40	7.5–45	Increased appetite, weight gain, somnolence	Increase dose slowly in patient with liver and renal impairment (CrCl < 40 ml/min)	When goals are increased appetite, improved oral intake and improved sleep

B. For Patients with Prognosis Measured in Days to Weeks:[b]

	Drug	Half-life	Dose (mg)	Adverse effects	Dose adjustment	Comments
Psychostimulants	Methylphenidate	3–5	10–30 in divided dose, typically 8am and 12pm	Tachyarrhythmia, decrease in appetite	Tolerance and dependence are possible	As adjuvant in patient with life expectancy less than 6–12 weeks and when rapid onset of action is required To countereffect the excess sedation from opioids and other medications
	Modafinil	15	100–400	Headache, nausea, insomnia	Decrease dose to 50% in severe hepatic failure Less potential for tolerance and dependence	As adjuvant in patient with life expectancy less than 6–12 weeks and when rapid onset of action is required To countereffect the excess sedation from opioids

[a] Psychostimulants may initially be offered simultaneously with longer-acting ones to accelerate the onset of treatment effect in patients with limited life expectancy.
[b] Mirtazapine at low dose of 7.5mg–15 mg has substantial effect on insomnia and appetite that occurs within a few days. These features make mirtazapine a desirable treatment for patients with prognosis measured in days to weeks.

- Consider psychiatry referral and/or hospitalization if patient is actively suicidal, has life-threatening weight loss, or limited oral intake or dehydration.

REFERENCES

1. Periyakoil VJ, Hallenback J. Identifying and managing preparatory grief and depression in end of life. *Am FamPhysician*. 2002;*65*:883–890.
2. Grudzen CR, Richardson LD, Morrison M, et al. Palliative care needs of seriously ill, older adults presenting to the emergency department. *Acad Emerg Med*. Nov 2010;*17*(11):1253–1257.
3. Schoevers RA, Geerlings MI, Beekman AT, et al. Association of depression and gender with mortality in old age. Results from the Amsterdam Study of the Elderly (AMSTEL). *Br J Psychiatry*. Oct 2000;*177*:336–342.
4. Cole GM, Dendukuri N. Risk factors for depression among elderly community subjects: a systematic review and meta-analysis. *Am J Psychiatry*. 2003;*160*:1147–1156.
5. Wilson KG, Chochinov HM, de Faye BJ, Breitbart W. Diagnosis and management of depression in palliative care. In: Chochinov HM, Breitbart W, eds. *Handbook of Psychiatry in Palliative Medicine*. New York NY: Oxford. University Press; 2000;25–49.
6. Akechi T, Okamura H, Kugaya A, et al. Suicidal ideation in cancer patients with major depression. *Jpn J Clin Oncol*. 2000;*30*(5):221–224.
7. Baile WF, DiMaggio JR, Schapira DV, Janofsky JS. The request for assistance in dying—the need for psychiatric consultation. *Cancer*. 1993;*72*:2786–91.
8. Severson KT. Dying cancer patients: choices at the end of life. *J Pain Symptom Manage*. 1997;*14*:94–98.
9. Breitbart W, Rosenfeld B, Pessin H, et al. Depression, hopelessness and desire for hastened death in terminally ill patients with cancer. *J Am Med Assoc*. 2000;*284*:2907–2911.
10. Wilson KG, Scott JF, Graham ID, et al. Attitudes of terminally ill patients toward euthanasia and physician-assisted suicide. *Arch Intern Med*. 2000;*160*:2454–60.
11. Clinical Factors Associated with Suicidality in Cancer Patients. *Jpn. J Clin Oncol*. 2002;*32*(12):506–551.
12. Block SD. Assessing and managing depression in the terminally ill patient. *Ann Intern Med*. 2000;*132*:209–221.
13. Lloyd-Williams M. Difficulties in diagnosing and treating depression in the terminally ill cancer patient. *Postgrad Med J*. 2000;*76*:555–558.
14. Passik SD, Lundberg J, Rosenfeld B, et al. Factor analysis of the Zung Self-Rating Depression Scales in a large ambulatory sample of oncology patients. *Psychosomatics*. 2002;*41*:121–127.
15. Massie MJ, Shakin EJ. Management of depression and anxiety in cancer patients. *Psychiatric Aspects of Symptom Management in Cancer Patients*. Washington, DC: American Psychiatric Press; 1993;1–21.
16. Endicott J. Measurement of depression in patients with cancer. *Cancer*. 1984;*53*:2243–2248.
17. Wilson KG, Chochinov HM. Diagnosis and management of depression in palliative care. *Handbook of Psychiatry in Palliative Medicine*. New York, Oxford University Press; 2000;25–49.
18. Chochinov HM, Kristjanson LJ, Breitbart W, et al. Effect of dignity therapy on distress and end-of-life experience in terminally ill patients: a randomised controlled trial. *Lancet Oncol*. Aug 2011;*12*(8):753–762. Epub 2011 Jul 6.
19. Mulder ME, Verwey B, van Waarde JA. Electroconvulsive therapy in a terminally ill patient: when every day of improvement counts. *J ECT*. Mar 2012;*28*(1):52–53.
20. Rasmussen KG, Richardson JW. Electroconvulsive therapy in palliative care. *Am J Hosp Palliat Care*. Aug 2011;*28*(5):375–377. Epub 2010 Nov 17.
21. Weiner RD. *The Practice of Electroconvulsive Therapy, Recommendations for Treatment, Training and Privileging*. 2nd Edition. American Psychiatric Pub; 2001;27–30.
22. Weiner RD, Krystal AD. (2009) Electroconvulsive Therapy. In Blazer DG, Steffens DC. (Eds), *The American Psychiatric Publishing Textbook of Geriatric Psychiatry*, 4th Edition. Arlington, VA: American Psychiatric Publishing, Inc. doi:0.1176/appi.books.9781585623754.397112
23. Manly DT, Oakley SP Jr, Bloch RM. Electroconvulsive therapy in old-old patients. *Am J Geriatr Psychiatry*. 2000;*8*:232–236.
24. Block SD. Assessing and managing depression in the terminally ill patient. ACP-ASIM End-of-Life Care Consensus Panel. American College of Physicians—American Society of Internal Medicine. *Ann Intern Med*. Feb 1, 2000;*132*(3): 209–218.
25. Temel JS, Greer JA, Muzikansky A, et al. Early palliative care for patients with metastatic non-small-cell lung cancer. *N Engl J Med*. 2010;*363*: 733–742.

65

Anxiety

CASE

You are called by the floor nurse to see Mrs. J, a 75-year-old woman with metastatic colon cancer who is complaining of new onset of acute abdominal pain, nausea, palpitations, and shortness of breath. You are in the middle of examining another patient, and you ask the nurse to check Mrs. J's vital signs and administer an EKG and oxygen. When you reach her room, you find Mrs. J sitting calmly.

Mrs. J mentions that out of nowhere, she had a feeling that she was about to die that was accompanied with acute abdominal pain, nausea, palpitations, and shortness of breath. She notes that the feelings lasted for about 20 minutes and then dissipated on their own, with no intervention. She notes that this has never happened before but does report that she has been quite anxious.

Mrs. J has removed the nasal canula, and the RN tells you her vital signs were normal throughout the event and gives you a normal EKG.

DEFINITION

Anxiety, or excessive worry, is common among patients with advanced illnesses. Anxiety becomes pathological when the patient's responses are exaggerated, when the anxiety prevents needed interventions, or when the anxiety causes significant distress to the patient. Anxiety can exacerbate chronic medical conditions.

PREVALENCE

The one-year prevalence of anxiety in the general population is 3% to 8%. In the palliative care setting, the prevalence can be as high as 25%.

LIKELY ETIOLOGIES

The etiology of anxiety can be multifactorial:
1. Underlying anxiety disorders noted prior to illness:
   - Patients who suffer from an anxiety disorder prior to their illness may suffer from acute exacerbations of the illness.

2. The disease/condition itself:
   - Thyroid disease, pulmonary disease, neurological disorders, including stroke.
3. Medications given/discontinued:
   - Medications including hormone, antiviral medications, psychostimulants, corticosteroids, and antineoplastic agents.
   - Abrupt or rapid discontinuation of sedatives, opiates, alcohol, and tobacco can cause withdrawal that can present as anxiety.
4. A natural response to illness:
   - Uncertainty regarding diagnosis/prognosis.
   - Fear of death.
   - Worry about the impact of illness on identity, finances, family, and social relationships.
   - Worry about body image (fear of amputation—fear of loss of function).
   - Fear of hospitalization with unfamiliar clinicians.
5. Other psychiatric illnesses:
   - Depression, delirium, and somatic disorders can also present with anxiety.

DIAGNOSIS

History

- The signs and symptoms of anxiety can be both psychological and somatic:
  Psychological symptoms:
  - Apprehension
  - Worry
  - Fear
  - Nervousness
  - Vigilance
  Somatic manifestations:
  - Autonomic hyperactivity (tachycardia, tachypnea)
  - Diarrhea
    - Shortness of breath/feeling of choking
    - Nausea/Abdominal pain

- Diaphoresis
- Insomnia
- Tremulousness
- Palpitations
- Parasthesias
- These signs and symptoms can occur alone or in combination with the other symptoms. Somatic complaints are often the first symptoms noted.
- Panic attacks are discrete episodes of severe anxiety that are accompanied by a sense of impending doom and several of the somatic symptoms listed above. They occur and resolve spontaneously.

Exam

- Diagnosing anxiety requires familiarity with the above signs and symptoms. Maguire et al. described an algorithmic approach to the diagnosis and treatment of anxiety in the setting of advancing disease.[1] The algorithm begins with the recognition of the anxiety and the exclusion of any iatrogenic causes (medication side effects/withdrawal). From there, a trial of benzodiazepines is warranted unless the patient exhibits severely disorganized thinking, in which case an antipsychotic medication would be more appropriate.
- If the patient does not respond to initial therapeutic options or is exhibiting psychosis (paranoia, hallucinations), referral to psychiatry should be strongly considered.

CONSEQUENCES OF UNTREATED ANXIETY

While untreated or undertreated anxiety is not fatal, it is quite uncomfortable for the patient and is detrimental to the patient's quality of life. Patients who suffer from anxiety may also refuse medical care at a higher rate than those who are not anxious.

Mrs. J's symptoms and test results indicate a diagnosis of anxiety, specifically a panic attack. Upon further discussion, she tells you that she has always been a nervous person, but since she received her diagnosis, she has been much more anxious. She worries about the possibility of becoming a burden to her family and that she will not be able to enjoy travel plans that she is looking forward to.

TREATMENT OPTIONS

Nonpharmacologic Treatment

- If the patient's anxiety is not alleviated by the elimination of possible iatrogenic causes, then nonpharmacological approaches for treating anxiety should be employed first.
- Relaxation techniques and exercises can be taught and employed. One such technique is progressive muscle relaxation. In this technique, ask the patient to focus on slowly tensing and then relaxing each muscle group, starting from the feet and working toward the head, tensing the muscles for at least five seconds and then relaxing for 30 seconds, with one repetition. (For other techniques, see Chapter 17: Complementary and Alternative Medicine.)
- Exploration of the natural responses to illness in a supportive way that focuses on disclosure of concerns and finding possible solutions may also be helpful. This approach may necessitate referral to a psychologist or other mental health practitioner.

Pharmacologic Treatment

- If the above techniques do not help alleviate anxiety, medications can be employed (Table 65.1). Of note, a Cochrane Review of drug therapy for anxiety in adult palliative care patients by Jackson and Lipman found no studies that met the author's criteria for inclusion in the review.[2]
- Multiple classes of medications, including benzodiazepines, antidepressants, antipsychotic medications, and beta blockers, are used to treat anxiety, but there is little evidence available about which medication is better for treating anxiety in the geriatric palliative care patient population.[3]

Since Mrs. J's thoughts are well organized and she is not exhibiting symptoms of psychosis, you order 0.5 mg of lorazepam every six hours as needed and make a referral to the social worker for therapy and training in relaxation techniques.

PALLIATIVE CARE ISSUES

- With the progression of a serious illness, the choice of medication to treat anxiety may be dictated by the available delivery routes and the time needed to achieve to anxiolytic effect rather than by medication class.
- The care setting may also define the choice of medication.

TABLE 65.1: PHARMACOLOGIC OPTIONS[4]

Class of Medication	Examples and Suggested Oral Dosing	Comments
Benzodiazepines[a]	Alprazolam 0.5 mg–1 mg; 3–4 times daily Lorazepam 0.5 mg–1 mg, 2–3 times daily Oxazepam 10 mg–30 mg, 3–4 times daily Clonazepam 0.25 mg–1 mg; 1–2 times daily	*Formulations:* Oral (tablets, liquid, sublingual tablets) IV/IM *Side effects:* Excess sedation Decreased cognitive function Decreased perceptomotor performance *Anxiolytic effect*: first line of treatment due to rapid onset; anxiolytic power *Toxicity:* Side effects include hypotension, confusion, falls, respiratory depression and coma Can be reversed with flumazenil *Potential for tolerance/addiction:* Benefit outweighs risk for terminal patients. Withdrawal symptoms include insomnia, agitation, somatic disturbance Rebound anxiety can occur after discontinuing *Administer with caution to:* Frail or elderly patients Patients with respiratory problems
Buspirone (Useful for treating anxiety in pts where sedation could be dangerous)	5–15 mg; 2–3 times a day	*Formulations*: oral preparation only *Side effects*: minimal Low potential for abuse Tolerance does not develop No withdrawal effects No effect on respiration *Time to anxiolytic effect*: 4–6 weeks
Beta blocker (Not FDA approved for treating anxiety)	Propranolol 10 mg to 320 mg daily	*Formulations*: oral, IV *Indications*: beneficial for somatic symptoms (palpitations, tremor) *Side effects*: cardiac effects (hypotension, bradycardia), fatigue, dizziness, weakness
SSRI antidepressants (Selective Serotonin Reuptake Inhibitor) Antidepressants also FDA approved for anxiety	Fluoxetine 10 mg–80 mg daily Fluvoxamine 150 mg–300 mg; 1–2 times daily Sertraline 25 mg–200 mg daily Paroletine 10 mg–50 mg daily Citalopram 10 mg–40 mg daily Escitalopram 5 mg–20 mg daily	*Formulations*: oral preparation only *Side effects*: generally well tolerated; side effects of all six medications may include: restlessness, GI effects, sedation, drowsiness, sexual dysfunction, some drug-drug interactions Time to anxiolytic effect: 2–6 weeks
SNRI antidepressants (Selective Serotonin Norepinepherine Reuptake Inhibitors)	Venlafaxine ER 150 mg–225 mg daily Duloxetine 20 mg–60 mg daily Desvenlafaxine 50 mg–100 mg daily	*Formulations*: oral preparations only *Side effects*: not as well tolerated as SSRIs Time to anxiolytic effect: 2–6 weeks; also takes longer to reach therapeutic dose

(continued)

TABLE 65.1: (CONTINUED)

Class of Medication	Examples and Suggested Oral Dosing	Comments
NaSSA (Noradrenergic and Specific Serotonergic) Antidepressant—not FDA approved for anxiety	Mirtazapine 7.5 mg–45 mg nightly	*Formulations:* oral preparation only *Side effects:* stimulates appetite and causes sedation; may help terminal patients *Time to anxiolytic effect:* 2–6 weeks Usually given at night
Tricyclic antidepressants/ MAO inhibitors	Amitriptyline Imipramine– Referral to psychiatrist is recommended if these medications are suggested	*Formulations:* oral preparations only *Times to anxiolytic effect:* 4–12 weeks to see effects; 3–6 months constitutes a fair trial *Side effects:* usually prohibitive for elderly population due to significant side effects; drug-drug interactions, anticholinergic side effects, and MAOI dietary restrictions usually prohibitive for elderly population
Anticonvulsants (Not FDA approved for anxiety)	Gabapentin 100 mg–500 mg; 2–3 times daily Pregabalin: 75 to 300 mg/day in 2–3 divided doses; adjust for renal impairment	*Formulations:* oral preparation only *Side effects:* Most well tolerated of this class of medications Minimal side effects Few drug-drug interactions Wide therapeutic dose range *Time to anxiolytic effect:* 1–3 days. Fair trials may last months with weekly escalation of doses.
	Carbamazepine Valproate—Referral to psychiatrist is recommended if you plan on suggesting these medications	*Formulations:* oral preparations only *Side effects:* significant side effects; blood tests required to monitor therapeutic dosing and side effects
Antipsychotics (Not FDA approved for anxiety) Can be helpful if patient shows signs of delirium or psychosis	Quetiapine 12.5 mg–50 mg; 1–2 times a day Olanzapine 2.5 mg–5 mg at bedtime Haloperidol 0.25 mg–1 mg; 1–3 times daily	*Formulations:* oral (sublingual, IV are available for selected medications) *Side effects:* many side effects, including black box warning for increased risk of death in demented elders. Use with caution *Anxiolytic effect:* These medications usually take effect in minutes and can last hours

[a] Although generally safe and effective for reducing anxiety, benzodiazepines can elicit a paradoxical reaction (also known as a disinhibitory reaction) in approximately 1% of the population.[4] Predisposing factors include increased age, psychiatric/aggressive personality disorders, or alcohol abuse problems. Should a paradoxical reaction occur, early identification and management is important for patient safety. Management options include providing support and reassurance to patient and caregivers, selecting an alternative treatment for anxiety, and treating the disinhibitory reaction or agitation with haloperidol.[5] For severe agitation that threatens patient safety and cannot be managed by readily available measures, clinicians may consider administration of additional doses of benzodiazepine. (The rationale for this approach is based on the fact that the initial benzodiazepine dose can bind to GABA receptors at the inhibitory neurons causing the central nervous system excitement. The additional dose will increase blood concentrations to bind at the excitory neurons, thus dampening the excitory effects.) Additional doses of benzodiazepine should be used with extreme caution in older adults, given the risk of unintended central nervous system and respiratory depression that can be fatal.[4]

TAKE-HOME POINTS

- Anxiety can take many forms, with both psychological and somatic symptoms.
- The etiology of anxiety is multifactorial and should be treated, as it is distressing and uncomfortable for the patient and family and can interfere with care.
- Various nonpharmacologic and family interventions can be employed prior to, and simultaneously with, pharmacologic interventions.

- There are many different classes of medications that can be used to treat anxiety, but as with all medications, the risks and benefits should be reviewed in the context of the individual patient.

REFERENCES

1. Maguire P, Faulkner A, Regnard C. Managing the anxious patient with advancing disease- a flow diagram. *Palliat Med.* 1993;7:239–244.
2. Jackson KC, Lipman AG. Drug therapy for anxiety in adult palliative care patients. *Cochrane Database of Systemic Reviews.* 2004, Issue 1. Art. No.: CD004596. doi:10.1002/14651858.CD004596.
3. Bezchlibnyk-Butler KZ, Jeffries JJ. *Clinical Handbook of Psychotropic Drugs, 12th revised edition.* Seattle, Washington: Hogrefe & Huber Publishers; 2002.
4. McKenzie WS, Rosenberg M. Paradoxical reaction following administration of a benzodiazepine. *J Oral Maxillofac Surg.* 2010;68:3034–3036.
5. Khan LC, Lustik SJ. Treatment of a paradoxical reaction to midazolam with haloperidol. *Anesth Analg.* 1997;85:213.

66

Alcohol Abuse and Dependence

CASE

Mr. RF is a 78-year-old male patient who presented to the emergency room after falling and sustaining a contusion and possible subdural hematoma. His clothing is disheveled and ill-fitting, suggesting marked weight loss. He is restless and agitated and appears both frightened and confused. His daughter and her husband have brought Mr. RF into the hospital after finding him on the bathroom floor in his apartment. They live several hours away but often visit on the weekend. He's been living alone for the past two years following the death of his wife of 55 years.

DEFINITION

Substance abuse disorders are a category of disorders in which pathological behavioral changes are associated with the regular use of substances that affect the central nervous system. Alcohol is the substance most commonly abused by the elderly, and therefore alcohol abuse and dependence will be the primary focus of this section.

Substance abuse disorders can be divided into two classes (Table 66.1).

1. Substance USE Disorders
   - Substance abuse
   - Substance dependence
2. Substance INDUCED Disorders
   - Intoxication
   - Withdrawal
   - Delirium
   - Persisting dementia
   - Psychotic disorder
   - Mood disorder
   - Anxiety disorder
   - Sleep disorder
   - Sexual disorder

PREVALENCE[2,3,4]

- Substance abuse among older adults is one of the fastest growing public health problems in the United States. It is estimated that the number of adults age 50 and older with substance problems will rise from 1.7 million in 2000/2001 to 4.4 million in the year 2020.
- Data from substance abuse programs treating older adults report that 48% abuse alcohol only; 52% abuse alcohol and illicit substances (40% cocaine, 29% marijuana, 16% opioids, 5% stimulants, and 10% other).
- Psychoactive medications with potential for abuse are used by 1 in 4 older adults.
- The baby-boom cohort has higher rates of illicit substance use and heavier alcohol use (including binge drinking) than any other aging cohort to date.

LIKELY ETIOLOGIES AND RISK FACTORS

- Increased rates of alcohol dependence are associated with:
  - Male sex
  - Younger age
  - Being single
  - Lower income
  - Genetic factors such as white or Native American ethnicity
- Sensible limits for weekly alcohol intake may not apply to older people due to age-related changes in metabolism, advancing ill health, and increased sensitivity to the effects.
- As lean body mass decreases with age, total body water decreases while body fat increases. Alcohol is water soluble, so the concentration of alcohol in the blood system is greater in older persons compared to younger ones, and the amount of alcohol previously tolerated may now be associated with intoxication.

DIAGNOSIS

History

- Alcoholism in older adults is commonly one of two types:

TABLE 66.1: SUBSTANCE ABUSE VS. DEPENDENCE[1]

Substance Abuse	Substance Dependence or Addiction

A maladaptive pattern of substance use leading to clinically significant impairment or distress as manifested by one (or more) of the following, occurring within a 12-month period:
Inability to fulfill major role obligations at work or home
Participation in physically hazardous situations while impaired
Recurrent legal or interpersonal problems
Continued use despite recurrent social and interpersonal problems
(These criteria may not be applicable to most older patients)
	A maladaptive pattern of substance use, leading to clinically significant impairment or distress, as manifested by three (or more) of the following at any time in the same 12-month period:
	Tolerance, as defined by either: a need for markedly increased amounts of the substance to achieve intoxication or desired effect, and/or markedly diminished effect with continued use of the same amount of substance
	Withdrawal, as manifested by either of the following:
	  a. the characteristic withdrawal syndrome for the substance
	  b. the substance (or a closely related) substance is taken to relieve or avoid withdrawal symptoms
	Substance is taken in larger amounts or for longer period of time than intended
	Persistent desire or unsuccessful efforts to cut down or control substance use
	A great deal of time is spent in activities necessary to obtain the substance, or recovering from its effects
	Important social, occupational, or recreational activities are given up or reduced because of substance use
	Substance use is continued despite knowledge of having persistent or recurrent physical or psychological problems likely to have been caused or exacerbated by the substance

- Early-onset or "hardy survivors" who have been drinking for many years.
- Late-onset drinkers whose patterns of abuse develop later in life and are most often related to lifestyle changes such as retirement, changes in independent function, and losses due to death or separation from friends, family, or even pets.
- Symptoms most often associated with substance abuse or addiction include:
  - Pain
  - Anorexia/Cachexia
  - Gastritis
  - Fatigue
  - Ataxia
  - Confusion/Delirium/Dementia
  - Ascites
  - Neuropathy
  - SOB/dyspnea
  - Seizures
  - Anxiety
  - Depression (hopelessness/helplessness/despair)
  - Withdrawal
  - Isolation

Exam

1. Diagnostic interview should be based on the DSM-IV-TR criteria, screening tools, and/or validated questionnaires. Assessment, diagnosis, treatment, and evaluation should always be substance-specific.
2. Screening:
   - Current data suggest there is both an increase in drinking among the baby-boom cohort and a reluctance to discuss abuse of alcohol or other drugs with health care providers.[5]
   - Substance use disorder among older adults is routinely misdiagnosed, underdiagnosed, undertreated, or left untreated because symptoms are often confused with other aspects of aging.[5]

- Valid and reliable screening tools can help to identify persons at risk. Generally, there are two kinds of appraisal tools: brief, often self-reporting, questionnaires used for screening, and more comprehensive tools used for assessment.[6]

1. **The CAGE questionnaire**: Widely used tool with four questions that identify usage patterns that reflect problems with alcohol.[7] A score of two or more positive responses is considered the cut-off for probable alcoholism. Recommended by the American Geriatrics Society as a screening tool for misuse of alcohol.

2. **Short Michigan Alcoholism Screening Test-Geriatric Version (SMAST-G):**[8] The SMAST-G is the first short-form screening tool developed specifically for use with older adults (Table 66.2). It is more likely than the CAGE to identify those at risk for negative outcomes of alcohol use. Scoring two or more "yes" responses is indicative of an alcohol problem.

Tests

- If prescription or illicit drugs are suspected, it is best to identify the specific drug(s) to be assayed on a toxicology request.
- Breathalyzers approximate blood alcohol levels; serum alcohol and toxicology tests provide direct measures.
- See Table 66.3 for relevant labwork that may be helpful in diagnosis of alcohol abuse.

On examination, Mr. RF is disoriented and does not remember falling; he is tachycardic (P = 104), hypertensive 160/100, and hyperthermic T = 38.4C (101.12F). He appears to be tremulous and is suspicious of the intent and motives of the people providing his care. He pushes your hand away from his abdomen and says, "Hey, watch it; that hurts."

CONSEQUENCES OF SUBSTANCE ABUSE

- Specific complications are determined by the substance(s) being used or abused (e.g., opioids, alcohol, benzodiazepines, tobacco) and the clinical circumstances (e.g., acute intoxication versus sequelae of long-term use).
- Multiple organ involvement is associated with both acute and chronic alcohol use (Table 66.4).

EXPECTED DISEASE COURSE

Persons with substance abuse and addictive disorders, particularly the elderly, are at increased risk for trauma falls, accidents and their sequelae, liver disease, pancreatitis, gastritis, cancer (including hepatocellular, pancreatic, lung, oral/head and neck, bladder), alcohol-related dementias, and increased risk for HIV related to IV drug use.

Mr. RF's daughter reports concern that her father's ability to care for himself has been declining, particularly over the last year. She is worried that he may not be able to care for himself independently.

TABLE 66.2: SHORT MICHIGAN ALCOHOLISM SCREENING TEST-GERIATRIC VERSION (SMAST-G)[8]

---

1. When talking with others, do you ever underestimate how much you drink?
2. After a few drinks, have you sometimes not eaten or been able to skip a meal because you didn't feel hungry?
3. Does having a few drinks help decrease your shakiness or tremors?
4. Does alcohol sometimes make it hard for you to remember parts of the day or night?
5. Do you usually take a drink to relax or calm your nerves?
6. Do you drink to take your mind off your problems?
7. Have you ever increased your drinking after experiencing a loss in your life?
8. Has a doctor or nurse ever said they were worried or concerned about your drinking?
9. Have you ever made rules to manage your drinking?
10. When you feel lonely, does having a drink help?

YES (1) NO (0)

TOTAL SMAST-G-SCORE (0–10) _____

TABLE 66.3: RELEVANT LABWORK FOR ALCOHOL ABUSE

Test	Rationale	Common Findings
Carbohydrate-deficient transferrin (CDT)	Alcohol inhibition of transfer of sugar to glycoproteins Highly sensitive for heavy drinking	Reduced concentration after excessive drinking Less sensitive in women
Complete blood count	Alcohol has bone-marrow suppressant effects Differential diagnosis	Decreased RBC Elevated MCV Elevated corpuscular Hgb Decreased WBC Decreased polymorpho-nuclear leukocytes Decreased lymphocytes Decreased leukocytes Decreased thrombocytes
Hepatic enzymes (GGT, ALT, AST) Aspartate aminotransferase	Closely correlated with alcohol consumption; especially GGT	Elevated ALT Elevated AST (higher than ALT) Elevated GGT Alanine aminotranserase Gamma glutamyl transpeptidase
Folic acid (Vit B9)	Deficiency may be associated with mega-loblastic anemia	Decrease related to drinking and poor diet
Thiamine (Vit B12)	Wernicke encephalopathy Korsakoff psychosis Peripheral neuropathy	Decreased Timely replacement to improve cognitive function

TABLE 66.4: EFFECT OF ACUTE AND CHRONIC ALCOHOL USE ON MAJOR ORGAN SYSTEMS

Organ System	Complication
Gastrointestinal	Gastritis and acid peptic disease Malabsorption syndrome Pancreatitis Alcoholic liver disease (ALD)
Cardiovascular	Cardiomyopathy Scarred/collapsed veins with IV drug use
Hematological	Megaloblastic anemia
Neurological and neuromuscular	Peripheral neuropathy Blackouts (anterograde amnesia) Wernicke's encephalopathy Dementia
Endocrine	Sexual dysfunction
Psychiatric complications of alcohol use	Mood disorders and suicide Alcohol-induced psychotic disorder (Korsakoff's psychosis) Social impact: increased social isolation; fixed income may be spent on alcohol or substance rather than rent, food

TREATMENT OPTIONS

Nonpharmacologic

- Prevention and early intervention should be the treatment goal for patients who exhibit problem drinking behavior that does not meet criteria for abuse or dependence[9,10]
- Brief alcohol counseling (BAC) has been shown to be effective intervention with a senior population. Varying definitions of BAC exist, but a typical intervention would consist of two 10- to 15-minute counseling sessions by primary health care provider; then two follow-up phone calls by clinic staff with advice, education, and reinforcement.
- Historically, most controlled studies comparing efficacy of structured treatment options for alcohol dependence have not included older adults in their demographics.[9]
- Although structured in-patient programs designed specifically for older adults are not widely available, there are data suggesting that:
  - Seniors will enter and respond positively to age-specific, supportive, and nonconfrontational group treatment.[11]
  - Programs addressing the stresses of aging, social isolation, and treatment of underlying depression are more effective than alcohol-specific approaches commonly used with younger adults.[9]
  - Older adults have favorable long-term outcomes following inpatient treatment relative to younger patients, possibly due to longer retention in treatment. They are also less likely to have family members or friends who encourage post-discharge alcohol use.[12]
- Outpatient approaches to treatment for the elderly include groups that meet at senior centers, assisted living, or local churches. Emphasis is placed on age-appropriate developmental tasks, using life experiences to help others with similar problems, forming friendships with other members, and participating in activities outside the group. While eliminating the use of alcohol is suggested and supported by the group, it is not the primary focus of the program.[13]
- Cognitive behavioral therapy and attendance at self-help groups such as Alcoholics Anonymous are effective, in conjunction with pharmacologic treatment.[14]

Pharmacologic[14]

- **Detoxification:** The incidence of medical and neurological complications during alcohol withdrawal syndrome is greater in older alcoholics:
  - Hospitalization is indicated for acute detoxification
  - Correct fluid and electrolyte imbalances
  - Give thiamine/niacin to prevent Wernicke-Korsakoff syndromes
  - Administer short-acting benzodiazepines on first day, then tapering by 50% on days 2 and 3 (taper to prevent withdrawal should be managed carefully due to increased susceptibility to adverse effects).
- **Rehabilitation:** The focus of rehabilitation should be encouraging positive attitude and motivation for recovery, while reducing the risk of relapse:
  - Disulfiram should be used cautiously and only for the short term because of the risk of precipitating a confusional state.
  - Naltrexone is safe for use as relapse prevention in older adults; has been shown to extend time to relapse and lower alcohol intake on drinking days.

PALLIATIVE CARE ISSUES

- Due to trauma and accidents associated with acute abuse, or the organ failure and life-limiting changes secondary to chronic abuse and dependence, the palliative care needs for the elderly at risk for substance abuse are significant.
- Prevention and early intervention strategies are highly recommended:
  - Improved screening to provide earlier, more appropriate care
  - Earlier detection and treatment of underlying psychiatric illness
  - Awareness of significant social stressors associated with serious illness, family caregiving, and bereavement; referral to resources designed to promote behavioral change, reduce isolation, and enhance supportive networking.
- For patients who are substance-dependent, careful attention should be paid to assessment and management of symptoms associated with acute substance abuse and the illnesses associated with chronic use or dependence, e.g., pain, nausea, vomiting, delirium, confusion, dyspnea, insomnia, anxiety, and depression.

- Periodic review of current medications (including over-the-counter) should be conducted, with vigilance surrounding medications with a high risk for abuse or hazardous interactions. Particularly important at points of transition between care settings.
- Attention to advance care planning is essential, particularly the designation of a health care proxy or surrogate decision-maker.
- Pain management for patients with a history of substance abuse can be particularly challenging. (See Chapter 29: Management of Pain in Older Adults.)

TAKE-HOME POINTS

- Although it is one of the fastest growing public health problems in the United States, substance use disorder among older adults is routinely misdiagnosed, undertreated, or left untreated.
- Symptoms of self-neglect, falls, cognitive and affective impairment, and social withdrawal are red flags and should trigger screening for substance abuse.
- Assessment, diagnosis, treatment, and evaluation should always be substance-specific.
- Health problems related to substance abuse/dependence in the elderly are exacerbated by age-related illness, social isolation, physical decline, and concomitant psychiatric illness.
- Brief alcohol counseling (BAC) has been shown to be effective for patients who exhibit problem drinking behavior that does not meet criteria for abuse or dependence.
- Seniors will enter and respond positively to age-specific, supportive, and nonconfrontational group treatment programs.
- Treatment programs that address the stresses of aging, social isolation, and treatment of underlying depression are more effective for elders than the alcohol-specific approaches commonly used with younger alcohol abusers.

REFERENCES

1. APA. *Diagnostic and Statistical Manual of Mental Disorders*, Fourth Edition, Text Revision. Washington, DC: American Psychiatric Association; 2000;105–151.
2. Rosen D, Smith ML, et al. The prevalence of mental and physical health disorders among older methadone patients. *Am J Geriatr Psychiatry.* 2008; 16(6):488–497.
3. Gfroerer JC, Penne MA, et al. Substance abuse treatment among older adults in 2020: The impact of the aging Baby-Boom cohort. *Drug and Alcohol Dependence.* 2003;69:127–135.
4. Simoni-Wastila L, Yang KA. Psychoactive drug abuse in older adults. *The Am J Geriatr Pharmacother.* 2006;4(4):380–394.
5. Han B, Gfroerer JC, Colliver JD, Penne MA. Substance use disorder among older adults in the United States in 2020. *Addiction.* 2009;104:88–96.
6. O'Connell H, Chin AV, et al. A systematic review of the utility of self-report alcohol screening instruments in the elderly. *Int J Geriatr Psychiatry.* 2004;19:1074–1086.
7. Bush B, Shaw S, Clearly P, et al. Screening for alcohol abuse using the CAGE questionnaire. *Am J Med.* Feb 1987;82(2):231–235.
8. University of Michigan Alcohol Research Center, Michigan Alcohol Screening Test (MAST-G). © The Regents of the University of Michigan, 1991.
9. Oslin DW. Evidence-based treatment of geriatric substance abuse. *Psychiatr Clin N Am.* 2005;28: 897–911.
10. Kaner EF, Dickinson HO, Beyer FR, et al. Effectiveness of brief alcohol interventions in primary care populations. *Cochrane Database of Systematic Reviews.* 2007, Issue 2. Art. No.: CD004148.
11. Lemke S, Moos RH. Prognosis of older patients in mixed-age alcoholism treatment programs. *Journal of Substance Abuse Treatment.* 2002;22: 33–43.
12. Satre DD, Mertens JR, Arean PA, Weisner C. Five-year alcohol and drug treatment outcomes of older adults versus middle-aged and younger adults in a managed care program. *Addiction* 2004;99:1296–1297.
13. Peterson M, Zimberg S. Treating alcoholism: an age-specific intervention that works for older patients. *Geriatrics.* 1996;51:45–49.
14. Caputo F, Vignoli T, Leggio L, et al. Alcohol use disorders in the elderly: a brief overview from epidemiology to treatment options. *Exp Gerontol.* 2012;47:411–416.

67

Dementia

CASE

Mrs. BR is an 82-year-old woman who has a history of hypertension, mild osteoarthritis of her knees, and hypothyroidism. She lives on her own and manages all her daily activities independently. One of her two daughters lives close by, and she is very concerned about her mother. On more than a few occasions, she has noticed that her mother is becoming forgetful. Her telephone line has recently been cut off, as she hasn't been paying her bills. She also repeatedly asks the same questions and is always misplacing things. The daughter would like her mother to be evaluated.

DEFINITION

Dementia can be defined as progressive deterioration of the brain characterized by loss of memory and impairment of at least one other cognitive function:[2]

- Communication (aphasia)
- Recognizing objects, persons, sounds, shapes, or smells (agnosia)
- Recognition and manipulation of objects in space (apraxia)
- Executive function, i.e., reasoning and planning
- Regulation of emotion and aggression

Diagnosis requires a decline from baseline these areas and resulting interference with daily function and independence. In the case study presented here, Mrs. BR's functional decline (e.g., inability to pay her bills) may be suggestive of dementia.

PREVALENCE

- The prevalence of dementia increases exponentially, doubling every 5 years at least to age 85. It affects about 8% of people over 65 and 50% of those over 85 years.
- Approximately 4.5 million Americans suffer from this disorder, and it is projected that within the next 50 years, between

11 million and 16 million people will be affected in the United States.[1]

LIKELY ETIOLOGIES

The most common cause of dementia is Alzheimer's disease, but there are many other types of dementia, some of which are reversible (Table 67.1).

DIAGNOSIS

History

1. **Assess cognitive history:** This information should be obtained from the patient, family, and caregivers by asking about the following symptoms:
   - Short-term memory loss:
     - Increased repetition of questions or comments
     - Difficulty remembering recent conversations, appointments, events
     - Misplacement of objects
     - Difficulty discussing current events in an area of interest
   - Ability to handle complex tasks:
     - Balancing a checkbook and paying bills
     - Cooking a meal
   - Reasoning ability:
     - Inability to respond with a reasonable plan to solve problems at work or at home
     - Uncharacteristic disregard for rules of social conduct
   - Spatial ability and orientation:
     - Difficulty driving
     - Difficulty organizing objects around the house
     - Difficulty navigating in familiar places
   - Language:
     - Difficulty finding words
2. **Assess drug history:** Be alert for drugs that impair cognition (e.g., analgesics,

TABLE 67.1: LIKELY ETIOLOGIES

Cause	Proportion	Distinguishing Features
Alzheimer's disease	60–80%	Insidious onset Smooth, inexorable decline Early stages: loss of short-term memory Middle stages: psychosis and behavioral disturbance Late stages: dependence in basic activities of daily living such as feeding, toileting
Vascular dementia	10–20%	Sudden onset associated with a stroke Stepwise deterioration Focal neurological exam Infarcts seen on cerebral imaging History of cardiovascular disease and risk factors
Lewy body dementia	5%	Gradually progressive Fluctuations in cognitive function Well-defined visual and occasional auditory hallucinations Parkinsonian motor features
Fronto-temporal dementia		Begins at a young age Personality changes and behavioral disturbances are prominent early symptoms Dis-inhibition and impaired executive function Memory may be relatively spared Progression rapid
Reversible dementias	1–2%	Medication induced (analgesics, anticholinergics, psychotropic medications, sedative-hypnotics, and steroids) Metabolic disorders (thyroid disease, vitamin B12 deficiency, hyponatremia, hypercalcemia, hepatic and renal dysfunction) Depression (known as pseudodementia) Central nervous system neoplasm, chronic subdural hematomas, chronic meningitis, Creutzfeldt-Jakob disease Normal pressure hydrocephalus

antidepressants, anticholinergics, psychotropic medications, sedative-hypnotics, and any over-the-counter agents such as antihistamines).

In the case of Mrs. BR, both her forgetfulness and her inability to pay her bills are indicative of dementia.

Exam
During the exam, the following domains should be assessed (Table 67.2):

- Physical: A thorough physical examination should be conducted to rule out other disease processes:

  - Acute disorders and exacerbations of chronic comorbidities that may be affecting cognitive function
  - Neurological findings suggestive of cerebrovascular disease
  - Extrapyramidal signs indicating parkinsonism
  - Symptoms of other neurodegenerative disorders
  - Symptoms of neuropathies or myopathies suggesting a treatable systemic disorder
- Functional status: Assess using "Get up and Go" assessment tool or "3 Chair Rise." (See Chapter 2: Principles of Geriatric Palliative Care.)

TABLE 67.2: ASSESSMENT OF COGNITIVE STATUS

Test	Description	Scoring	Limitations
Mini-cog	Consists of a clock drawing test and recall of 3 unrelated words	If all numbers on the clock are presented in the correct sequence and the hands display the correct time=NORMAL (no dementia) If no words recalled=DEMENTIA If 1–2 words recalled, look at the clock draw test. If abnormal=DEMENTIA	Quick initial screening test Needs to be followed by other tests such as the MMSE
Clock drawing test	Patient asked to draw a clock face with all the numbers and place hands at a stated time	12 must appear on top (3 points) 12 numbers must be present (1 point) 2 distinguishable hands (1 point) Time must be correctly identified for full credit Score of < 4/6 = impaired	Good screening test; however, not diagnostic
Mini-Mental State Exam (MMSE)	Tests a broad range of cognitive functions including orientation, recall, attention, calculation, language manipulation, and constructional praxis	Maximal score is 30 <24 = DEMENTIA (need to make adjustments for educational level, language, and age of patient)	Good diagnostic test Limited by educational level, literacy, and language
Neuropsychological testing	Extensive evaluation of multiple, cognitive domains (attention, orientation, executive function, verbal memory, spatial memory, language, calculations, mental flexibility, and conceptualization) Used when MMSE is limited by education or when MMSE result doesn't match clinical suspicion Helpful in distinguishing between cognitive impairment and depression	Complicated scoring	Very long (3 hours) and expensive Needs to be performed by a psychologist

- Depression: Assess using the Geriatric Depression Scale in Older Adults.

TESTS

Labs

- CBC
- Complete metabolic panel: electrolytes, liver and kidney function tests, serum calcium, albumin
- Thyroid functions
- Vitamin B12
- Folate
- Serological test for syphilis (selectively)
- Apolipoprotein E epsilon 4 allele. This controversial form of the gene is increased in familial and sporadic late-onset Alzheimer's disease, but its prevalence in non-Alzheimer dementias in Caucasian populations is unknown

Imaging

Non-contrast CT or MRI: performed routinely to exclude a secondary cause of dementia such as tumors, abscess, or NPH (normal pressure hydrocephalus) if there is a strong clinical suspicion. However, not often found to be positive in absence of abnormalities on the neurological exam.

EXPECTED DISEASE COURSE

- The majority of dementia patients die as a consequence of progressive brain deterioration leading to difficulty moving, eating, and swallowing, with consequent risk of pneumonia, pressure ulcers, wound infection, and urosepsis.
- Although dementia is a progressive disease, death is often not anticipated or expected because the onset of infectious etiology is may be sudden.

CARE PLANNING

- Dementia is a disease that affects both the patient and family, and clinicians should therefore understand the patient's values and the family's dynamics in order to guide the process of advance care planning (ACP).
- Ideally, advance care planning with patient and family (to address finances, long-term care insurance, and health care preferences) should take place in the early phases of the disease, when the patient still has capacity to participate.

- This is not a one-time discussion but rather an extended series of conversations that should be initiated as soon as the patient is diagnosed and while the patient retains decisional capacity.
- If possible, the planning process should involve a multidisciplinary team comprising a physician, nurse, social worker, and psychologist to provide comprehensive support for the patient-family-caregiver unit.[3] A planning approach based on disease severity is described below in Table 67.3.[4]

Mrs. BR most likely has mild dementia, so for short-term goals consider starting a cholinesterase inhibitor and ordering a home safety evaluation. Mid-range issues to recommend to the patient and family include appointing a health care proxy, writing a will, and financial planning. Long-term issues would be initiating discussions about advance directives and exploring patient and family preferences about artificial feeding and treatment of acute disorders should the patient become severely demented and unable to make these decisions.

TREATMENT OPTIONS

- Currently there is no treatment available for restoration of mental function. Correction of contributing factors should be attempted as follows:[5]
  - Identify and treat comorbid physical illnesses (e.g., HTN, DM)
  - Assess and treat for depression—improves attention, concentration, and energy levels and reduces disability; SSRIs recommended
  - Avoid anticholinergic medications (e.g., benzotropine, diphenhydramine, hydroxyzine, tricyclic antidepressants, etc.)
  - Limit psychotropic medication[6]
- Employ a multifactorial and multidisciplinary approach to manage comorbidities, optimize planning for the future, and provide family support.
- Agitation and disruptive behaviors are common; nonpharmacological treatment interventions should be explored first. (See Chapter 33: Behavioral Disorders in Dementia.)

Nonpharmacologic Treatment

- Behavior modification, e.g., scheduled toileting. Encourage the use of the toilet

every couple of hours to prevent accidents from occurring.
- Graded assistance (least restrictive alternative for ADL supports). Allow the patient to perform the ADL, offering help as needed.

- Practice with activities, e.g., exercise programs. Encourage physical activity in structured exercise programs.
- Positive reinforcements to increase independence. Encourage patient to carry out ADLs and IADLs and reward these attempts.

TABLE 67.3: ADVANCE CARE PLANNING

	Mild Dementia	Moderate Dementia	Severe or End-Stage Dementia
Common clinical manifestations	Mild cognitive decline May have gotten lost or confused May forget the name of a recent dinner guest or lose their keys often May have progressive difficulty with moderately complex daily activities such as paying bills, handling finances, preparing meals, and housekeeping Very emotionally labile; may become irritable, hostile and agitated Usually can compensate well and follow routine	Ability to perform simple daily activities of living such as bathing, dressing, toileting becomes impaired Cannot learn new information Becomes lost in familiar surroundings like own home Remains ambulatory but at increased risk of falls and accidents due to confusion and poor judgment Psychotic symptoms may occur May wander May become physically aggressive Sleep is disorganized	Cannot perform the most basic activities such as eating, walking Totally dependent on others Long- and short-term memory completely lost May become incontinent Reflex motor function such as swallowing is lost, putting patient at risk of aspiration pneumonia
Short-term (< 1 year) issues	Consider pharmacological treatments— cholinesterase inhibitors (described below) Home safety evaluation[1] Assess and offer resources to reduce family and caregiver burden[4]	Consider adding namenda to cholinesterase inhibitors May need some antipsychotic medication Register in a Safe Return program for wandering[2] Follow a routine in familiar surroundings[3] Assess and offer resources to help reduce family and caregiver burden[4]	Consider discontinuation of all pharmacological treatments such as cholinesterase inhibitors and namenda May need to continue with antipsychotics Assess and offer resources to help reduce family and caregiver burden[4] Consider long-term care facility or similar support at home
Mid-range (1–5 years) issues	Appoint a HCP[5] Write a will[6] Financial planning[6] Assess driving[7] Assess for family and caregiver burden	Consider more help at home (e.g., home health aide) or admission to a long-term care facility[4] Appoint an HCP if still able to do so[5] Assess and offer resources to help reduce family and caregiver burden	

(continued)

TABLE 67.3: (CONTINUED)

	Mild Dementia	Moderate Dementia	Severe or End-Stage Dementia
Long-term (> 5 years) issues	Complete advance directives[5] Make decisions about artificial feeding and treatment of acute disorders Discuss issues of family and caregiver burden Explore options for long-term care facility or 24-hour help at home		

[1] **Obtain a home safety evaluation.** Cue patients in the kitchen and bathrooms with signs, monitor use of appliances, utilize automatic shut-off features, ensure bright lighting, remove dangerous items.

[2] **If wandering is an issue,** register in the Safe Return program and have patients wear an identification bracelet or necklace.

[3] **Provide a safe and supportive environment** in a familiar surrounding; encourage routines.

[4] **Assess need for help with ADLs and IADLs** in the home. An assessment by a professional who is knowledgeable about dementia and is familiar with the patient's community can help match needs to resources and care options.

[5] **Appointing a health care proxy or a durable power of attorney for health care** who can make medical decisions on the patient's behalf when the patient is unable to make his/her own decision. State-specific advance directive forms can be found at www.caringinfo.org.

[6] **Appoint a power of attorney** so that finances are properly managed, bills paid; prepare a will or other estate planning documents; if under 65 years old, explore Social Security disability benefits to ensure a source of income. The Alzheimer's Association is a good place to start for resources.

[7] **Counsel patients and families about driving,** which is often a difficult issue to resolve. Refer patient and families to AARP Driving Safety Program regarding tips on talking about this issue, limiting driving, and retesting.

[8] **Encourage both physical and mental activity; avoid stress.**

Pharmacologic Options

- Consider pharmacological treatments that may be helpful in slowing the disease process. None of these medications restores memory or halts the disease process. However, they may slow progression of dementia (Table 67.4).

CAREGIVER SUPPORT

- Caregivers of patients with dementia can suffer significant stress. Of those caregivers reporting emotional stress, over 50% suffer depression, increased morbidity, or mortality.[7]
- Isolation, exhaustion, physical illness, burnout leading to anger, and resentment are common. As a result, clinicians should identify and respond appropriately to indications of caregiver stress in order to protect the family from undue physical and emotional burden, and patients from maltreatment and institutionalization. Suggested instruments to assess caregiver burden include the Zarit Burden Interview and the Modified Caregiver Strain Index (CSI).
- Caregiver support strategies and resources may include:
  - Education about the disease process
  - Providing information about support groups for caregivers, community services, respite care, adult day care for patients, and programs available through faith-based organizations
- Encouraging use of Internet for information on resources and services. Helpful internet sites include:
  - Alzheimer's Association (www.alz.org)
  - Well Spouse Foundation (www.wellspouse.org)
  - National Hospice Organization (www.nho.org)
  - Health Care Financing Administration (www.medicare.gov)
- Referral to interdisciplinary health care professionals as indicated, e.g. social work, chaplaincy, psychiatry. (See

TABLE 67.4: PHARMACOLOGICAL OPTIONS

Generic Name	Mechanism of Action	Dosing	Side Effects
Donepezil (Aricept)	Cholinesterase inhibitors	Start at 5 mg once daily, increasing to 10 mg daily after 1 month	GI: nausea, vomiting, diarrhea CVS: AV block, HTN
Galantamine (Razadyne) Razadyne ER (extended release)	Cholinesterase inhibitors	Start at 4 mg every 12 hours increasing to 8 mg every 12 hours after 4 weeks Recommended dose 8–12 mg every 12 hours Start at 1 capsule daily	GI: nausea, vomiting, diarrhea Headache, dizziness, brady arrhythmias
Rivastigmine (Exelon)	Cholinesterase inhibitors	Start at 1.5 mg every 12 hours and titrate up to 3 mg every 12 hours If tolerated, continue to 6 mg every 12 hours	GI: nausea, vomiting, diarrhea
Memantine (Namenda) (moderate to severe Alzheimer's dementia)	Noncompetitive N-methyl-D-aspartate (NMDA) receptor antagonist	Start at 5 mg daily and increase by 5 mg at weekly intervals to a maximum of 10 mg every 12 hours (reduced dose in renal impairment) Can be used alone or in combination with a cholinesterase inhibitor	HTN, syncope, dizziness, headache, constipation, vomiting
Vitamin E	Found to delay functional decline; however, also shown to increase mortality in high doses		Increased mortality in high doses
Gingko biloba	Although proponents claim gingko biloba stabilizes or improves mental and social function, there is no data to support this result		Has side effects, so not recommended

Chapter 4: Special Issues in Caregiving, and Chapter 28: Caregivers.)

PALLIATIVE CARE ISSUES

• Most patients with end-stage dementia die of infectious complications such as aspiration pneumonia, urinary tract infections, and skin breakdown. The patient's and family's ability to understand the expected course of the disease will often dictate the type of care the patient receives as dementia progresses to advanced stages.

• Treatment decisions about artificial hydration and nutrition, resuscitation, intubation, and the use of antibiotics should be discussed at appropriate stages of the disease.

• As dementia worsens, highly aggressive interventions and acute care in the hospital may cause more harm than good; therefore, the possible benefits of hospitalization should be weighed against associated discomfort, burdens, and risks.

- Palliative care should be offered as an optimal approach at any point in the trajectory of the disease.
- Clinicians should explore the following issues with family members/caregivers:
  - The importance and meaning of comfort to the patient.
  - The types of support and resources that are available for families; anticipate the family's need for supportive services before a crisis develops.
  - Financial planning.
  - The importance of appropriate care settings (discuss home, hospitalization, and nursing home placements).
  - The potential for increased family and caregiver burden as disease progresses.

TAKE-HOME POINTS

- Dementia is one of the most common causes of institutionalization, morbidity, and mortality in the elderly.
- Both nonpharmacological and pharmacological treatment options should be used.
- Behavioral symptoms are common and very disturbing for both patients and their families, and should be treated.
- Advance care planning should take place in the early phases of the disease when the patient still has capacity to participate.

- Clinicians should seek to identify indications of caregiver stress and offer resources for education, respite care, and psychosocial support.
- Palliative care should be offered as an optimal approach as the disease progresses.

REFERENCES

1. Cleusa PF, et al. Global prevalence of dementia: a Delphi consensus study. *Lancet.* 2001;*366*(9503): 2112–2117.
2. Beers M. (Ed.) Merck Manual of Health and Aging. Chapter 27. Whitehorse Station, NJ: Merck and Co, Inc. 2004.
3. Callahan CM, Boustani M, Sachs GA, Hendrie HC. Integrating care for older adults with cognitive impairment. *Curr. Alzheimer Res.* Aug 2009;*6*(4): 368–374.
4. Hogan, et al. Diagnosis and treatment of dementia. Approach to management of mild to moderate dementia. *CMAJ.* Oct 2008;*179*(8):787–793.
5. Kester MI, Scheltens P. Dementia: the bare essentials. *Pract Neruol.* Aug 2009;*9*(4):241–251.
6. Doherty D, Collier E. Caring for people with dementia in specific settings. *Nurs Older People.* Jul 2009;*21*:28–31.
7. Caregiving in the U.S. National Alliance for Caregiving and AARP. 2004.

68

Seizure

CASE

Mrs. T is a 47-year-old woman recently diagnosed with glioblastoma multiforme after a seizure. She has undergone resection of her tumor along with a course of radiation therapy. Despite treatment, her tumor continues to progress. She now suffers from recurrent seizures in which she develops a rhythmic contraction of her left arm, which gradually increases in intensity. It causes her to become inconsolable and anxious followed by shouts of obscenities and then extreme fatigue. Her family expresses distress at this behavior as previously she was a happy, positive, and gentle individual. Following these episodes, which typically last about 10 minutes, she becomes calm and will rest for several hours. In the past two weeks she has experienced a generalized seizure lasting for greater than 10 minutes requiring intervention with intravenous medication.

DEFINITION

Epileptic seizure is defined by the International League Against Epilepsy (ILAE) as a transient occurrence of signs and/or symptoms due to abnormal, synchronous neuronal activity in the brain.[1] This in turn may lead to abnormal neurological function such as alteration in consciousness or convulsion. Epilepsy is the syndrome defined by recurrent, unprovoked seizures.

- Secondary seizure disorders are related to a focal abnormality such as a mass lesion (e.g., tumor, hemorrhage), stroke, or infection.

- Convulsion, representing the motor manifestation of a seizure, is defined as a contortion of the body caused by violent, involuntary muscular contractions of the extremities, trunk, and head.

CLASSIFICATION

- Major seizure categories include[1]:
  - Partial seizures: simple or complex
  - Primary generalized seizures
  - Secondary generalized seizures
- Seizures are also classified by the scope of their effect—those that remain confined to a single hemisphere, with or without a change in consciousness, and those that affect both hemispheres. Table 68.1 illustrates the most common physical findings seen in the three major categories of seizures.

Mrs. T suffers from recurrent complex partial epilepsy as described by her alteration in consciousness and appearance of focal clonic movements of her right arm.

PREVALENCE

Epilepsy occurs in approximately 1% to 3% of the population. As much as 10% of the population will experience a seizure in their lifetime.[3]

LIKELY ETIOLOGIES

- Seizures may be either provoked or unprovoked. Abnormalities such

---

TABLE 68.1: CLASSIFICATION ACCORDING TO SYMPTOMS

	Partial Seizures		Generalized Seizures
	(Simple)	*(Complex Partial)*	
Consciousness	Unchanged	Altered	Lost
Focal neurological signs during seizure	Common	Common	None

Note. Adapted from Shneker BF, Fountain NB. Epilepsy. *Dis Mon.* 2003;49:426–478.

as metabolic derangement (e.g., hyponatremia), mass lesion, or injury may lead to the occurrence of a focal or generalized seizure.

- Generalized seizures may also arise from congenital abnormalities resulting in structural anomalies; these patients usually present earlier than their geriatric years.
- More common in the geriatric population, and perhaps most relevant for non-neurologists, are secondary seizure disorders. The most common form of secondary seizure disorders includes partial seizures whose impact is limited to one cerebral hemisphere. Partial seizures may result from a variety of causes:[2]
  - Stroke
  - Trauma
  - Mass lesion (tumor/AVM)
  - Hemorrhage
  - Metabolic abnormality
  - Toxic/metabolic encephalopathy:
    - Hyperglycemia
    - Hypoglycemia
    - Hyponatremia
    - Hypocalcemia
  - Neurodegenerative disorders (such as Alzheimer's disease)
  - Alcohol withdrawal

Mrs. T's seizure disorder is secondary to the presence of an infiltrating glioblastoma, which is now causing mass effect from vasogenic edema.

REFRACTORY EPILEPSY

- Refractory seizures, either recurrent within a short period of time (minutes to hours) or persistent without remittance, require immediate intervention. The most serious of refractory seizure conditions is generalized convulsive status epilepticus

(GCSE or "status"). This condition represents a medical emergency, requiring immediate intervention to reduce serious morbidity or mortality. Table 68.5 outlines recommended protocols for termination of seizures in the setting of status epilepticus.

- Non-convulsive status epilepticus (NCSE) should be considered in a patient with unexplained depressed level of consciousness who is at risk for a seizure disorder. This condition often requires bedside EEG monitoring.

Mrs. T experienced one episode of generalized status epilepticus in which convulsions persisted for more than 10 minutes. The seizure was terminated by using lorazepam followed by a loading dose of phenytoin.

DIAGNOSIS

Exam

- A patient first initially presents with an alteration in level of consciousness. This may or may not be associated with movements suggesting convulsion.
- The descriptive history provides clues as to likelihood of a diagnosis of seizure or other neurological abnormality, such as transient ischemic attack (TIA), stroke, or syncope. Table 68.2 lists common distinguishing features between syncope, stroke, and seizure.[4]
- The medical history, including stroke, malignancy, or metabolic abnormalities (e.g., diabetes) in addition to medication usage, may provide useful information leading to accurate diagnosis.
- The neurological examination, with attention to the region in which the seizure manifests, allows for assessment of both the

TABLE 68.2: DISTINGUISHING FEATURES OF SYNCOPE, TIA, SEIZURE

	Syncope	TIA/Stroke	Seizure
Prodrome	Autonomic, prolonged	Any	Any, short
LOC duration	Brief	Rare	Varies
Postictal confusion	Rare	Varies	Common
Related to posture	Common	Rare	Rare
Urinary incontinence	Rare	Rare	Varies
Preceding injury	Rare	Varies	Common

Note. Adapted from Shneker BF, Fountain NB. Epilepsy. *Dis Mon.* 2003;49:426–478.

pre-seizure state and the period following the seizure, known as the post-ictal state. As an example, a motor seizure may result in a post-ictal neurological dysfunction known as Todd's paralysis, which resolves over a short time. Such abnormalities may result in difficulty distinguishing seizure from TIA or stroke.

- Syncope is uncommon in stroke conditions unless blood supply is altered in both carotid arteries (as may be the case during hypotensive episode) or in the posterior circulation affecting the brainstem.

Tests

- Diagnostic testing should be undertaken only if treatment will change as a result of the findings. The burden of the evaluation must be considered in the context of prognosis, comorbidities, and goals of care.
- If a decision is made to pursue evaluation, the American Academy of Neurology endorses the following for the evaluation of seizure disorders: laboratory testing, neuroimaging, lumbar puncture, and electroencephalography.[5]
- Lab tests should include complete blood count, chemistry, serological abnormalities. Recurrent seizures in individuals on anticonvulsant therapy warrant testing serum levels of the respective agent when such is available.
- Neuroimaging plays a vital role in the determination of seizure disorders. Computerized axial tomography (CT) of the brain provides the most rapid assessment for gross structural abnormalities such as blood, as in the case of hematoma (epidural, subdural, subarachnoid, and intracerebral) or mass lesion such as tumor. Chronic changes associated with prior injury or stroke may also be visible assisting in clarification of the differential diagnosis.
- Magnetic resonance imaging (MRI) provides the greatest resolution of brain tissue. Small structural lesions such as heterotopic brain tissue or tumor may be visible on MRI and not other imaging modalities.
- Lumbar puncture may play role in the evaluation of a new seizure, especially if central nervous system infection is suspected. The lumbar puncture may

also be used to exclude a diagnosis of subarachnoid hemorrhage in the setting of a normal CT scan.

- Electroencephalography (EEG) examines electrical activity of the brain, which may be normal in seizure disorders. Extended trial of EEG monitoring may be helpful in severe cases of refractory epilepsy or when the diagnosis remains obscure.

Mrs. T's electroencephalogram demonstrated periodic epileptiform discharges in the temporal lobe, correlating with the site of her tumor.

EXPECTED DISEASE COURSE

Depending upon the etiology, seizure disorders can remit, remain the same, or worsen. In particular, evolving mass lesions tend to result in worsening seizure control.

TREATMENT OPTIONS

Pharmacologic

- The primary treatment of seizure disorders includes treatment of the underlying condition to the best extent possible to reduce or prevent provocation of additional seizures.
- The treatment of unprovoked seizures may require pharmacological intervention. Tables 68.3 lists agents commonly used with adults and elderly adults, respectively.[6]
- Popular regimens for seizure control include carbamazepine, phenytoin, and divalproex sodium, whose serum levels are also conveniently available to guide therapy.
- Clonazepam, with its long half-life as compared with other benzodiazepines, is another choice—especially when anxiolytic or sedative effects are also desired. For patients unable to tolerate oral medications, diazepam is available in a rectal gel preparation.
- In complex cases of seizure, clinicians are advised to seek a consultation with a neurologist for a seizure management plan.
- In general, monotherapy should be attempted for seizure control. Should monotherapy fail, an additional agent may be considered. Table 68.4 includes agents included in the practice parameter from the American Association of Neurology.

TABLE 68.3: INITIAL MONOTHERAPY FOR ADULTS AND ELDERLY ADULTS WITH PARTIAL-ONSET SEIZURES

Name	Initial Dose	Increment	Daily Dose Range	Serum Level
Carbamazepine	200 mg bid	200 mg/d q wk	400 mg bid-tid	6–10
Phenytoin	15–20 mg/kg div		300–400 mg qd or div	10–20
Phenobarbital	15–20 mg/kg		60 mg bid-tid	
Primidone	100–125 mg qd	100–125 mg qd q3d	250 mg tid	
Divalproex sodium	10–15 mg/kg div	5–10 mg/kg/d q7d	30–60 mg/kg div	50–100
Lamotrigine	See mfr titration		100–400 mg div	
Topiramate	25 mg bid	50 mg/d q wk	200 mg bid	
Gabapentin	300 mg tid		300–1200 mg tid	
Clonazepam	0.5 mg tid	0.5–1 mg/d q 3d	0.5–5 mg tid	
Oxcarbazepine	300 mg bid	300 mg/d/q 3d	600 mg bid	

Surgical Options

- In severe cases of refractory epilepsy (either partial or generalized), surgery may be considered a curative or, more generally, palliative option to reduce seizure frequency and intensity.
- Referral to a comprehensive epilepsy program that offers surgical options may result in recommendations for cortical resection or lobectomy.

STATUS EPILEPTICUS

- Treatment of prolonged seizures (status epilepticus) requires immediate intervention with parenteral agents for inpatients, or sublingual (SL) or subcutaneous (SQ) if at home. Table 68.5 lists commonly used agents.
- Diazepam or lorazepam are often the first agents utilized to terminate status epilepticus, followed by an anticonvulsant such as fosphenytoin or valproic acid.
- These agents are commonly limited to use in a hospital setting; the rectal gel preparation of diazepam may be a satisfactory option in an ambulatory or home setting.
- In extreme situations, and in the event of inadequate control even with these agents, general anesthesia may be considered.

As Mrs. T's condition worsened, her seizures became more frequent and intense, requiring continuous infusion with lorazepam to remain seizure-free.

PALLIATIVE CARE ISSUES

- Seizure disorders presenting as primary or secondary illness may detract from quality of life due to the uncertainty of occurrence as well as severity in effect.

TABLE 68.4: ADJUNCTIVE TREATMENT

Name	Initial Dose	Increment	Daily Dose Range
Tiagabine	4 mg qd	4 mg/d q wk	32–56 mg/d
Levetiracetam	500 mg q12h	1000 mg/d q 2wk	500–1500 mg q12h
Lamotrigine	See mfr titration		200 mg/d
Topiramate	25 mg qd-bid	25–50 mg/d q wk	100–200 mg bid
Gabapentin	300 mg tid		300–1200 mg tid
Zonisamide	100 mg qd	Q 2 wks	100–600 mg/d
Oxcarbazepine	300 mg bid	600 mg/d q wk	600 mg bid

TABLE 68.5: TREATMENT OF STATUS EPILEPTICUS

Name	Initial or Loading Dose	Average Dose (70 kg adult)	Increment
Diazepam	0.2–0.5 mg/kg	5–10 mg IV (2–5mg/minute)	2–5 mg/min
Diazepam rectal gel	0.2–0.5 mg/kg	5–10 mg PR	As tolerated
Fosphenytoin	20 mg/kg	1400 mg IV (< 150 mg/minute)	
Lorazepam	0.05–0.1 mg/kg	4–8 mg (2 mg/minute)	
Midazolam	0.2 mg/kg IV or IM	14 mg (2–5 mg/minute)	
Valproic Acid	25 mg/kg	20–500 mg/minute	

- Control of seizures is important to maximize quality of life. Consideration should be given to patient's care setting when developing a treatment plan because some medications require IV administration and could not be used at home.
- Benzodiazepines are often the drug of choice in seizure patients with advanced cerebral malignancy who are near the end of life, because of benzodiazepines' immediate control of seizures along with anxiolytic, sedative, and muscle-relaxing properties.
- In a scenario of worsening underlying conditions, such as advancing cerebral malignancy, effective treatment of seizures may lead to side effects of sedation, especially with use of benzodiazepines.
- Discussions about goals of care may assist in achieving an acceptable balance between treatment efficacy and desirable or undesirable side effects of available medications.
- For patients requiring longer-term control of seizures, an anticonvulsant may be the best choice of agent to reduce seizure frequency.

TAKE-HOME POINTS

- Seizures should be considered in the differential diagnosis of an alteration in consciousness, whether or not convulsive movements are observed.
- Seizures may significantly detract from quality of life due to the uncertainty of occurrence as well as severity in effect.

- Seizure control can be highly variable. It is best defined as a satisfactory level of control, as determined by the patient and his or her physician.
- Status epilepticus is a medical emergency requiring immediate intervention. If IV access is not an option, consider diazepam, which is available in a rectal preparation.

REFERENCES

1. Fisher RS, van Emde Boas W, Blume W, et al. Epileptic seizures and epilepsy. Definitions proposed by the International League Against Epilepsy (ILAE) and the International Bureau for Epilepsy (IBE). *Epilepsia.* 2005;*46*:470–472.
2. Engel J. A proposed diagnostic scheme for people with epileptic seizures and epilepsy Report of the ILAE Task Force on classification and terminology. *Epilepsia.* 2001;*42*(6):796–803.
3. Hauser WA, Annegers JF, Rocca WA. Descriptive epidemiology of epilepsy: contributions of population-based stiudies from Rochester, Minnesota. *Mayo Clin Proc.* 1996;*71*(6):576–586.
4. Shneker BF, Fountain NB. Epilepsy. *Dis Mon.* 2003;*49*:426–478.
5. Krumholz A, Wiebe S, Gronseth G, et al. Practice parameter: Evaluating an apparent unprovoked first seizure in adults (an evidence-based review). *Neurology.* 2007;*69*:1996–2007.
6. Glauser T, Ben-Menachem E, Bourgeois B, et al. ILAE treatment guidelines: Evidence-based analysis of antiepileptic drug efficacy and effectiveness as initial monotherapy for epileptic seizures and syndromes. *Epilepsia.* 2006;*47*(7): 1094–1120.

69

Stroke

CASE

Mrs. N is a 74-year-old, right-handed woman with a 17-year history of hypertension. She is a heavy drinker and also smokes cigarettes. She has not maintained contact with a primary care doctor or the medical system since her diagnosis of hypertension. She experienced sudden weakness of the right side of her body and slurring of her speech. Her husband called 911 to have her treated at the local hospital. She was diagnosed with a new stroke in the cerebral cortex of the left hemisphere, in the vascular territory of the left middle cerebral artery. After four days, she continues to experience aphasia, dysphagia, dysarthria, and right hemiparesis. The medical team has raised the question of whether or not a feeding tube should be placed. Mrs. N has a living will that specifies her wishes to forgo CPR, intubation, and artificial nutrition and hydration in the setting of terminal illness.

DEFINITION

Stroke is defined as sudden neurological dysfunction resulting from loss of blood supply to one or more vascular territories of the brain.

- Loss of blood supply can occur on a global scale, as in the case of profound hypotension, or may be localized as in the case of thrombosis, embolism, or hemorrhage.
- Focal neurological symptoms persist longer than 24 hours and are associated with signs of tissue ischemia.
- Transient ischemic attack (TIA) is the term used when neurological symptoms completely resolve within 24 hours. A TIA may not be associated with obvious brain injury on imaging.

Mrs. N was diagnosed with a left middle cerebral artery stroke affecting the parietal cortex resulting in right hemiparesis, aphasia, dysarthria, and dysphagia.

CLASSIFICATION

- Stroke is often classified as hemorrhagic, in which blood escapes from the vasculature, usually entering the brain parenchyma, ventricles, or subarachnoid space, or non-hemorrhagic. Non-hemorrhagic strokes may convert to secondary hemorrhagic strokes after the initial event.
- Major categories of stroke include:
  Hemorrhagic infarction
  - Subararachnoid
  - Intracerebral
  - Primary
  - Secondary
  Non-hemorrhagic infarction
  - Cardioembolic
  - Lacunar (small vessel)
  - Atherothrombotic (medium-large)
  - Watershed (hypoperfusion)
- Stroke may also be defined anatomically (by vascular distribution or brain region) and functionally. Clinical signs of neurological dysfunction tend to localize to the region rendered ischemic. The neurological history and physical examination may thus be quite predictive of both the type of stroke and the anatomical region affected.

PREVALENCE

- The prevalence of stroke among U.S. adults aged 20 and over in 2004 was estimated at 5,700,000, or approximately 1.9% of the general population.
- From 2005–2006, the prevalence of stroke was approximately 7.8% among men aged 60–79 and approximately 7.6% among women, aged 60–79.
- In people aged 80 years and older, prevalence increases to 17.1% of men and 13.5% of women.
- New or recurrent stroke occurs in about 700,000 people in the United States each year.[1] Of these strokes, 87% are ischemic or embolic in nature; intracerebral and

subarachnoid hemorrhage account for the remainder of all other strokes.

LIKELY ETIOLOGIES

- Stroke can be attributed to a number of different causes as outlined in Table 69.1, with the most common disease risk factors being atrial fibrillation, hypertension, hyperlipidemia, and diabetes.
- Hypertension contributes to atherothrombotic events, while atrial fibrillation tends to contribute to

TABLE 69.1: CAUSES OF STROKE

Stroke Type	Risk Factors
Cardioembolic	Atrial fibrillation
	Valvular heart disease including prosthetic valve
	Structural heart disease (e.g., PFO)
	Acute MI and left ventricular thrombus
	Cardiomyopathy
Large artery atherosclerosis	Extracranial carotid disease
	Extracranial vertebrobasilar disease
	Intracranial atherosclerosis
Atherothrombotic	Hypertension*
	Hyperlipidemia
	Diabetes mellitus
	Alcohol
	Tobacco
Hypercoagulable state	Factor V Leiden
	Protein C/S deficiency
	Paraneoplastic
	Inflammatory
Other	Hypotension
	Toxic/Metabolic (carbon monoxide, cyanide)
	Trauma
	Sickle-cell disease
	Arterial dissection (carotid/vertebral)
	Coagulopathy*
	Thrombocytopenia*
	Tumor*
	Arteriovenous malformation (AVM)

* Risk factors for hemorrhagic stroke

thromboembolic events, especially in the case of cortical infarction.
- The category of lacunar infarction includes strokes often resulting from atherothrombotic events, localized to subcortical regions.

In Mrs. N's case, likely etiologies include her longstanding, untreated hypertension and tobacco and alcohol use. Her newly identified atrial fibrillation may also have contributed to her stroke.

DIAGNOSIS

Exam

- The neurological examination remains the mainstay of initial diagnosis and serves to predict the region or territory of brain affected (Tables 69.2A, 69.2B). The neurological examination also serves to specify the functional deficit resulting from the event.
- Ongoing, serial examination helps to quantify the degree of deficit and the course of recovery or decline. In the immediate phases of stroke, neurological function may decline as edema worsens or, as in the case of hemorrhage, mass effect worsens. Over time, however, function may improve as edema and mass effect resolve, or on a longer time scale, neural plasticity may allow regional compensation for lost function.

Mrs. N presented with cortical findings of aphasia, along with hemiparesis. These findings point to a dominant hemisphere stroke in the (L) parietal cortex.

- Localization of stroke has important clinical significance. It often allows clinicians to predict the potential neurological deficits and can be helpful in conceptualizing the resulting functional impact. For example, a cortical stroke resulting in hemiparesis may also present with a cognitive deficits such as aphasia or neglect. A corresponding subcortical stroke resulting in similar hemiparesis may present with no cognitive deficits whatsoever. The presence of cognitive deficits often compounds the quality of life impairments and may limit potential for rehabilitation.

TABLE 69.2A: LOCALIZATION OF STROKE—CORTICAL INFARCTION SYNDROMES

Vascular	Neurological Symptoms
(L) Middle cerebral artery (MCA) dominant hemisphere, anterior division	Expressive aphasia, right hemiparesis
MCA (dominant hemisphere), posterior division	Receptive aphasia
MCA (non-dominant)	Neglect
Anterior cerebral artery (ACA)	Contralateral lower extremity hemiparesis
Posterior cerebral artery	Unilateral hemianopsia

TABLE 69.2B: LOCALIZATION OF STROKE—LACUNAR SYNDROMES

Syndrome	Location	Symptoms
Pure motor stroke	Pons, or internal capsule	Hemiparesis of face, arm, or leg
Pure sensory stroke	Lateral thalamus and/or posterior limb internal capsule	Hemisensory loss of face, arm, or leg
Ataxic hemiparesis	Subcortical white matter, pons	Incoordination and hemiparesis
Clumsy hand-dysarthria	Pons	Dysarthria and incoordination of hand

TESTS

Imaging

- Neuroimaging serves to rapidly distinguish hemorrhagic from non-hemorrhagic stroke. Computerized axial tomography (CT) provides the most rapid assessment and can be used in the presence of implanted devices such as pacemakers and defibrillators. Findings on CT scan may remain elusive for up to 24 hours, especially in the case of small, non-hemorrhagic strokes, or those occurring in the brainstem or cerebellum.
- Magnetic resonance imaging (MRI) offers a substantial clinical advantage over CT scan by revealing stroke in its earliest stages. Newer scanning sequences such as diffusion weighted imaging (DWI) offer the most rapid confirmation of ischemic stroke. Additional scanning sequences such as T2 and FLAIR provide indications of chronic processes such as underlying demyelinating processes.
- Magnetic resonance angiography (MRA) can be used to identify stenosis or occlusion of both intracranial and extracranial vessels.
- Ultrasound imaging is used to identify the presence of stenosis in the large arteries. Doppler studies of the carotid arteries can rapidly assess for carotid stenosis. Transcranial techniques may also be used to further assess the intracranial portion of the carotid system as well as the vertebrobasilar system.
- Transthoracic (TTE) and transesophageal (TEE) echocardiogram are best used to assess cardiogenic causes of stroke. While TEE offers greater resolution and the opportunity to better assess structural abnormalities, its use requires concomitant endoscopy increasing the technical difficulty of the study.

Labs

- When etiology of stroke remains obscure, laboratory studies may be helpful. In such cases, information gained may also be helpful to identify inherited risk factors.
- Laboratory markers may be used to identify factors leading to hypercoagulability. The Factor V-Leiden abnormality is the most prevalent of the commonly available serological markers of hypercoagulability. Uncommon causes of stroke including hyperhomocysteinemia, protein C/S deficiency, or antiphospholipid antibody syndrome are also assessed with lab studies.

EXPECTED DISEASE COURSE

- Following development of initial symptoms, overall function may deteriorate as infarcted tissue experiences edema, leading to further extension of dysfunction. Symptoms tend to improve most rapidly over the next four weeks, followed by continued improvement for up to six months to two years.

- Complications depend upon the disability experienced. For example, dysphagia may limit adequate oral intake, leading clinicians to refer patients for gastrostomy tubes. Hemiparesis or neglect may lead to a loss of ability to live independently. Aphasia may result in social isolation from loss of communicative abilities.

TREATMENT OPTIONS

Non-Pharmacologic

- Treatment of completed stroke with potential for functional recovery typically focuses on three main areas: supportive care during the initial phases, rehabilitation of lost function, and secondary prevention.
- Supportive care in the immediate post-stroke setting serves to reduce morbidity from complications following the initial event. Prophylaxis against deep venous thrombosis, urinary tract infection, pneumonia, and decubitus ulcers is paramount and now recognized as a quality indicator in acute hospital care. [Note: "Supportive care" is the traditional terminology used to denote care of the individual in the immediate post-stroke period. Supportive care is palliative in nature, with attention paid to preventing complications, managing active symptoms, and reducing the burden of new symptoms that may arise as a consequence of functional deficits.]
- Restorative care focuses on rehabilitation of lost function and is recommended for those with a prognosis of improvement. Such care may occur in a variety of settings, including acute inpatient rehabilitation, skilled nursing facilities, outpatient rehabilitation, or home.
- Rehabilitative strategies for selected deficits include:[2]
  - Hemiparesis: physical and occupational therapy
  - Neglect: occupational and cognitive therapy
  - Aphasia: speech therapy
  - Dysphagia: speech therapy

Pharmacologic

- Preventive care often necessitates the use of pharmacologic therapy to reduce the chances of recurrent stroke. Table 69.3 illustrates recommended interventions based on likely etiology for all stroke types.[3]
- Agents available to reduce occurrence of subsequent strokes of non-cardioembolic origin include combinational or individual use of aspirin, clopidogrel, and dipyridamole.[4] When considering pharmacologic interventions, especially combination anticoagulation, clinicians should weigh the benefits of treatment against the risk of bleeding and falls.

PALLIATIVE CARE ISSUES

- Because stroke can vary greatly in its symptomatic and temporal manifestations, determining prognosis is a dynamic process requiring frequent reassessment.
- In the case of catastrophic event such as whole hemisphere infarction, or massive intracranial hemorrhage, discussions about overall survival tend to dominate over predictions about recovery of function. In the more typical setting of non-life-threatening stroke, discussions about expected complications and recovery in the post-stroke period are more germane.
- Function can change rapidly in the early phases of stroke (either improving or worsening), and reassessment of goals of care is often required. Assessment and prognosis should be characterized (and revised) according to the acute (hours-days), subacute (weeks-months),

---

TABLE 69.3: PHARMACOLOGIC INTERVENTIONS FOR SECONDARY STROKE PREVENTION BY STROKE TYPE

Etiology	Recommendation
Atrial fibrillation	Anticoagulation (warfarin)
Hypertension/Diabetes	Anti-platelet therapy (aspirin)
Carotid stenosis	Surgery, anti-platelet therapy
Congestive heart failure	Anticoagulation
Anti-phospholipid antibody syndrome	Anticoagulation (warfarin)

and chronic (months-years) phases of the stroke.

Mrs. N initially presented with complete dysphagia, necessitating treatment with intravenous fluids. Her previously stated wishes were to forgo artificial feeding, even temporarily, leading her family to choose a plan of care in accordance with her wishes. Over several days, she regained the ability to tolerate pureed consistency, and her care plan was revised to add speech therapy to help her achieve improved function.

- When addressing goals of care with patient and family, it is important not only to provide prognostic information about survival but also to explore whether the expected recovery of function provides a quality of life that is acceptable to the patient. (See Chapter 7: Prognostication.)
- While some patients may accept short- and long-term assistance with basic needs required to sustain life, others may decline. The final care plan should take into consideration the patient's current or past expression of goals for care, prognosis of the disease in the context of comorbidities, the patient's expectations for quality of life, and the resources available to the patient and family.

SETTING OF CARE
- Individuals who have experienced severe functional deficit and are not expected to make significant functional improvement will require long-term care. Home-based care often requires extensive support from either family or licensed care providers (e.g. certified nursing aide). When such care is impractical or unavailable, the long-term care facility should be considered at the completion of a rehabilitative course of treatment.
- Hospice-level care is available for individuals with life expectancy of six months or less and who wish to forgo aggressive restorative treatment. Hospice care includes rehabilitative services (PT, OT, speech) and can be provided in the home setting if there are sufficient supplementary resources, a long-term care facility, or a dedicated hospice facility.

Mrs. N received supportive care consisting of intravenous fluids while she remained NPO (i.e., nothing-by-mouth) for severe dysphagia. After discussion with her family, she declined placement of a feeding tube, opting instead for comfort care and permissive feeding, recognizing and accepting the risk of aspiration. Over the next several days, however, she was able to swallow a pureed consistency and was transferred to a short-term rehabilitation facility.

TAKE-HOME POINTS
- Stroke represents a serious condition that not only can lead to morbidity but also can result in significant loss of function and quality of life.
- Determining prognosis is often a dynamic process in the early stages of a stroke and may vary greatly, depending on comorbidities, functional status, and cognition, as well as development of complications.
- Complications resulting in significant functional decline (e.g., new myocardial infarction, aspiration pneumonia, infection) are likely to interfere with improvement and suggest a poor prognosis when compared with the patient who proceeds to rehabilitation without complication.
- Discussions of goals of care are essential throughout the initial and subacute stages to guide appropriate choices for care and to make decisions about further interventions.

REFERENCES
1. American Heart Association. *Heart and Stroke Statistical Update-2007.* Dallas, Tex: American Heart Association; 2007.
2. Duncan PW, et al. Management of adult stroke rehabilitation care: a clinical practice guideline. *Stroke.* 2005;36:e100–e143.
3. Sacco RL, et al. Guidelines for prevention of stroke in patients with ischemic stroke or transient ischemic attack: a statement for healthcare professionals from the American Heart Association/American Stroke Association Council on Stroke. *Stroke.* 2006;37:577–617.
4. Adams HP. Secondary prevention of atherothrombotic events after ischemic stroke. *Mayo Clin Proc.* 2009;84(1):43–51.

70

Parkinson's Disease

CASE

Mr. R, an 85-year-old male with a 15-year history of Parkinson's disease (PD), presents to the clinic because of gait instability and cognitive impairment. He was initially diagnosed with PD when he presented with a rest tremor in the left hand and slowness of movements and rigidity of the left side. He was treated then with carbidopa/levodopa, with a dramatic improvement in his symptoms. As his PD progressed, Mr. R's primary care physician added pramipexole to his levodopa regimen. His family notes that he is sedated in the daytime and is experiencing visual hallucinations in which he sees cats or strangers in his house. However, he does report that he knows they are not real. On exam, Mr. R is oriented to person, place, and time, and is able to follow simple commands. He scores a 25/30 on the Mini-Mental State Exam (MMSE). He is noted to have a masked facies, with hypophonia. He has a mild chin tremor and a mild rest tremor in the left more than the right hand. Cogwheel rigidity is elicited in his left more than right extremities, and a moderate slowing of movements is seen in his left more than right side. He needs to use his arms to get up from a chair. He has a mildly stooped posture, with a slow shuffling gait. He has intermittent freezing and moderate postural instability.

DEFINITION

Parkinson's disease (PD) is a neurodegenerative disorder characterized by a variable combination of the cardinal clinical features:

- Tremor at rest
- Bradykinesia (slowness of movement)
- Cogwheel rigidity
- Postural instability

Pathologically, there is nigrostriatal neuron degeneration in the substantia nigra pars compacta. This depletion of dopamine produces the characteristic motor abnormalities seen in PD.

The remaining neurons contain intracytoplasmic inclusion bodies called Lewy bodies.

PREVALENCE

- Increases with age
- Affects approximately 2% of those aged 65 and older[1]
- As high as 7% to 9%[2,3] in institutionalized elderly

LIKELY ETIOLOGIES

- The etiology of PD remains unknown, with the vast majority of cases (over 90%) occurring sporadically. A minority of cases are familial.
- Currently, it is felt that the etiology of PD may be multifactorial, involving an interplay of both genetic variations or predispositions that may render a person more susceptible to environmental factors that may increase risk.[4]

DIAGNOSIS
History and Exam

- Patients usually report a gradual onset of symptoms. In general, progression of disease tends to be slow, although the disease may progress at different rates in different individuals.
- At the onset of disease, the cardinal features are typically unilateral, with one side of the body affected predominantly with slowness, stiffness, or a tremor at rest.
- While tremor is the most common initial manifestation of PD, postural instability and gait difficulty (PIGD) are reported to be a more common initial presentation in the elderly.
- As the disease progresses, non-motor features as well as axial signs of the disease become more prominent. These features have been increasingly recognized as a

major source of disability and in general tend to be resistant to levodopa treatment.

Presentation of PD in the Elderly

Non-Motor Features:
- Neuropsychiatric complications: depression, anxiety, apathy
- Dementia
- Autonomic dysfunction: orthostatic hypotension, urinary urgency, constipation
- Sleep disorders

Axial, or Midline Features:
- Speech impairment: dysarthria, dysphagia
- Gait and postural impairments: freezing, postural instability, festination

EXPECTED DISEASE COURSE

- In the first few years of dopaminergic therapy, patients typically experience a "honeymoon" period, in which dopaminergic medications dramatically improve the motor symptoms and signs of PD. But as the disease advances, patients begin to develop motor complications, which limit the usefulness of levodopa as a treatment in advanced stage disease.
- "Wearing off" is the earliest motor complication; patients experience an earlier recurrence of parkinsonian symptoms prior to the next dosing interval.
- In time, patients typically develop motor fluctuations. They alternate throughout the day between being in an "ON" state, in which they are well controlled on anti-PD medications but experience *dyskinesias* (extra involuntary movements), and an "OFF" state, in which the patient is suboptimally controlled on medications and is experiencing recurrence of their parkinsonian symptoms.
- With advancing disease, patients experience non-motor and axial features that are less responsive to levodopa as well as progression of motor complications, which tend to lead to a poorer prognosis and worsening disability.
- Mortality is two to five times that of age- and sex-matched controls.[5] The leading cause of death in PD is pneumonia, typically due to aspiration.[6]
- In addition, PD patients with immobility and dementia often develop complications

such as fractures, thromboses, and infections.[7] As a result, goals of care conversations with focus on quality of life should be addressed simultaneously with treatments to minimize symptoms.

TREATMENT OPTIONS

Treatment strategies in PD focus on three goals:

- Control of motor symptoms and signs of the disease
- Reduction of disability
- Improving quality of life

While neuroprotection (to modify the course of disease or slow progression) is a goal of research, no such proven treatment is currently available. Making a decision as to which anti-PD therapy to employ in a particular patient will depend on several variables, including the functional status of the patient, the level of the patient's cognitive function, and the presence of other comorbidities.

Nonpharmacologic

- Movement disorders are best treated by a strong interdisciplinary team. Physical and occupational therapies can help to maintain and improve functional mobility, quality of life, and steadiness of ambulation.
- Exercising to maintain physical activity is highly encouraged. Stretching exercises should be suggested to improve flexibility and stooped posture. Physical therapists can provide patients with realistic exercises and movement strategies to improve ambulation that is consistent with their disease severity.
- Occupational therapy can assess and teach patients and their caregivers strategies and recommend assistive devices to enable the patient to remain as independent as possible. Therapists may also recommend home modifications.
- Family caregiver support is crucial to the ability to keep patients living at home. Social workers can help patients and families plan for future financial needs and may also offer supportive counseling and referral to individual and family therapy.
- Individuals with movement disorders may find themselves becoming socially isolated, resulting not only from mobility issues but also from self-consciousness

about difficulties with eating/feeding and drooling. A dietician and/or occupational therapist may offer the patient and family ideas about food choices and utensils that will minimize distress or discomfort.

Pharmacologic

- While dopamine replacement is the gold standard of symptomatic treatment, it is associated with an increased risk of motor complications as well as non-motor features. Dopamine agonists are less effective than levodopa and have a lower risk of motor complications such as dyskinesias. However, dopamine agonists are more likely than levodopa to cause visual hallucinations and confusion, which can be very distressing for older adults and caregivers.
- Other anti-PD pharmacological therapies include (Table 70.1):
  - MAO-B inhibitors can be used either as monotherapy in early stage disease, or as adjunctive therapy to levodopa in the treatment of motor fluctuations.
  - COMT inhibitors are used in conjunction with levodopa to extend the serum half-life of levodopa and are indicated to treat wearing-off in PD.
  - Other agents such as anticholinergics and amantadine may also be used but are generally mild symptomatic treatments. Amantadine is also used to treat dyskinesias in PD patients. Anticholinergics may be of use in treating tremor, i.e., in tremor-predominant PD, but given their side effect profile, should be used with caution particularly in elderly patients with dementia.

Special Pharmacologic Considerations in Older Adults

- Frail older adults with cognitive impairment and/or multiple medical comorbidities are more susceptible to the neuropsychiatric side effects such as visual hallucinations or confusional state that occur commonly with dopamine agonists.
- PD patients are also prone to develop these side effects with the other classes of anti-PD medications such as MAO-B or COMT

inhibitors, amantadine, and anticholinergic medications.
- Anticholinergic agents may cause other side effects in elderly patients such as urinary retention, glaucoma, constipation, orthostasis, and delirium.
- For these reasons, levodopa tends to be the most well-tolerated agent in the treatment of elderly patients. In contrast, a "levodopa sparing strategy" may be employed in a young, cognitively intact PD patient, by starting treatment with a non-levodopa agent such as a dopamine agonist (DA) as monotherapy.
- Visual hallucinations can be managed by reducing or eliminating the dopaminergic medications, in particular dopamine agonists. If unable to reduce the dopaminergic medications due to worsening of parkinsonian symptoms, a trial with an atypical antipsychotic, such as quetiapine, may control the hallucinations.

Treatment of Non-Motor Complications in PD

Non-motor features in PD are myriad and include neuropsychiatric disorders such as hallucinations and depression, dementia, delirium, autonomic dysfunction, and sleep disorders.

1. Depression:
   - Has been described in up to 70% of PD patients.[8]
   - May precede the onset of motor symptoms of PD and is thought to be a potential marker for development of the illness.
   - Tricyclic antidepressants and SSRIs may be effective (SSRI trials involved small number of patients). Exercise and behavioral approaches may also be beneficial. (See Chapter 64: Depression.)
2. Dementia:
   - PD-related dementia (PDD) affects up to approximately 40% of patients.[9]
   - Cholinesterase inhibitors, including donezepil and galantamine, have been studied for the treatment of PDD. A randomized double-blind, placebo-controlled crossover study of donezepil in patients with PDD showed a significant improvement in MMSE

(Mini-Mental State Examination) and CGI (Clinical Global Impression) scores, although ADAS-cog (AD Assessment Scale-Cognitive Subscale) scores did not improve.[10]

- Rivastigmine is FDA-approved for the treatment of PD-related dementia. An RCT noted cognitive improvement by the ADAS-cog score and overall change in clinical status by the

TABLE 70.1: MEDICATIONS USED TO TREAT PARKINSON'S DISEASE

Medication	Dosage	T1/2 (Half-Life)	Metabolism	Side Effects
DA replacement—most potent for symptomatic management				
Carbidopa/ levodopa	100 mg TID (available in immediate release: 10/100, 25/100, 25/250 and controlled release 25/100, 50/200 tablets)	1–11/2 hours	Hepatic	Visual hallucinations Confusion Nausea Vomiting Induction of motor complications Orthostasis
DA agonists				
Pramipexole	Initial dose: 0.125 mg TID Maximal dose: 4.5 mg per day	8–12 hours	Renal	Fewer motor complications than levodopa but more likely to cause visual hallucinations and confusion in older adults Peripheral edema Orthostasis Visual hallucinations Impulse control disorders
Ropinirole	Initial dose: 0.25 mg TID Maximal dose: 24 mg per day	4–6 hours	Hepatic	Fewer motor complications than levodopa but more likely to cause visual hallucinations and confusion in older adults Peripheral edema Orthostasis Visual hallucinations Impulse control disorders
Apomorphine	Initial dose: subcutaneous injection of 0.2 mL (2 mg), then 0.2 to 0.6 mL (2 to 6 mg) as needed for "OFF" episodes. Maximal is 1 dose/episode, with at least 2 hours between episodes. Do not dose more than 5 times a day or over 2 mL (20 mg) per day	40–90 minutes	Unclear	Take frequent vital signs during the initial treatment to ensure orthostasis does not develop Nausea is common: to reduce nausea, pre-treat with trimethobenzamide 300 mg po TID at least 3 days prior to apomorphine treatment Sweating Bradycardia Pallor Yawning Peripheral edema Local site reaction Impulse control disorders

(continued)

TABLE 70.1: (CONTINUED)

Medication	Dosage	T1/2 (Half-Life)	Metabolism	Side Effects
MAO inhibitors: act by inhibiting the enzymes that facilitate the metabolism of levodopa				
Selegiline	Initial dose: 5 mg po qd Maximal dose: 10 mg per day	0.5 to 1 hour	Hepatic	Nausea Orthostasis Hallucinations Insomnia Rarely, a "tyramine effect," ingestion of MAO-B inhibitor with food containing tyramine such as red wine or cheese can cause a hypertensive crisis
Rasagiline	Initial dose: 0.5 mg po qd Maximal dose: 1 mg po qd	3.5 hours	Hepatic	Nausea Orthostasis Hallucinations Insomnia Rarely, a "tyramine effect," ingestion of MAO-B inhibitor with food containing tyramine such as red wine or cheese can cause a hypertensive crisis
COMT inhibitors				
Entacapone	Initial dose: 200 mg given with each dose of levodopa Maximal dose: 1600 mg po qd	0.4–0.7 hour	Hepatic	Dopaminergic side effects from COMT inhibition include increased dyskinesias, hallucinations, orthostasis, nausea, constipation, diarrhea, urine discoloration (which is benign)
Tolcapone	Initial dose: 100 mg po given with each dose of levodopa Maximal dose: 600 mg po qd	2–3 hours	Hepatic	Rare: fulminant hepatotoxicity (monitor LFTs carefully) Dopaminergic side effects from COMT inhibition include increased dyskinesias, hallucinations, orthostasis, nausea, constipation, diarrhea
Other medications				
Amantadine	Initial dose: 100 mg po qd Maximal dose: 400 mg po qd	10–28.5 hours	90% is excreted in urine via glomerular filtration and tubular secretion	Confusion, dizziness, peripheral edema, congestive heart failure, orthostasis, livedo reticularis
Trihexyphenidyl	Initial dose: 1 mg po qd Maximal dose: 2–3 mg TID	3.3–4.1 hours	Excreted in the urine, probably as unchanged drug	Use with caution in elderly due to common side effects of sedation, confusion, dry mouth, memory impairment, orthostasis, urine retention, blurred vision

Clinical Global Impression (CGI).[11] (See Chapter 67: Dementia.)

3. Anxiety:
   - Also common in PD and can represent an "OFF" phenomenon. SSRIs or a short-term trial of benzodiazepines may be tried, taking into consideration the increased risk of falls, sleepiness, or confusion.

4. Autonomic dysfunction:
   - Prevalent in PD, typically in more advanced states.
   - Symptoms include orthostatic hypotension (OH), urinary urgency, constipation, increased drooling, dysphagia, and erectile dysfunction.
   - Botulinum toxin injections to the salivary glands may be used to control sialorrhea.
   - Urinary frequency and incontinence may be treated with agents such as oxybutinin and tolterodine, although the anticholinergic side effects may be prohibitive.

5. Orthostatic hypotension (OH):
   - Described in at least 20% of PD patients and correlates with disease duration.[12]
   - Orthostasis may be caused by anti-PD medications, particularly the dopaminergic agents, and may not always be symptomatic. Pharmacologic treatment should be considered when it is symptomatic, and may involve reducing the dose of the offending medications.
   - Nonpharmacologic measures including adequate hydration, liberalizing salt intake, and the use of compressive leg stockings.
   - If these measures do not elevate the blood pressure, options include the mineralocortoid, fludrocortisones 0.1 mg po once or twice a day, or the alpha-receptor agonist midodrine 10 mg po TID.

6. Sleep disorders:
   - Sleep disorders seen commonly in PD include REM behavior disorder (RBD), restless leg syndrome, and sleep apnea. PD patients may also have both sleep initiation and sleep maintenance insomnia.
   - Etiology is multifactorial and can be due to PD itself, to anti-PD medications, or to primary sleep disorders.

- Implementation of good sleep hygiene is important. Substances that may interfere with sleep, such as caffeine, should be avoided, and regular sleeping hours should be enforced.
- Sleep disruption may occur due to nocturnal onset of PD-related symptoms such as rigidity and akinesia. Using controlled-release levodopa before bedtime may help reduce nighttime PD symptoms.
- Nocturia is also a frequent symptom, and patients can be advised to reduce fluid intake prior to bedtime. Intranasal desmopressin may be used to reduce nocturia.
- PD patients may also have excessive daytime somnolence (EDS) that may be an effect of anti-parkinsonian medications. (Dopamine agonists have been implicated in "sleep attacks," or episodes of sudden onset of sleep.)[13]
- A trial with modafinil 100 to 400 mg per day or methylphenidate for EDS may be considered but should be used with caution in the elderly. Side effects of methylphenidate and modafinil include increased blood pressure or heart rate and cardiac arrthythmias, especially in patients with cardiac disease, as well as dizziness, insomnia, and anxiety.
- In summary, the causes of sleep disturbance in PD are numerous, and often patients may have several contributing factors. Careful evaluation of the sleep disturbances affecting a PD patient, including a polysomnogram when appropriate, can lead to specific treatments to consolidate nocturnal sleep and enhance daytime alertness. The burden of the evaluation, however, must be considered in the context of prognosis, comorbidities, and goals of care.

Deep Brain Stimulation (DBS)

DBS of the subthalamic nucleus (STN) is an FDA-approved surgical treatment for PD. Many investigators consider older age, i.e., older than 70 years of age, to be an indicator of poor outcome after DBS surgery, partly due to a higher incidence of cognitive impairment in this population.[14]

However, good outcomes have also been reported in elderly cohorts.[15]

SYMPTOM MANAGEMENT TO IMPROVE QUALITY OF LIFE

The case of Mr. R highlights several symptoms that should be managed to improve quality of life for the elderly PD patient population:

- Gait dysfunction is frequent, particularly as disease progresses. Complications of advanced PD, such as worsening of postural instability and freezing, are often not levodopa-responsive. Physical therapy and the use of assistive devices when needed may be of help.
- In an elderly cohort, cognitive dysfunction may be due to underlying PD-related dementia or may be a side effect of anti-PD medications. Memory impairment may also represent a pseudodementia due to depression, which is highly prevalent in PD. Withdrawal of medications that can cause confusion or cognitive dysfunction, such as the dopamine agonist in this case, may help.
- Visual hallucinations are often a dopaminergic side effect, and discontinuing the dopamine agonist will likely help in this instance.
- Daytime sedation is also a common problem in elderly PD patients, and can sometimes be improved with tapering of anti-PD medications. Taking a careful sleep history is also important to uncover any underlying sleep disorders.
- Difficulty eating and communicating are features that typically develop in the late stages of illness and are likely to contribute to reduced quality of life for patients.

PALLIATIVE CARE ISSUES

- Patients with PD and their families have care needs that will significantly benefit from a palliative care approach.[16,17]
- While the treatment options noted above can slow down the progression of functional limitations, there is currently no treatment to halt these eventual symptoms. Therefore, it is crucial that goals of care discussions with PD patients and family members be initiated early in the trajectory of the disease, prior to development of cognitive impairment or difficulty communicating.

- Discussions should address the patient's preferences for feeding when dysphagia develops (by parenteral route or with the aide of a feeding tube), as well as treatment preferences when medications and other modalities no longer maintain the patient in the physical condition previously expressed as acceptable to the patient.
- Pain is prevalent and undertreated, especially in patients with more advanced PD, and must be systematically assessed and managed. For diagnostic purposes, it is helpful to classify pain in PD into one or more of five categories: musculoskeletal pain; radicular, or neuropathic, pain; dystonia-related pain; akathitic discomfort; and primary or central pain.
- Clinical management of musculoskeletal and radicular pain may respond to physical and occupational therapy. A variety of pharmacologic agents may be helpful for dystonia (domaminergic agents), central pain (levodopa and dopaminergic agents; neuropathic pain agents), and akathisia (levodopa; dopamine agonists; opioids). The usual precautions concerning dosing and side effects should be exercised when prescribing these medications for older PD patients.[18]
- Because of the chronic nature of this progressively debilitating disease, the significant caregiver stress associated with the care of PD patients must be recognized and addressed. Early involvement of a social worker who is knowledgeable about counseling and other health care services and how to access community resources is an important component of the treatment plan.

TAKE-HOME POINTS

- Key features of idiopathic Parkinson's disease include unilateral onset of symptoms, the presence of rest tremor, asymmetry of findings on exam, slow progression of symptoms, and dramatic responsiveness to levodopa. It is important to accurately diagnose PD so that the patient can be informed regarding overall prognosis of disease and the likelihood of good response to dopaminergic medications.
- Non-motor features of PD are important and, in some cases, more disabling than the motor features of the illness. Therefore, it is important to inquire about and treat

the non-motor symptoms, i.e., pain, neuropsychologic issues, sleep disorders, autonomic dysfunction, etc.

- Levodopa is the most well tolerated and efficacious anti-PD medication for elderly patients. Dopamine agonists may be effective in some patients but may have a higher risk of visual hallucinations, orthostasis, and confusion, particularly in elderly patients with cognitive impairment.
- Early focus on advance care planning, continuing discussion of goals of care as functional independence declines, and management of physical and emotional symptom distress are critical components of comprehensive medical care for Parkinson's disease.

REFERENCES

1. de Rijk MC, Tzourio C, Breteler MM, et al. Prevalence of parkinsonism and Parkinson's disease in Europe: the Europarkinson Collaborative Study. European Community Concerted Action on the Epidemiology of Parkinson's disease. *J Neurol Neurosurg Psychiatry.* 1997;*62*:10–15.
2. Tse W, Libow LS, Neufeld R, et al. Prevalence of movement disorders in an elderly nursing home population. *Arch Gerontol Geriatr.* 2008;*6*(3): 359–366.
3. Moghal S, Rajput AH, Meleth R, D'Arcy C, Rajput R. Prevalence of movement disorders in institutionalized elderly. *Neuroepidemiology.* 1995;*14*: 297–300.
4. Przedborski S. Etiology and Pathogenesis of Parkinson's disease. In: *Parkinson's Disease and Movement Disorders.* Jankovic J, Tolosa E, eds. Fifth edition Lippincott Williams and Wilkins, Phila; 2007:78–92. FROM p 81.
5. Goy ER, Carter JH, Ganzini L. Parkinson disease at the end of life: caregiver perspectives. *Neurology.* 2007; *69*:611–612.
6. Poewe W. The natural history of Parkinson's disease. *J Neurol.* 2006;*253*(suppl 7):VII/2–VII/6.

7. Gorell JM, Johnson CC, Rybicki BA. Parkinson's disease and its comorbid disorders: an analysis of Michigan mortality data, 1970 to 1990. *Neurology.* 1994;*44*:1865–1868.
8. Diamond A, Jankovic J. Treatment of advanced Parkinson's disease. *Expert Rev Neurotherapeutics.* 2006;*6*(8):1181–1197.
9. Cummings JL. Intellectual impairment in Parkinson's disease: clinical, pathological and biochemical correlates. *J Geriatr Psychiatry Neurology.* 1988;*1*(1): 14–36.
10. Ravina B, Putt M, Siderowf A, et al. Donepezil for dementia in Parkinson's disease: a randomized, double-blind, placebo-controlled, crossover study. *J Neurol Neurosurg Psychiatry.* Jul 2005;*76*(7):934–9.
11. Emre M, Aarsland D, Albanese A, et al. Rivastigmine for dementia associated with Parkinson's disease. *N Engl J Med.* 2004;*351*:2509–2518.
12. Zesiewicz TA, Baker MJ, Wahba M, Hauser RA. Autonomic nervous system dysfunction in Parkinson's disease. *Curr Treatment Options Neurology.* 2003;*5*:149–160.
13. Frucht S, Rogers JD, Greene PE, Gordon MF, Fahn S. Falling asleep at the wheel: motor vehicle mishaps in persons taking pramipexole and ropinirole. *Neurology.* 1999;*52*(9):1908–1910.
14. Welter ML, Houeto JL, Tezenas du Montcel S, et al. Clinical predictive factors of subthalamic stimulation in Parkinson's disease. *Brain.* 2002;*125*: 575–583.
15. Tagliati M, Pourfar MH, Alterman RL. Subthalamic nucleus deep brain stimulation in Parkinson's disease patients over age 70 years. *Neurology.* 2005;*65*: 179–180.
16. Hudson PL, Kristjanson LJ. Would people with Parkinson's disease benefit from palliative care? *Palliative Med.* 2006;*20*:87–94.
17. Elman LB, Houghton DJ, Wu GF, Hurtig HI, Markowitz CE, McCluskey L. Palliative care in amyotrophic lateral sclerosis, Parkinson's disease and multiple sclerosis. *J Palliative Med.* 2007;*10*(2): 433–457.
18. Ford, B. Pain in Parkinson's disease. *Movement Disorders.* 2010;*25*(suppl 1):S98–S103.

71

Essential Tremor

CASE
Mrs. S is an 85-year-old female nursing home resident with a past medical history of diabetes and hypertension. She presented with bilateral hand tremors, which she had noticed when she was reaching for objects. She stated that the hand tremors had probably started in her 60s but had become progressively more disabling in the last 10 years. She had difficulty feeding herself, and said that she would often spill soup when eating from a spoon. In order to avoid spilling from a cup, she would use a straw to drink. Mrs. S also described impairment in her handwriting and complained of social embarrassment due to the tremors.

DEFINITION
Essential tremor (ET) is a clinical disorder consisting of isolated action and postural tremor that most commonly affects both upper extremities, but can also involve the head, voice, legs, and trunk.

PREVALENCE
Essential tremor increases with age; affects an estimated 5 in every 100 adults over 60 years of age.[1]

LIKELY ETIOLOGIES
- There is a strong hereditary component to ET. Familial ET is inherited in an autosomal dominant fashion.[2]
- The pathophysiology of ET is not known, although clinical data implicate a cerebellar abnormality in ET patients.

EXPECTED DISEASE COURSE
- ET is usually a slow, progressive disease, although the course may be variable in certain cases. Onset of symptoms may be earlier in patients with familial ET.
- Patients will often seek evaluation because of functional or social disability as a result of the tremor. They will complain of difficulty performing activities of daily living that involve their hands, such as feeding, drinking, writing, and dressing.

- Patients will often describe significant improvement of their tremor with small amounts of alcohol intake.

DIAGNOSIS
Exam
- The sole clinical presentation of ET is a postural and/or kinetic tremor. This commonly affects:[3]
  - Upper extremities (95%)
  - Head (34%)
  - Lower extremities (20%)
  - Voice (12%)
  - Face (5%)
  - Trunk (5%)
- During evaluation, it is important to take a detailed medication history in order to rule out a medication-induced tremor. Thyroid function tests should be performed if there is a suspicion of hyperthyroidism.

TREATMENT OPTIONS
- ET is a slowly progressive disease, and patients may not consult their doctor until they experience significant disability from the tremor.
- The case of Mrs. S illustrates the different side effect profiles of anti-tremor medications.
- The choice of medication should always be tailored specifically to the patient and his or her other medical comorbidities. Anti-tremor medications tend to have better efficacy in controlling hand tremors but are often not as effective in treating voice or head tremor.

Nonpharmacologic
- Patients can be advised to use heavier cups or cups with a heavy base to help steady their hands when drinking.
- Using weighted eating utensils can also help steady the tremor.

TABLE 71.1: PHARMACOLOGICAL OPTIONS FOR TREATMENT
OF ESSENTIAL TREMOR

Medication	Dosage	Effect	Tolerability	Side Effects
Propranolol (beta blocker)	40 mg to 320 mg per day (starting dose is 20 mg per day)	50–60% of patients will have good response[4]	Well tolerated	Dizziness Bradycardia Nausea Fatigue Depression
Primidone (antiepileptic)	25 to 1000 mg per day (starting dose is 25 mg per day)	May be the drug of choice in patients with cardiovascular disease	Side effects likely during initiation phase but tolerance to side effects sometimes develops over time	Ataxia Vertigo Nausea Vomiting Sedation Granulocytopenia Red cell hypoplasia

- Avoiding caffeine may help prevent exacerbation of the tremor.
- Printing rather than writing in script may also help to make handwriting more legible.

Many other useful tips for coping with ET can be found at www.essentialtremor.org

Pharmacologic

- The two most widely studied agents for the treatment of ET are propranolol and primidone. Treatment aims to decrease the tremor severity and improve functional ability (Table 71.1).
- Other medications that have been studied for ET include gabapentin, topiramate, levetiracetam, and benzodiazepines, with variable efficacy in controlling the tremor.
- Deep brain stimulation (DBS) of the ventral intermediate nucleus of the thalamus (Vim), an approved neurosurgical treatment for ET, is effective in medication-refractory, disabling ET.
- Botulinum toxin injections into the forearm muscles for hand tremors, or into the cervical neck muscles for head tremor, may be useful.

On exam, Mrs. S had a head tremor, which was side to side, as well as a mild voice tremor. She had a moderate postural and action tremor in both upper extremities. Mrs. S was started on low-dose propranolol for her tremor. She initially *noted mild improvement in her hand tremor and tolerated the medication well. As the dose of propranolol was titrated upward, the nursing home staff noted that the patient developed bradycardia and would complain of dizziness when standing up from a seated position. Propranolol was discontinued, and the patient was started on primidone. She initially experienced some sedation and confusion on low-dose primidone, but after a few days these side effects abated, and she was able to tolerate it. She noted improvement in her functional disability from the hand tremors, as well as in her handwriting and ability to feed herself, but she did not achieve much improvement in her head and voice tremor.*

TAKE-HOME POINTS

- Essential tremor (ET) is a common movement disorder, and prevalence increases with age.
- Primidone and propranolol are well studied and effective treatments for ET.
- The choice of anti-tremor medication for a particular patient depends on tolerability and medical comorbidities.
- Deep brain stimulation (DBS) of the ventral intermediate nucleus of the thalamus (Vim) can be effective in cases of medication refractory, disabling ET.

REFERENCES

1. Lyons KE, Pahwa R, Comella C. Benefits and risks of pharmacologic managements for essential tremor. *Drug Saf.* 2003;26:461–481.

2. Critchley M. Observations on essential (heredofamilial) tremor. *Brain.* 1949;*72*:113–139.

3. Lyons KE, Pahwa R. Pharmacotherapy of essential tremor. *CNS Drugs.* 2008;*22*(12): 1037–1045.

4. Calzetti S, Findley LJ, Perucca E, et al. The response of essential tremor to propranolol: evaluation of clinical variables governing its efficacy on prolonged administration. *J Neurol Neurosurg Psychiatry.* 1983;*46*:393–398.

72

Malignant Spinal Cord Compression

CASE

Mrs. AD is a 65-year-old female with stage IV breast cancer with metastases to the liver. She is currently being treated with chemotherapy and is very functional at home with an Eastern Cooperative Oncology Group performance status of 0. At her visit today she is complaining of new onset midlevel back pain for one month that is not relieved with NSAIDs.

DEFINITION

Cord compression refers to compression of the dural sac and its contents (spinal cord and/or cauda equina) by an extradural tumor mass. The minimum radiologic evidence for cord compression is indentation of the thecal sac at the level of clinical features. Approximately 70% of cases occur in the thoracic spine, 20% in the lumbosacral spine and 10% in the cervical spine. Many patients will have multilevel disease.

PREVALENCE

The prevalence of cord compression in metastatic cancer is between 0.2% and 7.9%, with autopsy studies showing cord compression in about 5% of patients with cancer.[1]

LIKELY ETIOLOGIES

- Breast cancer (15–20%)
- Prostate cancer (15–20%)
- Lung cancer (15–20%)
- Multiple myeloma (5–10%)
- Renal cell carcinoma (5–10%)
- Non-Hodgkin's lymphoma (5–10%)

DIAGNOSIS

Exam

- In a patient with cancer and back pain, malignant spinal cord compression must always be ruled out. The most common symptom is often pain without any neurologic sequelae.

- Back pain is the most common and earliest complaint before permanent neurological deficits develop. Other symptoms may include:
  - Weakness (decreased motor strength)
  - Lhermitte's sign: a tingling, electrical sensation in the arms or trunk occurring when the neck is flexed
  - Sensory deficits
  - Loss of bowel and bladder function and decreased rectal tone

Tests

- If cord compression is suspected, corticosteroids should be given immediately and not delayed until imaging can be obtained.
- Imaging options include MRI, CT myelogram, CT scan, and bone scan. MRI is considered the gold standard for diagnosing spinal cord compression and should be performed first. It provides high-resolution imaging of all aspects of the spine. It is superior to CT myelogram for evaluation of epidural and soft tissue diseases. MRI also avoids the invasive use of myelographic contrast to visualize the subarachnoid space.
- A bone scan can be used if the other scanning options are unavailable. However, a bone scan indicates only the presence or absence of vertebral metastases; it does not provide information about spinal cord involvement.

Mrs. AD undergoes an MRI of her thoracic spine. She is found to have vertebral metastases in multiple thoracic vertebrae with epidural extension and spinal cord compression at the level of T10.

EXPECTED DISEASE COURSE

- Cord compression is a medical and palliative care emergency. Failure to treat immediately may lead to neurological compromise including loss of bowel and bladder continence as well as the loss of lower extremity sensation and function.

- Pretreatment ambulatory status and time from development of motor deficits to treatment (surgery or radiotherapy) are the most important predictors of ambulation after treatment.
- Overall, the majority of patients who are ambulatory prior to diagnosis retain the ability to ambulate. Of those who are paraparetic and paralyzed, only a minority regain function after appropriate treatment.
- Median survival after spinal cord compression depends on the patient's tumor type, ambulatory status, and number and site of metastases. Patients with a single metastasis, a radiosensitive tumor, or with breast or prostate cancer have the longest survival. Patients with multiple metastases, visceral or brain metastases, or lung or gastrointestinal cancers have the shortest.

TREATMENT OPTIONS

The three main components of treatment are medical therapy with pharmacologic agents, radiation, and surgery.

Pharmacologic Therapy

- Glucocorticoids:
  - Glucocorticoids are used to improve neurologic function by decreasing edema and may have tumor regression (oncolytic) effects as well as analgesic effects. Glucocorticoids also may temporarily prevent the onset of cord ischemia.

- The dose and length of glucocorticoid therapy varies by institution. The randomized controlled trials (RCT) that have evaluated the use of dexamethasone (Table 72.1) have not established any one regimen as superior.[2,3,4]
- The most comprehensive evaluation of corticosteroid use in malignant spinal cord compression involved the use of a bolus dose of 96 mg.[2] There are no standard guidelines for the bolus dose or a maintenance standing dose. While there are few institutions that give a bolus dose of 96 mg of dexamethasone, the majority give either 10 mg or none at all.
- Additionally, most institutions use dexamethasone 16 mg daily in four divided doses, usually to be tapered over a two-week period.
- Opioids for treatment of pain (See Chapter 29: Management of Pain in Older Adults.)
- Neuropathic adjuvants for treatment of neuropathic pain.
- Laxatives for prevention of constipation (See Chapter 45: Constipation.)
- Physical therapy to maintain and improve function and prevent related complications.

Radiation

- The course of RT can be a short (hypo-fractionated) course or a long course. The short course consists of one fraction (given in one day) or five fractions (given daily for five days). The long course

---

TABLE 72.1: TRIALS OF DEXAMETHASONE FOR CORD COMPRESSION

Study Design	Reference	Description
RCT—Nothing vs. 96 mg dexamethasone IV bolus then 24 mg orally QID (in divided doses) for 3 days, then taper	Sorensen et al[2]	N = 57; 81% vs. 63% ambulatory after RT with 11% serious toxicity (psychoses, gastric ulcers requiring surgery)
RCT—Dexamethasone 100 mg IV bolus vs. 10 mg IV bolus followed by 16 mg orally daily in divided doses (tapered after radiation therapy)	Vecht et al[3]	N = 37; 25% (high dose) vs. 8% (moderate dose) improvement in motor status (p = 0.22); no differences in pain control
Case control—96 mg IV bolus followed by 24 mg orally QID compared to dexamethasone 10 mg IV bolus, then 4 mg IV QID	Heimdal et al[4]	N = 66; 14% of high dose group vs. 0% of mod dose with serious adverse effects (ulcers with hemorrhage, GI perforations); ambulatory outcomes not reported

consists of 10 to 20 fractions given over two to four weeks.

- Evidence suggests that patients with a higher probability of being alive at six months benefit the most from the longer course of radiation therapy, and that those with a shorter life expectancy benefit from the shorter course.[5]
- Patients who are ambulatory at the time of the diagnosis have a higher probability of obtaining good response to treatment and a longer survival.[5]

Surgery

- If the patient has a good performance status at the time of diagnosis, a neurosurgical evaluation should be performed.
- Newer surgical techniques that involve direct decompressive surgery as opposed to laminectomies have been shown in an RCT to be superior to radiation therapy in select patient populations.[6]
- In this trial, the surgical group experienced decreased glucocorticoid use and opiate use, as well as retaining and regaining the ability to ambulate.[6]

Mrs. AD was admitted to the hospital and started on dexamethasone 10 mg IV bolus, followed by 4 mg orally every 6 hours and pain management with opioids. Neurosurgery and radiation oncology were consulted. She underwent direct decompressive surgery and was discharged to an acute rehab facility, where she remains ambulatory with plans to start systemic chemotherapy once discharged.

TAKE-HOME POINTS

- Cord compression is a **medical emergency.**
- Back pain is the earliest and most reliable sign and symptom of incipient cord compression.

- Start steroids upon consideration of the diagnosis.
- The treatment of cord compression is multidisciplinary and involves the input of multiple members of the health care team.
- In a patient with a good performance status, a neurosurgical evaluation should be performed.
- The time course of radiation therapy should be dictated by prognosis.
- Patients with treatment-sensitive and good functional status prior to diagnosis have a better overall prognosis.

REFERENCES

1. Prasad D, Schiff D. Malignant spinal-cord compression. *Lancet Oncol.* 2005;6:15–24.
2. Sorensen S, Helweg-Larsen S, Mouridsen H, et al. Effect of high-dose dexamethasone in carcinomatous metastatic spinal cord compression treated with radiotherapy: A randomised trial. *Eur J Cancer.* 1994;30A:22–27.
3. Vecht CJ, Haaxma-Reiche H, van Putten WL, et al. Initial bolus of conventional versus high-dose dexamethasone in metastatic spinal cord compression. *Neurology.* 1989;39:1255–1257.
4. Heimdal K, Hirschberg H, Slettebo H: High incidence of serious side effects of high-dose dexamethasone treatment in patients with epidural spinal cord compression. *J Neurooncol.* 1992;12:141–14.
5. Rades D, Dunst J, Schild SE. The first score predicting overall survival in patients with metastatic spinal cord compression. *Cancer.* 2008;112:157–161.
6. Patchell RA, Tibbs PA, Regine WF, Payne R, et al. Direct decompressive surgical resection in the treatment of spinal cord compression caused by metastatic cancer: a randomised trial. *Lancet.* 2005;366:643–649.

73

Chronic Obstructive Pulmonary Disease

CASE
Mrs. O, a 75-year-old female ex-smoker (60 pack-years) is admitted to hospital with progressive dyspnea, worsening in the week prior to admission. Chest X-ray reveals diffuse bullous emphysema without infiltrates. She improves with steroids, antibiotics, bronchodilators, and supplemental oxygen. She has not been to a doctor in years and states she has never been told there is any problem with her lungs.

DEFINITION[1]
Chronic obstructive pulmonary disease (COPD) is characterized by chronic airflow limitation that is not fully reversible. Chronic small airway inflammation causes remodeling and/or parenchymal destruction. COPD is associated with an abnormal inflammatory response of the lungs to noxious particles or gases, primarily from cigarette smoking. Often preventable and treatable if caught early

- Usually progressive with significant systemic consequences over time
- Can overlap with asthma in some patients
- Traditional distinction into chronic bronchitis or emphysema is no longer emphasized, as these terms do not define the disease adequately. Chronic bronchitis is a clinical term describing chronic or recurrent increase in bronchial secretions that causes expectoration on most days for a minimum of three months per year for at least two successive years. Emphysema is a pathologic term describing destruction and irreversible enlargement of airspaces distal to the terminal bronchioles without fibrosis.

CLASSIFICATION OF SEVERITY
The GOLD (Global Initiative for Chronic Obstructive Lung Disease) report classifies the severity of COPD based on spirometric classification into four stages, using the ratio of FEV_1

(forced expiratory volume in one second) to FVC (volume of air at maximal inspiration).[1]

In patients with $FEV_1/FVC <0.70$, the stages of COPD are:

Stage I: Mild—$FEV_1 \geq 80\%$ predicted
Stage II: Moderate—$50\% \leq FEV_1 < 80\%$ predicted
Stage III: Severe—$30\% \leq FEV_1 <50\%$ predicted
Stage IV: Very Severe—$FEV_1< 30\%$ predicted or $FEV_1 <50\%$ predicted, plus chronic respiratory failure (*Note*: Chronic respiratory failure defined as $PaO_2 < 60$ mmHg +/– $PaCO_2 > 50$ mmHg while breathing at sea level)

For COPD symptoms based on severity, please see Table 73.1. (See also Chapter 41: Dyspnea.)

PREVALENCE
- Wide range of prevalence estimates due to variable definitions of COPD. Studies estimate a prevalence of 0.2–18.3% worldwide.[1,2] Up to 25% of adults ≥ 40 years of age may have airflow limitation classified as Stage I.
- Higher prevalence found among:
  - Smokers and ex-smokers than non-smokers
  - Age > 40 years
  - Men more than women, though prevalence and COPD deaths have been increasing in women[1,2]

LIKELY ETIOLOGIES[1,2]
- Tobacco smoke: most common risk factor worldwide
- Indoor/outdoor pollution:
  - Biomass cooking (wood, animal dung, crop residues, or coal for fuel) in developing countries
  - Women and children at high risk for respiratory problems and COPD

TABLE 73.1: COPD SYMPTOMS BASED ON SEVERITY

Severity	Symptoms
I (Mild)	Chronic cough and sputum production May not have functional impairment or airflow limitation
II (Moderate)	Dyspnea with exertion and may interfere with daily activities Typical stage at which medical attention is sought and patients are diagnosed with COPD
III (Severe)	Reduced exercise tolerance; repeated exacerbations
IV (Very Severe)	Quality of life is appreciably impaired Exacerbations may be life-threatening.

- Fossil fuel combustion
- Motor vehicle emissions
- Particulate matter, nitrogen oxide, carbon monoxide, biological allergens
- Genetic factor: á$_1$-antitrypsin deficiency— only 1% of COPD patients have severe deficiency; they are usually of Northern European origin.

DIAGNOSIS

Exam[1,2]

Patients with severe COPD may exhibit the following symptoms:

- Tachypnea
- Purse-lipped breathing to assist expiratory flow
- Central cyanosis—bluish discoloration of mucosal membranes
- "Barrel-shaped" chest—horizontal ribs due to hyperinflation
- Use of accessory respiratory muscles (scalene and sternocleidomastoid)
- Cachexia
- Reduced breath sounds
- Wheezing during quiet breathing; absence of wheezing does not indicate absence of obstructive lung defect
- Signs/symptoms of pulmonary hypertension or right heart failure (cor pulmonale):
  - Pronounced P2
  - Lower extremity edema
  - Raised jugular venous pressure
  - Hepatomegaly

Once Mrs. O's condition is stabilized, she will need pulmonary function testing (PFT) to evaluate the severity of her COPD.

Tests[1,10]

- **Pulmonary function testing**
  1. Spirometry: gold standard for diagnosis and monitoring progression of airflow limitation:
     - Airflow limitation: post-bronchodilator $FEV_1/FVC < 0.70$
     - Measurements are compared with reference values based on age, height, sex, and race. Declines in ratio with aging may lead to misdiagnosis of COPD. Results used from best of three trials.
  2. Bronchodilator reversibility testing— FEV_1 measured 10 to 15 minutes after administration of short-acting â-agonist or anticholinergic. Increase in FEV_1 > 200 mL with ≥ 12% improvement above pre-bronchodilator FEV_1 is considered significant.
  3. Lung volumes: hyperinflation (increased total lung capacity, TLC); airtrapping (increased residual volume, RV).
  4. Diffusing capacity of carbon monoxide (DLCO)—reflects gas exchange; decreased in patients with emphysema, pulmonary fibrosis, pulmonary hypertension, or pulmonary vascular disease.

- **Six-minute walk test:**
  - Measures distance walked in six minutes; monitors oxygen saturation to assess for the need for and titration of supplemental oxygen.

Imaging

- Chest X-ray: Exclude alternative diagnoses and establish presence of significant comorbidities (pneumonia, cardiac failure). Classic findings: hyperinflation (flattened diaphragm on lateral chest film, increased air in retrosternal space), hyperlucency of lungs, rapid tapering of vascular markings.

- Computed Tomography (CT) of chest: Consider if concern for malignancy, or high-resolution CT (HRCT) scan for other diagnoses, such as bronchiectasis or interstitial lung disease.

Labs

1. Arterial blood gas
   - Check in patients with FEV1 < 50% predicted or with clinical signs suggestive of respiratory failure or right heart failure while breathing room air (FiO2 21% at sea level).
   - Patients with PaO2 < 55 mmHg should be provided with home oxygen therapy to reduce risk of pulmonary hypertension.
2. á$_1$-antitrypsin deficiency screening
   - Consider testing in patients of caucasian descent, or with strong family history of the disease. For patients less than 45 years old, consider testing if appropriate.
   - Serum concentration of á$_1$-antitrypsin < 15% to –20% of normal value is highly suggestive of homozygous deficiency.

EXPECTED DISEASE COURSE[1,2]

- Natural history of COPD is variable. It is generally progressive, especially with continued exposure to noxious agents.
- Symptoms usually progress with time and include chronic and progressive dyspnea, cough with or without sputum production, and airflow limitation.
- Patients with moderate-severe COPD or less severe stage but significant symptoms or frequent exacerbations should be referred to a pulmonologist.
- Main causes of death: cardiovascular disease, lung cancer, and respiratory failure.
- Most patients have existing comorbid illnesses: DM, HTN, obesity, hyperlipidemia, cardiac arrhythmias, atherosclerosis, pulmonary embolism, CHF, lung cancer, renal disease, depression.
- Determinants of prognosis include:
  - Severity of symptoms
  - Degree to which daily activities are affected

- Objectively measured exercise impairment
- Weight loss
- Reduced arterial oxygen tension
- BODE (Body mass index, Obstruction, Dyspnea and Exercise): Multidimensional 10-point staging scale that is used to predict risk of death in patients with COPD (See Chapter 7: Prognostication.)

END-STAGE COPD

No strict definition exists of end-stage COPD, but patients with high risk of morbidity and mortality usually exhibit one or more of following:[2,4,5]

- Decreased functional status: increasing visits to the emergency department or hospitalizations for pulmonary infections and/or respiratory failure
- Need for supplemental oxygen: either hypoxemia PO2 ≤ 55 mmHg) at rest on room air, or oxygen saturation ≤ 88% on supplemental oxygen or hypercapnia (PCO2 ≥ 50 mmHg)
- Severe airflow limitation with FEV1 < 30% predicted
- Right heart failure secondary to pulmonary disease (cor pulmonale)
- Unintentional progressive weight loss > 10% of body weight over the preceding six months

TREATMENT OPTIONS

Nonpharmacologic[2,6,7,10]

- Nonpharmacologic treatment strategies for COPD include patient education, improved nutrition, pulmonary rehabilitation, oxygen therapy, ventilatory support, and complementary and alternative therapies (Table 73.2).
- Surgical interventions may also be appropriate in carefully selected patients.

Pharmacologic[1,10]

- Medication is used to decrease symptoms and reduce frequency and severity of exacerbations, improve health status, and improve exercise tolerance (Table 73.3). No pharmacologic interventions have been shown to modify the long-term decline in lung function.

TABLE 73.2: NONPHARMACOLOGIC TREATMENT

Modality	Goal	Components	Outcomes
Patient Education (printed material, workshops, sessions, group discussions)	To provide information patient can use to improve quality of life	Reducing risk factors (such as smoking cessation) Nature of disease Proper use of inhalers and medications Recognizing and treating exacerbations Reducing dyspnea Potential complications Oxygen therapy Advance directive and end-of-life decisions	Improves patient adherence to medication and management Can improve patient's ability to cope with illness
Nutrition	To improve nutritional status; low body mass index is an independent risk factor for mortality in patients with COPD	Usually underweight due to low intake and high-energy needs Small, frequent meals in patients with severe dyspnea Increased caloric intake alone is not sufficient; should be with exercise Nutritional supplements (such as creatine) are not beneficial	Greater mortality rates in COPD patients who are underweight/normal weight rather than overweight[6]
Pulmonary rehabilitation	To reduce symptoms, improve quality of life, increase physical and emotional participation in everyday activities	Should incorporate patient education (see above), exercise training, nutrition counseling, psychological support/self-management, including breathing techniques Minimum duration of program should be six weeks; longer program provides more effective results Not appropriate for patients at the end of life	Improves exercise capacity Reduces perceived intensity of breathlessness Improves health-related quality of life Reduces number of hospitalizations and days in hospital Reduces anxiety and depression associated with COPD Improves survival Benefits extend well beyond immediate period of training

(continued)

TABLE 73.2: (CONTINUED)

Modality	Goal	Components	Outcomes
Oxygen therapy	To increase baseline PaO2 ≥ 60 mmHg and/or SaO2 ≥ 90% to ensure adequate oxygen delivery and prevent progression of pulmonary hypertension	Qualification requirements: PaO2 ≤ 55 mmHg or SaO2 ≤ 88% PaO2 55 mmHg–60 mmHg or SaO2 ≤ 88% with evidence of pulmonary hypertension, peripheral edema suggesting right heart failure, or polycythemia (hematocrit >55%) Delivery by nasal cannula should be ≤ 4 LPM, otherwise use facemask May require humidification of oxygen if nasal mucosal dryness or epistaxis Fixed oxygen concentrator may be more cost-effective than cylinder delivery systems Air travel with oxygen: increase the flow by 1–2 LPM during flight Patients with PaO2>70 mmHg at sea level are likely to be safe without supplementary oxygen May provide symptomatic relief at the end of life Represents a powerful symbol of continued medical care	Long-term administration (>15 hours per day) increases survival vs. nocturnal use alone
Ventilatory support	To assist ventilation by improving inspiratory flow rate, correcting hypoventilation, and resting respiratory muscles	Non-invasive ventilation is used to treat acute exacerbations of COPD Not recommended for routine treatment of patients with chronic respiratory failure due to COPD Informed patient preference often dictates use of ventilatory support in end-stage disease	Non-invasive ventilation has not been shown to be beneficial for routine use in severe COPD patients with chronic respiratory failure but may avert need for intubation in acute exacerbations
Complementary and Alternative Modalities (CAM)	To improve symptoms of dyspnea	Neuroelectrical muscle stimulation, breathing training, chest wall vibration, use of walking aids have shown some benefit[11]	Insufficient evidence to recommend routine use of any herbal medicine,[7] relaxation, acupuncture, counseling, case management, psychotherapy;[11] more studies required Tai chi and yoga have been shown to improve perception of dyspnea[8, 9]

Surgical treatment	*Bullectomy* (To remove large area of dead space ventilation and decompress adjacent lung with effective gas exchange)	Likely beneficial for patients with normal–minimally reduced diffusing capacity: No hypoxemia Regional reduction in perfusion with good perfusion in remaining lung Bulla occupying ≥50% of hemithorax with definite displacement of adjacent lung	Improves lung function and symptoms of dyspnea in carefully selected patients May be associated with significant peri- and postoperative adverse outcomes, especially in elderly patients or those with end-stage pulmonary disease
	Lung volume reduction surgery (To reduce hyperinflation and restore mechanical efficiency of diaphragm)	Generally considered for patients < age 65 For patients with regional distribution of emphysema Clinical trials with bronchoscopic LVRS and endobronchial valve placement	Advanced age is a major risk factor for poor outcome Increased survival rate, work capacity and decreased frequency of exacerbations compared to medical therapy in patients with upper-lobe emphysema and low exercise capacity May be associated with significant peri- and postoperative adverse outcomes, especially in elderly patients and those with end-stage disease
Lung transplantation	To improve lung function, exercise capacity, survival, and quality of life in appropriately selected patients	Criteria for referral: Generally considered for patients < age 65 FEV1 <35% predicted PaO2 < 55–60 mmHg PaCO2 >50 mmHg Secondary pulmonary hypertension	Does not confer a survival benefit in patients with end-stage emphysema after two years Disadvantages/Complications: Shortage of donors, cost, operative mortality, acute and chronic rejection, opportunistic or bacterial infections, lymphoproliferative disease

TABLE 73.3: PHARMACOLOGIC TREATMENT OPTIONS

Class	Examples	Advantages	Disadvantages
Bronchodilator—B2-agonist (Stimulate B2 adrenergic receptors to increase cAMP resulting in smooth airway muscle relaxation)			
Short-acting	Albuterol, Levalbuterol Terbutaline	Rapid onset—rescue inhaler Improve airflow Increase exercise capacity PRN use for symptoms Duration of action 4–6 hours	No significant change in FEV1 Tachycardia, somatic tremors Inhaler may be technically challenging for elderly or debilitated patients Oral therapy slower onset and more side effects
Long-acting	Formoterol Salmeterol	Duration of action ≥ 12 hrs Reduces COPD exacerbations Initiate as needed for moderate/Stage II COPD	Potential hypokalemia and cardiac arrhythmias
Bronchodilator—Anticholinergic (Block acetylcholine effect)			
Short-acting	Ipratropium bromide	Rapid onset—rescue inhaler Improve airflow	Anticholinergic effects, such as dryness of mouth Bitter, metallic taste Reports of acute glaucoma with nebulizer solutions
Long-acting	Tiotropium	Duration of action > 24 hours; should improve compliance Reduces COPD exacerbations Improves effectiveness of pulmonary rehab Poorly absorbed systemically For moderate/Stage II COPD	Possible increase in cardiovascular events (needs further investigation) Tiotropium requires education to ensure proper use; may be difficult to coordinate for older patients
Bronchodilator—Methylxanthines (Exact mechanism unclear; may act as non-selective phosphodiesterase inhibitors)	Theophylline Aminophylline	Orally administered Efficacy in COPD with slow-release preparations (reduces exacerbations)	Narrow drug therapeutic window; dose-related toxicity Clearance of medication declines with age and certain meds (cytochrome P450) Cardiac arrhythmias Grand mal seizures Headaches, insomnia, nausea, heartburn, nausea, vomiting, seizures

Anti-inflammatory

Class	Examples	Effects/Indications	Side effects/Considerations
Inhaled glucocortico-steroids For patients with FEV1 <50% and frequent exacerbations	Beclomethasone, budesonide, fluticasone, triamcinolone	Reduces frequency of exacerbations in patients with FEV1 <50% predicted No effect on bone density and fracture rate	May have increased likelihood of pneumonia Does not reduce overall mortality or modify long-term decline of FEV1 Skin bruising Thrush
Combination inhalers			
Short-acting B2-agonist + anticholinergic	Albuterol/Ipratropium	Rapid onset—rescue inhaler Greater and more sustained FEV1 improvements over individual inhalers	See above for each medication class Increased costs with more medications
Long-acting B2-agonist + inhaled glucocorticosteroid	Formoterol/Budesonide, Salmeterol/Fluticasone	Reduces COPD exacerbations and improves lung function Reduces rate of decline in patients FEV1 <60% May increase compliance as only twice daily; decrease rescue inhaler use Fewer inhalers to cause confusion	May increase likelihood of pneumonia due to steroid inhaler component Dry-powder inhaler may be confusing or difficult to use
Systemic glucocortico-steroids (Decreases inflammation associated with acute exacerbations)	Prednisone, prednisolone, methylprednisolone, hydrocortisone	For treatment of acute exacerbations Recommended dose: Prednisolone 30–40 mg daily or equivalent for 7–10 days	Not recommended for long-term management of stable COPD Myopathy, skin bruising, diabetes mellitus, adrenal suppression, osteoporosis, glaucoma, hyperglycemia, mental status changes
Antibiotics	**For exacerbations:** Outpatient: B-lactam, B-lactamase inhibitor, tetracycline, bactrim, macrolides, 2nd/3rd generation cephalosporins, fluoroquinolone (levofloxacin) Inpatient: parenteral B-lactam/B-lactamase inhibitor (ampicillin/sulbactam), 2nd or 3rd generation cephalosporins, fluoroquinolone (levofloxacin) **For prophylaxis:**[12] Azithromycin 250 mg daily or 3 times/week can be considered in patients with ≥ 2 exacerbations/year despite maximal medical therapy Compared with placebo, macrolides have shown to decrease acute COPD exacerbations/year Reassess individual patient after 1 year to see if benefits outweigh risks	Recommended for treating infectious exacerbations of COPD	May lead to overgrowth of C. difficile May lead to resistant strains of bacteria Not recommended for prophylactic use by GOLD report Macrolides can prolong QTc interval: EKG must be monitored at baseline and while on therapy Avoid in patients with high risk of baseline cardiovascular disease Macrolides can cause ototoxicity; must monitor for hearing impairment Macrolides should not be used in patients with liver disease Monitor for drug-drug interactions; macrolides inhibit CYP3A4 isoenzyme

(continued)

TABLE 73.3: (CONTINUED)

Class	Examples	Advantages	Disadvantages
Mucolytic agents	Ambroxol, erdosteine, carbocysteine, iodinated glycerol	May benefit a few patients with viscous sputum	Routine use not recommended
Antioxidant agents	N-acetylcysteine	May reduce exacerbations in patients not using inhaled glucocorticosteroids	May be difficult for patients to use due to odor
Antitussives	Benzonatate, dextromethorphan, hydrocodone (see opioids)	Can be used in acute illness when cough is severe	Not recommended in stable COPD as cough has protective role
Opioids[6] (See also Chapter 29: Management of Pain in Older Adults)	Morphine: oral, parenteral and nebulized hydrocodone	Decreases central respiratory drive to reduce ventilatory demand Has no impact on PaO_2 Decreases minute ventilation at rest and submaximal exercise Reduces sensation of dyspnea and anxiety Use for patients with severe COPD	Nebulized opioids are not more effective than nebulized saline Constipation Transient confusion (tolerance develops after 1–2 days) Dry mouth
Benzodiazepines[6]	Diazepam, Alprazolam	Recommended for use in patients with anxiety on individual basis	Concern for respiratory suppression if overdosed Not more effective than placebo for improving dyspnea
Antidepressants[5]	Nortriptyline, SSRIs	Anxiety and depression in patients with COPD is under-recognized and undertreated Treatment can improve mood, depression, ratings of dyspnea and other physical symptoms in patients with COPD	For SSRIs: suicidial ideation, hyponatremia, serotonin syndrome See side effect profile for individual medications
Vaccines	Killed or live, inactivated influenza vaccines are recommended annually Pneumococcal polysaccharide vaccine recommended, especially COPD pts age ≥65	Strains adjusted each year for appropriate effectiveness Reduces incidence of community-acquired pneumonia in pts age <65, FEV1 <40% predicted	Avoid in patients with hypersensitivity or allergy to eggs

- Short-acting inhalers should be used as rescue inhalers for all stages of COPD. Long-acting inhalers should be initiated as needed for moderate or Stage II COPD. Inhaled corticosteroids should be used in patients with FEV1<50% and frequent exacerbations.
- Poor inhaler compliance in the elderly can be due to complexity caused by the number, frequency, and technique of different inhalers, and to functional decline and cognitive dysfunction due to comorbidities and progressive debility.
- Review and observe the patient's technique with inhaler use at each visit. Use combination inhalers, when appropriate, to help reduce patient's confusion caused by multiple inhalers. However, cost of combination inhalers may be higher.

Mrs. O's outpatient PFTs revealed an FEV$_1$ 50% predicted without bronchodilator response, but with mild air trapping and a moderate gas transfer defect. She walked a shorter distance than expected on her Six Minute Walk Test, but she did not desaturate or require oxygen during the study. Her primary care physician prescribed tiotropium and told her to continue her rescue combination inhaler (albuterol/atrovent) as needed. Influenza and pneumococcal vaccines were administered during her recent hospitalization.

Mrs. O was referred to a pulmonologist who added an inhaled corticosteroid plus long-acting beta-agonist to her regimen since her exercise tolerance was still limited, though improved, with tiotropium. The pulmonologist described the nature of COPD, reviewed the proper technique and use of her medications, and reinforced the importance of minimizing exposure to tobacco smoke.

PALLIATIVE CARE ISSUES

- While multiple options exist for management of end-stage COPD, the preferences of the patient and family should ultimately dictate the treatment plan. Patients and clinicians should establish goals and preferences for disease management, as well as the type and setting of care preferred when respiratory failure occurs. Clinicians should then make management recommendations that are consistent with the patient's goals. This future care planning process can be expected to involve several conversations. (See Chapter 8: Advance Care Planning, and Chapter 9: Communication Skills.)

- Discussions regarding advance care are especially important in patients with COPD because it is difficult to predict who may die within the next six months. Patients may have stable symptoms and then develop an unpredictable acute exacerbation that leaves them critically ill.[5] Before the discussion occurs, clinicians should determine the nature and amount of information that patients and families may want to receive, and be prepared to provide information on: diagnosis and disease process; prognosis; available treatments and the benefits and burdens associated with each; signs and symptoms of the dying process as the disease worsens; and approaches to controlling symptom distress and assuring patient comfort throughout the course of the illness. (See Chapter 7: Prognostication.)
- While these goals of care decisions are being formulated, burdensome symptoms such as dyspnea, anxiety, and secretions should be monitored and aggressively managed to optimize the patient's quality of life.
- The use of noninvasive mechanical ventilation during critical care treatment should be considered in the larger context of agreed-upon and achievable goals of care. (See Chapter 26: Mechanical Ventilation.)

TAKE-HOME POINTS

- Recognition of COPD may not occur until the disease has already progressed due to late manifestation of symptoms.
- Smoking cessation is one of the most important things patients can do to reduce severity of disease.
- Though long-term decline in lung function is inevitable, medications and therapies can improve symptoms and exercise tolerance and can reduce exacerbations.
- For patients who meet end-stage lung disease criteria, clinicians should initiate discussions on advance care planning to define achievable goals for future medical care, including the options for ventilation support during episodes of critical care, and the role of hospice.
- Burdensome symptoms such as dyspnea, anxiety, and secretions should always be monitored and aggressively managed to optimize the patient's quality of life.

REFERENCES

1. Global Initiative for Chronic Obstructive Lung Disease. Global strategy for the diagnosis, management, and prevention of chronic obstructive pulmonary disease: Updated 2009. www.goldcopd.com. Date last accessed: September 2010.
2. Viegi G, Pistelli F, Sherrill DL, Maio S, Baldacci S, Carrozzi L. Definition, epidemiology and natural history of COPD. *Eur Respir J.* 2007;*30*:993–1013.
3. Celli BR. Predictors of mortality in COPD. *Respir Med.* Jun 2010;*104*:773–779.
4. Dean MM. End-of-life care for COPD patients. *Prim Care Resp J.* 2008;*12*(1):46–50.
5. Curtis JR. Palliative and end-of-life care for patients with severe COPD. *Eur Respir J.* 2008;*32*: 796–803.
6. Clini EM, Ambrosino N. Nonpharmacological treatment and relief of symptoms in COPD. *Eur Respir J.* 2008;*32*:218–228.
7. Guo R, Pittler MH, Ernst E. Herbal medicines for the treatment of COPD: a systematic review. *Eur Respir J.* 2006;*28*(2):330–338.
8. Yeh GY, Roberts DH, Wayne PM, Davis RB, Quilty MT, Phillips RS. Tai chi exercise for patients with chronic obstructive pulmonary disease: a pilot study. *Respir Care.* 2010;*55*(11):1475–1482.
9. Donesky-Cueno D, Nguyen HQ, Paul S, Carrieri-Kohlman V. Yoga therapy decreases dyspnea-related distress and improves functional performance in people with chronic obstructive pulmonary disease: a pilot study. *J Altern Complement Med.* 2009;*15*(3):225–234.
10. Hanania NA, Sharma G, Sharafkhaneh A. COPD in the elderly patient. *Seminars in Respiratory and Critical Care Medicine.* 2010;*31*(5):596–606.
11. Bausewein C, Booth S, Gysels M, Higginson I. Non-pharmacologic interventions for breathlessness in advanced stages of malignant and non-malignant diseases. *Cochrane Database Syst Rev.* 2008, CD005623.
12. Wenzel RP, Fowler AA, Edmond MB. Antibiotic prevention of acute exacerbations of COPD. *N Engl J Med.* 2012;*367*:340–347.

74

Aspiration Pneumonia

CASE

Mr. K is an 84-year-old male with a history of dementia, hypertension, coronary artery disease, diabetes mellitus, and pneumonia, transferred to the emergency room with increased confusion and somnolence. He has resided in a long-term care facility for the past six months following a seven-day hospitalization with pneumonia. When interviewed, he denies any distress including cough, shortness of breath, or chest pain. He is oriented to person. He is tachypneic and his breathing is mildly labored. His examination is significant for poor dentition with retained food particles, halitosis, and diffuse coarse rhonchi.

DEFINITION

The lack of a precise definition of aspiration pneumonia has contributed to difficulty in clinical management. *Aspiration* generally refers to the entry into the tracheobronchial tree of oropharyngeal secretions, gastric contents, or exogenous matter (frequently nutrients). *Pneumonitis* refers to the resulting inflammatory response in the distal airways and alveoli that occurs when the aspirated material overcomes the innate defenses of the lung against such invasion.

- The lack of a "gold standard" for diagnosis of aspiration pneumonia also contributes to the paucity of studies offering high-quality evidence to guide clinical decision making. Two distinct syndromes can occur:
  - *Aspiration pneumonitis:* Aspiration of gastric contents of low pH resulting in an inflammatory response in the absence of ongoing infection of the lung parenchyma is commonly termed "aspiration pneumonitis" or "chemical pneumonitis."
  - *Aspiration pneumonia:* Aspiration of a sufficient microbial load to result in sustained infection of the lung parenchyma is commonly referred to as "aspiration pneumonia."

- An imprecise yet practical definition of aspiration pneumonia may be: *infection of the lung occurring in patients at increased risk for aspiration of oropharyngeal contents.*

PREVALENCE

- Although aspiration pneumonia is commonly encountered, prevalence statistics are not precisely known. Several studies have reported the incidence of pneumonia specifically in patients with dysphagia following stroke variously from 7% to 33%.[1]
- One large epidemiologic study of community-acquired pneumonia (CAP) reported that about 10% of all cases of CAP were considered to be cases of aspiration pneumonia.[2]

LIKELY ETIOLOGIES

Identification and management of aspiration pneumonia requires recognition of patients predisposed to aspiration as well as the likely microbiologic agents responsible for the acute infection.

1. Risk factors for aspiration pneumonia include:
   - Dysphagia due to:
     - Neurologic disease: stroke, dementia, Parkinson's disease, neuromuscular disease (such as ALS)
     - Cancer of the head and neck, and esophagus (and associated therapy such as radiation)
     - General debility
   - Ineffective cough
   - Impaired immunity related to malnutrition, medication, chronic disease
   - Poor oral hygiene due to poor dentition, drying of oral secretions (medication, dehydration)
   - Poor functional status associated with residence in a long-term care facility

- Medications that can alter mental status, e.g., sedatives, sleeping medications, opioids, neuroleptics
- Risk factors for readmission with recurrent aspiration pneumonia include (case-control study):[3]
  - Swallowing difficulty
  - Current smoking
  - Use of tranquilizers
  - Lower ADL scores

2. Likely responsible microbiologic agents
   - An accurate understanding of the bacteria responsible for aspiration pneumonia is limited by the difficulty in isolating specific causative organisms.
   - For patients with risk factors for health care-associated pneumonia, responsible bacteria include gram negative bacteria and Staphylococcus aureus.
   - The most commonly implicated organisms for anaerobic bacteria in aspiration pneumonia are Prevotella spp., Fusobacterium spp., Bacteroides spp., and Peptostreptococcus spp.

DIAGNOSIS

Typical signs and symptoms of pneumonia and sepsis may be less prevalent in the elderly population. Recognition of aspiration pneumonia therefore requires a sufficient index of suspicion.

History
- Look for a history of pneumonia and conditions associated with dysphagia. Ask about clues to dysphagia and aspiration: difficulty swallowing food or medication; cough associated with eating/drinking.
- Fever, pleuritic chest pain, cough, sputum production, and dyspnea may be absent or subtle.
- Look for nonspecific symptoms such as decreased activity, anorexia, confusion, change in personality.
- Review medications, looking particularly for those with sedative effects and immunosuppressives.

Exam
- Lung exam may be difficult, as patients may be unable to cooperate. Listen for crackles, bronchial breath sounds, or less specific rhonchi or wheezing.
- Examine the oropharynx for poor dentition, xerostomia, retained food.

- Look for signs of systemic inflammatory response (fever/hypothermia, tachypnea, tachycardia, hypotension) and signs of organ dysfunction (altered mental status, cardiac dysfunction).
- Assess for respiratory compromise (increased work of breathing, hypoxia, respiratory acidosis, use of accessory muscles).
- Explore any other aspect that may be related to the patient's self-report of symptoms.

Tests
- Given the frequency of subtle presentations and the highly associated morbidity and mortality, suspicion of aspiration pneumonia warrants imaging and testing with focus on rapid assessment for evidence of sepsis and organ dysfunction in patients with signs of instability.
- Labs: Look for evidence of systemic inflammation (leukocytosis/leucopenia) and signs of organ dysfunction secondary to sepsis (such as renal failure). Obtain blood cultures.
- Chest X-ray: A lower threshold for obtaining imaging is generally prudent given the frequency of atypical presentations. Look for evidence described in Table 74.1.

Laboratory tests obtained include a white blood cell count of 12.1, BUN of 43, and creatinine of 2.2 (baseline creatinine 1.4). Chest X-ray reveals a new area of patchy density in the right lower lobe.

EXPECTED DISEASE COURSE
- Elderly patients with aspiration pneumonia are at increased risk for complications of pneumonia, including sepsis, respiratory failure, multiorgan failure, and death. Specific data regarding morbidity and mortality is hampered by a lack of precise definitions in studies.
- Factors such as normal age-related decline in vital capacity and respiratory muscle endurance, along with frequent comorbid illness (particularly chronic cardiopulmonary disease), contribute to impaired cardiopulmonary reserve in elderly patients.
- Mortality in one large study was 23.5%. Another recent study found one-year mortality for those with pneumonia and

TABLE 74.1: CHEST X-RAY FINDINGS IN ASPIRATION PNEUMONIA

Pulmonary Conditions	CXR Findings
Pneumonia/consolidation	Densities with or without air bronchograms, frequently in dependent lung zones: superior segments of lower lobes or posterior segments of upper lobes in a supine patient; basal segments of lower lobes
Cavitation/lung abscess	Air fluid levels may be present in subacute cases (fluid level within an area of density on CXR or cavitation on CT)
ARDS/acute lung injury	Diffuse/patchy bilateral density
Fibrosis	Increased reticular/streaky densities at bases may indicate fibrosis associated with chronic aspiration
Effusions	Dependent homogenous opacity may indicate parapneumonic effusion or emphysema

dysphagia to be 55% (more than twice the mortality of those with pneumonia without dysphagia).[4]

- Although little data are available regarding the prognosis of aspiration pneumonia specifically, studies of elderly patients with pneumonia generally are helpful in discussing prognosis.
  - Mortality of pneumonia in the elderly: 10%
  - Mortality of pneumonia in the elderly requiring mechanical ventilation: 55%
  - One-year mortality of pneumonia in the elderly with poor functional status (multiple dependencies): 60%[5]
  - Six-month mortality rate for nursing home residents with advanced dementia with pneumonia: 46.7%[6]

TREATMENT OPTIONS

- Treatment of aspiration pneumonia should address appropriate antibiotic therapy, management of respiratory failure and sepsis, and management of symptoms such as dyspnea, cough, anxiety, secretions, and pain.
- Appropriate antibiotic therapy for aspiration pneumonia should generally be the same as those given for "conventional" pneumonia, based on risk factors for drug-resistant gram negative bacteria and MRSA (Table 74.2).
- Management of respiratory failure and sepsis: Treatment of sepsis, organ dysfunction, and respiratory insufficiency should include prompt initiation with appropriate fluid resuscitation and

hemodynamic or ventilatory support as indicated, and in context of achievable goals for care, prognosis, and patient and family preferences.

PALLIATIVE CARE ISSUES

- The type and extent of treatment for aspiration pneumonia should be based on discussions regarding prognosis and the patient's goals for care. In the absence of previously established decisions regarding treatment interventions, a discussion should be undertaken with the patient and proxy/family members if there is adequate time for informed decision-making.
- In the absence of previous decisions, and if life-sustaining therapy is required emergently, it is often appropriate to undertake a defined "trial" of critical care with frequent reassessment and discussion with the patient/proxy/family regarding ongoing critical care.
- Previously executed advance directives regarding mechanical ventilatory support, cardiopulmonary resuscitation, and artificial nutrition and hydration should be elicited from the patient (or health care proxy or next of kin if the patient is unable to communicate). (See Chapter 26: Mechanical Ventilation and Chapter 27: Artificial Nutrition and Hydration.)
- Although "curative" interventions may or may not be life-prolonging, they may increase and prolong discomfort. An observational cohort study of pneumonia in patients with advanced dementia found

TABLE 74.2: ANTIBIOTIC THERAPY FOR PNEUMONIA

Community Acquired Pneumonia

Previously healthy	Macrolide
No risk factors for drug-resistant Strep pneumoniae	
Patients with comorbidities	Respiratory fluoroquinolone
Inpatient treatment	OR
	B lactam + macrolide

Health Care-Associated Pneumonia (HCAP)/Hospital-Acquired Pneumonia

Pts at risk for multi-drug resistant pathogens:	Antipseudomonal cephalosporin (cefepime, ceftazidime)
Hospitalization within 90 days	OR
Long-term care facility residence	Antipseudomonal carbapemen (imipenem, meropenem)
Hemodialysis	OR
Home infusions or wound care	B-lactam/B-lactamase inhibitor (piperacillin/tazobactam)
Exposure to a family member infected with MDR pathogen	PLUS
Other risks:	Antipseudomonal fluoroquinolone (levofloxacin, ciprofloxacin)
Prior antibiotic therapy within six months	OR
Poor functional status	Aminoglycoside (amikacin, gentamicin, tobramycin)
Immunocompromise	PLUS
Severe pneumonia	Vancomycin or linezolid (for MRSA)

Pneumonia Requiring Anaerobic Coverage

Indicated in patients with:	Clindamycin
Clear history of loss of consciousness associated	Ampicillin/sulbactam
with overdose or seizure and concomitant gingival	Amoxicillin/clavulanate
or esophageal motility disorders	Piperacillin/tazobactam
	Imipemen, meropenem

Note: Although frequently administered, specific antibiotic therapy to treat anaerobic bacteria is likely overutilized.[8]

that patients treated with antibiotics had improved survival but more discomfort on a standardized scale than patients who did not receive antibiotics. Scores indicating greater discomfort correlated with aggressiveness of care.[7]

- Symptom management is essential. Whether the goal is maximal possible prolongation of life, or if intervention is no longer the objective because of comorbidities, prognosis, or previously expressed wishes, aggressive symptom management is always indicated. The common symptoms listed in Table 74.3 are extremely distressing to patients and family members, and can be managed optimally with the recommended options.

Mr. K was treated with antibiotics, intravenous fluids, and intravenous morphine for dyspnea. Over the subsequent 48 hours, he was hemodynamically stable, his breathing became less labored, serum *creatinine decreased to 1.4, and white blood cell count decreased to 8.5. He remained somnolent and disoriented with intermittent agitation.*

REDUCING RISK OF ASPIRATION

- The prognosis for patients diagnosed with aspiration pneumonia, and for those with risk factors for aspiration pneumonia, may be improved by appropriate preventive care. Bedside swallow evaluation, along with adjunctive studies as indicated (such as videofluoroscopy), is effective at diagnosing dysphagia, and appropriate precautions and therapy can then be instituted.
- Swallowing studies are also used to evaluate a patient's ability to safely ingest oral food and oral secretions. Assessment of swallowing function can aid in developing feeding strategies, including appropriate food consistencies, positioning of the head

TABLE 74.3: SYMPTOM MANAGEMENT

Symptom	Management Options
Cough	Tessalon perles Dextromethorphan hbr with or without Guaifenesin Hydrocodone with homatropine Opioid Management of GERD
Secretions	Scopolamine Glycopyrrolate Atropine eye drops Reduce or hold IV infusions of fluid or nutrition, both of which can increase secretions
Anxiety	See Chapter 65: Anxiety
Dyspnea	See Chapter 41: Dyspnea
Pain	See Chapter 29: Management of Pain in Older Adults
Delirium (apathetic or agitated)	See Chapter 34: Delirium

and neck, timing of meals, and strategies for family involvement.

- Patients who may benefit from swallowing evaluation include those with risk factors for aspiration who recover from pneumonia as well as those who have not yet experienced an episode but are judged to be at risk.
- For palliative care patients at risk for aspiration pneumonia, the decision to perform a swallowing evaluation should take into consideration the burden of evaluation, achievable goals of care, prognosis, and patient/family wishes. If the decision is made to forgo a swallowing evaluation, aspiration precautions should nevertheless be instituted.
- The following measures are also likely to decrease the risk of recurrent aspiration pneumonia:
  - Oral hygiene
  - Pneumococcal and influenza vaccination
  - Smoking cessation
  - Adequate nutrition
- While the following therapies are employed to prevent recurrent aspiration pneumonia, there is little to no evidence to support their use.

- **Drug therapy**: Various medications have been studied in predominantly small, nonrandomized studies to assess for the prevention of aspiration pneumonia. Data are inadequate to recommend ACE inhibitors (one trial showed reduced rates in an Asian population only), amantadine, capsaicin, or any other drugs.[9]
- **Percutaneous gastrostomy tube (PEG)**: In patients with advanced neurodegenerative disease such as dementia, there is no evidence that percutaneous gastrostomy tube feeding is effective at preventing aspiration pneumonia or prolonging survival. Furthermore, there is no evidence that post pyloric or jejunostomy tube feeding reduces risk of aspiration pneumonia.
- **Tracheotomy**: Although potentially useful in weaning from mechanical ventilation and in allowing a conduit for suction of the lower airways, placement of a tracheotomy tube does not prevent aspiration.

After extensive discussions between the clinical team and Mr. K's family, it was decided to pursue a palliative course of treatment, including decisions to not institute mechanical ventilation or perform cardiopulmonary resuscitation. After evidence of significant aspiration on bedside evaluation, a percutaneous gastrostomy tube was placed at the insistence of his family for enteral feeding. On hospital day nine, while awaiting transfer to a long-term care facility, Mr. K was found obtunded with tachypnea, tachycardia, and labored breathing. Appropriate medications were given to ensure his comfort, and he passed away with his family at the bedside.

TAKE-HOME POINTS
- Goals of care discussions and symptom management are essential components in the care and treatment of aspiration pneumonia.
- The immediate management of aspiration pneumonia is generally the same as management of pneumonia, including the selection of appropriate antibiotic therapy.
- Patients diagnosed with aspiration pneumonia should be evaluated for dysphagia and/or aspiration. Dysphagia and aspiration are associated with

significantly higher mortality in elderly patients diagnosed with pneumonia.

- In palliative care patients at risk for aspiration pneumonia, the decision to perform a swallow evaluation should take into consideration the burden of evaluation, achievable goals of care, prognosis, and patient/family wishes.
- In patients with advanced dementia, there is no evidence that placement of a tracheotomy tube or placement of a gastrostomy (PEG) tube for enteral feeding will prevent aspiration pneumonia.
- When the underlying cause of aspiration pneumonia is irreversible and progressive (most frequently in patients with dementia), the episode presents an opportunity for the discussion of prognosis, goals of care, and the initiation of palliative care focused on maximizing quality of life, if these issues have not previously addressed comprehensively.

REFERENCES

1. Martino R, Foley N, et al. Dyphagia after stroke: incidence, diagnosis, and pulmonary complications. *Stroke.* 2005;36:2756–2763.
2. Shariatzadeh MR, Huang JQ, et al. Differences in the features of aspiration pneumonia according to site of acquisition: community or continuing care facility. *JAGS.* 2006;54:296–302.
3. El Solh AA, Brewer T, et al. Indicators of recurrent hospitalization for pneumonia in the elderly. *J Am Geriatr Soc.* 2004;52:2010–2015.
4. Cabre M, Serra-Prat M, et al. Prevalence and prognostic implications of dysphagia in elderly patients with pneumonia. *Age and Ageing.* 2009;39(1): 39–45.
5. Muder RR, Brennen C, et al. Pneumonia in a long-term care facility: a prospective study of outcome. *Arch Intern Med.* 1996;156:2365–2370.
6. Mitchell SL, Teno JM, et al. The clinical course of advance dementia. *N Engl J Med.* 2009;361: 1529–1538.
7. Givens JL, Jones RN, et al. Survival and comfort after treatment of pneumonia in advanced dementia. *Arch Intern Med.* 2010;170:1102–1107.
8. Mandell LA, Wunderlink RG, et al. Infectious Diseases Society of America/American Thoracic Society consensus guidelines on the management of community-acquired pneumonia in adults. *Clinical Infectious Diseases.* 2007;44:S27–S72.
9. El Solh AA, Saliba R. Pharmacologic prevention of aspiration pneumonia: a systematic review. *Am J Geriatr Pharmacother.* 2007;5:352–362.

75

Colonic Diverticulitis

CASE

Mrs. Z, an 82-year-old female with history of hypertension and diabetes, presents with complaints of left lower quadrant abdominal pain, constipation for last three days, and chills. Her previous surgical history is significant for abdominal hysterectomy for fibroids in remote past. Physical examination reveals temperature of 101.1 and left lower quadrant tenderness with some guarding in the left lower quadrant. Urinalysis shows numerous white blood cells and polymicrobial flora.

DEFINITION

Colonic diverticulosis describes presence of false diverticula in the colon. They represent acquired outpouchings of the colonic mucosa through defects in the muscularis layer of the colonic wall. *Diverticulitis* refers to the inflammatory process associated with colonic diverticula.

PREVALENCE

- Colonic diverticulosis is extremely common in the western hemisphere. Diverticula can be found in > 80% of adult population older than 80 years.
- About 10% to 20% of persons with diverticulosis will develop symptoms, and 10% to 20% of those individuals will require hospital admission. Less than 1% with diverticulosis will ultimately require surgical intervention.[1]
- It is unclear whether diverticula without inflammation can cause symptoms, because many of these patients have been diagnosed with irritable bowel syndrome.

LIKELY ETIOLOGIES

Although the etiology and pathogenesis of diverticulitis still remain poorly understood, several important observations have been made:

- Diverticular disease is prevalent in countries with lower fiber content in diet.

- The condition was uncommon until late 19th century, when milled flour was introduced.
- The sigmoid colon is the most common site of diverticular disease. Diverticular disease occurs in the area of highest intraluminal pressures during segmental colonic contractions where there is significant hypertrophy of the muscular layer of the colon.

CLASSIFICATION

Classifying acute disease into broad categories such as complicated vs. uncomplicated disease can aid clinical management.[2]

- Uncomplicated disease (localized inflammatory process without identifiable abscess on CT) can usually be treated with oral or parenteral antibiotics.
- Complicated disease most often requires hospital admission and possible radiologic or surgical intervention. Complicated diverticulitis can be divided into categories of severity based on the Hinchey classification system. Classification may assist in communication with surgical consultants on radiographic findings and clinical findings:
  - Perforated (Hinchey classification):
    - I: Localized pericolic or mesenteric abscess
    - II: Confined pelvic abscess
    - III: Generalized purulent peritonitis resulting from perforation of an abscess
    - IV: Generalized fecal peritonitis secondary to free colonic perforation
  - Phlegmon: large inflammatory mass without identifiable abscess on CT
  - Fistula: colovesical, colovaginal, colocutaneous, coloenteric

- Stricture: with or without large bowel obstruction
- Ureteral obstruction

DIAGNOSIS

Exam

- Acute diverticulitis may present with guiaic positive stool but is not usually associated with acute massive diverticular bleeding.
- Uncomplicated diverticulitis presents with:
  - Left lower quadrant pain, localized tenderness, fever, and mild leucocytosis.
  - Mild diarrhea or constipation is also common.
  - While redundant inflamed sigmoid colon can be located in the right lower quadrant with corresponding tenderness, leading to an initial diagnosis of acute appendicitis, this scenario is quite uncommon in the geriatric patient.
- Perforated diverticulitis can present as:
  - Localized left lower quadrant tenderness
  - Diffuse tenderness with frank peritoneal signs
  - Tender palpable abdominal mass or fullness
- Colovesical fistula presents with fecaluria, pneumaturia, recurrent UTIs with enteric flora as clues.
- Large bowel obstruction (of subacute presentation) can occur in patients with diverticular stricture.

Imaging

- Clinical diagnosis alone may be unreliable, especially in geriatric populations, and may underestimate the severity of intra-abdominal pathology. CT scan of abdomen and pelvis is the mainstay in diagnosis.[3] The value of CT scanning:
  - Identifies colonic wall thickening, diverticula, surrounding inflammation, and possibly extraluminal air.
  - Also visualizes colovesical fistula, pelvic abscess, diverticular phlegmon, or ureteral obstruction.
  - Sometimes identifies metastatic disease in the liver from underlying colonic neoplasm.
- Abdominal X-ray has limited value. Contrast enema has been largely supplanted by CT scans and colonoscopy.

- Colonoscopy is contraindicated while acute symptoms are present because of fear of perforation. However, once acute episode resolves, it is mandatory to perform colonoscopy to rule out underlying colon cancer.

EXPECTED DISEASE COURSE

- It is speculated that the initiating event for colonic diverticulitis is microperforation of the diverticulum, often associated with hard stool. The perforated area quickly becomes sealed off by surrounding tissues. This generally leads to a localized inflammatory response with the typical clinical picture of localized left lower quadrant pain associated tenderness with fever and leucocytosis.
- If surrounding tissues are unable to localize the perforation, diffuse purulent or even fecal peritonitis can ensue with the development of a generalized septic picture.
- The inflammatory process around the perforated area of the colon may also erode into surrounding structures with formation of fistula (fistula between sigmoid colon and urinary bladder is most common).
- Inflammation or abscess may resolve with nonoperative treatment with minimal consequences. Occasionally, inflamed areas may scar down with development of colonic stricture and present with a large bowel obstruction.
- Of note, colon cancer with perforation or obstruction can be clinically confused with diverticulitis, hence the importance of diagnostic colonoscopy once acute inflammatory symptoms subside.

TREATMENT OPTIONS

Treatment is tailored to the clinical stage of the disease and options include nonoperative (medical and percutaneous) modalities as well as surgical interventions.

Medical Management

Outpatient

Mild cases of uncomplicated diverticulitis can be treated with:

- Clear liquid diet
- A 10- to 14-day course of oral antibiotics (amoxicillin/clavulanate or fluoroquinolone/metronidazole)

Mrs. Z is admitted to the hospital for intravenous antibiotics and fluid resuscitation. A CT scan of the abdomen and pelvis is performed and reveals inflammatory stranding of the sigmoid colon with a small localized and contained 2.0 cm abscess without significant free air present. Air is noted in her bladder without recent catheter insertion, which is suggestive of a colocutaneous fistula.

Inpatient

For those patients who fail outpatient treatment, or who have initial toxic appearance, hospital admission and treatment recommendations are as follows:

- Patients are placed on full bowel rest, using intravenous fluid replacement.
- After a period of five to seven days without resolution of symptoms, and if concordant with goals of care, initiate parenteral nutritional support.
- Obtain CBC, chemistry, coagulation profile, type, and cross drawn in anticipation of possible diagnostic imaging with IV contrast and invasive procedure or even surgery.
- Start intravenous antibiotics covering most of enteric gram-negative and anaerobic flora. Common combinations include quinolone (ciprofloxacin or levofloxacin) with metronidazole, or monotherapy with ampicillin/sulbactam (Unasyn), or piperacillin/tazobactam (Zosyn) for more severe cases.
- Order CT scan of abdomen and pelvis to determine whether there are complications. Patients with no evidence of complications should be treated with course of intravenous antibiotics until resolution of fever and normalization of white blood cell count.
- Most patients with stage II per Hinchey classification, and some patients with stage I, are appropriate candidates for CT guided percutaneous drainage.
- Small abscesses (less than 3 cm), especially those covered by adjacent loops of intestines, may not be amenable for percutaneous drainage. These patients should continue IV antibiotics and be re-imaged in few days, provided their clinical condition is not worsening. Small abscesses often will respond well to antibiotic treatment alone and sometimes will become amenable to percutaneous drainage on repeated imaging.

- Pain should be treated while waiting for disease to resolve.
- Once acute inflammatory symptoms subside, diet can be gradually restarted and advanced as tolerated.

Mrs. Z undergoes percutaneous CT guided drainage within 12 hours of admission; her symptoms improve and she recovers. After five days of intravenous antibiotics as an inpatient, she is discharged to home on oral antibiotics for seven to ten days, with follow-up in three to four weeks. She is advised about the need for colonoscopy as an outpatient in four to six weeks.

Follow-Up

- There is little evidence regarding the appropriate amount of dietary fiber consumption immediately following an acute episode. A high-fiber diet is recommended, however, following resolution of acute symptoms.
- Four to six weeks after resolution of acute episode, patients should undergo colonoscopy to rule out underlying colon cancer.

At her follow-up appointment, Mrs. Z is feeling much improved and has no specific complaints. The possibility of a colo-vesical fistula from diverticular disease is discussed, and a colonoscopy is scheduled.

Surgical Management

- Fewer than 1% of patients with asymptomatic diverticula will require surgery. However, 20% to 50% of patients hospitalized for diverticulitis may require surgery. Specific indications for surgery include[4]:
  - No response or symptoms worsening within 24 to 48 hours of nonoperative treatment
  - Abscess not amenable to percutaneous drainage and fails antibiotic therapy
  - Initial presentation with Hinchey III or IV perforated diverticulitis
  - Fistula; stricture with large bowel obstruction
  - Recurrent (two or more) episodes of uncomplicated diverticulitis
  - Unsuccessful nonoperative treatment of Hinchey I and II stage
  - Attack of diverticulitis in immunocompromised patient (AIDS, chronic glucocorticoid treatment, chemotherapy, radiation)

- Historically, elective sigmoidectomy was advised after two or more episodes of uncomplicated diverticulitis because recurrent disease was thought to carry a higher risk of complicated diverticulitis and increased incidence of morbidity and mortality. Recent evidence has caused a shift in emphasis away from this position, and the number of attacks of uncomplicated diverticulitis is no longer considered an overriding indication for surgical intervention.[2]
- Most operative interventions now include resection of affected segment of colon during first operation. Usually the part of the colon with most dense diverticular disease is removed. This portion is most often the sigmoid colon to the level of the upper rectum.
- Decision about performing primary anastomosis or diverting stoma is tailored to specific clinical scenario and local tissue quality in the operating room and is beyond the scope of this text.
- Advanced age alone should not be used as an indication or contraindication for colostomy. Rather, the patient's baseline sphincter function, bowel habits, comorbidities, and cognitive and functional status should be assessed preoperatively to guide decision-making.
- The role of laparoscopic surgery for diverticular disease is well established in elective settings but continues to evolve for emergent management of acute complicated diverticulitis.[5]

Mrs. Z's colonoscopy reveals the presence of a colo-vesicular fistula, and she is offered a sigmoid resection with primary anastomosis. The benefits of the surgical intervention include reduction of urinary tract infection and inflammation due to the fistula and prevention of recurrent attacks of diverticulitis.

PALLIATIVE CARE ISSUES
- While immunocompromised and transplant patients and those with Hinchey I and II disease have relative indications for surgical intervention, the expected benefit of elective surgery (especially in geriatric patient) should be weighed against risk of major surgical intervention and overall life expectancy.[6]

- Recent evidence offers support for this individualized approach to choice of operative vs. nonoperative treatment of complicated diverticular disease.[7] The benefit-burden analysis should weigh many factors, including the patient's operative risk, comorbidities, and patient preferences.
- When exploring the option of nonoperative management, consideration should also be given to burdens associated with the prospect of multiple recurrences, i.e., interruption of lifestyle, repeated exposure to CT scans, multiple hospital admissions, and frequent courses of antibiotics.[7]
- The role of age in the management of diverticular disease remains a source of debate in the field. The risks for both colostomy and diverticular disease-associated morbidity/mortality in the geriatric population with recurrent uncomplicated disease remain unclear. Evaluating risk on a case-by-case basis is thus critical in assessing which geriatric patients are likely to benefit from surgical intervention. Consideration should include current and predicted comorbidities, functional status, cognition, and anticipated quality of life.
- Colostomy may have a negative impact on quality of life, but it has been shown to be well tolerated in most patients. For some geriatric patients with moderate to severe fecal incontinence at baseline, colostomy may be more acceptable when compared with reconstruction. The decision should be individualized, with careful consideration given to patient preferences and goals, including an informed discussion of what may be an acceptable quality of life from the patient's perspective.

SYMPTOM MANAGEMENT TO IMPROVE QUALITY OF LIFE
- Nonoperative candidates may benefit from a fiber diet, particularly cellulose.
- Physical activity and weight management may also be helpful.
- Patient education may also result in early recognition of symptoms and timely initiation of antibiotics or guided drainage to optimize nonsurgical therapy.

TAKE-HOME POINTS
- Few patients with colonic diverticula require surgical intervention.

- Acute diverticulitis can often be managed with a multidisciplinary approach without acute surgical intervention.
- Follow-up colonoscopy is essential to exclude malignancy because diverticulitis can present similarly in the geriatric population.
- Two or more attacks of uncomplicated diverticulitis are no longer considered an overriding indication for surgical intervention.
- Data regarding the risks of recurrent disease in the geriatric population and nonoperative management after percutaneous drainage are unclear.
- Decisions for surgical intervention should be weighed carefully based on patient's perioperative risk and severity of disease.

REFERENCES

1. Wolff B et al. *The ASCRS Textbook of Colon and Rectal Surgery*. New York: Springer; 2007.
2. Rafferty J et al. Practice parameters for sigmoid diverticulitis. Standards Committee of American Society of Colon and Rectal Surgeons. *Dis Colon Rectum*. Jul 2006;*49*(7):939–944.
3. Kaiser AM et al. The management of complicated diverticulitis and the role of computed tomography. *Am J Gastroenterol*. Apr 2005;*100*(4):910–917.
4. Collins D, Winter DC. Elective resection for diverticular disease: an evidence-based review. *World J Surg*. Nov 2008;*32*(11):2429–2433.
5. Senagore AJ. Laparoscopic sigmoid colectomy for diverticular disease. *Surg Clin North Am*. Feb 2005;*85*(1):19–24, vii.
6. Stocchi L. Current indications and role of surgery in the management of sigmoid diverticulitis. *World J of Gastroenterol*. Feb 21, 2010;*16*(70):804–817.
7. Nelson RS, Ewing BM, Wengart TJ, Thorson AG. Clinical outcomes of complicated diverticulitis managed non-operatively. *Am J Surg*. 2008;*196*:969–974.

76

Mesenteric Ischemia

CASE

Mrs. X is a 65-year-old female with a history of hypertension and atrial fibrillation who presents to the emergency room at 8 p.m. complaining of severe abdominal pain and nausea. She has had no prior surgeries except for a myocardial infarction 20 years ago for which she received coronary artery stents.

DEFINITION

Mesenteric ischemia occurs as the result of inadequate perfusion via the mesenteric circulation, which may lead to local small bowel tissue inflammation, injury, and necrosis. This often involves the three major branch vessels of the abdominal aorta that supply the abdominal viscera: the celiac artery (CA), the superior mesenteric artery (SMA), and the inferior mesenteric artery (IMA), but it may also involve the cascades of small collateral vessels.

PREVALENCE

- Mesenteric ischemia accounts for 1 out of every 1000 hospital admissions. The prevalence of increases with age.
- In patients on hemodialysis, the incidence is much higher, occurring at a frequency of 0.3% to 1.9% per patient year.[1]

CONSEQUENCES OF UNTREATED MESENTERIC ISCHEMIA

- Arterial insufficiency leads to tissue hypoxia. The injury to the affected bowel may range from reversible ischemia to transmural infarction.
- Mucosal sloughing can cause bleeding into the gastrointestinal tract. However, if ischemia persists, the mucosal layer of the bowel wall loses its integrity, releasing toxins and inflammatory cells, thereby causing bacterial translocation and perforation. As a result, multisystem organ failure can occur with eventual bowel wall necrosis within 8 to 12 hours from the onset of symptoms.

CLASSIFICATION

Mesenteric ischemia can either be acute or chronic (Figure 76.1):

- Acute mesenteric ischemia (AMI) can be catastrophic unless there is early diagnosis and intervention, with reported mortalities as high as 70%.
- Chronic mesenteric ischemia (CMI) accounts for 5% of all intestinal ischemic events and is rarely life-threatening. It is usually a manifestation of chronic, flow-limiting atherosclerotic disease.[2]

ACUTE MESENTERIC ISCHEMIA

Acute mesenteric ischemia (AMI) is divided into four different primary clinical presentations:

1. AMI from a superior mesenteric artery (SMA) embolus:
   - Accounts for 50% of all cases
   - Source: Cardiac in origin
   - Risk factors: Atrial fibrillation, myocardial infarction, cardiac valve disease, and hypercholesterolemia
   - Usually lodges 6 to 8 cm distal to the origin of the SMA before the takeoff of the middle colic artery
   - Vascular occlusion is sudden
   - Presentation: Severe ischemia and abdominal pain out of proportion to their physical exam findings
   - Prognosis: Mortality rate after surgery for acute mesenteric ischemia from an SMA embolus is high, emphasizing the importance of early surgery
2. AMI from an SMA thrombosis:
   - Accounts for 25% of cases
   - Source: Pre-existing chronic mesenteric ischemia from atherosclerosis
   - Risk factors: Coronary artery disease, stroke, CHF, and peripheral vascular disease

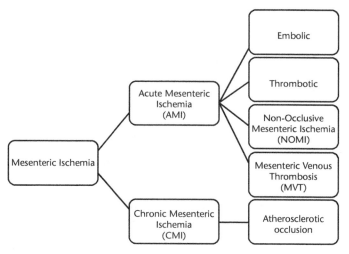

FIGURE 76.1: Classification of Mesenteric Ischemia.

- May also be a complication of arterial aneurysm or other vascular pathologies, including an aortic dissection and traumatic injuries
- Thrombosis tends to occur at the origin of the SMA, causing widespread infarction
- Presentation: Postprandial pain, weight loss, nausea, and an abnormal aversion to food
- Prognosis: Mortality after surgery for acute mesenteric ischemia from a SMA thrombosis is high, emphasizing the importance of early diagnosis and intervention

3. Non-occlusive mesenteric ischemia (NOMI):
   - Accounts for 20% of cases
   - Source: Severe reduction in mesenteric perfusion usually from vasoconstriction secondary to cardiac failure, septic shock, hypovolemia, or the use of medications such as digitalis, cocaine, diuretics, vasopressin, and other medications that may lead to vasoconstriction
   - Gross pathologic arterial or venous occlusions are not observed in patients with NOMI
   - Presentation: The severity and location of abdominal pain associated with NOMI can be more variable than with AMI. In fact, abdominal pain is absent in up to 25% of patients with NOMI, but patients are usually elderly with precipitating disorders including

hypotension, congestive heart failure, hypovolemia, and cardiac arrhythmias.
   - Prognosis: Mortality rates for NOMI have been reported to be as high as 70%, mostly due to the difficulty in diagnosis and the significant comorbidities of this patient population. Often mesenteric ischemia is a late complication of underlying disease and associated global hypoperfusion.

4. Mesenteric venous thrombosis (MVT):
   - Accounts for 5% of cases
   - Often affects a much younger population
   - Sources: hypercoagulable states, sickle cell disease, cirrhosis, pancreatitis, cancer, trauma, or intra-abdominal inflammatory processes
   - Presentation: Can have subclinical and insidious onset with crampy abdominal pain, nausea, anorexia, and malaise for days to weeks
   - Prognosis: Improved survival can be seen in up to 80% of patients treated promptly with beta blockade and anticoagulation

DIAGNOSIS

History and Exam

- A thorough history and physical exam is crucial in the diagnosis of AMI. Despite the different etiologies for AMI, physical examination findings are similar. The most important finding is pain out of proportion to exam.

- Early in the course of the disease, in the absence of peritonitis, physical signs are few and nonspecific. Bowel sounds are variable and have not been found to be a useful diagnostic tool.
- Presenting symptoms include:
  - Nausea and vomiting: 75% of patients
  - Abdominal distension and GI bleeding: 25% of patients
  - Peritoneal signs or hematochezia (bloody stools): often a late and ominous sign of infarction and mucosal sloughing
  - Bowel necrosis: associated with fever, hypotension, tachycardia, tachypnea, and altered mental status
- Early recognition of acute mesenteric ischemia is critical to maximizing patient outcome. AMI has a catastrophic outcome if not properly and rapidly treated. It should be considered in any patient with abdominal pain disproportionate to physical findings, gut emptying in the form of vomiting or diarrhea, and the presence of risk factors, especially age older than 50 years.

Mrs. X's physical exam reveals minimal tenderness to deep palpation at her mid-abdomen without any rebound or guarding. She still complains of a severe, intermittent abdominal pain.

Tests

There are no pathognomic laboratory tests for the diagnosis of AMI.

- Leukocytosis: > 15,000 cells/mm^3 occurs in approximately 75% of patients with AMI.
- Metabolic acidosis is present in approximately 50% of patients.
- May have elevations of serum and peritoneal fluid amylase, alkaline phosphatase, and inorganic phosphate values.

Mrs. X has a leukocytosis of 15,000 cells/ mm^3 and a lactate of 3.5 but no other laboratory abnormalities.

Imaging

- The diagnosis of AMI usually depends on clinical exam and anatomic findings seen on computed tomography (CT) scan, angiography, or by ultrasound.
- Waiting for laboratory results should not delay radiographic studies if serious suspicion of AMI exists (Table 76.1).

At 11 p.m. Mrs. X has a CTA (computed tomographic angiography) of her abdomen and pelvis that reveals no free peritoneal air, free fluid, or signs of bowel obstruction. There is a cut-off sign at the distal superior mesenteric artery.

- Plain abdominal films are generally nonspecific in the diagnosis of mesenteric ischemia, but are most useful in ruling out other abdominal etiology like a small bowel obstruction (SBO) or perforation.
- Ultrasonography is used to demonstrate an obstruction to blood flow in the celiac artery or SMA, but visualization may be obstructed by dilated loops of bowel.
- Non-contrast CT scan can be obtained in patients with renal insufficiency or with contrast allergies to detect a narrowing of the intestinal blood vessels but cannot clearly visualize mesenteric obstruction without the administration of contrast.
- Computed tomographic angiography (CTA) is the optimal diagnostic study for patients without contrast allergies or renal insufficiency. It is becoming more readily available and is highly sensitive for the diagnosis of mesenteric ischemia.
- Mesenteric angiography is the gold standard for diagnosis of mesenteric ischemia. It involves a contrast dye being injected into the blood vessels, producing three-dimensional views of the mesenteric circulation. While mesenteric angiography is an invasive procedure, it does carry the benefit of providing pharmacological therapy (thrombolysis, papaverine), angioplasty, and stenting directly at the site of vascular obstruction.
- Magnetic resonance imaging (MRI) and magnetic resonance angiography (MRA) provide findings similar to CTA but are not so readily available and are expensive and time-sensitive.

EXPECTED DISEASE COURSE

- The prognosis of AMI of any type is sobering, with mortality rates in the range of 50% to 80%. Survivors of extensive bowel resection may face lifelong disability.
- Individual decision-making regarding realistic outcomes should be openly discussed between members of the family, physicians, and palliative care practitioners. This is especially important in cases

TABLE 76.1: DIAGNOSTIC TESTING IN MESENTERIC ISCHEMIA

	Plain Abdominal Film	Ultrasound	CTA	Angiography/ Arteriography	MRI/MRA
Invasive	No	No	No	Yes	No
Sensitivity	Low	Moderate	High	Highest	Highest
Cost	$	$	$	$$	$$
Complications	Minimal	Minimal	Nephrotoxicity*	Nephrotoxicity Bleeding Pseudoaneurysms	May not be readily available

* CT without contrast can reduce contrast nephrotoxicity but with much less diagnostic sensitivity.

of complete bowel necrosis, where the prognosis is grim with or without surgery.

TREATMENT OPTIONS

Medical Management

- Medical management should begin with correction of plasma volume deficits with aggressive fluid resuscitation, nasogastric tube decompression, and broad-spectrum antibiotics.[4] (Figure 76.2)
- Early recognition of AMI before permanent tissue damage occurs is the best way to improve patient survival, and only angiography or exploratory surgery makes early diagnosis possible.
- The use of angiography in the absence of peritonitis can allow for early pharamacologic therapy, such as the infusion of thrombolytics and papaverine. Systemic anticoagulation with use of heparin can also be used to treat AMI, especially in the treatment of mesenteric venous thrombosis (MVT). The drawback to these interventions is that they carry a risk of bleeding.

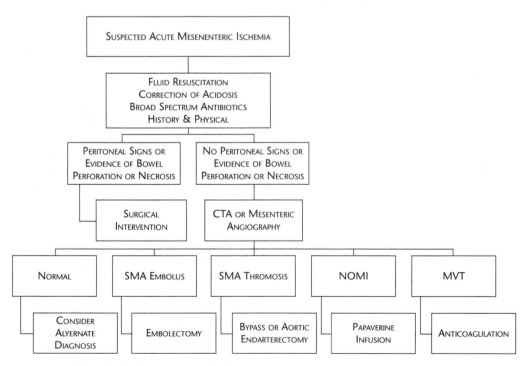

FIGURE 76.2: Algorithm for the treatment of AMI.

- AMI carries a mortality rate as high as 70%, and thus it is very important to treat the patient's pain and symptoms and support the family while workup and curative treatment options are being pursued.

Mrs. X is admitted to the ICU for observation. She is started on isotonic fluid resuscitation and given a Foley catheter and nasogastric tube. An urgent surgery consult is placed.

Surgical Management

Mrs. X receives a surgical evaluation at 1 a.m. She is now tachycardic, disoriented, and peritoneal on physical examination. Discussions are undertaken with the family and her care team about the prognosis of suspected mesenteric ischemia. Her family is informed that although early surgical intervention carries the best prognosis for survival, several complications may result from surgical resection and alter a patient's long-term quality of life. Alternatively, medical therapy may include intravenous rehydration, anticoagulation, and pain control, but is associated with very poor survival. Based on their understanding of the patient's wishes, the family decides to proceed with surgery.

- The surgical management for AMI is individualized to the cause of the ischemic event, but nonetheless follows four general surgical principles:
  - Resection of affected bowel
  - Identification of ischemic source
  - Revascularization of end organ
  - Reassessment of tissue viability, usually in 24 to 48 hours
- Surgical decision-making should always include an assessment of patient's long-term quality of life preferences because patients who survive surgical resection often have significant limitations.
- Some potential consequences of extensive bowel resection may include short bowel syndrome, malnutrition, diarrhea, steatorrhea, malabsorption, anemia, fluid and electrolyte disturbances, hypergastrinemia, gastric hypersecretion, and a lifelong need for total parenteral nutrition and enterostomy.

Prognosis

Mrs. X undergoes a laparotomy, small bowel resection, and superior mesenteric artery embolectomy. She returns to the operating room for second-look procedure and is found to have viable remaining small bowel. An anastomosis is created. She requires a prolonged inpatient hospitalization.

- After initial medical and/or surgical stabilization, patients with AMI typically have a prolonged inpatient recovery time. This is especially true when resection of necrotic bowel is performed.
- These patients may require supplemental nutrition with total parenteral nutrition (TPN). One of the most important predictors of outcome is the extent of bowel resection. Some patients may have mild functional changes such as increased bowel frequency, while patients with extensive resection may require lifelong TPN and possible small bowel transplant.
- During the inpatient stay, efforts must be made to find and, if possible, treat any predisposing cause(s) of AMI. For example, patients who have had MVT need warfarin therapy for at least six months or for life if a hypercoagulable state was discovered during treatment. Patients with atrial fibrillation should also be discharged on warfarin.

CHRONIC MESENTERIC ISCHEMIA

Mr. X is a 63-year-old man who smokes one pack of cigarettes a day and has a known history of coronary artery disease. He weighs 112 pounds and presents to the emergency room complaining of intermittent abdominal pain over the last year. His pain is worst one hour after eating but then subsides.

- Chronic mesenteric ischemia (CMI) or intestinal angina is a disease of the aging population and is characterized by recurrent episodes of insufficient blood flow to the bowel during digestion. It is most commonly associated with atherosclerotic disease in the celiac, superior mesenteric, and inferior mesenteric arteries.
- Patients with CMI complain of crampy, postprandial abdominal pain and increased aversion to food. This "food fear" can eventually lead to severe weight loss. Patients usually present in their 50s or 60s, with a stronger female predominance. Physical findings are limited and nonspecific in the absence of late peritoneal signs.

- Similar to the diagnosis of AMI, CT scans and duplex ultrasonography support the diagnosis of CMI, but the study of choice is biplanar mesenteric angiography. In CMI, angiography shows stenosis or occlusion of at least two of the major vessels, the celiac, SMA, or IMA.
- Surgical revascularization has been the mainstay of therapy for patients with CMI. Several procedures, including aortic reimplantation of the superior mesenteric artery, transarterial and transaortic mesenteric endarterectomy, and antegrade or retrograde bypass, have been advocated for restoring normal blood flow distal to an occlusion of the superior mesenteric or celiac arteries.
- Percutaneous transluminal angioplasty has become an alternative to surgery for the many patients with CMI who are poor surgical candidates, and for patients in whom the diagnosis remains uncertain. Often, angioplasty may be combined with the placement of a stent to prevent further stenosis or occlusion of the affected blood vessel. At many hospitals the treatment of choice depends on the availability of experienced vascular surgeons or interventional radiologists.
- The decision to perform open surgery versus angioplasty and stenting is based upon the patient's age, comorbidities, the number and severity of occluded vessels, and the ease of vascular access to the stenosed vessels. In most patients, angioplasty is preferred, with surgery reserved for younger patients with fewer comorbid conditions.

Mr. X undergoes a CT angiogram that shows 80% occlusion of his SMA. He is seen by a vascular surgeon and agrees to proceed with a surgical end-arterectomy (removal of plaque). He tolerates the procedure well and is discharged home on postoperative day 7 without any further postprandial pain or symptoms.

Prognosis
- Reported surgical outcomes have varied depending on the nature of the operation employed and the number of vessels revascularized, but in general success rates are greater than 90%, with low operative mortality and recurrence rates of less than 10% in selected patients.[3]

- The experience with percutaneous angioplasty with or without stenting is limited, although success rates have been similar to those of conventional surgery, but with higher recurrence rates.
- Current recommendations suggest that patients with CMI who are good surgical candidates should have an attempt at surgical revascularization; patients at higher surgical risk may be appropriate candidates for percutaneous transluminal mesenteric angioplasty with or without stenting.

PALLIATIVE CARE ISSUES
- Measures to improve quality of life for patients with mesenteric ischemia include early assessment at the primary care level for symptoms and signs, risk factor modification, and early involvement with palliative care specialists to maximize patients' overall quality of life regardless of goals of care or surgical candidacy.
- In both acute and chronic mesenteric ischemia, pain and other burdensome symptoms should be should be aggressively managed regardless of disease outcome.
- While surgical intervention for AMI may improve survival rates, quality of life is often severely impacted. An open and direct discussion with the patient and family members can ensure that the treatment provided is consistent with the patient and family's overall short- and long-term quality of life preferences and achievable goals for care.
- In cases of complete bowel necrosis, where the prognosis is grim with or without surgery, clinicians should intitiate discussions regarding realistic outcomes with patients, members of the family, and other involved health care providers.
- For CMI patients who are not candidates for any invasive intervention, medical management includes anticoagulation with blood thinners, pain management, optimizing treatment of atherosclerotic disease, and consideration of long-term parenteral nutrition.

TAKE-HOME POINTS
- Acute mesenteric ischemia should be considered in all elderly patients with abdominal pain, especially if the pain is disproportionate to physical examination findings (Figure 76.2).

- The greatest predictor of mortality from AMI is the time between the onset of symptoms and intervention.
- For chronic mesenteric ischemia, demonstration of stenosis with intestinal angina and weight loss is highly diagnostic.
- For suitable surgical candidates, surgical revascularization is the mainstay of therapy.
- Angioplasty and stenting have been shown to have decreased morbidity and mortality in selected patients, although their long-term outcomes do not approach those of open surgery.
- Medical and surgical management of severe mesenteric ischemia should always involve open communication with family members and address patient's quality of life preferences and achievable goals of care.
- Symptoms of pain in both acute and chronic mesenteric ischemia should be managed regardless of disease outcome.

- Measures to improve quality of life include early assessment at the primary care level for symptoms and signs of mesenteric ischemia, risk factor modification, and early involvement with palliative care specialists to maximize patients' overall quality of life regardless of goals of care or surgical candidacy.

REFRENCES

1. Yu CC, Hsu HJ, et al. Factors associated with mortality from non-occlusive mesenteric ischemia in dialysis patients. *Ren Fail.* 2009;31(9):802–806.
2. Chang JB, Stein TA. Mesenteric ischemia: acute and chronic. *Ann Vasc Surg.* 2003;17:323–328.
3. Sreenarasimhaiah J. Chronic mesenteric ischemia. *Best Pract Res Clin Gastroenterol.* 2005;19: 283–295.
4. Fazio VW et al. *Current Therapy in Colon and Rectal Surgery.* Philadelphia, PA: Mosby, Inc.; 2005.

77

End-Stage Liver Disease

CASE

Mr. M is a 67-year-old man who presents for an initial visit complaining of fatigue, increased abdominal distension associated with pain, and yellowing of the skin for about a month. He notes a history of drinking a pint of vodka daily for more than 20 years. He is still drinking daily. You suspect advanced liver disease. What other findings would indicate advanced liver disease? If he does have advanced liver disease, what are possible treatment options for the underlying liver disease as well as the symptoms he is presenting with?

DEFINITION

End-stage liver disease can be defined as a pathologic finding of cirrhosis associated with signs of clinical decompensation. Markers of liver decompensation in cirrhotic patients are encephalopathy, variceal bleeding, hepatorenal syndrome, hepatopulmonary syndrome, hepatocellular carcinoma, and ascites.

PREVALENCE

- About 5.5 million people, or 2% of the U.S. population, have chronic liver disease.[1]
- In 2007, more than 29,000 Americans died from liver diseases. Chronic liver disease and cirrhosis are the 12th leading cause of death in the United States.[1]
- Sixty percent of all newly diagnosed chronic liver disease occurs in the elderly.[2]
- In 2008, liver disease was the 10th leading primary diagnosis for hospice admission and accounted for 1.5% of all hospice admissions.[3]

LIKELY ETIOLOGIES

Common causes of chronic liver disease include:

- Hepatitis C (57%)
- Alcohol (24%)
- Nonalcoholic fatty liver disease (9.1%)
- Hepatitis B (4.4%)

- Other (<2%): primary biliary cirrhosis, primary sclerosing cholangitis, hereditary hemochromatosis, autoimmune hepatitis, alpha1 antitrypsin deficiency, and liver cancer.[4]

RISK FACTORS

- Intravenous drug use (associated with hepatitis C and B)
- Alcohol consumption
- Unprotected sexual activity (associated with hepatitis B)
- Obesity (associated with nonalcoholic fatty liver disease)
- Asian descent (associated with high prevalence of chronic hepatitis B)

DIAGNOSIS

History

Patients with advanced liver disease present with complaints of jaundice, fatigue, and ascites. Because early cirrhosis is often asymptomatic, other patients are identified due to abnormalities in routine lab tests that indicate liver dysfunction.

Mr. M had more than 20 years of heavy alcohol consumption but only recently had symptoms of advanced liver disease such as jaundice and ascites.

Exam

The physical manifestations of advanced liver disease are often related to portal hypertension or abnormalities in nutrient and hormone metabolism, which is normally the key function of the liver. Physical exam findings that may indicate chronic liver disease are listed in Table 77.1.

Tests

- A comprehensive metabolic profile that includes liver function tests is important in helping to diagnose liver disease. In a

TABLE 77.1: CHRONIC LIVER DISEASE: PHYSICAL EXAMINATION FINDINGS

Vital signs	In advanced liver disease blood pressure can be low due to decreased systemic vascular resistance and decreased effective circulating volume, although the patient may have extravascular volume overload and increased cardiac output The systolic blood pressure is often less than 100 The respiratory rate may be increased
General	Cachexia
Thorax and lungs	Gynecomastia Decreased breath sounds or rales in the bottom portions of the lungs
Cardiac	Systolic flow murmur that is related to anemia, tricuspid regurgitation
Abdominal	Caput medusa (varicose veins radiating from the umbilicus) Ascites The liver may be small, normal sized, or enlarged. If palpated, it is usually nodular Splenomegaly
Extremities	Palmar erythema Edema can be debilitating, so ambulation is difficult
Genital-urinary	Testicular atrophy, which may result in decreased libido
Dermatologic	Spider telangiectasias: the size and number of the lesions correlate with disease severity Jaundice
Neurological	The patient may be lethargic or confused from hepatic encephalopathy Asterixis is a flapping tremor associated with encephalopathy

patient who has risk factors and physical exam findings consistent with liver disease, blood work can help to differentiate from other diseases such as congestive heart failure that can have similar presentation of edema, ascites, and fatigue. Any lab abnormalities also help to gauge the severity of the liver disease.

- Liver function tests including bilirubin, albumin, alkaline phosphatase, GGTP (gamma-glutamyltransferase), ALT (alanine aminotransaminase), and AST (aspartate aminotransferase) should be ordered if liver disease is suspected.
- Albumin is an indicator of synthetic function of the liver as well as nutritional status.
- Prothrombin time is related to the synthetic function of the liver since clotting factors are produced in the liver.
- Chemistry profile is helpful because hyponatremia is often a harbinger of end-stage cirrhosis. Assessment of renal function is crucial if the patient is on diuretics as well as to diagnose hepatorenal syndrome.
- Hematologic abnormalities are common, and they include anemia, thrombrocytopenia, and leukopenia. These

abnormalities result from hypersplenism and malnutrition.

Imaging

- Ultrasound is usually the initial radiographic test in the evaluation of hepatic disease. Cirrhosis can be inferred from a small nodular liver on ultrasound associated with the appropriate history, physical, and lab tests. Ultrasound examination can also detect ascites, portal vein thrombosis, hepatocellular carcinoma, and splenomegaly.
- MRI and CT scans are helpful in noninvasive assessment of masses picked up on ultrasounds that may be hepatocellular carcinoma.
- Elastography is a noninvasive measurement of liver fibrosis using ultrasound probes that has a high correlation with liver biopsy results. In addition to making the initial diagnosis of cirrhosis, this technique is useful for following pathologic progression of fibrosis previously possible only by repeat biopsies. This new technique has been studied mostly in patients with viral hepatitis, particularly in those with hepatitis C. In patients with obesity there is decreased accuracy.[5]

Biopsy

- Biopsy is the gold standard to diagnose cirrhosis but is associated with significant cost, requires the expertise of a specialist, and carries a rare but serious risk of injury or death (mortality approximately 1 in 10,000). There may also be sampling errors in the range of 15% to 30%.[6]
- In advanced liver disease, biopsy is associated with more complications due to increased tendency to bleed, so the benefits must be weighed against the burdens. However, many centers will require a biopsy if treatment is contemplated.

EXPECTED DISEASE COURSE

- Hepatic injury leading to fibrosis of the liver usually occurs over decades. In patients who have hepatitis C and heavy alcohol use, however, cirrhosis can occur in 10 years.
- Older patients who get infected with hepatitis C and B are more likely to progress to cirrhosis and to have more serious disease, which may be a function of their immune system.[2]
- Once a patient has developed cirrhosis, the median survival is 10 years for those with compensated disease. Even though there may be ongoing damage to the liver from continued alcohol consumption or untreated viral causes, many patients are relatively asymptomatic until there are signs of decompensation.

DISEASE STAGING

- As with many non-cancer diagnoses, there is often uncertainty about when patients should be referred to hospice. (See Chapter 7 Prognostication.) The hospice eligibility criteria for liver disease developed by Centers for Medicare and Medicaid Services is a helpful guideline to determine if a patient has a limited prognosis from end-stage liver disease (Table 77.2).
- The Model for End-Stage Liver Disease, (MELD) score is another prognostic tool used for patients with cirrhosis. MELD is used by the United Network for Organ Sharing (UNOS) for allocating livers for transplantation. It has been validated in many studies to accurately predict three-month survival. The MELD score is calculated using a formula based on INR, bilirubin, and creatinine.

TABLE 77.2: HOSPICE ELIGIBILITY CRITERIA FOR LIVER DISEASE

---

1. Prothrombin time (PT) more than 5 seconds over control, or International Normalized Ratio (INR) > 1.5 **AND**
2. Serum albumin < 2.5 gm/dl **AND**
3. One or more of the following conditions:
   a. Ascites, refractory to treatment or patient noncompliant
   b. Spontaneous bacterial peritonitis
   c. Hepatorenal syndrome; elevated creatinine and BUN; oliguria (< 400 ml/day); urine sodium concentration < 10 mEq/L
   d. Hepatic encephalopathy, refractory to treatment or patient noncompliance
   e. Recurrent variceal bleeding, despite intensive therapy
4. Supporting documentation for hospice eligibility:
   a. Progressive malnutrition
   b. Muscle wasting with reduced strength and endurance
   c. Continued active alcoholism
   d. Hepatocellular carcinoma
   e. HbsAg (Hepatitis B) positivity
   f. Hepatitis C refractory to interferon treatment

- In one large prospective study with 3437 patients awaiting liver transplant, mortality was directly proportional to the MELD score at the time of listing.[7] Three-month mortality was 1.9% for patients with MELD scores < 9, and 71% for patients with MELD scores ≥40.[4]

TREATMENT OPTIONS

- Transplantation has become a viable treatment for patients with end-stage liver disease. The 7- to 10 -year survival rate after transplantation is 60% to 80%, depending on the etiology of liver disease.[8] While transplantation does not necessarily cure the patient, it is treatment for the complications of end-stage liver disease.
- The benefits of transplantation should be weighed against the burdens, i.e. the risk of surgery itself, immunosuppression, and a complicated medical regimen after the surgery.
- The major barrier to liver transplantation is that there are not enough organs for those needing transplants. In 2006, there were 16,861 patients awaiting liver

transplantation; however, there were only 6,362 transplantations that year.[9] In addition, older patients often have comorbidities that exclude transplantation as an option.

- Contraindications to transplantation include active substance abuse (most centers require six months of abstinence before listing for transplant), severe cardiopulmonary disease, and non-hepatic malignancy within five years. Hepatocellular carcinoma is not a contraindication as long as a solitary lesion is no more than 5 or 10 centimeters (depending on the transplant center) or, if there are multiple lesions, as long as there are no more than 3 lesions, and none more than 3 centimeters in size. Older age itself is no longer an absolute contraindication.[10]

PALLIATIVE CARE ISSUES

- Advance directives, especially the appointment of a health care agent, should be addressed early in the disease trajectory because hepatic encephalopathy often causes cognitive impairment and it becomes challenging to engage the patient in meaningful conversation.
- Palliative care should be offered to patients with advanced liver disease even while the patients pursue aggressive life-prolonging treatments. In such cases, palliative care can alleviate the high symptom burden and assist with difficult issues regarding care goals in the setting of potential transplantation. Please refer to Table 77.3 for recommended symptom management options.
- Due to impaired drug metabolism, benefits and burdens of medications for symptom management should be discussed with the patient, family, and the involved hepatologist before initiation, and then reviewed throughout the course of treatment.
- Opioids may be used to treat a number of the symptoms of end stage liver disease, but barriers to use include: 1) opioids are metabolized in the liver; 2) these patients are often medically fragile and at high risk for encephalopathy; and 3) many of the patients have a history of substance abuse that prompts concerns about psychological

dependence. If using opioids for this patient population, therefore, clinicians should use caution and give smaller doses at longer intervals. (See Chapter 29: Management of Pain in Older Adults.)

- For patients seeking liver transplants and their families, palliative care is especially appropriate for assistance with communication about goals of care, advance directives, patient and family support, and symptom management.
- When there is a shortage of organs, or if the patient is not appropriate for transplantation, the patient faces a limited prognosis; if the patient agrees to a comfort-oriented approach, referral to hospice should be considered.

Mr. M is counseled to discontinue alcohol use because the resulting decrease in portal hypertension associated with alcohol cessation may help decrease ascites and prevent complications such as variceal bleeding. Cessation of alcohol use and improved nutrition may also be beneficial for his fatigue. Additional treatment options for his ascites are fluid restriction, diuretics, and periodic large volume paracentesis. If Mr. M's abdominal pain does not improve with treatment of his ascites and does not respond to acetaminophen, a low-dose opioid such as oxycodone 2.5 mg to 5 mg every 6 hours standing with 2.5 mg to 5 mg every 2 hours as needed for breakthrough should be considered. Referral to hospice should be discussed, especially if Mr. M is unable to cease alcohol. Ongoing alcohol consumption in the setting of cirrhosis portends poor prognosis, and liver transplantation is not an option.

TAKE-HOME POINTS

- End-stage liver is a geriatric disease, and older patients may have increased morbidity and mortality from the disease.
- Patients may pursue aggressive life-prolonging treatments including transplantation and still have palliative care to address goals of treatment, advance directives, family support, and symptom management.
- Appropriate pharmacologic treatments should not be withheld because of fear of side effects or psychological dependence, but use caution and give smaller doses at longer intervals.

TABLE 77.3: SYMPTOM MANAGEMENT IN END-STAGE LIVER DISEASE

Symptom	Management
Ascites	Stopping alcohol use will immediately decrease portal pressures Sodium restriction to 2 grams a day Fluid restriction, especially if serum sodium is low Diuretics Consider transjugular intrahepatic portosystemic shunt (TIPS), including risk/benefit analysis Large volume paracentesis Indwelling catheters (See Chapter 43: Ascites)
Pain	Acetaminophen is first line for mild pain, but no more than 2 grams a day Avoid NSAIDs, as they may precipitate renal failure or increase ascites Low-dose opioids given at longer intervals Avoid codeine, which requires hepatic activation (See Chapter 29: Management of Pain in Older Adults)
Dyspnea	Oxygen Nonpharmacologic strategies such as fans and relaxation techniques Low-dose opioid given at longer intervals If anxiety is a component, low-dose medium half-life benzodiazepine (See Chapter 41: Dyspnea)
Encephalopathy	Lactulose 30 mL starting at twice a day and titrate to four stools a day Neomycin 500 mg twice a day to 1 gm four times a day Avoid medications that can worsen encephalopathy Manage and avoid risk factors such as constipation, large protein intake, electrolyte abnormalities, and gastrointestinal bleeding (See Chapter 50: Hepatic Encephalopathy)
Malnutrition	Education about disease process Exercise Consider a nutrition consultation
Fatigue	Proper nutrition Consider physical therapy Low dose of psychostimulant such as methylphenidate Steroids (See Chapter 30: Fatigue)
Pruritis	Antihistamines are usually ineffective and sedating Cholestyramine, but monitor for constipation Rifampin Naltrexone For cholestatic liver disease, consider endoscopic or percutaneous drainage (See Chapter 60: Pruritis)
Depression	Selective serotonin reuptake inhibitors Counseling Low dose of a psychostimulant such methylphenidate (See Chapter 64: Depression)

REFERENCES

1. Xu J, Kochanek KD, Murphy SL, et al. Deaths: Final Data for 2007. *National Vital Statistics Reports*; 2010:58(19).
2. Junaidi O, Di Bisceglie AM. Aging liver and hepatitis. *Clin Geriatr Med.* 2007;23:889–903.
3. NHPCO Facts and Figures: Hospice Care in America 2009 edition. www.nhpco.org/files/public/Statistics_Research/NHPCO_facts_and_figures.pdf.
4. Sanchez W, Talwalker JA. Palliative care for patients with end-stage liver disease ineligible

for liver transplantation. *Gastroenterol Clin North Am.* 2006;*23*:201–219.

5. Castera L, et al. Non-invasive evaluation of liver fibrosis using transient elastography. *J Hepatol.* 2008;*48*:835–847.

6. Carlson JJ, Kowdley JV, Sullivan SD, et al. An evaluation of the potential cost-effectiveness of non-invasive testing strategies in the diagnosis of significant liver fibrosis. *J Gastroenterol Hepatol.* 2009;*24*:786–791.

7. Weisner R, Edwards E, Freeman R, et al. Model for end-stage liver disease (MELD) and allocation of donor livers. *Gastroenterology.* 2003;*124*:91–97.

8. Larson A, Curtis R. Integrating palliative care for liver transplant candidates. *JAMA.* 2006;*295*: 2168–2176.

9. *2007 Annual Report of the US Organ Procurement and Transplantation Network and the Scientific Registry of Transplant Recipients: Transplant Data 1994–2007.* Rockville (MD): Department of Health and Human Services, Health Resources and Services Administration, Healthcare Systems Bureau, Division of Transplantation; Richmond (VA): United Network for Organ Sharing; Ann Arbor (MI): University Renal Research and Education Association; 2007.

10. Cross TJ, Antoniades CG, Muiesan P, et al. Liver transplantation in patients over 60 and 65 years: An evaluation of long-term outcomes and survival. *Liver Transpl.* 2007;*13*:1382–1388.

78

Feeding Tube Management

CASE

Mrs. A is an 87-year-old woman with advanced dementia, depression, hypertension, and diabetes who had a percutaneous gastrostomy placement five months ago. She is wheelchair-bound and dependent on assistance for all of her activities of daily living. Her family reports that leakage of feeds occurs around the gastrostomy tube. On examination the feeding tube is intact, but tension placed on the tube by the dressing has led to tube dilation and orifice ulceration.

DEFINITION

A *feeding tube* is usually a 12 to 20 French-sized tube that is inserted into the stomach or jejunum. The most common method of tube placement is a percutaneous endoscopic gastrostomy (PEG). Gastrosotomy tubes can also be inserted surgically by an interventional radiologist using fluoroscopy. Jejunostomy tubes are usually placed surgically but can be placed endoscopically as well.

WHEN TO CONSIDER A FEEDING TUBE

- Feeding tubes are placed to provide nutrition when eating by mouth is not an option.
- Feeding tube placement is commonly performed for patients who have impaired swallow mechanisms or inadequate oral intake.
- The most common clinical settings for feeding tubes are neurologic disorders (58%) and cancer (25.3%).[1]
- For short-term access to the digestive tract, a nasogastric tube can be placed, but long-term access usually requires a gastrostomy tube or a jejunostomy tube. Placement of gastrostomy tube vs. jejunostomy depends upon the location of the disease.

INDICATIONS FOR PLACEMENT

- The data is mixed on benefit of feeding tube placement in patients who have dysphagia without complications.

- The placement of a feeding tube for non-volitional enteral feeding for other indications, such as advanced dementia and aspiration pneumonia, has not been shown to improve survival, nutritional status, quality of life, or function.
- Overall mortality for older patients after PEG placement is approximately 25% at 30 days and 50% at one year. The median survival after PEG tube placement is 7.5 months.[2,3]
- Because feeding tube placement is associated with risk of complications (see below), decisions about placement should be based on careful analysis of the expected benefits and burdens for the individual patient. Figure 78.1 proposes an evidence-based medical decision-making algorithm for PEG tube placement.[4]

ENTERAL TUBES FOR SYMPTOM MANAGEMENT

- Enteral tubes can also be placed as a palliative measure to decrease gastric distension, nausea, and vomiting in patients with gastric outlet or small bowel obstruction.
- The tubes may be left open and allowed to drain into a collection device such as a urinary catheter bag. These tubes are often larger-caliber and are placed by surgery or interventional radiology.
- Depending on the patient's goals of care and life expectancy, monitoring of volume and electrolyte loss may be necessary.

MANAGEMENT OF ENTERAL TUBES

- Once a feeding tube has been placed, the length of the tube beneath the skin should be carefully noted. Most feeding tubes

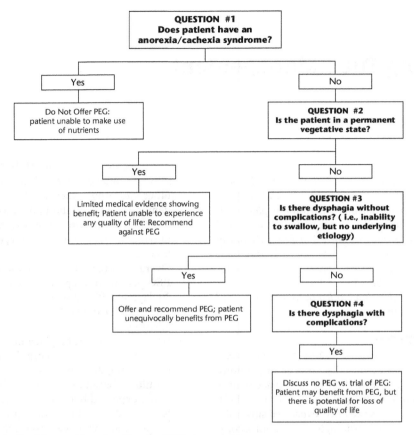

FIGURE 78.1: Decision-making algorithm for PEG placement.[4]

will have length markers on the lumen of the tube.

- The positioning of the external bolster should be recorded, as this will be helpful if any issues arise in the future about whether or not the tube has been moved.
- For patients who are cognitively impaired, the external length of the tube should be kept short to reduce the likelihood of the patient pulling on the tube and causing inadvertent removal.

COMPLICATIONS

The incidence of immediate complications associated with PEG placement is approximately 1.5% to 4% of cases. The incidence of post-procedure complications is 4.9% to 10.8% overall. Commonly encountered issues include.

Obstruction of the Lumen

- Obstruction is a common issue that arises with feeding tubes. Most cases are related

to medications administered through the feeding tube. Prevention is the best method of addressing the problem of obstruction:

- Review medications administered through the tube.
- Make sure that medications formulated as sustained-release granules (e.g., Kadian, a long-acting morphine medication) are diluted in large amounts of fluid so that they do not cake when administered.
- Do not crush nongranular sustained-release medications (e.g., oxycodone SR, morphine LA tablets) for administration via the feeding tube, as they will become "immediate release" and likely result in a medication overdose.
- Pills that can be crushed should be crushed very finely and then diluted in a large volume of fluid into a thin solution/suspension.

- Administered medication should not be a slurry consistency.
- Management tips for obstructed feeding tube:
  - The caregiver at home can first instill a colored carbonated beverage (e.g., cola) to fill the tube. The combination of the phosphoric acid in the cola in conjunction with the carbon dioxide gas that is released when the cola heats up may dissolve and clear the obstruction.
  - If this does not work, a catheter tip syringe can be used to unclog the tube. The syringe should be filled with water and the water injected through the port at the top of the feeding tube. The feeding port should be held very tightly against the tip of the syringe to allow high pressure to be applied to the plunger.
  - If available, an endoscopy cleaning brush or long pipe cleaner can be used to mechanically push through the blockage.
  - Finally, if the blockage cannot be dislodged, a non-endoscopic replacement of the tube can be performed.

Infection

- Infection and cellulitis at the feeding tube site is a common late complication, with incidence ranging from 4% to 30%. Signs and symptoms of infection include:
  - Erythematous, edematous, and painful site around the feeding tube abdominal wall entrance
  - An infectious exudate may be present around the tube.
  - Exam should involve a careful inspection of the site to rule out an abdominal wall abscess.
- Management of feeding tube site infections:
  - Most cases of feeding tube site infections can be treated as a cellulitis with enterally administered antibiotics covering skin and enteric organisms.
  - Small collections can often be drained by applying direct pressure to milk the pus from the collection, which usually communicates with the feeding tube tract.
  - Formal surgical incision and drainage may be required for larger collections.
  - Feeding can be continued unless there is a concomitant leak.

- Topical antibiotics are neither necessary nor helpful.

Leaks

- Management of a leak from the tube:
  - Examine the tube to determine if it has a detachable feeding port.
  - If the feeding port can be removed, the tube should be cut below the level of the leak and the feeding adaptor reinserted.
  - If the feeding tube is a single-piece design, the entire feeding tube must be replaced. Refer to the gastroenterologist, surgeon, or interventional radiologist who originally placed the tube.
- Management of a leak from around the tract:
  - Determine the underlying etiology, which may include infection, widening of the tract caused by traction forces, or poor wound healing. A leak due to mechanical forces rather than infection will lack the other signs of infection, e.g., exudate, foul smell, erythema, and induration.
  - Treat the patient with high-dose proton pump inhibitors to decrease the volume of gastric secretions and the acid content of the leaked fluid, which together can decrease the volume of the leak and facilitate closure.
  - Make a small hill of gauze around the feeding tube to ensure that the position of the tube entry is directly perpendicular to the skin. Minimize any pressure on the skin caused by traction on the feeding tube to allow maximal healing of the tract.
  - Replace the tube by a larger caliber tube if the leak persists. However, if leakage persists after replacement, the problem may worsen if the underlying cause has not been accurately identified and addressed.

Inadvertent Tube Removal

- If the tube is inadvertently removed less than 30 days after placement:
  - Nothing should be placed into the lumen, as there is no stable tract between the skin and lumen of the stomach.
  - The site should be allowed to heal.
  - Alternate methods of hydration or feeding should be employed, if indicated.

- New feeding tube should be placed, if indicated.
- If the tube is inadvertently removed more than 30 days after placement:
  - Existing tract may be kept open by the insertion of a urinary catheter of approximately the same caliber through the matured tract.
  - This should be performed within 24 hours of the tube becoming dislodged.
  - A replacement feeding tube should then be inserted, if indicated.
- In both cases of inadvertent tube removal, verification of tube replacement is ideally performed by obtaining an abdominal flat plate X-ray immediately after flushing the newly replaced tube with a water-soluble radiopaque contrast.
- If radiographic confirmation cannot be obtained, a bulb syringe can be used to determine if gastric contents can be withdrawn through the tube. Water can also be infused and then withdrawn to see if the water becomes bile tinged. While auscultation of the stomach as air is insufflated using a bulb syringe can also help confirm placement, it is considered the least accurate approach.

Buried Bumper Syndrome

- Buried bumper syndrome is a **medical emergency** that occurs when the feeding tube has been partially dislodged and then sits between the wall of the stomach and the abdominal wall. Signs and symptoms include an intermittently functioning tube or a tube that is difficult to flush.
- If buried bumper syndrome is suspected, the feeding tube should not be used for any purpose in order to reduce the risk of peritonitis. The patient should be immediately evaluated by a physician.

Discoloration of the Tubing

- Discoloration is a common occurrence with feeding tubes that have been in place for one year or more. The discoloration of the tubing is due to fungal colonization of the tubing material and does not pose any threat to the patient.
- Replacement of the tube is not necessary as long as it remains functional. The problem is a cosmetic one only.

PALLIATIVE CARE ISSUES

- Clinicians should keep in mind that decisions about feeding tube placement are not solely based on available medical evidence. Patient's values, culture, and religion, as well as family attitudes and beliefs, are factors that may exert more influence on feeding tube placement decisions than the evidence provided by the medical literature.
- It is important, therefore, that decisions regarding feeding tube placement involve conversations between clinicians and the patient-family unit to make sure that decisions are fully informed and consistent with the expressed wishes, achievable goals of care and values of the patient and family.
- In advanced neurodegenerative disease, refusal of food or inability to swallow food and fluids is a part of the natural history of end-stage disease. Patients do not benefit from feeding tubes in terms either of quality or length of life under these circumstances.
- Once a decision is made to place a feeding tube, discussion with the patient and family should continue at regular intervals to assure that this medical treatment remains consistent with achievable medical goals. Some patients and families opt for a time-limited trial.

TAKE-HOME POINTS

- Clinicians should be familiar with the relevant data in order to have a meaningful discussion with patient and family before placing enteral feeding tubes.
- Complications from enteral feeding tubes are common and can often be addressed by the primary care provider without hospitalization.
- A feeding tube does not always mean the patient cannot eat. Clinicians should understand why a feeding tube was placed and allow the patient to have oral intake whenever possible.

REFERENCES

1. Kadakia S, Sullivan H, Starnes E. Percutaneous endoscopic gastrostomy or jejunostomy and the incidence of aspiration in 79 patients. *Am J Surg.* 1992;*164*:114–118.

2. Grant MD, Rudberg MA, Brody JA. Gastrostomy placement and mortality among hospitalized Medicare beneficiaries. *JAMA*. 1998;*279*: 1973–1976.

3. Mitchell S, Kiely D, Lipsitz L. The risk factors and impact on survival of feeding tube placement in nursing home residents with severe cognitive impairment. *Arch Intern Med*. 1997;*157*:327–332.

4. Rabeneck L, McCullough L, Wray N. Ethically justified, clinically comprehensive guidelines for percutaneous endoscopic gastrostomy tube placement. *Lancet*. 1997;*349*:496–498.

79

End-Stage Renal Disease

CASE

Dr. S is a 94-year-old retired surgeon with congestive heart failure, peripheral artery disease, peripheral neuropathy, and end-stage renal disease (eGFR 12mL/min/1.73m²) who is referred for symptom management and dialysis discussions. Dr. S is frail, has been home/wheelchair-bound for two years, and scores 22 on the Mini-Mental State Exam (MMSE). His main complaints are that he has right hip pain that does not respond to acetaminophen, but he cannot tolerate codeine, has restless legs at night, and insomnia. His wife and daughter are his health care proxies, and they are present at this office visit to participate in the dialysis discussions and to explore how his symptoms will be treated.

DEFINITION

Chronic kidney disease can be defined as the presence of kidney damage or decreased kidney function that lasts for three or more months.

- Glomerular filtration rate (GFR) is considered to be the best index of overall kidney function. Declining GFR is an indication of progressive kidney disease. *End-stage renal disease* (ESRD) is defined as an eGFR < 15 mL/min/1.73m.[1]
- The most commonly used methods to estimate GFR in the United States are measurement of the creatinine clearance or the use of estimation equations based upon creatinine clearance, e.g., Cockcroft-Gault equation or the Chronic Kidney Disease Epidemiology Collaboration (CKD-EPI) equation).

PREVALENCE

- At the end of 2009, more than 871,000 people were being treated for ESRD in the United States.[2]
- Between 1980 and 2009, the prevalence rate for ESRD increased nearly 600 percent, from 290 to 1,738 cases per million.

- Dialysis is a form of artificial renal replacement for patients with ESRD. The fastest growing population of individuals initiating dialysis in the United States is people over 75 years old.

LIKELY ETIOLOGIES

- Diabetes and hypertension (most common)
- Cardiorenal syndrome
- Obstructive uropathy
- Chronic glomerulopathy: nephrotic syndrome, previous vasculitis/rapidly progressive glomerulonephritis (RPGN), systemic lupus erythematosis (SLE)
- Chronic interstitial nephritis/drug toxicity, e.g., analgesics and nonsteroidal anti-inflammatory drugs (NSAIDs)
- Acute kidney injury (AKI) is a significant risk factor for ESRD in older chronic kidney disease (CKD) patients.[3]

DIAGNOSIS

Exam

- Determine "functional age," i.e., classify as healthy vs. vulnerable vs. frail (Table 79.1)
- Functional status: ability to ambulate or transfer, degree of dependency for activities of daily living (ADLs)
- Presence and degree of dementia
- Depression screen
- Uremia screen (delirium, asterixis, ankle clonus, twitching, pericardial rub)
- Volume status (fluid overload)
- Skin exam (excoriations, calciphylaxis)

Tests

- Electrolytes include BUN, creatinine
- Urinanalysis w/micro
- Spot urine protein/creatinine ratio
- Complete blood count
- Iron studies
- eGFR-MDRD or eCrCl-CG (www.kidney.com)

TABLE 79.1: FUNCTIONAL AGE CLASSIFICATION

An elderly patient with advanced kidney disease or who is on dialysis can be classified into one of the following general "functional age" categories using a comprehensive or modified geriatric assessment. This classification is useful to frame treatment decisions and management issues.[1,4]

Healthy/usual: The most optimal dialysis patient who might also be a transplant candidate

Vulnerable: Typical dialysis candidate. Geriatric assessment and intervention plans (e.g., rehabilitation, pain control, treatment of cognitive deficits and depression, limiting poly-pharmacy, preventing falls, instituting home services) may slow the progression of geriatric susceptibility factors that will adversely affect prognosis, quality of life, and the dialysis experience.

Frail: Suboptimal dialysis candidate and should be considered for a non-dialysis medical treatment (NDT) plan, or a time-limited dialysis trial. Final decisions will hinge on prognosis, patient preferences, quality of life, and contextual issues.

- Albumin
- Calcium and PO^4
- Intact PTH
- 25 Hydroxy Vitamin D
- Renal ultrasound

Note: Patients with an eGFR < 30 mL/min/m2 should be referred to a nephrologist.

TREATMENT OPTIONS

Dialysis

- Dialysis is a life-sustaining therapy for patients with ESRD in the form of artificial renal replacement.
- Dialysis for an older person, especially for frail patients, has many attributes of a chronic progressive illness (reduced lifespan, progressive disability, repeated hospitalization, significant comorbidity, high symptom burden, and caregiver stress).

Non-Dialysis Medical Therapy (NDT)

- Non-dialysis medical therapy (NDT) is reoriented comprehensive care for patients with ESRD who forego initiation of dialysis.
- NDT focuses on quality of life and symptom control. Active medical treatment of renal complications (e.g., fluid/electrolyte disorders, renal anemia, fluid overload, CKD, and mineral bone disease) is continued simultaneously with evaluation and treatment of geriatric syndromes and symptoms (e.g., pain, depression, fatigue, insomnia, pruritus, constipation) to maximize function and quality of life.

- In selected subgroups of patients (those with multiple comorbid conditions, ischemic heart disease, or frailty), life expectancy may be similar to those on dialysis.[5]
- An NDT approach can result in fewer hospitalizations, more time spent at home and with family, and ultimately less suffering.
- Opting for non-dialysis medical therapy should be a decision made in the context of informed consent based on patient-centered goals for care.

EXPECTED DISEASE COURSE

For Dialysis Patients in General[6]

- Functional decline over months to years
- Episodes of acute (and serious) complications
- Common causes of death include cardiovascular conditions, infection, and discontinuation of dialysis.

For Geriatric Dialysis Patients

- One-year probability of death in dialysis patients ≥ 85 years is twice that of death in the general dialysis population.[7,8]
- The following signs and symptoms can progress over time, especially if present at earlier stages of CKD, and are associated with adverse outcomes:
  - Frailty syndrome: Frailty in dialysis patients is associated with death (adj. HR 2.24) and combined death or hospitalization (adj. HR 1.63) outcome.[9]
  - Functional limitations

- Cognitive dysfunction: Dialysis patients with dementia have a two-year 50% reduction in life expectancy compared with non-demented ESRD patients.[10]
- Falls and fall-related injuries
- Increasing hospital admissions
- Increasing symptom burden

For Nursing Home (NH) Dialysis Patients

- Yearly death rate of NH dialysis patients is double that of the general > 65-year-old ESRD population.
- Impact of cognitive impairment is significant, with approximately 60% of NR patients showing moderate to severely impaired decision-making skills, with no advanced directives in 60% to 65% of these patients and no DNR in 25% to 30%.[10]
- Dialysis does not prevent functional decline in NH patients, with significant loss of ADL functional level and death at one year following dialysis initiation.[11]

PROGNOSIS

- Geriatric susceptibility factors with accompanying Relative Risk (RR) associated with death in older dialysis patients:[8]
  - Older age, compared with 80–84 years: 85–89 years = RR 1.22; > 90 yrs = RR 1.56
  - Non-ambulatory status = RR 1.54
  - Serum albumin concentration <35 g/l = RR 1.28
  - Congestive heart failure = RR 1.21
  - Underweight (BMI < 18.5) = RR 1.2
  - Number of comorbid conditions** 2–3 = RR 1.31; ≥ 4 = RR 1.68
- One-year mortality in dialysis patients > 80 years old (46%)
- 5- and 10-year survival on dialysis—31% and 10%, respectively[7]
- Life expectancy of dialysis patients is approximately 17–20% of age-matched non-dialysis patients. Median survival of dialysis vs. non-dialysis general population:

- 80–84 yrs old—15.6 months vs. 105 months
- 85–89 yrs old—11.6 months vs. 78 months
- ≥ 90 yrs old—8.4 months vs. 7 months

CAUSES OF MORTALITY IN DIALYSIS PATIENTS

General

- More than 50% of patients will die from cardiovascular events (sudden death/arrhythmias, heart failure, myocardial infarction, peripheral vascular disease with gangrene, infection and amputation, stroke).
- Fifteen to twenty percent die from infection (pneumonia, access-related, post-renal transplant).
- Ten percent die from cancer.
- Twenty percent die following dialysis withdrawal (commonly due to increasing comorbid conditions and/or acute intercurrent illness, advancing debility, and failure to thrive; rarely because of technical problems).

After Dialysis Withdrawal

- The majority of chronic dialysis patients who stop dialysis will die within eight to 10 days or sooner if they are actively ill; almost 100% will expire by 30 days.
- For those patients who forgo or withdraw from dialysis, uremia is usually associated with a peaceful death, but close monitoring and treatment of symptoms (pain, dyspnea, twitching, delirium, nausea/vomiting, pruritus) is required. They will usually spend their remaining time in a hospital or nursing home, or less commonly at home with hospice.

Geriatric NDT Patients

- Older patients with ESRD who have not initiated dialysis have a more uncertain time course because they lose renal function more slowly than younger patients and die more often from non-renal causes, especially those ≥ 85.[12]
- In one study of ESRD patients treated medically without dialysis, the median age was 83 years, and the time to death starting from a GFR of 15 mL/min was 540 days (4-2193 days).[5] These patients are best

---

(**Albumin concentration <35 g/l, anemia, underweight, CHF, diabetes, ischemic heart disease, COPD, cancer, cerebrovascular disease, and PAD)

managed by a combined nephrology and geriatric palliative care approach.

MAKING THE DECISION ABOUT DIALYSIS[4]

- ESRD is medically managed without dialysis until uremic syndrome, hyperkalemia, acidosis, or fluid overload become refractory to medical therapy.
- The decision about whether to initiate renal replacement therapy should take into consideration medical indications, expected disease course, prognosis, patient preferences and goals of care, quality of life, and the context in which the decision takes place.
- The Four Topics method described below is a useful template to address the main components of a dialysis discussion and facilitate decision-making and planning for older CKD/ESRD/dialysis patients.[13]
- Each topic is framed by underlying ethical principles and their associated clinical considerations. Fully exploring and discussing each topic will enhance informed consent and contribute to more collaborative decisions.

"FOUR TOPICS" METHOD FOR DIALYSIS DISCUSSION AND DECISION-MAKING

Topic 1. Medical Indications for Dialysis

- Prognosis: benefits versus burdens
- What is the functional age ("healthy" "vulnerable" "frail") of this patient?
- What are the geriatric susceptibility factors?
- What are potential adverse geriatric outcomes or complications?
- What are the survival data?
- Based on the above: Is the patient a candidate for dialysis or non-dialysis medical treatment?

Topic 2. Patient Preferences

- Establish "big picture" goals and outcomes (e.g., "pain-free," stay at home, live as long as possible).
- Explore patient's personal narrative, i.e. patient's understanding of what dialysis requires and experiences with dialysis in friends or family members.

- Since there is increased prevalence of cognitive dysfunction and inability to make decisions in advanced kidney disease, substituted judgment will be more common. Engage the family on these issues.
- Be prepared for:
  - Preferences that may change over time and with new events
  - Patients who are not able to decide or express their preferences
  - Patients who may want to receive limited or no information at all, and who prefer to delegate the discussion to others

Topic 3. Quality of Life (QOL)

- There is no universal metric for QOL.
- What constitutes QOL is a value judgment and very personal.
- There are some objective criteria (end-stage dementia, cachexia, advanced cancer), but families may not see it that way.
- Significant symptom burden has impact.
- A time-limited trial to assess whether QOL would be acceptable on dialysis is an important option to explore.

Topic 4. Contextual Features

- Is the family supportive of the patient and in agreement with his or her decision?
- Are the descriptions of patient wishes consistent?
- Are adequate supports available to encourage adherence with the decided renal plan and ensure that the patient's daily needs are met?
- What is the cultural, ethnic, or religious belief background?
- Are there conflicts between family members, among health care providers ("mixed messages"), or between the medical team and the family?

Table 79.2 applies the "Four Topics" method to a discussion of dialysis with Dr. S and his family.

SPECIAL ISSUES IN END-STAGE RENAL DISEASE

Calciphylaxis (Calcific Uremic Arteriopathy)

- Calcific uremic arteriopathy (CUA) is a disabling skin disorder in patients with ESRD, characterized by painful necrotic

TABLE 79.2: APPLYING THE FOUR TOPICS METHOD TO THE DIALYSIS DISCUSSION

Topic 1. Medical indications for dialysis
Functional age: Frail
Survival data on dialysis:
Mortality 1 year 46%; life expectancy 8.4 months
Possible adverse geriatric outcomes:
Increasing frailty and loss of function
Worsening cognitive dysfunction
Increased risk for hospitalization/falls
Geriatric susceptibility factors associated with increased mortality:
Older age >90
Non-ambulatory status
Serum albumin <35 g/L
4 chronic conditions
Dr. S is a suboptimal or non-ideal candidate from a medical indications standpoint.

Topic 2. Dr. S's preferences:
Decisional capacity: Yes
Advance directives: Documented
Health care proxy support: Yes
Clear and convincing evidence that he preferred to live his remaining time without dialysis
Dr. S has an informed right to forgo dialysis therapy

Topic 3. Dr. S's quality of life
Deteriorating medical condition
Concerns about symptom burden
Strong desire to remain at home

Topic 4. Contextual features
Supportive and involved family
Consistent descriptions re: patient wishes
Outcome: **All four topics explored**
Treatment plan: **Non-dialysis medical therapy; referral for home hospice services**

lesions secondary to small vessel ischemic disease with vascular calcifications; associated with high morbidity and mortality.[14]
- Treatment options
  - Wound care
  - Treatment of hyperparathyroidism/Ca/phosphorous abnormalities
  - Trial of sodium thiosulfate, an antioxidant cation -chelator shown to have some efficacy in small series although there are no randomized studies currently.[15]

Restless Leg Syndrome (RLS)[16]

- Restless leg syndrome is a lower extremity sensory syndrome in ESRD and occurs in both NDT and dialysis patients. It is defined as repetitive episodes of uncomfortable sensation (crawling, itching) relieved by movement, prominent in evening and associated with insomnia, with potential relation to uremic neuropathy, anemia, low serum ferritin, inadequate dialysis, medications (antidepressants-SSRIs, TCA; neuroleptics), and caffeine.
- Treatment options:
  - Dopamine receptor agonists (pramipexole, ropinirole, pergolide) have fewer side effects (e.g., daytime sleepiness and augmentation) than carbi-levodopa.
  - Gabapentin
  - Benzodiazepines (clonazepam) for immediate relief and associated sleep issues

SYMPTOM MANAGEMENT TO IMPROVE QUALITY OF LIFE

Regular communication with the nephrology team, especially for advice on dialysis-related symptoms, will optimize medical management. The paucity of RCTs is a limitation when making recommendations for symptom management.

PAIN

- Pain may result from multiple and coexisting etiologies, including:
  - Bone/joint/muscle
  - Renal disease
  - Peripheral vascular disease
  - Neuropathy,[17] including restless leg syndrome
  - Dialysis procedure-related pain
- Treatment options for pain management:[18] Use general World Health Organization (WHO) analgesic ladder for chronic pain management.
- Employ geriatric drug prescribing principles, i.e., lower starting doses and longer dosing intervals, including the following caveats. (See also Chapter 29: Management of Pain in Older Adults.)

Non-Opioids
- Acetaminophen: use as in geriatric population.

- NSAIDs: if patient is on dialysis and not on anticoagulants, may consider short-term course with gastric protection. Do not use NSAIDs in NDT ESRD patients.
- In the context of ESRD or NDT, use tramadol with caution.

Opioids[19,20]
- Preferred: fentanyl and methadone (non-active metabolites; negligible removal by dialysis; consult specialist for methadone management).
- Acceptable but should be used with caution: hydromorphone (removed by dialysis) and possibly oxycodone at 25% to 50% normal starting dose and at q6–12h intervals.
- Avoid: morphine, meperidine, dextropropoxyphene, dihydrocodeine, codeine.
- Adjuvants for neuropathic pain:
  - Gabapentin 100–300 mgq post-dialysis
  - TCAs: despiramine (fewer side-effects) 10–40 mg qd
  - Tegretol 100–600 mg bid
  - Valproic acid 250–500mg bid

MUSCLE CRAMPS
Treatment options include:

- Dialysis sodium/ultrafiltration profiling
- Midodrine for blood pressure support during dialysis
- Oxazepam—10 mg tid prn (short-term use the elderly; avoid if history of falls)
- Vitamin E—400 IU qd
- Intradialytic carnitine (10–20 mg/kg q post-dialysis)

PRURITUS
(See Chapter 60: Pruritus.)

FATIGUE
Treatment options include:[21]

- Erythropoetin therapy
- Adequacy of dialysis
- Intradialytic carnitine
- Regular exercise
- Yoga
- Acupressure
- Empiric trial of methylphenidate or other psychostimulants (See Chapter 30: Fatigue.)

SYMPTOMS OF ADVANCED CKD AT THE END OF LIFE[22]
Consider anticipatory prescribing for optimal symptom control near the end of life:

- Nausea/vomiting (See Chapter 53: Nausea and Vomiting)
- Dyspnea (See Chapter 48: Dyspnea)
- Delirium (See Chapter 34: Delirium and Chapter 35: Terminal Delirium)
- Retained respiratory secretions (See Chapter 40: Cough and Secretions)
- Myoclonic jerking: Decrease or rotate opioids; decrease or discontinue gabapentin and metopropamide; use lorazepam for control
- Uremic seizures: IV lorazepam/midazolam

Dr. S's hip X-ray was negative for fracture and showed severe osteoarthritis. Since he opted for non-dialysis medical therapy, NSAIDs were not used. Using the WHO ladder approach, his pain was controlled on fentanyl patch 25 mcg q72hrs and oxycodone 2.5 mg q8h prn with a bowel regimen. His restless leg syndrome was treated by switching from desipramine to gabapentin. Dr. S received home hospice services for ongoing symptom management, assistance with ADLs, patient and family support, and counseling regarding disease progression.

TAKE-HOME POINTS
- ESRD is medically managed without dialysis until uremic syndrome, hyperkalemia, acidosis, or fluid overload become refractory to medical therapy.
- Dialysis is life-sustaining therapy for patients with ESRD in the form of artificial renal replacement. Dialysis for an elderly person, especially for frail patients, has the attributes of a chronic progressive illness (e.g., reduced lifespan, progressive disability, repeated hospitalization, significant comorbidity, high symptom burden, and caregiver stress).
- The decision about whether to initiate renal replacement therapy should take into consideration medical indications, expected disease course, prognosis, patient preferences and goals of care, quality of life, and the context in which the decision takes place.
- Non-dialysis medical therapy (NDT) is a realistic alternative treatment that should be explored, especially in selected older

patients with serious comorbidities and frailty, since in these cases dialysis may not prolong life but may increase symptom burden and cause suffering.

- NDT prioritizes quality of life and symptom control combined with active medical treatment of renal complications. It is continued simultaneously with evaluation and treatment of geriatric syndromes and symptoms to maximize function and quality of life.
- In selected subgroups of patients (those with multiple comorbid conditions, ischemic heart disease, frailty), life expectancy of NDT patients may be similar to those on dialysis, but with fewer hospitalizations, more time spent at home and with family, and ultimately with less suffering.
- Symptom assessment and treatment must take into account special issues related to ESRD and dialysis including: effects of uremia and fluid excess, associated comorbidities and geriatric syndromes, proper renal dosing, and sensitivity to palliative medications.

REFERENCES

1. Rodin MB, Mohile SG. A practical approach to geriatric assessment in oncology. *J Clin Oncol.* 2007;*25*(14):1936–1944.
2. National Kidney and Urologic Diseases Information Clearinghouse. Kidney disease statistics for the United States. Retrieved from http://kidney. niddk.nih.gov/kudiseases/pubs/kustats/#7.
3. Ishani A et al. Acute kidney injury increases risk of ESRD among elderly. *J Am Soc Nephrol.* 2009; *20*(1):223–228.
4. Swidler MA. Dialysis Decisions in the Elderly Patient with Advanced CKD and the Role of Nondialytic Therapy, Chapter 37 in Geriatric Nephrology Curriculum. American Society of Nephrology: Washington, DC, 2009.
5. Murtagh FE et al. Dialysis or not? A comparative survival study of patients over 75 years with chronic kidney disease stage 5. *Nephrol Dial Transplant.* 2007;*22*(7):1955–1962.
6. Lorenz KA et al. Evidence for improving palliative care at the end of life: a systematic review. *Ann Intern Med.* 2008;*148*(2):147–159.
7. U.S. Renal Data System, USRDS 2007 Annual Data Report: Atlas of End-Stage Renal Disease in the United States, National Institutes of Health, National Institute of Diabetes and Digestive and Kidney Diseases, Bethesda, MD, 2007.
8. Kurella M, Covinsky KE, Collins AJ. Octogenarians and nonagenarians starting dialysis in the United States. *Ann Intern Med.* 2007;*146*(3):177–183.
9. Johansen KL, Chertow GM, Jin C, Kutner NG. Significance of frailty among dialysis patients. *J Am Soc Nephrol.* 2007;*18*(11): 2960–2967.
10. U.S. Renal Data System, USRDS 2007 Annual Data Report: Atlas of End-Stage Renal Disease in the United States, National Institutes of Health, National Institute of Diabetes and Digestive and Kidney Diseases, Bethesda, MD, 2004.
11. Kurella Tamura M, Covinsky KE, Chertow GM et al. Functional status of elderly adults before and after initiation of dialysis. *N Engl J Med.* 2009;*361*(16):1539–1547.
12. O'Hare AM, Choi A, Bertenthal D et al. Age affects outcomes in chronic kidney disease. *J Am Soc Nephrol.* 2007;*18*(10): 2758–2765.
13. Jonsen AR, Seigler M, Winsade WJ. *Clinical Ethics.* 2006. New York: McGrawHill, Medical Pub Division.
14. Rogers NM, Coates PT. Calcific uraemic arteriolopathy: an update. *Curr Opin Nephrol Hypertens.* 2008;*17*(6):629–634.
15. Schlieper G, Brandenberg V, Kettler M et al. Sodium thiosulfate in the treatment of calcific uremic arteriolopathy. *Nat Rev Nephrol.* 2009;*5*(9): 539–543.
16. Novak M, Mendelssohn D, Shapiro CM. Diagnosis and management of sleep apnea syndrome and restless legs syndrome in dialysis patients. *Semin Dial.* 2006;*19*(3):210–216.
17. Krishnan AV, Kiernan MC. Neurological complications of chronic kidney disease. *Nat Rev Neurol.* 2009;*5*(10):542–551.
18. Kurella M, Bennett WM, Chertow GM. Analgesia in patients with ESRD: a review of available evidence. *Am J Kidney Dis.* 2003;*42*(2):217–228.
19. Dean M. Opioids in renal failure and dialysis patients. *J Pain Symptom Manage.* 2004;*28*(5): 497–504.
20. Niscola P, Scaramucci L, Vischini G et al. The use of major analgesics in patients with renal dysfunction. *Curr Drug Targets.* 2010;*11*(6):752–758.
21. Jhamb M, Weisford SD, Steel JL, Unruh M. Fatigue in patients receiving maintenance dialysis: a review of definitions, measures, and contributing factors. *Am J Kidney Dis.* 2008;*52*(2):353–365.
22. Douglas C, Murtagh FE, Chambers EJ et al. Symptom management for the adult patient dying with advanced chronic kidney disease: a review of the literature and development of evidence-based guidelines by a United Kingdom Expert Consensus Group. *Palliat Med.* 2009;*23*(2):103–110.

80

Recurrent Urinary Tract Infection (RUTI)

CASE
Mrs. J, an 82-year-old, wheelchair-bound female with an indwelling Foley and moderate dementia, is admitted to the hospital from a long-term care facility (LTC) with her third episode of urosepsis in six months. Review of records reveals two previous urine cultures with E. coli, treated with trimethoprim-sulfazoxazole (TMP-SX), and two episodes of Clostridium difficile-related diarrhea (CDD) treated with vancomycin.

DEFINITION
Recurrent urinary tract infection can be defined as two or more episodes of symptomatic health care-associated (nursing home, hospital) urinary tract infections (UTIs) during the last six months; for symptomatic community-associated UTIs, three or more episodes during the last six months.

- Includes cystitis and chronic prostatitis (lower tract), pyelonephritis and renal/peri-renal abscess (upper tract), and urosepsis (systemic signs and bacteremia). Recurrent urinary tract infections (RUTIs) are further divided into two categories:[1,2]
  - "Relapse" type: Symptomatic infection after therapy, resulting from persistence of pre-therapy isolate in the urinary tract; should prompt a urological evaluation and will require prolonged antibiotic therapy
  - "Reinfection" type: Symptomatic infection with a bacterial strain originating from outside of the urinary tract enters the bladder during or after treatment; can be either a new or previously identified organism
- Other important categories when assessing for RUTIs include:[1,3]
  - **Complicated urinary tract infection (UTI):**
    - In geriatric palliative care, RUTIs may be viewed as a form of complicated UTI.
    - Implies functional or structural abnormality; can lead to serious complications (local and metastatic abscesses) and repeated treatment failure.[4]
- **Asymptomatic bacteriuria and asymptomatic urinary tract infection (positive urine cultures):**
  - In the absence of UTI symptoms, screening for and treatment of asymptomatic bacteriuria is not recommended in long-term care patients, unless undergoing urologic procedure where mucosal bleeding is anticipated.
  - Studies on antibiotic usage have not demonstrated improvement in symptom management or mortality but have shown increased adverse drug effects and antibiotic resistance.[5]
- **Pyuria:**
  - Presence of increased numbers of urinary polymorphonuclear leukocytes; reflects local urinary tract host inflammatory response
  - Presence or absence of pyuria does not differentiate symptomatic from asymptomatic UTI, nor is it relevant to selection of appropriate antibiotic therapy.[5]
  - Increased incidence of pyuria with asymptomatic bacteriuria in diabetic women (70%), elderly LTC patients (90%), hemodialysis (90%), short-term catheters (30–75%), and long-term catheters (50–100%)[5]
- **Chronic urinary catheter-related bacteriuria:**
  - 100% of patients with chronic indwelling catheter will have positive urine studies.
  - Evidence does not support treating asymptomatic UTI, except before a planned genito-urinary (GU)

intervention, since treatment will increase adverse drug effects and resistant organisms, and will not sterilize the bladder.

PATHOGENESIS

- Perineal and gastrointestinal flora colonize vagina and peri-urethral orifice, ascend to bladder, and may localize in prostate.
- Obstruction or reflux increases probability of upper tract involvement.
- Foreign bodies including catheters, stents, and nephrostomy tubes provide entryway and nidus for RUTIs.
- Prolonged antibiotic treatment will change resident flora, leading to increased incidence of MRSA (methicillin-resistant Staphylococcus aureus), VRE (vancomycin-resistant enterococci), and CDD (Clostridium difficile disease).
- Less commonly, UTI occurs through hematogenous spread.

PREVALENCE

- Asymptomatic bacteriuria: For patients over 65 years, the prevalence in females is 10% to 20% in the community (higher range for patients > 80 years old) and 25% to 55% in long term care facilities (LTCs). Prevalence in males is 5% to 15% (higher range for patients > 75 yrs. old) and 15% to 40% in LTCs.
- Symptomatic UTI: For women, ranges from 7% in community up to 14% in LTC settings. For men, range is up to 17% in the community and 14% in long-term care.[5]
- For patients with chronic indwelling catheter, prevalence of asymptomatic bacteriuria is 100%. Patients with short-term catheters develop bacteriuria at a rate of 2% to 7% per day.[5]

RISK FACTORS

- Functional and structural abnormalities that cause incomplete voiding, stasis, and retention. The presence of a post-void residual (PVR)
- Foreign bodies, struvite stones, prostatic calculi that provide a nidus for bacteria
- History of UTI before menopause in outpatient females
- Poor functional status and catheterization in long-term care females increase susceptibility[6]
- Prostate enlargement is the most important determinant in men

- Comorbidities: Advanced age, debilitation, prolonged hospitalization, urinary and rectal incontinence, diabetes, estrogen deficiency
- Prolonged and repetitive courses of antibiotics, with resulting change in resident flora

LIKELY ETIOLOGIES[3]

- Indwelling or intermittent urinary catheters, nephrostomy tube, ureteral stent
- External condom catheters, ileal conduits
- Bladder stones, diverticulae, cystocele
- Bladder dysfunction in setting of neurological disease (dementia, Parkinson's disease, stroke, paraplegia)
- Prostatic hypertrophy, prostatic calculi
- Ureteral stones, stricture, clot
- Cancer-associated UTI from obstruction by tumor (pelvic, prostate, bladder), malfunctioning stent, nephrostomy tube, or fungal ball

DIAGNOSIS

Exam

- Atypical symptoms: New or increased (not chronic) urinary incontinence, delirium, respiratory symptoms, fever, GU symptoms/signs such as dysuria, urgency, frequency
- Signs: Costovertebral angle (CVA)/flank tenderness, palpable or tender bladder, signs of neuropathy, urethral catheter, ileal conduit
- Localizing GU symptoms and signs are most predictive of a UTI in a long-term care patient presenting with acute change in status and no catheter
- Absence of local GU findings makes interpretation more difficult, especially given high prevalence of asymptomatic bacteriuria in long-term care patients. If patients with indwelling Foley present with fever and with no other likely sources of infection, then patient should be treated for presumed UTI

Tests[1]

- Urine dipstick: Absence of nitrates and leukocyte esterase have high reliability to rule out UTI. Presence of nitrite and leukocyte esterase is not useful in long-term care patients with or without indwelling catheter given chronic asymptomatic UTI.

- Urinalysis with micro exam: Absence of pyuria is useful to exclude UTI but has low specificity for infection since it is common with and without bacteriuria in long-term care patients.
- Urine culture and sensitivity:
  - Specimen collection:
    - Non-catheter mid-stream clean catch or straight cath sterile catheterized specimen
    - If indwelling catheter, replace, then get a urine C/S, since these specimens tend to be more accurate.[1,7,8] Do not use specimens from bedpan or used Foley bag, condom catheter, or legbag.
  - Colony count general guidelines for UTI:
    - $\geq 10^5$ cfu/mL in voided specimen; lower in men, renal dysfunction, diuresis, fastidious organisms, urethral catheterization
    - 10^4 cfu/mL if clinical criteria are consistent with acute pyelonephritis
    - $\geq 10^2$ "in and out" straight catheter specimen
    - $\geq 10^5$ external condom catheter

Imaging

- Imaging should be done if there is delayed response to antibiotics, flank pain, systemic toxicity, diabetes, acute renal failure, or if patient is immunocompromised.
- Renal and bladder ultrasound: Assess for stones, obstruction, pyelonephritis, renal abscess, cysts (including polycystic kidney disease), anatomic abnormality.
- CT scan with thin cuts or renal stone protocol (non-contrast) is more sensitive.

Microbiology[1,3]

- See Table 80.1 for percent (%) prevalence of organisms in community-based (C) and long-term care (LTC) geriatric patients with symptomatic UTIs and no chronic catheter. (Listed in order of most to least common: 4+ > 50%, 3+ 20%–49%, 2+ 10%–19%, 1+ < 10%.) (Table 80.1).
- E. coli is most common organism in females; in men, both gram-negative and gram-positive
- Higher incidence of resistant and poly-microbial infection in long-term care setting
- Catheter-related organisms: Endogenous bowel flora, exogenous

TABLE 80.1: MICROBIOLOGY OF UTIS

	Women		Men	
	C	LTC	C	LTC
E. coli	4+	4+	2–3+	2+
K. pneumoniae	1–2+	1–2+	1+	1+
P. mirabilis	1+	1–3+	1+	3+
Pseudomonas	–	1+	1+	2+
Other gram-neg	1+	2+	1+	2+
Coag-neg staph	1+	1+	1–3+	3+
Enterococcus	1+	1+	2–3+	1–3+
Staph aureus	–	1+	1+	1+
Group B strep	2+	1–2+	–	1+
Other gram-pos		2+		1+

(cross-contamination from other patients and personnel) organisms, VRE, and MDR
- In ICU setting, suspect highly resistant organisms (P. aeruginosa, Candida) (associated with use of broad spectrum antibiotics and indwelling catheters)[9]

EXPECTED DISEASE COURSE

- Unless a reversible cause is found, RUTIs and the adverse effects of repetitive infection and antibiotic exposure with antimicrobial resistance will contribute to increasing frailty and functional decline in the geriatric palliative care population.
- RUTI-associated delirium will contribute to the progression of dementia and is a significant source of distress for patients, families, and clinical staff.

TREATMENT OPTIONS

Nonpharmacologic/Preventive

- Maximize unrestricted urine flow (avoid or relieve obstruction) and regular complete voiding.
- Use bladder scanners for residual urine, and assess need for catheterization.
- Implement prompted scheduled toileting in demented patient q 2–3h during day.
- Chronic-indwelling catheters should be avoided except for:
  - Symptomatic relief of obstruction or urinary retention not amenable to medical management
  - Sacral decubitus wound care

- Symptomatic incontinence during active dying.
- Supra-pubic catheters do not reduce infection but may be used to relieve meatal/penile trauma/discomfort.
- Condom catheters reduce risk of infection but are associated with discomfort and penile ulceration.
- Cranberry juice and lactobacillus may be of some preventive benefit in females.

Pharmacologic[6]

- Topical treatment (for women):
  - Topically applied intravaginal estrogen can reduce the incidence of RUTI by reducing vaginal colonization and pH-increasing resident lactobacillus.
  - Topical estrogens include estrogen creams (Premarin, Ogen, Estrace), estradiol vaginal ring (Estring), and intravaginal tablets (Vagifem).
- Antibiotic guidelines for treatment of RUTIs[1,3]:
  - If clinical status permits, delay antibiotic initiation until urine culture and sensitivity testing (C/S) are available.
  - If starting empiric therapy, use prior urine C/S to guide choice of antibiotic. If test results are not available, then use common local community, hospital, or LTC organism susceptibilities and reevaluate antibiotics at 48 hours when C/S is available.
  - Every geriatric patient should have a serum creatinine-based GFR (MDRD) or CrC (CG) to appropriately dose antibiotics. (Calculate as follows: Glomerular filtration rate (GFR) $\times$ serum creatinine clearance (SCr) = Urine creatinine concentration (UCr) $\times$ Urine volume (V))
  - If patient has received trimetheprim-sulfazoxazole or a fluoroquinolone in the last three to six months, antibiotic resistance is more likely.
  - Duration of therapy: Seven days for lower tract and 10 to 14 days for upper tract or bacteremia. Four to six weeks for chronic bacterial prostatitis
- Suppressive low-dose therapy:
  - May be warranted for selected non-catheter-related RUTI situations (chronic struvite stones, ureteral stent, immuno-suppressed host/renal transplant).

- Not recommended for LTC-related RUTIs because of increased incidence of adverse drug effects, bacterial resistance, and Clostridium difficile-related diarrhea.
- Indwelling Foley, stent, or nephrostomy tube should be changed or removed.
- If there is no clinical response to antibiotic therapy by 48 to 72 hours, then evaluate for obstruction or abscess, check for antibiotic resistance, or rule out non-urinary tract source as a source of deterioration.
- If the underlying functional or structural abnormality persists or recurs, UTI may recur within six weeks in up to 50% of patients.

PALLIATIVE CARE ISSUES

- A short course of phenazopyridine (for up to two days) for infection-associated dysuria may be used if renal function is adequate. Avoid if GFR < 50 mL/minute.
- In the context of end-stage dementia affecting long-term survival, the topic of antibiotic therapy when burdens of therapy outweigh benefits should be included in discussisons about goals of care and the focus of a shared-decision-making process.

Mrs. J meets criteria for "relapse" RUTI. Her risk factors include indwelling Foley, poor functional status, and dementia in a long-term care setting. The catheter should be replaced immediately with cultures taken on insertion of the new catheter. TMP-SX resistant E. coli urosepsis should be presumed. Patient should be treated with a fluoroquinolone or third-generation cephalosporin with additional gram-positive coverage for possible enterococccus, S aureus, and coagulase-negative staphylococci until results of C/S are known.

Documentation of reason for chronic indwelling catheter and prior urological workup should be reviewed. If no clinical response within 48 to 72 hours, then consider treatment for possible vancomycin-resistant enterococci and Candida. Remove catheter if possible.

The most important preventive intervention would be to discontinue chronic catheter use, institute a program of scheduled voiding, and review catheter care techniques with LTC staff. Hand hygiene, aseptic technique, maintaining a closed urinary drainage system, and never allowing backward flow of urine into the bladder are imperative in catheter care. There are no accepted guidelines regarding the use of coated catheters or scheduled catheter replacement.

TAKE-HOME POINTS

- Symptomatic recurrent urinary tract infections (RUTIs) are a form of complicated UTI and require urological assessment, attention to pathogen susceptibility, and consideration of prior treatment history when choosing antibiotics.
- Be alert for atypical presentations in patients with dementia and poor functional status.
- Avoid indwelling catheters and condom catheters in long-term care patients.
- There should be a valid reason to get a urine analysis or urine C/S in a chronically ill, long-term care patient, or patient at the end of life, with or without chronic dwelling urethral catheter.
- Unless a reversible cause is found, RUTIs may contribute to increasing frailty and functional decline in the geriatric palliative care population.

REFERENCES

1. Nicolle LE. Urinary tract infections in older people. *Reviews in Clinical Gerontology.* 2008;*18*:103–114.
2. Nicolle LE, ed. Urinary Tract Infections. In: Halter JB et al., eds. *Hazzard's Geriatric Medicine and Gerontology.* New York: McGraw-Hill Medical; 2009:1547–1559.
3. Nicolle LE. Complicated urinary tract infection in adults. *Can J Infect Dis Med.* 2005;*16*(6):499–504.
4. Lichtenberger P, Hooton TM. Complicated urinary tract infections. *Curr Infect Dis Rep.* 2008;*10*(6): 499–504.
5. Nicolle LE et al. Infectious Diseases Society of America guidelines for the diagnosis and treatment of asymptomatic bacteriuria in adults. *Clin Infect Dis.* 2005;*40*(5):643–654.
6. Raz R, Stamm W. Optimal treatment of UTI in postmenopausal women. *J Am Med Dir Assoc.* 2000;*1*(4):172–174.
7. Trautner BW. Management of catheter-associated urinary tract infection. *Curr Opin Infect Dis.* 2010;*23*(1):76–82.
8. Raz R, Schiller D, Nicolle LE. Chronic indwelling catheter replacement before antimicrobial therapy for symptomatic urinary tract infection. *J Urol.* 2000;*164*(4):1254–1258.
9. Nicolle LE. Urinary tract pathogens in complicated infection and in elderly individuals. *J Infect Dis.* 2001;*183*(suppl 1):S5–S8.

81

Diabetic Management in Advanced Illness

CASE

Mrs. R, is a 78-year-old woman who comes in for a follow-up appointment with her primary care doctor. She has long-standing type 2 diabetes mellitus, complicated by retinopathy and stage 4 chronic kidney disease (CKD). She also suffers from hypertension, hyperlipidemia, coronary artery disease, and increasing debility. She tests her blood sugar once daily before breakfast and is concerned today about a recent rise in her blood sugar. To control her blood sugar, Mrs. R takes a combination of once-daily basal insulin as well as a mealtime insulin secretagogue.

DEFINITION

Diabetes mellitus occurs when blood glucose levels become elevated because of one or more of the following defects in glucose homeostasis (Table 81.1):

- Decreased insulin secretion
- Increased insulin resistance
- Impaired insulin signaling

Type 1 diabetes (historically referred to as "juvenile-type diabetes") is primarily a disease of insulin deficiency; it is typically caused by progressive autoimmune injury in individuals with a genetic susceptibility, although it can occur with pancreatic injury from other causes such as medications or trauma. It is typically thought to be a disease of children and adolescents, but adults with newly diagnosed diabetes can also present with evidence of insulin deficiency. Approximately 10% of all diabetes cases can be classified as type 1 diabetes.

Type 2 diabetes (historically referred to as "adult onset diabetes") is a more heterogeneous disease arising out of a complex interplay between environmental and genetic factors. The beginning stages are defined by increased insulin resistance, but over time beta cell failure also occurs, leading to either relative or absolute insulin deficiency.

PREVALENCE

- Dramatic increase in the number of cases of diabetes over the past 30 years in the United States. Currently, at least 10% of adults in the United States and more than 20% of those over 60 years of age suffer from diabetes.
- A much larger percentage of the population has disrupted glucose metabolism. Estimates suggest that one-fourth of the adult population has impaired fasting glucose or prediabetes.[2]

LIKELY ETIOLOGIES

- Autoimmune
- Genetic
- Environmental: Overweight/obesity, sedentary lifestyle, calorie-rich/nutrient-poor diet
- Medications: Steroids, atypical antipsychotic (clozapine, olanzapine), thiazide diuretics, immunosuppressants

TABLE 81.1: BLOOD GLUCOSE LEVELS

	Normal	Prediabetes	Diabetes
Fasting plasma glucose	<100 mg/dL	100–125 mg/dL	126 mg/dL or greater
Post 2 hr OGTT	<126	126–199 mg/dL	200 mg/dL or greater
"Casual" or random plasma glucose	***	***	200 mg/dL or greater

OGTT = oral glucose tolerance test (75 gram)[1]

(tacrolimus, cyclosporine), HIV protease inhibitors, nicotinic acid.

DIAGNOSIS

History

History-taking should attempt to identify symptoms of cardiac and vascular ischemia, peripheral neuropathy, autonomic dysfunction, and visual complaints. Episodes of hypoglycemia should be discussed; if such episodes have occurred without associated symptoms, then "hypoglycemia unawareness" should be suspected and noted.

Exam

In addition to a general medical examination, special attention should be paid to the lower extremities for evidence of ulcers, neuropathy, and arterial/vascular insufficiency.

Tests

Lab tests should include:
- Comprehensive metabolic panel
- Lipid profile
- Urine microalbumin
- Hemoglobin A1c
- Thyroid-stimulating hormone (TSH)

EXPECTED DISEASE COURSE

Chronic diabetes is associated with an increase in vascular disease leading to associated morbidities such as myocardial infarction, stroke, lower extremity ulcers, amputations, end-stage renal disease, and visual impairment. Cardiovascular disease is the leading cause of death in diabetic individuals.

- Microvascular diseases: Retinopathy, neuropathy, nephropathy
- Macrosvascular diseases: Cerebral vascular disease, coronary heart disease, peripheral vascular disease.

TREATMENT OPTIONS

Nonpharmacologic

- The mainstay of diabetes treatment is the management of blood glucose levels through changes in diet, increased physical activity when possible, weight management, self-monitored blood glucose testing in selected individuals, and the use of anti-hyperglycemic medications as needed (See Tables 81.1 and 81.2).
- It is important to note, however, that diabetes management requires more than glucose control in order to prevent or delay diabetes-associated complications. Diabetes risk reduction strategies include:
- Blood pressure management (<130/80)
- LDL lowering (<100 mg/dL or <70 mg/dL with overt CHD)
- Smoking cessation
- Dilated eye exams

TABLE 81.2: ORAL ANTI-HYPERGLYCEMIC MEDICATIONS

Medication	Examples	Indications	Advantages	Disadvantages
Biguanides	Metformin	Normal renal function No heart failure	Weight neutral	GI side effects
Sulfonylureas	Glimepiride, Glipizide Glyburide	Consistent PO intake	Rapidly effective	Hypoglycemia Weight gain
Glinides	Repaglinide Nateglinide	Sporadic PO intake	Rapid action	Hypoglycemia Weight gain Frequent dosing
α—Glucosidase inhibitors	Acarbose, miglitol	2nd–3rd line agent	Weight neutral	Frequent GI side effects
Thiazolidinediones	Pioglitazone Rosiglitazone	Younger patients Non-obese	Less hypoglycaemia	Fluid retention CHF/MI risk Fracture risk
DPP-4 inhibitors	Sitagliptin	Can renally dose	Weight neutral	Cost Long-term risk

- Lower extremity inspection
- Urine microalbumin monitoring
- Hemoglobin A1c monitoring
- Use of aspirin, statins, ACE-inhibitors[3]
- Diabetic therapy must be tailored to the individual patient. Treatment algorithms can assist the practitioner but cannot take the place of customizing a treatment plan. Important issues to be considered include:
  - Renal function
  - Presence of congestive heart failure
  - Ability to administer injections
  - Vision problems that may hamper injections or glucose meter use
  - Presence of "hypoglycemic unawareness"
  - Nutritional status
  - Cost of medications

Glycemic control:
- Large studies such as the Diabetes Control and Complications Trial (DCCT: Type 1 Diabetes) and the United Kingdom Prospective Diabetes Study (UKPDS: Type 2 Diabetes) have demonstrated the importance of lowering blood glucose levels in the chronic management of diabetes in order to prevent diabetes-associated complications.
- In the outpatient setting, the hemoglobin A1c (which gives an estimate of the average blood glucose level over the past two to

three months) is a useful tool for assessing chronic glycemic control. Currently, the American Diabetes Association (ADA) recommends a target hemoglobin A1c of less than 7.0% for many nonpregnant adults with diabetes.
- The target HgA1c should be individualized. Patients with frequent hypoglycemia, advanced disease, or shortened life expectancy may not benefit from "tight" glycemic control (see discussion below).
- There are also significant limitations to the use of HgA1 as a monitoring tool. Anemia and other erythrocyte disruptions can "falsely" lower the measured HgA1c. Also, extreme swings in blood glucose may be overlooked because the reported HgA1c reflects "average" glucose levels.

Pharmacologic[4]

Anti-hyperglycemic medications are available in oral and injectable formulations (Tables 81.2 and 81.3).

GLYCEMIC CONTROL FOR OLDER AND SERIOUSLY ILL PATIENTS

- The benefits and burdens of glycemic control must be weighed in context of functional and cognitive capacity,

TABLE 81.3: INJECTABLE ANTI-HYPERGLYCEMIC MEDICATIONS

	Examples	Indications	Advantages	Disadvantages
Insulins	Prandial: regular, aspart, lispro, glulisine	Type 1s Type 2s with postprandial elevations	Rapidly effective	Hypoglycemia Weight gain Injections
	Intermediate: NPH	Prednisone-induced hyperglycemia Tube feeds		
	Basal: glargine, detemir	Type 1s Type 2s failing orals		
	Fixed-mix: 70/30, 75/25, 50/50	Some type 1s Type 2s failing orals		
Glp-1 agonists	Exenatide	Obese type 2s	Weight loss	GI side effects Frequent injections Cost
Amylin agonists	Pramlintide	Type 1s: 2nd to 3rd line agent in addition to prandial insulin	Weight loss	GI side effects Frequent injections Cost

comorbidities, prognosis, and patient and family goals for care.

- Hyperglycemia can lead to dehydration and increased risk of infection, as well as other serious metabolic morbidities. Uncontrolled diabetes has also been associated with increased cardiovascular risk.
- Because of data supporting the association of long-term control of blood glucose in both type 1 and type 2 diabetics with decreased morbidity and mortality, recent studies have examined whether "tighter" glycemic control in both inpatients and outpatients would lead to further improvements in outcomes.
- The recently reported outcomes from the VADT, ACCORD, and ADVANCE trials seem to suggest that in older outpatients with longstanding diabetes and associated complications, attempts at "normalizing" glucose levels may cause more harm than benefit. Inpatient and ICU glycemic targets remain an area of active debate, and individualized glycemic targets should be considered for individuals of advanced age or with significant disease burden.[5,6,7,8]
- Recently the American Association of Clinical Endocrinologists (AACE) and the American Diabetes Association (ADA) issued the following new glycemic targets for hospitalized patients:
  - ICU setting: 140–180 mg/dL
  - Hospital wards: 100–180 mg/dL
- There have been few published guidelines regarding appropriate target HgA1c's and glucose levels in elderly or palliative care populations, but it is reasonable to suggest slightly higher HgA1c's of 7–8. This would correlate approximately to a blood glucose range of 100–200 mg/dL.

For Mrs. R, a higher target HgA1c goal would be appropriate because she has already developed several end organ complications from her diabetes. This can be a challenging discussion for a care provider to have because it may mark a shift from counseling the patient has received from other providers in the past. It is important to explain the risks of strict glycemic goals vs. the limited benefit of achieving such goals.

HYPOGLYCEMIA MANAGEMENT

- Because of concern regarding the association between hypoglycemia and cardiovascular risk, falls, and possibly

dementia, it is important to try to avoid significant hypoglycemia in both the inpatient and outpatient settings. This is particularly true in elderly and seriously ill populations.

- For those on insulin and sulfonylurea, monitor closely for signs/symptoms of hypoglycemia and adjust dosages accordingly.
- Use insulin sensitizers or the newer DPP-4 inhibitors for those in whom hypoglycemia could cause significant morbidity.
- Hypoglycemia is more likely to occur if oral intake is interrupted or sporadic. Declining renal function can also result in decreased clearance of insulin, thus predisposing to hypoglycemia.
- Individuals who are being treated with hypoglycemic agents (insulin, sulfonylureas, other insulin secretagogues, exanetide) should have routine blood glucose monitoring.
- The frequency of such monitoring depends on the individual, but monitoring should be increased in times of acute illness, perioperative setting, or change in nutritional status.
- Strategies to reduce the risk of significant hypoglycemia include:
  - Self-monitoring of blood glucose levels by the patient or caregiver
  - Educating the patient/caregiver about the signs and symptoms of hypoglycemia
  - Counseling the patient/caregiver about the need for prompt treatment of hypoglycemia
  - Scheduled and coordinated delivery of nutrition and diabetic therapy
  - Active titration of diabetic medication

For Mrs. R, the risk of hypoglycemia may increase as her renal function further declines. A nutritional history to understand how consistently she is eating will guide education about the symptoms and treatment of hypoglycemia.

PALLIATIVE CARE ISSUES

- While there is little guidance on how diabetes should be managed in patients at the end of life, it is quite clear that HgA1C and tight control of blood sugar to prevent end organ damage is no longer the primary goal.
- Diabetic management should be guided by the patient's goals for care, maintenance

TABLE 81.4: APPROACH TO DIABETIC MANAGEMENT AT THE END OF LIFE

	Diabetes Type 1	Diabetes Type 2
Goal of treatment	Avoid hypoglycemia and diabetic ketoacidosis	Avoid hypoglycemia and hyperglycemia
Frequency of glucose testing/ monitoring	Once daily or as needed based upon the individual	As needed, based on symptoms of hypoglycemia or hyperglycemia
Medication Management options for:		
Patient who is eating	Continue once-daily basal insulin in addition to bolus mealtime insulin. If oral intake is consistent, twice daily pre-mix insulin may be an option. There are currently no alternatives to daily insulin therapy for individuals with type 1 diabetes.	If possible, once-daily oral medications should be attempted. The choice of agent needs to take into account individual patient's kidney function, cardiac status, and risk of hypoglycemia. If needed, a once-daily dose of basal insulin can be added to an oral regimen.
Patient on feeding tube: a) continuous b) bolus feeding	Patients with type 1 require continuous insulin therapy. Once-daily basal insulin with scheduled correction/bolus doses can be tailored for both continuous or bolus feeding.	Either once-daily basal insulin or NPH q 6 hrs may be sufficient with continuous feeding. NPH or a shorter-acting insulin such as regular insulin may be given at the start of bolus feeding and titrated as needed.

of physical and cognitive function, and minimizing burdensome testing and symptoms (Table 81.4). The goal during late stages of disease, or among patients with multiple chronic conditions and functional impairment, is focused on improving the patient's quality of life.

- Frequency of fingerstick should be adapted to the individual and take into account patient preference. Some patients who have been on tight glucose control all their lives may need to maintain that control and way of life. While it is important to educate patients and their families that the goal of blood glucose management has changed, it is also important to allow for it if the patient insists.
- Diabetic management for those who wish to forgo the need for frequent testing should focus instead on short-term goals of avoiding symptoms of hypoglycemia such as lethargy and symptoms of hyperglycemia such as polydipsia, polyuria, polyphagia, and weakness.
- When the burdens of diabetic control outweigh its benefits, clinicians may give patients permission to miss meals, stop or

decrease glucose testing frequency, or stop or simplify medication regimen.

TAKE-HOME POINTS

- The mainstay of diabetes treatment is the management of blood glucose levels through diet, increased physical activity, weight management, blood glucose testing, and anti-hyperglycemic medications.
- Diabetes management needs to be flexible and responsive to the changing care needs, achievable goals, and comorbidities of an individual patient. Target glucose goals that were appropriate in the past for a specific patient may no longer be appropriate.
- While all individuals with type 1 DM and many with type 2 DM require daily insulin to safely manage their disease, these regimens may be simplified to accommodate a patient's preference or a changing clinical situation.
- Hypoglycemia poses a serious risk in the elderly. Recognizing which diabetic therapies or clinical situations may predispose to hypoglycemia is important in safely managing these patients.

REFERENCES

1. Standards of medical care in diabetes—2009. *Diabetes Care.* 2009;*32*(suppl 1):S13–S61.
2. Centers for Disease Control and Prevention. *National diabetes fact sheet: general information and national estimates on diabetes in the United States, 2007.* Atlanta, GA: Centers for Disease Control and Prevention, U.S. Department of Health and Human Services; s.n. 2008.
3. Buse JB et al. Primary Prevention of cardiovascular diseases in people with diabetes mellitus: a scientific statement from the American Heart Association and the American Diabetes Association. *Circulation.* Jan 2, 2007;*115*(1): 114–126.
4. Nathan, DM. Medical management of hyperglycemia in type 2 diabetes: A consensus algorithm for the initiation and adjustment of therapy: A consensus statement of the American Diabetes Association and the European Association for the Study of Diabetes. *Diabetes Care.* Jan 1, 2009;*32*: 193–203.
5. Skyler JS. Intensive glycemic control and the prevention of cardiovascular events. *Diabetes Care.* Jan 1, 2009;*32*:187–192.
6. Action to Control Cardiovascular Risk in Diabetes Study Group. Effects of intensive glucose lowering in type 2 diabetes. *N Engl J Med.* Jun 12, 2008;*358*: 2545–2559.
7. ADVANCE Collaborative Group. Intensive blood glucose control and vascular outcomes in patients with type 2 diabetes. *N Engl J Med.* Jun 12, 2008;*358*: 2560–2572.
8. VADT Investigators. Glucose control and vascular complications in veterans with type 2 diabetes. *N Engl J Med.* Jan 8, 2009;*360*:129–139.

82

End-Stage Heart Failure

CASE

Mr. W is a 79-year-old man with hypertension, dia-betes, osteoarthritis, and ischemic cardiomyopathy. His ejection fraction is 20%. He has an ICD, which has never fired. He is admitted with his third episode in the past six months of acute decompensated heart failure, after developing subacute onset of worsening dyspnea. At his best, Mr. W is able to walk to the mailbox. He has been homebound for two weeks due to weakness and dyspnea. The night prior to admis-sion, he could not sleep because he was unable to lie down and was dyspneic at rest. He has been care-fully taking his prescribed medication regimen.

DEFINITION

Heart failure (HF) is a complex clinical syndrome that can result from any structural or functional cardiac disorder that impairs the ability of the ventricle to fill with or eject blood.

- Patients may have this clinical syndrome with low or preserved ejection fraction (EF).[1] HF with normal EF is more common in older women. Disease course and optimal management are better elucidated for HF with low EF.
- The ACC/AHA Classification scheme emphasizes that HF is preventable when risk factors are optimally treated (Box 82.1).
- There is no universally accepted definition of *end-stage heart failure*. The Heart Failure Society of America defines patients with end-stage heart failure as those with advanced, persistent HF with symptoms at rest despite repeated attempts to optimize pharmacologic and nonpharmacologic therapy. Under this definition, "advanced/persistent" HF is evidenced by one or more of the following:[3]
  - Frequent hospitalization (three or more per year)
  - Chronic poor quality of life with inability to accomplish activities of daily living

- Need for intermittent or continuous intravenous support
- Consideration of assist devices as destination therapy

Mr. W has at least stage C heart failure. If treat-ment of this acute exacerbation does not result in improvement in symptoms and clinical stability, he would be considered to have stage D heart failure. He currently has functional class IV symptoms.

PREVALENCE[2]

- There are 5.8 million people in the United States with HF; 670,000 new cases are diagnosed annually.
- Heart failure is a disease of older adults. The prevalence of HF in the 60–79-year age group is 9% of men and 5% of women. In the 80-and-over age group, this rises to 15% of men and 13% of women. The prevalence of heart failure in people over 80 years old is 13%.
- Heart failure accounts for over 1.1 million hospital admissions annually; 75% of heart failure hospitalizations are for patients 65 or older.
- The significant increase in the prevalence of HF among older adults is due to both increased incidence and improved survival.

LIKELY ETIOLOGIES

Major causes of heart failure in the United States are:

- Coronary artery disease
- Hypertension
- Non-ischemic dilated cardiomyopathy
- Valvular disease

DIAGNOSIS

History and Exam

A comprehensive history and physical exam should confirm the diagnosis of heart failure,

---

BOX 82.1 ACC/AHA CLASSIFICATION OF HEART FAILURE

American College of Cardiology/American Heart Association Classification of HF[1]

Stage	Definition
A	Presence of a condition (e.g., hypertension) that puts patient at risk for HF, but without structural heart disease or symptoms of HF
B	Presence of structural heart disease but no symptoms
C	Presence of structural heart disease and current or prior symptoms of HF
D	Refractory HF, requiring specialized interventions. These patients have symptoms at rest despite maximal medical therapy.

This classification scheme is complementary to the New York Heart Association Functional Classification, which describes degree of symptoms with activity or rest for patients with Class C or D heart failure.

New York Heart Association Functional Classification

Class	Patient Symptoms
Class I	No functional limitation; no symptoms of heart failure (dyspnea, fatigue) with ordinary physical activity
Class II	Some functional limitation with heart failure symptoms with ordinary physical activity; no symptoms at rest
Class III	Significant functional limitation with heart failure symptoms with less than ordinary activity; no symptoms at rest
Class IV	Severe functional limitation with symptoms with any physical activity; symptoms even at rest

---

assess symptom severity, determine volume status, and determine degree of hemodynamic compromise.

1. For the patient with acute decompensated heart failure (ADHF), the goal of the evaluation is to determine:
   - Presence and severity of symptoms
   - Volume status
   - Adequacy of systemic perfusion
   - Degree of organ dysfunction
   - Need for intravenous vasodilators, inotropes, and/or pressors
   - Presence of common precipitating factors: acute coronary syndrome, uncontrolled hypertension, arrhythmia, infection, pulmonary emboli, renal failure, change in medication/non-adherence to regimen, change in diet
   - Prognosis
2. For the stable patient with chronic heart failure, the focus of the evaluation is to assess:
   - Volume status
   - Adequacy and tolerance of medical regimen
   - Presence of ischemia and/or valvular disease, which may be amenable to intervention
   - Candidacy for advanced therapies such as ICD or cardiac resynchronization therapy
   - Understanding of diagnosis, prognosis, treatment regimen

Symptom Assessment

Heart failure patients may experience a wide variety of distressing symptoms and should have a comprehensive symptom assessment, with special attention to fatigue, dizziness/lightheadedness, palpitations, chest pain, dyspnea, anorexia, edema, pain, depression, sleep disturbance, and skin breakdown.

Tests

- Full chemistry panel, CBC, ECG, Chest X-ray, BNP (Brain natriuretic peptide) testing as appropriate.
- Other cardiac imaging or hemodynamic monitoring as appropriate in context of

prognosis, function, comorbid disease, and goals of care.

Upon presentation, Mr. W is severely volume overloaded with evidence of impaired systemic perfusion. He has severe dyspnea at rest, severe orthopnea, mild nausea, moderate pain in his legs and feet, increased abdominal girth, and edema. His blood pressure is 82/65, pulse is 110, SaO2 90% on 2L NC O2. His weight is up eight pounds from his last outpatient visit. He has elevated jugular venous pressure to the angle of the jaw, an S3 gallop, a holosystolic murmur, normal lung exam and 2+ pedal edema. Pertinent lab values include serum sodium 128, BUN 48, creatinine 2.8 (his usual creatinine is 1.7), BNP 1000 pg/mL. ECG shows sinus tachycardia and Left Bundle Branch Block (LBBB) (old). He is admitted to an HF unit and placed on telemetry monitoring. Serial cardiac enzymes are obtained and found to be negative.

EXPECTED DISEASE COURSE
- Progression of disease is variable with wide spectrum of symptoms, ability to tolerate medical therapy, and complications.
- The severe end of the spectrum is characterized by recurrent episodes of decompensated heart failure with symptoms of congestion and/or low cardiac output.
- Death occurs due to:
  - Progressive pump failure, usually preceded by severe symptoms and hospitalization
  - Arrhythmia: Incidence of sudden cardiac death is decreasing with increasing use of ICDs, but 20% to 50% of deaths of patients with HF are sudden.[3]

PROGNOSIS
- Many factors have been shown to correlate with worse prognosis of HF, including:[1,3,4,5,6,7]
  - Poor functional status
  - Impaired renal function (BUN > 30)
  - Hypotension (SBP <120)
  - Hyponatremia (Na < 135)
  - Frequent hospitalizations despite optimal medical therapy
  - Inability to tolerate medical therapy with angiotensin-converting enzyme inhibitors (ACEI) or beta blockers (BB), especially when previously tolerated and associated with failure of improvement in systolic function on medical therapy

- Severe systolic dysfunction
- Presence of peripheral arterial disease
- Appropriate shocks from ICD
- Six-minute walk distance
- Brain natriuretic peptide
- Significant weight loss or poor nutritional status
- Models have been developed that incorporate these factors and patient comorbidities to estimate mortality. For geriatric patients with comorbid conditions, the mortality rate at one year after first HF hospitalization approaches 50%.[8,9]
- While the likelihood of death in a given time period may be estimated for an individual patient, it is nonetheless difficult to determine, during an episode of decompensation, how close death may be.[10]

Mr. W has many markers of poor prognosis, including hypotension, severe systolic dysfunction, poor renal function, high BNP, poor functional status, and frequent hospitalizations.

TREATMENT OPTIONS
- Treatment plans should be individualized for each patient through a process of shared and fully informed decision-making. This process should include a thorough exploration of the benefits and burdens of each treatment option (e.g., hospitalization, intravenous inotropes, ICU care, or device therapy) in the context of each patient's functional and cognitive status, comorbidities, prognosis, preferences, values, and achievable goals of care.
- The uncertain nature of prognosis in heart failure can present communication challenges. It is important to acknowledge the uncertainty, but to clearly explain that disease progression should be expected; to explore the patient's attitude about balancing risks of treatments with uncertain benefits; and to keep lines of communication open as new data modifies the prognosis.[10]
- Contemporary medical therapy for heart failure has disease-modifying and life-prolonging benefits, and also provides symptom relief, so it is important that the treatment regimen be optimized.[3] Reversible factors must also be identified and treated.
- Some patients will be unable to tolerate optimal medical management because

of side effects or the impact of comorbid illnesses. Comprehensive care, including collaboration with a cardiologist when appropriate, will ensure that each patient receives the optimal treatment regimen.[1]

Nonpharmacologic

Clinicians should provide the following interventions to all their advanced HF patients:[5]

- Educate patient and family about diagnosis, course, prognosis, and disease management, including monitoring of weight and symptoms.
- Discuss advance care plans especially in periods of clinical stability, as acute exacerbations may be complicated by delirium and compromised decision-making capacity.
- Assess for appropriateness of invasive cardiac therapies that are aligned with goals of care, such as:
  - Coronary revascularization
  - Surgical correction of valvular disease
  - Cardiac resynchronization therapy (CRT)
  - Implantable cardioverter defibrillator (ICD)
  - Advanced therapies such as transplantation or left ventricular assist device
- Reassess treatment preferences and goals and values on a regular basis, especially after changes in clinical status or significant life events.
- Comprehensively assess symptoms, including functional status, quality of life, role, function.
- Monitor needs of family and loved ones.
- Assess for hospice eligibility; if not hospice-appropriate, assess need for home health care.
- Discuss deactivation of implantable cardiac devices.
- Coordinate care among involved specialists and across care settings.
- Palliative therapies aimed at relieving sources of suffering in multiple domains are appropriate for advanced HF patients regardless of other therapies chosen.

Pharmacologic

- Optimum treatment for stable, chronic heart failure includes:

- Ace inhibitor or angiotensin receptor blocker at target or maximally tolerated doses
- Beta blocker at target or maximally tolerated doses
- Aldosterone antagonist in selected patients
- Adequate treatment of hypertension, ischemia, arrhythmia, diabetes, exacerbating or underlying comorbid conditions
- Diuretic as required to control congestion
- Oxygen as indicated for hypoxia
- Opioids for persistent dyspnea
- Optimum treatment for acute decompensated heart failure may include:
  - Oxygen
  - Intravenous therapies
  - Diuretics
  - Vasodilators (nesiritide, nitroglycerin, nitroprusside)
  - Inotropic agents (dobutamine, milrinone)
  - Pressors (dopamine, vasopressin)
  - Ultrafiltration
  - Adjustment of oral medication regimen
  - Opioids for dyspnea

Mr. W is treated for acute decompensated HF. He requires inotrope support for two weeks and ultrafiltration. His course has been complicated by delirium with agitation. Although his volume status and delirium have improved, and he is weaned off inotropic agents, he can no longer tolerate an ACE inhibitor or beta blocker due to symptomatic hypotension. Aldosterone antagonist has been stopped due to worsening renal function.

His primary clinician notices that Mr. W seems sad, despite improvement in HF symptoms. A comprehensive discussion about sources of suffering for Mr. Walters reveals that he is frightened by his recent hospitalizations and feeling less hopeful about his future. He is bothered by chronic moderate pain in his knees and shoulders, and even though he is less short of breath, he lacks energy to do basic tasks like walking to the bathroom. It has been months since he was able to participate in his weekly card game. His wife tries to help him at home but is unable to bathe him. In order to properly address Mr. Walters' suffering and concerns, and to help him choose treatment options that achieve his goals of care, a meeting is arranged with the cardiologist, the primary care provider, Mr. W, and his family.

SYMPTOM MANAGEMENT TO IMPROVE QUALITY OF LIFE

In general, HF symptoms should be managed as in other conditions, but taking into account these HF-specific issues:

- Nonsteroidal anti-inflammatory agents should be avoided, as they promote fluid retention and may worsen renal function.
- Chronic ischemic chest pain may respond to nitrates or beta blockers. The newer antianginal agent, ranolazine, may be considered in appropriate patients.[11]
- Dyspnea may respond to diuretics. Thoracenteses may relieve dyspnea in the setting of pleural effusion refractory to diuretic therapy.[9] For persistent dyspnea, consider opioids. (See Chapter 41: Dyspnea.)
- Treatment of sleep-disordered breathing, common in HF patients, with CPAP may improve fatigue.[12]
- Sodium phosphate and magnesium citrate containing preparations used to treat constipation should not be used in HF patients because salt absorption is increased.
- Methylphenidate, used to treat depression, may potentiate arrhythmia and ischemia.[9]

REFERRAL TO HOSPICE

In the context of the following clinical conditions, referral to hospice is appropriate:

- NYHA functional class IV symptoms persist despite maximally tolerated medical therapy.
- Patient is dependent on inotropic support.
- Multiple markers of poor prognosis
- Recent clinical decline without reversible cause:
  - Two or more hospital admissions in within six months
  - Worsening functional status/inability to perform ADLs
  - Progression of organ dysfunction (renal, hepatic, CNS)[9]

Mr. W qualifies for hospice care. At a family meeting, Mr. W, his family, and medical providers decide that referral to hospice is the best option to achieve his goals of care, which are to avoid any further hospitalizations, avoid being bed-bound for a prolonged period, remain at home until death, and have home care for help with daily bathing.

BARRIERS TO TIMELY HOSPICE REFERRAL

Barriers to timely hospice referral and acceptance of hospice by heart failure patients include:

- Difficulty in determining prognosis
- No clear distinction between disease-modifying and palliative treatment (unlike cancer care)
- Fear that HF treatments may be stopped
- Fear that hospitalization for exacerbations may not be permitted
- For an individual patient, prognosis, even during the last days of life, is often overestimated[9]
- Some hospices may lack familiarity with HF management
- Preference for continuing IV inotropic therapy for symptom relief and inability of some hospices to offer costly long-term IV inotrope therapy

PALLIATIVE CARE ISSUES

1. **Care setting considerations:**
   - While maximal medical therapy should be continued as tolerated regardless of setting, it is important to realize that regulations in certain care settings may not allow for all the patient's desired treatments for decompensated heart failure. For example, most nursing homes would not administer inotropes or pressors.
   - Setting considerations should therefore be addressed together with the benefits and burdens of the treatment options when establishing goals of care and clarifying the plan of care.
2. **Refining HF oral medication regimen at end of life:**
   - There are little data to provide guidance about discontinuing HF medications near the end of life. When tailoring the medical regimen, therefore, careful consideration should be given to the palliative benefits and risks of abrupt withdrawal.
   - Medications used in the treatment of heart failure may provide symptomatic

relief and palliative benefit in the short term, in addition to modifying the course of the disease in the longer term. Considerations include:

- Beta blockers may provide palliation by controlling angina, tachyarrhythmia, ventricular response of atrial fibrillation/flutter, and palpitations, but should be stopped in the event of symptomatic bradycardia, hypotension, refractory volume overload, and severe fatigue.
- Abrupt discontinuation of ACE inhibitors and angiotensin receptor blockers, as well as the combination of hydralazine/isosorbide dinitrate, may precipitate hemodymanic decompensation. Indications to discontinue ACEI/ARB include hypotension, renal failure, and hyperkalemia.
- Spironolactone should be used with great caution in patients with creatinine 1.5 or above and should be avoided in patients with worsening renal function or potassium above 5.[1]
- Long-acting nitrates provide anti-anginal effect.
- The benefits of digoxin as a rate control agent and oral inotrope must be balanced against the risks of toxicity in patients with changing and/or compromised renal function.
- Diuretic dose should be reevaluated as the patient's oral intake and volume status fluctuates. Torsemide is better and more predictably absorbed after oral administration.[13]
- Statin therapy may have some short-term benefits for patients with active acute coronary syndromes, but the primary outcomes are longer term. Statin therapy should be discontinued for Stage C-D or FC III-IV heart failure.[14]

3. **Intravenous inotropes at end of life:**
   - Patients are inotrope-dependent if withdrawal of the agent results in symptomatic hypotension, worsening renal function, or pulmonary congestion that requires restarting of the drug.
   - Intravenous inotropes may provide symptomatic relief, but likely shorten life expectancy, increasing the risk for arrhythmic death.
   - Clinical use is to maximize quality of life in the face of limited life expectancy for patients who are inotrope dependent.
   - With adequate home care support, intravenous inotropes can be administered in the home.

4. **Deactivation of implantable cardiac devices:**
   - Implantable cardiac devices are used very successfully for treatment of cardiac rhythm problems, but most patients are not made aware of the possibility of future burden at the time of implantation. Two commonly used devices are implantable cardiac defibrillators (ICDs) and implantable pacemakers.
   - As with other medical therapies, the benefits and burdens of these cardiac devices should be explored and reevaluated with advanced heart failure patients and their families.
   - As the end of life approaches, it is appropriate to reassess whether prevention of sudden cardiac death from conduction or rhythm abnormalities remains consistent with the patient's prognosis and goals of care. For example, although the ICD may prevent fatal arrhythmia, deactivating the ICD may provide benefits for the terminally ill patient, including:
     - Avoiding the physical pain of repeated shocks
     - Relief of anticipatory anxiety wondering if and when shock will come
     - Avoiding the prolongation of the dying process
   - Patients and families should be engaged in conversations about wishes/preferences in advance of the need to make a decision about deactivation. These discussions should ideally be initiated before the placement of the device.
   - Deactivation of cardiac devices should also be readdressed during any advance directive or DNR discussions about preferences and achievable goals of care. It should be explained that

deactivation is not painful and does not require surgical removal of the device. Applying a magnet over the generator will disable the shock function of most defibrillators.[15]

- If the patient's implantable cardiac device has multiple functions, consider each one separately:
  - Pacing
  - Arrhythmia therapy (defibrillation and anti-tachycardia pacing)
  - Arrhythmia detection and monitoring
- Deactivating a pacemaker entails a benefit/burden analysis that is separate from the question of deactivating an ICD:
  - Because pacing it is not effective under the conditions of imminent death (metabolic derangement, tissue hypoxia), pacing is not likely to prolong dying.
  - Withdrawal of pacing may lead to dyspnea, lightheadedness, syncope, or worsening HF symptoms, which may impact quality of life in more functional HF patients.
  - Depending on the outcome of benefit/burden discussions, the monitoring, pacing, and anti-tachycardia pacing functions of an implantable device may remain activated even after the shock function is deactivated.
- The Heart Rhythm Society has published guidelines for managing patients with cardiovascular implantable electronic devices when they are nearing the end of life, or who are requesting withdrawal of device therapy. This document will provide further guidance about defibrillators and pacemakers. Ethical, legal, practical, and communication issues are discussed.[16]

After discharge from the hospital, Mr. Walters meets with the hospice team in his home. He is asked about changing the settings of his defibrillator so that it will not deliver a shock in the event of ventricular tachycardia or ventricular fibrillation. He has never experienced a shock before, but understands that it can be life-saving. He wants to consider that decision further and not deactivate the ICD now. He instructs his wife, who is his health care proxy, to deactivate the ICD in the event his condition worsens and his is unable to make his own medical decisions.

5. Left Ventricular Assist Device (LVAD)
   - An LVAD is an implanted mechanical pump that does the work of the left ventricle. The device has been shown to prolong survival and improve quality of life in patients with severe heart failure who are not candidates for heart transplantation.
   - Complications associated with LVAD treatment include:
     - Infection
     - Bleeding
     - Thromboembolic event, including stroke
     - Mechanical failure
     - Psychological distress from high level of care/maintenance, living with risk of failure of device
   - Other burdens of LVADs include caregiver burden, pain/discomfort related to the device, and intense follow-up care
   - While initially used as a bridge to transplant, LVADs are increasingly used as destination therapy. While LVAD as destination therapy improves mortality in this critically ill population, survival is poor, with estimates of mortality of 30% in hospital and 50% at 1 year, and with a heavy therapy-related burden.
   - All patients considered for or treated with LVAD are appropriate for palliative care because of the high symptom burden and mortality risk.

TAKE-HOME POINTS
- Heart failure is a common disease in older adults and is associated with high morbidity and mortality.
- Reversible factors should be identified and treated. Sources of suffering should also be addressed.
- Individualized treatment plans should be based on the benefits and burdens of each treatment option, taking into account the patient's functional and cognitive status, comorbidities and prognosis, preferences and values, and achievable goals of care.
- Contemporary medical therapy for heart failure has disease-modifying and

life-prolonging benefits and provides symptom relief, so it is important that the treatment regimen be optimized.

- Goals of care should be reviewed and adjusted along the trajectory of the disease.
- The benefits and burdens of implantable cardiac devices should be explored with advanced heart failure patients and their families.
- All patients considered for or treated with LVAD are appropriate for palliative care because of the high symptom burden and mortality risk.

Mr. Walters does well on the hospice program. With close attention to symptoms and volume status and with support from the hospice team, he is able to enjoy visiting with his family, sit in a chair, and use a bedside commode. After three months on the hospice program, his condition worsens and he becomes weaker, bed-bound, and confused. His prior decision to forgo any further hospitalizations and to die at home is honored.

REFERENCES

1. Hunt SA, Baker DW, Chin MH et al. 2009 Focused Update Incorporated Into the ACC/AHA 2005 Guidelines for the Diagnosis and Management of Heart Failure in Adults. *J Am Coll Cardiol.* 2009;*53*: e1–e90.
2. Lloyd-Jones D, Adams RJ, Brown TM et al. Heart Disease and Stroke Statistics 2010 Update: a report from the American Heart Association. *Circulation.* 2010;*121*:e46–e215.
3. Heart Failure Society of America. Heart Failure Guidelines. Section 8: disease management in heart failure, education and counseling. *J Card Fail.* 2006;*12*:e58–e69.
4. Huynh BC, Rovner A, Rich MW. Identification of older patients with heart failure who may be candidates for hospice care: development of a simple four-item risk score. *J Am Geriatr Soc.* 2008;*56*: 1111–1115.
5. Hauptman PJ, Havranek EP. Integrating palliative care into heart failure care. *Arch Intern Med.* 2005;*165*:374–378.
6. Poole JE, Johnson GW, Hellkamp AS, et al. Prognostic importance of defibrillator shocks in patients with heart failure. *N Engl J Med.* 2008;*359*: 1009–1017.
7. Adler ED, Goldfinger JZ, Kalman J, Park ME, Meier DE. Palliative care in the treatment of advanced heart failure. *Circulation.* 2009;*120*:2597–2606.
8. Jong P, Vowinckel E, Liu PP, Gong Y, Tu JV. Prognosis and determinants of survival in patients newly hospitalized for heart failure. *Arch Intern Med.* 2002;*162*:1689–1694.
9. Stuart B. Palliative care and hospice in advanced heart failure. *J Palliat Med.* 2007;*10*: 210–228.
10. Goodlin SJ, Quill TE, Arnold RM. Communication and decision-making about prognosis in heart failure care. *J Card Fail.* 2008;*14*:106e–113.
11. Eid F, Boden WE. The evolving role of medical therapy for chronic stable angina. *Current Cardiol Rep.* 2008;*10*:263–271.
12. Goodlin SJ. Palliative care for end-stage heart failure. *Curr Heart Fail Rep.* 2005;*2*:155–160.
13. Sica DA, Gehr TWB, Frishman WH. Use of diuretics in the treatment of heart failure in the elderly. *Clin Geriatr Med.* 2007;*23*:107–121.
14. Vollrath AM, Sinclair C, Hallenback J. Discontinuing cardiovascular medications at the end of life: lipid-lowering agents. *J Palliat Med.* 2005;*8*(4): 876–881.
15. Wilkoff BL, Auricchio A, Brugada J, et al. Expert consensus on the monitoring of cardiovascular implantable electronic devices (CIEDs): description of techniques, indications, personnel, frequency and ethical considerations. *Europace.* 2008;*10*: 707–725.
16. Lampert R, Hayes DL, Annas GJ, Farley MA, Goldstein NE. HRS Expert Consensus Statement on the Management of Cardiovascular Implantable Electronic Devices (CIEDs) inpatients nearing end of life or requesting withdrawal of therapy. *Heart Rhythm.* July 2010;*7*(7):1008–1026.

83

Arrhythmias

Cardiac arrhythmias are common in older adults as a result of changes in cardiac conduction associated with aging and concomitant cardiovascular diseases. Atrial fibrillation (AF) and conduction system disease leading to symptomatic bradycardia commonly coexist.[1]

PART A: ATRIAL FIBRILLATION (AF)

Case

Ms. A is an 83-year-old woman with a history of hypertension and osteoporosis who presents with palpitations for the past week. She has no history of heart disease, diabetes mellitus, or stroke. Her blood pressure is 142/86 mmHg, her pulse is rapid, and irregularly irregular, and there is no evidence of congestive heart failure. The electrocardiogram demonstrates atrial fibrillation with a rapid ventricular response at 110 beats per minute.

Ms. A started therapy with metoprolol succinate, 100 mg daily. After a discussion with her health care team about the benefits and risks of anticoagulant therapy to prevent thromboembolism, she started warfarin with a target INR of 2-3. She remained in AF with a ventricular rate of 70 beats per minute and was asymptomatic with an unlimited exercise tolerance.

Definition

Atrial fibrillation is caused by irregular electrical activation and contraction of the atria, resulting in potentially accelerated ventricular rates and uncoordinated atrial and ventricular contraction.

Prevalence

AF occurs in three to four percent of the population older than age 60, and 10% of the population older than 80.[2,3]

Likely Etiologies

AF is often idiopathic but three reversible causes should be excluded:

- Hyperthyroidism
- Pulmonary embolism
- Ischemia (uncommon)

Diagnosis

Exam

- Beat-to-beat variation in blood pressure
- Irregularly irregular ventricular rhythm and pulse, variable intensity of S1
- Disappearance of A wave in jugular venous pulse contour
- If hemodynamically significant, AF may result in congestive heart failure.

Tests

- Electrocardiogram: Irregularly irregular atrial rhythm with variable atrioventricular conduction; may show signs of atrial enlargement, left ventricular hypertrophy, conduction abnormalities or cardiomyopathy.
- Echocardiogram: To evaluate for the presence of structural heart disease including valvular heart disease and left ventricular hypertrophy; to assess thromboembolic risk and guide appropriate medical therapy.
- Labs: to evaluate etiology and guide choice of therapy:
  - Thyroid function tests
  - Kidney function tests
  - Liver chemistries

Expected Disease Course

- Atrial fibrillation in older adults is commonly associated with comorbid cardiovascular conditions such as valvular heart disease, hypertensive heart disease, and coronary artery disease.
- As age advances, so does morbidity, including stroke, cognitive impairment, and heart failure. Medication intolerance and the risk of bleeding associated with anticoagulant therapy also increase with age.

Prognosis

AF is usually a chronic disease requiring long-term treatment. Once treated, the prognosis of patients with AF is closely related to status of other underlying comorbid conditions.

Treatment Options

A range of nonpharmacologic and pharmacologic therapies are available to achieve control of heart rate and/or rhythm in AF.[4] Choice of treatment should be based on patient's goals, values, and existing comorbidities.

Nonpharmacologic

- Direct Current Cardioversion (DCCV):[5]
  - Effective in restoring normal sinus rhythm, at least temporarily, in the majority of patients with AF.
  - Conversion from AF to normal sinus rhythm is associated with increased thromboembolic risk; appropriate candidates should be therapeutically anticoagulated at the time of cardioversion.[6] (See Thromoembolsm Prophylaxis below.)
  - Anticoagulation should be maintained in the therapeutic range for four weeks before and after cardioversion (electrical or chemical) if AF is greater than 24 to 48 hours in duration.
  - Transesophageal echocardiogram should be performed prior to cardioversion to exclude left atrial or left atrial appendage or thrombus in those who have not been adequately anticoagulated.
  - Cardioversion may be hazardous or unsuccessful in presence of digitalis toxicity, hypokalemia, and multifocal atrial tachycardia.
- Other nonpharmacologic options for the treatment of AF may be considered in selected patients who do not achieve adequate rate control or symptom relief with conventional measures. These involve consultation with cardiology and include:
  - Catheter-based atrial fibrillation ablation
  - AV node ablation and PPM placement

Pharmacologic

Pharmacologic strategies to control ventricular rate or maintain sinus rhythm should be tailored to the patient's clinical condition. The most common agents for rate control are:

- **Beta-adrenergic blocker:** Use with caution or avoid in patients with bradycardia or CHF.
- **Calcium channel blockers:** Use with caution or avoid in patients with bradycardia or CHF.
- **Digoxin:** Enhances vagal tone and is more effective at rest than with activity; adjust dose according to age and kidney function.
- **Anti-arrhythmic drugs:**
  - May be used in consultation with a cardiologist if there are no contraindications in terms of coronary artery disease and heart failure.
  - Amiodarone is the most effective agent available but carries a risk of long-term toxicities including lung, liver, ocular, and thyroid.

Thromboembolism prophylaxis

- In AF, the risk of thromboembolic complications such as stroke increases with advancing age and can be reduced with anticoagulant therapy.[6] Older adults with AF with no contraindications, and who are at risk of stroke, should be anticoagulated with warfarin to a target international normalized ratio of 2–3, or with a direct thrombin inhibitor such as dabigatran or rivaroxaban. (Note: Aspirin is also commonly used as an alternative anticoagulant.)
- In older adults, the benefits associated with anticoagulation to prevent thromboembolic complications are increased, but so are the risks.[7] Assessing the risk-to-benefit ratio of anticoagulant therapy requires consideration of the following issues:
  - Risk of stroke
  - Risk of bleeding (i.e., gastrointestinal, genitourinary, or intracranial)[7]
  - Use of concurrent medications that may increase bleeding risk (i.e., aspirin and nonsteroidal anti-inflammatory drugs) or that affect warfarin dose requirement (i.e., erythromycin and amiodarone— lower dose requirement)
  - Medical conditions that affect warfarin dose requirement (i.e., liver disease and CHF—lower dose)
  - Care support system, ability to follow up for regular monitoring and dose adjustment.
- The presence of cognitive impairment or disability is not an absolute contraindication to anticoagulation.

PART B: BRADYCARDIA

Case

Mr. B, a 76-year-old man with hypertension, presents to his geriatrician with progressive dyspnea on exertion, dizziness, and syncope. Electrocardiogram demonstrates sinus bradycardia at 35 beats per minute with first-degree AV block; ambulatory monitoring correlates the patient's symptoms with bradycardic episodes. Mr. B's quality of life and functional status are excellent. He is not taking any medications that cause bradycardia. After discussion with his physician, he decides to undergo permanent pacemaker implantation. Transtelephonic monitoring is arranged by his cardiologist in order to minimize office visits.

Definition

- *Bradycardia* is defined as a heart rate of less than 60 beats per minute. In the tachycardia-bradycardia syndrome, periods of tachycardia and bradycardia alternate; bradycardia may be particularly pronounced after conversion from AF to normal sinus rhythm.
- Conduction system abnormalities may occur at the level of the sinus node, the atrioventricular (AV) node, and/or His-Purkinje system.

Prevalence

Prevalence of bradycardia increases after the age of 65.

Likely Etiologies

- Medications that cause bradycardia include beta blockers and non-dihydropyridine calcium channels blockers such as diltiazem and veramapil.
- Medical conditions that cause bradycardia include Lyme disease and endocarditis.
- Age-related slowing of the conduction system is also a contributing factor.

Diagnosis

History

Signs of congestive heart failure or hypoperfusion include dizziness, dyspnea, altered mental status, hypotension, or kidney dysfunction.

Exam

- Slow pulse
- Cannon a-waves in the case of complete heart block
- Wide pulse pressure
- Soft S1 or beat-to-beat variation in intensity of S1

Tests

- Electrocardiogram: to assess baseline conduction properties
- Echocardiogram: to establish ventricular function

Expected Disease Course

- Bradycardia may be asymptomatic, or associated with symptoms including pre-syncope, syncope, dyspnea, confusion, hypotension, or heart failure.
- Untreated symptomatic bradycardia may lead to hypoperfusion, bradyarrhythmic arrest, and death.

Prognosis

- Isolated sinus bradycardia progresses slowly to complete heart block.
- Severe bradycardia may lead to congestive heart failure and asystole.

Treatment Options

Consider treatment options based on patient's goals for care and values, and take into consideration the impact of comorbidities. Reverse any medical etiologies and stop any contributing medications immediately.

Nonpharmacologic

- If symptomatic bradycardia persists, consult a cardiologist to evaluate for permanent pacemaker (PPM) placement.
- A PPM is indicated in selected patients who experience symptomatic bradycardia that does not have a reversible cause, or advanced conduction system disease (second degree type II AV block, associated bundle branch block, complete heart block).

Pharmacologic

- Use caution with any pharmacologic agent that lowers blood pressure (which may be elevated as a compensatory response to maintain cardiac output) in a symptomatic patient until the bradycardia has been evaluated.
- Intravenous atropine, dopamine, and percutaneous or transvenous pacing may be used as temporary measures in symptomatic patients.
- The tachycardia-bradycardia syndrome is often treated with drug therapy for

tachyarrhythmia and, if accompanied by symptomatic bradycardia, PPM placement.

PART C: VENTRICULAR ARRHYTHMIAS AND SUDDEN CARDIAC DEATH

Case

Ms. C is an 86-year-old woman with diabetes mellitus, hypertension, hyperlipidemia, chronic renal insufficiency, breast cancer, dementia, and osteoarthritis. She suffered from a myocardial infarction six months prior, and a recent echocardiogram demonstrated a left ventricular ejection fraction of 30%. She is home-bound due to dementia and joint pain.

Definition

Ventricular tachycardia (VT) is an arrhythmia originating in the ventricle. Non-sustained VT (NSVT) lasts more than three beats but less than 30 seconds. Sustained VT lasts more than 30 seconds or leads to hemodynamic instability.

Prevalence

Prevalence of VT is increased in patients with cardiomyopathy, a condition which becomes more prevalent with age.

Likely Etiologies

- Cardiomyopathy
- Idiopathic VT is more common in younger individuals.

Diagnosis

Exam

Hemodynamic instability may be present.

Tests

- Electrocardiogram is used to differentiate supraventricular from ventricular tachycardia.
- Echocardiogram evaluates for the presence of structural heart disease.

Expected Disease Course

Frequent or hemodynamically significant VT may lead to CHF, syncope, and death.

Prognosis

Sustained ventricular tachycardia and ventricular fibrillation are associated with high mortality due to underlying heart disease.

Treatment Options

Treatment options for VT should be based on patient's goals, values, and existing comorbidities.

Nonpharmacologic

- Implantable cardiac defibrillators (ICDs) are used in selected patients for prevention of sudden cardiac death if such therapy is appropriate in context of cognitive and physical function, comorbidities, and achievable goals for care.
- A discussion of medical prognosis and achievable goals of care should be part of the decision to recommend ICD therapy. Patient should also be informed of the option to deactivate shock therapy once an ICD is in place.
- Appropriate patients should be referred for an ICD evaluation if they have a significantly reduced ejection fraction (<35%) and congestive heart failure, or if they have experienced sustained VT or survived cardiac arrest.
- Contraindications to ICD therapy include NYHA class IV heart failure symptoms and a life expectancy of less than one year.

Pharmacologic

Pharmacologic therapies include beta blockers and anti-arrhythmic agents.

A discussion takes place between Ms. C's heath care proxy and her physician about the benefits (prevention of sudden arrhythmic death) and risk of an implantable ICD (related to the procedure as well as shocks thereafter). The decision is made not to place an implantable cardioverter-defibrillator, consistent with the patient's stated wishes.

Making Decisions about ICD Therapy

- Discussions regarding circumstances that might trigger a decision to disable an ICD should be initiated prior to implantation. The topic of disabling defibrillation therapy should be readdressed frequently during the course of the illness.
- As patient and family priority shifts from prolongation of life to maximizing comfort, the option to disable defibrillation therapy should be discussed with the goal of

avoiding repeated shocks during the final stage of a terminal illness.

- During advance directive discussions, the patient's preferences regarding ICD deactivation should always be explored and documented.
- When considering DNR status, the option to deactivate an ICD should be addressed as well. If a DNR order is issued based on the goals of care, the ICD would be turned off in conjunction with the DNR decision. If a decision is made to deactivate an ICD, the factors underlying this choice would also support a DNR order.
- The defibrillation function can be deactivated in a clinic, hospice, or at home.
- There is no clear palliative benefit to disabling pacing therapies, which also raises more complex ethical concerns than disabling defibrillation therapy. In general, consider pacing therapy as you would any medical treatment, and determine if it meets patient's goals of care and is in alignment with cultural/spiritual considerations.
- If patients are not candidates for ICD therapy and cannot tolerate pharmacological treatment, the symptoms related to CHF (e.g., shortness of breath and anxiety) should be aggressively addressed and managed. (See Chapter 41: Dyspnea, and Chapter 65: Anxiety.)

TAKE-HOME POINTS

- Atrial fibrillation (AF) and conduction system disease leading to symptomatic bradycardia commonly coexist in older adults.
- In AF, strategies to 1) maintain sinus rhythm or control ventricular rate and 2) prevent thromboembolic events should be tailored to the patient's clinical condition.
- A permanent pacemaker is indicated in selected patients who experience bradycardia associated with symptoms not attributable to medication, or signs of advanced conduction system disease (second degree type II AV block, associated bundle branch block, complete heart block).
- Patients should be referred to a cardiologist for ICD evaluation if they have experienced sustained VT, survived cardiac arrest,

or have a significantly reduced ejection fraction and congestive heart failure, and if a good quality of life and functional capacity are achievable.

- A discussion of medical prognosis and achievable goals of care should be part of the decision to recommend ICD therapy. Patient should also be informed of the option to deactivate shock therapy once an ICD is in place.
- As patient priority shifts from prolongation of life to maximizing comfort, the physician should offer the option of disabling defibrillation therapy.

REFERENCES

1. Rodriguez RD, Schocken DD. Update on sick sinus syndrome, a cardiac disorder of aging. *Geriatrics* 1990;*45*:26–30.
2. Feinberg WM, Blackshear JL, Laupacis A, Kronmal R, Hart RG. Prevalence, age distribution, and gender of patients with atrial fibrillation. Analysis and implications. *Arch Intern Med.* 1995;*155*:469–473. [PMID: 7864703]
3. Lakatta EG, Levy D. Arterial and cardiac aging: major shareholders in cardiovascular disease enterprises: Part II: the aging heart in health: links to heart disease. *Circulation.* Jan 21, 2003;*107*(2):346–354. [PMID: 12538439]
4. ACC/AHA/ESC 2006 Guidelines for the Management of Patients with Atrial Fibrillation: a report of the American College of Cardiology/American Heart Association Task Force on Practice Guidelines and the European Society of Cardiology Committee for Practice Guidelines (Writing Committee to Revise the 2001 Guidelines for the Management of Patients With Atrial Fibrillation): developed in collaboration with the European Heart Rhythm Association and the Heart Rhythm Society. Fuster V, Rydén LE, Cannom DS, et al. American College of Cardiology/American Heart Association Task Force on Practice Guidelines; European Society of Cardiology Committee for Practice Guidelines; European Heart Rhythm Association; Heart Rhythm Society. *Circulation.* Aug 15, 2006;*114*(7):e257–354.
5. ACC/AHA/HRS 2008 Guidelines for Device-Based Therapy of Cardiac Rhythm Abnormalities: a report of the American College of Cardiology/American Heart Association Task Force on Practice Guidelines (Writing Committee to Revise the ACC/AHA/NASPE 2002 Guideline Update for Implantation of Cardiac Pacemakers and Antiarrhythmia Devices) developed in collaboration with the American Association for Thoracic Surgery and Society of Thoracic Surgeons. Epstein AE, DiMarco JP, Ellenbogen KA, et al.

American College of Cardiology/American Heart Association Task Force on Practice Guidelines (Writing Committee to Revise the ACC/AHA/NASPE 2002 Guideline Update for Implantation of Cardiac Pacemakers and Antiarrhythmia Devices); American Association for Thoracic Surgery; Society of Thoracic Surgeons. *J Am Coll Cardiol*. May 27, 2008;*51*(21):e1–62. No abstract available. Erratum in: *J Am Coll Cardiol*. Apr 21, 2009;*53*(16):1473. *J Am Coll Cardiol*. Jan 6, 2009;*53*(1):147. [PMID: 18498951]

6. Singer DE, Albers GW, Dalen JE, et al. American College of Chest Physicians. Antithrombotic therapy in atrial fibrillation: American College of Chest Physicians Evidence-Based Clinical Practice Guidelines (8th Edition). *Chest*. Jun 2008;*133*(suppl 6):546S–592S. [PMID: 18574273]

7. Poli D, Antonucci E, Grifoni E, Abbate R, Gensini GF, Prisco D. Bleeding Risk During Oral Anticoagulation in Atrial Fibrillation Patients Older Than 80 Years. *J Am Coll Cardiol*. Sep 8, 2009;*54*(11):999–1002.

84

Valvular Heart Disease

CASE

Mrs. A is an independent, 86-year-old woman with no significant past medical history who presents to the office complaining of dyspnea when she walks two blocks. She denies any previous history of heart disease but has been told that she had a murmur. She denies palpitations, chest pain, dizziness, syncope, or cough. Examination is notable for a systolic murmur loudest at the right upper sternal border, radiating to the neck and across the precordium. The carotid pulse is delayed and diminished in amplitude. An echocardiogram shows a calcified aortic valve with a calculated valve area of 0.6 cm² and a gradient of 65 mmHg.

DEFINITION

Patients with **valvular heart disease** have a malfunction of one or more of the valves that regulate blood flow through the heart. More than one valve may be dysfunctional at the same time. Common valvular disorders in elderly adults include aortic stenosis, aortic regurgitation, mitral stenosis, mitral regurgitation, and tricuspid regurgitation.

- In elderly patients, valvular heart disease is often complicated by other cardiovascular problems, such as coronary disease, systolic or diastolic heart failure, hypertension, pulmonary hypertension, or arrhythmias.
- *Note on antibiotic prophylaxis:* Indicated only for patients with prosthetic heart valves, history of endocarditis, or certain congenital heart conditions.[1] Not routinely recommended for stenosis or regurgitation of a native heart valve without one of the complications noted above.

AORTIC STENOSIS[1,2]

Definition

Failure of the leaflets of the aortic valve to open, resulting in a pressure gradient between the left ventricle and the aorta during systole.

Prevalence

Estimated at about 3% of adults over 75 years.

Likely Etiologies

- Usually due to calcification of the valve
- May be a late presentation of rheumatic heart disease
- Congenital bicuspid aortic valves usually come to medical attention and require intervention before the age of 65.

Diagnosis

Exam

- Blowing crescendo-decrescendo systolic murmur loudest at the right upper sternal border, radiating to both carotid arteries.
- Murmur will peak later in systole as the severity of AS worsens.
- Second heart sound may be diminished or absent with worsening AS.
- Hemodynamically significant AS will produce a carotid pulsus parvus et tardus, a small amplitude, delayed pulse.

Tests

- Electrocardiogram may show signs of left ventricular hypertrophy.
- Echocardiogram confirms diagnosis and grade severity.
- Left and right heart catheterization is indicated if intervention (surgery or valvuloplasty) is being considered, or to exclude coronary disease as a contributor to symptoms.

Expected Disease Course

- Asymptomatic AS has a low incidence of sudden death but becomes symptomatic commensurate with the degree of stenosis.

TABLE 84.1: AORTIC STENOSIS PROGNOSIS[2]

	Valve Area (cm²)	Prognosis
Aortic stenosis	Mild > 1.5	Low risk of death within 5 years
	Moderate 1.0–1.5	Up to 40% progress to aortic valve surgery or death within 5 years
	Severe < 1.0	> 50% risk of death within 5 years if untreated once symptoms develop

- Symptoms of severe AS include syncope, angina, and clinical heart failure
- Time to 50% mortality if untreated: syncope (5 years); angina (3 years); clinical heart failure (2 years)
- Aortic stenosis with a valve area of 0.6 cm² or less has a poor prognosis even for asymptomatic patients (Table 84.1).

Treatment Options

- Cardiology consultation should be considered for any patient with symptomatic AS, or for asymptomatic patients with moderate or greater severity of stenosis.
- Discussion and selection of treatment options should be based on patient's goals, values, and prognosis associated with existing comorbidities.
- Surgical valve replacement is the treatment of choice for appropriate patients (Table 84.2).
- Pharmacological treatments focus on volume optimization with diuretics and control of blood pressure, usually with ACE inhibitors as first choice. Nitrates can be used with caution but may cause hypotension and syncope.

- For management of dyspnea, see Chapter 41: Dyspnea.

Mrs. A states that she would like to be as independent as possible. As hesitant as she is about surgery, she is willing to take the risk if she can improve her function and quality of life.

AORTIC REGURGITATION (AR)[1,2,3]

Definition

Aortic regurgitation, also called aortic insufficiency, failure of the leaflets of the aortic valve to close effectively, resulting in retrograde flow of blood from the aorta to the left ventricle during diastole.

Prevalence

For moderate AR or worse, about 2% in adults over 70.

Likely Etiologies

Causes include rheumatic heart disease, endocarditis, dilation of the aortic root. Acute AR can also be due to endocarditis or retrograde aortic dissection.

TABLE 84.2: SURGICAL OPTIONS

	Aortic Stenosis	Aortic Regurgitation
Surgical valve replacement	Treatment of choice (Even age >80 should be considered)	Treatment of choice (Even age >80 should be considered)
Percutaneous valve replacement	May be an alternative in the near future; in clinical trials in the United States, approved in Europe/Canada	May be an alternative in the near future; in clinical trials in the United States, approved in Europe/Canada
Balloon valvuloplasty (Reasonable efficacy and safety in experienced hands)	Can be offered to palliate AS symptoms in selected patients; lower risk than surgery but high rate of restenosis	

Diagnosis

Exam

- Diastolic decrescendo murmur usually heard best over the left sternal border.
- Associated with a wide pulse pressure, which can be associated with multiple clinical findings, including a bounding carotid pulse and abnormal amplification of blood pressure in the lower extremities (> 60 mmHg above arm pressure).

Tests

- Electrocardiogram, which may show signs of left ventricular hypertrophy
- Echocardiogram to confirm diagnosis and grade severity
- Left and right heart catheterization if surgery is being considered

Expected Disease Course

- Progressive dyspnea and clinical heart failure
- Asymptomatic patients with ejection fraction (EF) > 55%
- AR may be indolent for several years; symptoms become more prevalent with heart failure.
- Untreated symptomatic AR has an annual mortality of over 10%. Acute AR is poorly tolerated and if untreated is frequently fatal.

Treatment Options

- Consider treatment options based on patient's goals, values, and existing comorbidities.
- For surgical options, see Table 84.2.
- Pharmacologic treatments focus on volume optimization with diuretics and control of blood pressure, usually with vasodilators such as calcium channel blockers or nitrates.
- Beta blockers should be used with caution, as they may worsen hemodynamics by prolonging diastole.
- For management of progressive dyspnea, see Chapter 41: Dyspnea.

MITRAL STENOSIS (MS)[1,2]

Definition

Failure of the leaflets of the mitral valve to open, resulting in a pressure gradient between the left atrium and the left ventricle during systole and incomplete emptying of the left atrium.

Prevalence

- Occurs in fewer than 1% of geriatric patients
- Twice as common in females
- Has declined in Western countries due to antibiotic treatment of streptococcal infections in childhood and reduced incidence of rheumatic heart disease.

Likely Etiologies

- Usually due to rheumatic heart disease
- Severe annular calcification may contribute to functional mitral stenosis.

Diagnosis

Exam

Opening snap after S2 with a low-pitched rumbling diastolic murmur heard along the left axilla.

Tests

- Electrocardiogram may show signs of left atrial enlargement or atrial fibrillation
- Echocardiogram confirms diagnosis and grade severity (Table 84.3)
- Left and right heart catheterization if intervention (surgery or valvuloplasty) is being considered, or to exclude coronary disease as a contributor to symptoms

Prognosis[2]

	Valve Area	Prognosis
Mitral stenosis	Mild > 1.5	Asymptomatic, variable progression
	Moderate 1.0–1.5	Increased risk of dyspnea and atrial fibrillation
	Severe < 1.0	High risk of dyspnea and atrial fibrillation

Expected Disease Course

- Significant MS presents with progressive exertional dyspnea.
- Atrial fibrillation is common, may precede other symptoms, and carries a significant risk for stroke or thromboembolism in the absence of systemic anticoagulation.
- Stroke may be the presenting symptom.
- Pulmonary hypertension and right-sided heart failure signs are later manifestations of more severe MS and predictors of mortality.

TABLE 84.3: SURGICAL OPTIONS

	Mitral Stenosis	Mitral Regurgitation
Surgical valve replacement	Definitive treatment in MS patients when repair is not technically possible	Bioprosthetic replacement for MR if repair is not technically possible
Surgical valve repair	Definitive treatment in selected MS patients	Definitive treatment for symptomatic MR
Percutaneous valvuloplasty	Definitive treatment in those with favorable morphology; lower procedural risk than valve surgery*	

*Success and complication rates are less favorable in older adults.

Treatment Options

- Treatment should be based on patient's goals, values, and existing comorbidities. Cardiology consultation should be considered for any patient with symptomatic MS, or for asymptomatic patients with moderate or greater severity of stenosis.
- Surgical procedures are available for appropriate patients. (See Table 84.3.)
- Medical therapy is focused on anticoagulation if indicated for atrial fibrillation, history, or high-risk features for thromboembolism, and hemodynamic factors.
- Tachycardia is detrimental either in sinus rhythm or in atrial fibrillation, and beta blockers are thus usually the medication of first choice.
- Careful volume optimization to avoid pulmonary vascular congestion is important, but overdiuresis is also harmful.
- For management of dyspnea, see Chapter 41: Dyspnea.

MITRAL REGURGITATION (MR)[1,2]

Definition

Also called mitral insufficiency, failure of the leaflets of the mitral valve to close effectively, resulting in retrograde flow of blood from the left ventricle to the left atrium during diastole.

Prevalence

As high as 33% in elderly populations, though only a small subset will have severe regurgitation.

Likely Etiologies

- Progression of myxomatous degeneration and prolapse
- Mitral annular calcification
- Structural heart disease including ischemic and dilated cardiomyopathies
- Endocarditis
- Rheumatic heart disease.

Exam

Holosystolic murmur best heard at the apex. There may be enlargement of the left ventricle on palpation.

Tests

- Electrocardiogram, which may show signs of left atrial enlargement and/or left ventricular hypertrophy
- Echocardiogram to confirm diagnosis and grade severity
- Left and right heart catheterization if surgery is being considered, or to exclude coronary disease as a contributor to symptoms.

Expected Disease Course

- Once left ventricular dysfunction or exertional dyspnea are present, progression to refractory heart failure and death are increased, and the outcome of surgery is worse at this stage than in patients who undergo surgery before these features occur.
- For patients with severe MR without symptoms and with preserved left ventricular function, there is a variable and often indolent progression to symptoms of heart failure, most frequently exertional

dyspnea. This latent period may last for several years in some individuals.

Treatment Options
- Consider treatment options based on patient's goals, values, and existing comorbidities. Surgical options are shown in Table 84.3.
- For patients who are not surgical candidates, pharmacological treatments focus on volume optimization with diuretics and control of blood pressure, usually with ACE inhibitors and beta blockers, especially if systolic left ventricular dysfunction is present.
- For management of dyspnea, see Chapter 41: Dyspnea.

TRICUSPID REGURGITATION (TR)[1,2]

Definition
Also called tricuspid insufficiency, TR is a failure of the leaflets of the mitral valve to close effectively, resulting in retrograde flow of blood from the right ventricle to the right atrium during diastole.

Prevalence
Not well characterized.

Likely Etiologies
- Left ventricular systolic heart failure
- Pulmonary disease; endocarditis
- Right ventricular pacemaker or defibrillator wire in situ

Diagnosis
Exam
- Holosystolic murmur best heard at the apex or lower left sternal border. The murmur should increase in intensity with inhalation.
- V waves may be seen during systole at the jugular veins.
- Volume overload may produce jugular distension, lower extremity edema, and occasionally ascites.

Tests
- Electrocardiogram, which may show signs of right atrial enlargement or pulmonary disease
- Echocardiogram to confirm diagnosis and grade severity
- Left and right heart catheterization if surgery is being considered

Expected Disease Course
TR is frequently a consequence of left-sided heart disease or lung disease, and the underlying problem determines the disease course.

Treatment Options
- The treatment of choice is volume optimization with diuretics.
- TR by itself is rarely an indication for surgery, unless surgery is planned for another indication such as mitral valve or coronary artery disease.
- Management of underlying conditions such as heart failure or sleep apnea is important.

TAKE-HOME POINTS
- Severity of valve disease generally (but not always) correlates with symptoms.
- Severity of valve disease, in combination with symptoms, helps determine the natural history if untreated, as well as the potential benefit of intervention.
- Cardiology consultation should be considered for any patient with symptomatic valve disease, or for asymptomatic patients with moderate or greater severity of disease.
- The natural history of severe valvular heart disease is such that intervention should be considered even in the oldest patients.
- The benefits and burdens of intervention must be weighed in the context of patient and family goals for care, comorbidities and their associated prognoses, cognitive and functional status, and ability to comply with postoperative treatment regimen.

REFERENCES
1. Aronow WS. Heart disease and aging. *Med Clin North Am*. 2006;90:849–862.
2. Bonow RO, Carabello BA, Chatterjee K, et al. 2008 focused update incorporated into the ACC/AHA 2006 guidelines for the management of patients with valvular heart disease: a report of the American College of Cardiology/American Heart Association Task Force on Practice Guidelines (Writing Committee to Develop Guidelines for the Management of Patients with Valvular Heart Disease. *J Am Coll Cardiol*. 2008;52:e1–142.
3. Bekeredjian R, Grayburn PA. Valvular heart disease: Aortic regurgitation. *Circulation*. 2005;112:125–134.

85

Peripheral Arterial Disease

CASE

Mrs. R is a 76-year-old, cognitively intact female with diabetes, hypertension, and peripheral arterial disease complaining of a non-healing wound on her left first toe. She reports this started approximately two months ago after she accidentally stepped on a nail. She currently lives alone but finds it increasingly difficult to ambulate and perform her daily activities secondary to the pain.

DEFINITION

Peripheral arterial disease (PAD) is an increasingly prevalent condition affecting the elderly. The majority of PAD cases fall into the categories of atherosclerotic occlusive disease, aneurysmal disease, and vasculitic disorders. The focus of this chapter will be on arterial atherosclerotic occlusive disease. Common presentations of occlusive disease include intermittent claudication, rest pain, non-healing ulcers, and gangrene. However, most patients are asymptomatic.

PREVALENCE

The prevalence of PAD increases with age and is greater than 20% in those over age 75. Fewer than 1/3 of individuals with PAD are symptomatic.

LIKELY ETIOLOGIES

PAD is mainly atherosclerotic in the geriatric population. Atherosclerosis is caused by hypertension, dyslipidemia, diabetes, cigarette smoking, and high homocysteine.

- Strong association with coronary artery and cerebrovascular disease, given the similar risk factors; most patients with PAD will die from cardiac events or stroke.
- Other causes include atheroemboli and vasculitis, which will not be addressed in detail in this section. Treatment for atheroemboli disease usually involves thromboembolectomy and long-term anticoagulation. Vasculitis is treated

with steroids, immunosuppressants, and revascularization in severe cases.

CLASSIFICATION

PAD is categorized according to the Rutherford Classification system (Table 85.1).

On physical exam, Mrs. R has a 1 cm wound on the tip of her left first toe. It appears dry with no drainage or surrounding erythema. There is minimal tenderness at rest. No swelling is seen. Pedal pulses are not palpable. Only femoral pulses are palpable. Motor and sensation are intact distally. Capillary refill time is less than two seconds bilaterally.

DIAGNOSIS

History

Presenting signs and symptoms vary depending on Rutherford classification on presentation (Table 85.1).

- Intermittent claudication: Patients present with reproducible pain or muscle fatigue in specific muscle groups after walking a certain distance that will resolve with resting.
- Non-healing wounds: Patients present with distal wounds that do not close, or they have had a history of infection.
- Gangrene: Patients report ischemia that will usually start distally and can progress proximally. Dry gangrene has a mummified appearance. Wet gangrene is accompanied by a moist appearance and/or infection. Both forms may or may not be painful.

Exam

A focused vascular physical exam should always include:

- Visual examination of the skin for breaks and wounds (The presence of hair in a distal extremity is a sign of good perfusion.)

TABLE 85.1: RUTHERFORD CLASSIFICATION OF PAD[1]

Category	Signs and Symptoms	Intervention
0	Asymptomatic	No
1	Mild claudication	No
2	Moderate claudication	No
3	Severe claudication	Maybe
4	Ischemic rest pain	Yes
5	Mild tissue ulceration	Yes
6	Tissue loss/Gangrene	Yes

TABLE 85.2: ABI INDICES FOR INITIAL PAD EVALUATION AND PROGNOSIS[2]

Index	Assessment	5-Year Cumulative Survival Rate for Lower Extremity PAD Based on Resting ABI
> 1.30	Incompressible	
0.90–1.30	Normal	
0.70–0.89	Mild disease	91%
0.50–0.69	Moderate disease	71%
0.40–0.50		63%
< 0.39	Severe disease	

- Capillary refill
- Color and warmth of the extremities
- Thorough palpation of pulses throughout the extremities
- An assessment for bruits

Mrs. R has significant lower extremity PAD with Rutherford classification category 5. ABI/PVRs are obtained that show decreased waveforms bilaterally, left more than right. Distal indices are 0.8 on the right and 0.5 on the left. Vascular surgery consultation is discussed with the patient. She wants to proceed given her severe symptoms, which significantly compromise her daily activities, independence, and quality of life.

Tests
- Ankle brachial indices and pulses volume recordings (ABI/PVRs) should be obtained whenever the diagnosis of PAD is suspected. ABI/PVRs provide a physiologic assessment of the extremity's arterial supply (Table 85.2). These should include segmental pressures and waveforms at several levels. An ABI of less than 0.9 is consistent with underlying PAD. If the index is greater than 1.3 and/or incompressible as in calcified arteries of diabetic patients, the PVR waveforms can provide a qualitative assessment of the degree of occlusive disease.
- A secondary test such as a duplex ultrasound, angioplasty, or angiography is usually necessary if intervention is contemplated (Table 85.3).
- Duplex ultrasound is useful for a vascular specialist to identify specific areas of disease in preparation for an intervention. Routine use of this test is not useful for the primary physician.

- Computed tomography angioplasty (CTA) and magnetic resonance angiography (MRA) will be ordered by the vascular specialist when an intervention is under consideration. Both tests provide an anatomic assessment of the arterial disease. There are advantages and disadvantages to each, and the vascular specialist can decide on which to order based on his or her assessment. Distal small vessel imaging is currently suboptimal in both but will improve with evolving technology.
- Digital subtraction angiography is the gold standard for evaluating the arterial system. It is invasive, but an endovascular intervention can be performed in the same setting. There are risks involved, and it is contraindicated in those with renal insufficiency.

Mrs. R sees the vascular surgeon in consultation for her severe lower extremity PAD. CT angiography is obtained that shows bilateral multilevel arterial occlusive disease. Multiple mild and moderate stenoses are seen in the right femoral-popliteal and in the tibial arteries. Severe stenoses are in the left femoral-popliteal artery, and mild stenoses are in the left tibial vessels. The risks and benefits of the possible interventions are discussed with Mrs. R and her family, including the fact that the underlying vascular disease cannot be cured.

EXPECTED DISEASE COURSE
The life expectancy for a patient with PAD is 50% in 10 years, which is significantly lower than for control patients. The goal of treatment in a patient with PAD is dependent on the presenting issues. Some examples of specific goals include

TABLE 85.3: AVAILABLE TESTS FOR PAD

Test	Advantages	Disadvantages
ABI/PVRs	Done in office Not invasive Low cost	Arteries not imaged
Arterial duplex	Done in office Not invasive Low cost	Time consuming Technician dependent
CTA	Good imaging Not invasive	High cost Contraindicated in renal insufficiency Radiation
MRA	Good imaging Not invasive	High cost Contraindicated in renal insufficiency if intravenous contrast used
Conventional angiography	Best imaging and intervention possible at same time Good imaging of distal vessels	Very high cost Contraindicated in renal insufficiency Invasive

maximizing walking distance in claudication, alleviating symptoms in rest pain; promoting wound healing in ulcers; and "limb" salvage in gangrene.

- Patients with severe claudication should be considered for revascularization if symptoms significantly affect their lifestyle, if they are good surgical candidates, and if they are likely to benefit significantly from the intervention. All patients with severe disease in categories 4–6 should be offered surgical intervention if their cognitive and medical comorbidities, prognosis, and goals for care do not preclude surgery.
- Endovascular and open vascular surgeries are both limb-sparing attempts to treat PAD. If these interventions are not possible secondary to medical or surgical reasons, alternative goals of care should be discussed. While amputation is an alternative option for severe infections or gangrene that could result in sepsis and death, it does require patients to accept the fact that they will be losing part of their bodies. Amputation of a limb may be as devastating, or even more devastating, as death itself to some. Thus it is important for clinicians to have goals of care discussions with patients and families prior to surgical interventions, to make sure that all concerned understand the risk and extent of expected benefits, as well as the potential quality of life impact associated with the intervention.

- In general, patients in Grade 4–6 who are not candidates for revascularization may face a decision about life-saving amputation within several months. The extent of gangrene will often determine how long before sepsis and death will occur without the amputation.
- Survival for patients with critical limb ischemia is poor, and much of their care will be palliative in nature. Mortality reaches 70% at 5 years and 85% at 10 years. Multiple risk factors increase the long-term mortality, including advanced age, continued tobacco use, diabetes, and renal failure on dialysis.[1]
- For patients with gangrene who decide not to undergo amputation, treatment should focus on pain relief, management of non-pain symptoms such as fever and wound odor, and wound care. (See Chapter 29: Management of Pain in Older Adults, Chapter 32: Sweating and Fever, and Chapter 61: Malodorous Wounds.)

TREATMENT OPTIONS[3,4]

Nonpharmacologic

Management of risk factors is essential to prevent further progression of disease. Management strategies include:

- Control of hypertension, diabetes, and lipids
- Smoking cessation

- Weight loss in obese patients
- Foot care
- Supervised exercise regimen for those with intermittent claudication to increase patient's pain-free walking distance.

Pharmacologic

Few drugs have been shown to have a benefit in patients with PAD. Of those, the benefits are small or not well studied. Cilostazol (phosphodiesterase inhibitor) offers a small benefit in those with intermittent claudication by increasing pain-free walking distances, but it is contraindicated in congestive heart failure.

- While antiplatelet therapy (such as aspirin, clopidogrel, etc.) is usually initiated to help with pain, increase walking distances, and prevent cardiovascular death, more studies are needed to determine benefits such as preventing progression of atherosclerotic disease.
- For those patients who are not candidates for intervention, or who have decided against intervention, ischemic pain should be aggressively treated. (See Chapter 29: Management of Pain in Older Adults.)

Mrs. R agrees to undergo a percutaneous intervention to revascularize her left leg. A left leg angiogram confirms the findings on CT. The femoral artery is treated via balloon angioplasty and a stent

is placed. She is started on clopidogrel 75 mg daily. She tolerates the procedure well and is discharged with home nursing and physical therapy.

SURGICAL OPTIONS

Surgical interventions are available for patients with severe disease (Table 85.4). The risks and benefits of revascularization or amputation should be weighed against a patient's cognitive and functional status, life expectancy, ability to understand what can and cannot be accomplished with surgery, and goals for care.

- **Endovascular interventions (limb sparing):** There has been an increase in the use of percutaneous techniques for revascularization of the ischemic extremity. Balloon angioplasty, stenting, cryoplasty, mechanical atherectomy, and laser atherectomy are now available. Patency rates for these methods are not as good as open surgical interventions, but the risks are lower. More long-term studies are needed to determine the long-term patency rates of these modalities.
- **Open surgical revascularization (limb sparing):** Remains the gold standard for treatment in most cases. Arterial bypass can be done using autogenous or synthetic conduit. Endarterectomy can also be utilized, depending on the nature of the occlusive disease.

TABLE 85.4: INTERVENTIONS FOR PAD

Intervention	Advantages	Disadvantages
Endovascular: angioplasty, stenting, atherectomy	Lower risk Shorter hospital stay Local anesthesia Percutaneous access	Lower long-term patency rates Need for repeat interventions in future
Surgical: bypass, endarterectomy	Higher long-term patency rates	Higher risk Longer hospital stay General or regional anesthesia Infection Pain Rehabilitation
Surgical: amputation	Definitive treatment Alleviates ischemic pain Removes infected/gangrenous tissue	Limb loss Operative risks including infection, bleeding, respiratory and cardiac issues Phantom limb pain Rehabilitation Altered function, independence, and quality of life

- **Amputation:** While amputation is the only definitive treatment for removal of infected and gangrenous tissue to prevent mortality, this intervention has the most significant adverse impact on patients' quality of life. Older adults with amputations typically do not qualify for prosthesis because of comorbidities. This will alter their lifestyle and increase dependency and care needs. Conversations with the patient and caregivers regarding treatment goals, prognosis, and the realities of post-amputation care should therefore take place before amputation occurs.

Mrs. R's pain has improved, and she can now perform her daily activities better. Her toe wound appears to be healing and is getting smaller. She will follow up with the vascular surgeon for vascular monitoring and wound care.

TAKE-HOME POINTS

- Treatment decisions should not be based solely on age or disease classification, but should occur in the context of achievable patient-determined goals for care, cognitive and functional status, and prognosis.
- A careful, comprehensive assessment of a patient's overall medical condition, functional status, mental status, surgical risk, and life expectancy, as well as quality of life, is essential to developing a treatment plan that is consistent with the patient's goals of care.
- While an endovascular treatment approach should be considered to improve arterial inflow, alleviate ischemic pain, and promote wound healing, amputation may be the only definitive treatment available to minimize mortality.

REFERENCES

1. Rutherford RB, ed. *Vascular Surgery*, 6th edition. Philadelphia: WB Saunders, 2005.
2. Sikkink CJ, van Asten WN, van't Hof MA, et al. Decreased ankle/brachial indices in relation to morbidity and mortality in patients with peripheral arterial disease. *Vasc Med.* 1997;2:169–173.
3. Hirsch AT et al. ACC/AHA 2005 practice guidelines for the management of patients with peripheral arterial disease. *Circulation.* Mar 21, 2006;*113*(11): e463–e654.
4. Scottish Intercollegiate Guidelines Network. Diagnosis and management of peripheral arterial disease. *A national clinical guideline.* Oct 2006;*89*: 1–24.

86

Hip Fracture Management

CASE
Mrs. S is a 90-year-old woman with hypertension, osteoporosis, advanced Alzheimer's disease, and recurrent aspiration pneumonia. She resides in a long-term care facility and has been wheelchair-bound for three years due to debility and cognitive decline. She is fully dependent in activities of daily living. She presents to the emergency room after an observed fall while trying to get up from her wheelchair unassisted. On physical exam, her right leg appears shortened and externally rotated, and she appears to be in pain.

DEFINITION
Hip fracture most commonly refers to any fracture in the femur bone at the head, neck, or trochanteric regions of the femur.

INCIDENCE
- Approximately 250,000 hip fractures occur annually in the United States. This number is expected to grow to 650,000 by 2040. Ninety percent hip fractures result from a fall.
- The average age of a patient with hip fracture is 82. The incidence of fracture increases exponentially with advancing age. Women are two to three times more likely than men to fracture a hip.

CLASSIFICATION
- **Femoral head fracture:**
  - Usually occurs with dislocations of the hip
  - May be caused by impaction or shearing injuries
  - High risk for nonunion and avascular necrosis (AVN) of the femoral head
- **Femoral neck fracture:**
  - Also known as "subcapital" or "intracapsular"
  - Common in elderly population

- Located within the capsule of the hip joint; occurs between the femoral head and trochanters
- Blood supply to femoral head runs along femoral neck; blood supply may be disrupted in femoral neck fracture leading to AVN of femoral head and increased incidence of non-union of fracture fragments.
- **Intertrochanteric fracture:**
  - Common in elderly population
  - Intertrochanteric fractures are lateral to the femoral neck; occur in a line between greater and lesser trochanter
  - Extracapsular
  - Range in severity from non-displaced to highly comminuted
- **Lesser trochanteric fracture**: Rare avulsion fracture at insertion site of iliopsoas muscle
- **Greater trochanteric fracture:**
  - Rare on its own; may be a component of intertrochanteric fracture
  - May be caused by direct injury or avulsion force of gluteus muscles.

RISK FACTORS
- Female sex; Caucasian
- Osteoporosis; low body weight; visual impairment; physical inactivity
- History of falls; gait disorder
- Previous fracture; maternal history of hip fracture
- Nursing home residence
- Psychotropic medication; alcohol use
- Cognitive impairment

Diagnosis
Exam
- Pain in affected leg
- Shortening of leg
- External rotation of leg
- Inability to bear weight on affected leg

Note: In non-displaced or impacted fractures, pain may be elicited only in extremes of range of motion but may not be elicited with weight-bearing.

Tests

See Table 86.1 for imaging studies that are used to detect hip fracture.[1]

EXPECTED DISEASE COURSE

- After hip fracture up to 50% of previously mobile patients may be dependent on assistive devices for ambulation for up to one year. Most patients will require rehabilitation in an acute care setting, subacute rehabilitation, or at-home physical therapy.
- Up to 25% of previously community-dwelling older adults who sustain a hip fracture will remain in a health care or long-term care facility for one year after fracture.
- While surgery improves likelihood of ambulation, it does not lead to better pain control.
- Mortality at six months after fracture is over 50% in patients with end-stage dementia.[2]

Mrs. S's initial AP pelvis radiograph demonstrates a right-sided, comminuted fracture of the femoral neck. Orthopedic consultation offers surgery with probable hemiarthroplasty, followed by an inpatient stay and then transfer to a rehabilitation facility. Mrs. S appears to be in pain and begins pulling out the IV and Foley catheter that have been placed. Her daughter, who has been approached for consent for surgery, asks if there are non-surgical options. She remembers that her mother had expressed in the past that if her dementia progressed she would not want to undergo major procedures.

TREATMENT OPTIONS

- There are very few well-conducted randomized trials that compare conservative and operative treatment of hip fracture in older patients. One small study found no difference in medical complications, mortality, and long term pain.[3] However, operative intervention did result in healing without leg shortening, a shorter hospital stay, and a statistically non-significant increase in ability of patients to return to their original residence.[3]
- Definite conclusions about treatment options cannot be made from limited information available. Making the surgical vs. non-surgical management decision requires a conversation about achievable goals of care between the patient, the family, and physician.

Non-Surgical Management

- Given the risks and benefits of surgery, non-surgical options should be explored in the following patient populations:
  - Non-ambulatory patients
  - Patients with end-stage dementia
  - Patients with decreased life expectancy from other diseases
  - Patients at high surgical risk
- For those patients who decline surgical intervention after considering benefits and burdens, medical management may include:
  - Careful positioning measures to promote healing and prevent further dislocation
  - Pain management
  - Protected weight-bearing when tolerated, using assistive devices
- Prophylaxis against complications caused by the fracture (DVT, pressure ulcers)

TABLE 86.1: RADIOGRAPHIC DETECTION OF HIP FRACTURE

Imaging	Comment
X-ray	AP pelvis view AP and lateral ("frog legged") views of affected hip (Stress fracture and valgus impaction may not be seen on X-ray)
MRI	Use if X-ray is equivocal and there is high clinical suspicion of fracture May show bone bruising, edema, other signs of acute fracture
Technetium-99m Bone Scan	Consider if X-ray is equivocal Less sensitive than MRI, as it may look normal in the first 72 hours of fracture After 72 hours, sensitivity is 90%

TABLE 86.2: NON-SURGICAL MANAGEMENT OF HIP FRACTURE

Complications of Fracture	Preventive Measures	Additional Management Information
Pain	Adequately assess and treat pain	See Chapter 29: Management of Pain in Older Adults
DVT	Prophylaxis in both surgical and non-surgical patients	
Delirium	Treat underlying causes	See Chapter 34: Delirium
Deconditioning	PT/OT; early mobilization	
Pressure ulcers	Frequent turning, avoid immobilization	See Chapter 59: Pressure Ulcers

should also be carefully considered (Table 86.2).

Surgical Intervention

- Although the evidence is limited on the question of conservative versus operative intervention for older patients, variation in practice has declined and most hip fracture patients currently do elect to undergo one of the following surgical interventions:[3]
  - Hemiarthroplasty: May be performed for displaced femoral neck fractures with disrupted blood supply and risk of nonunion or avascular necrosis.
  - Open reduction and internal fixation (ORIF) with screw: May be performed in intertrochanteric fractures, which are less likely to be associated with disruption of blood supply and its complications, or in non-displaced or minimally displaced femoral neck fractures.
  - Total hip replacement: For joints severely damaged by prior disease (i.e., osteoarthritis), total hip replacement may be indicated when hemiarthroplasty might be otherwise performed.
- Complications of surgery:
  - Dislocation (the most common complication may occur in up to 5% of patients).
  - Other complications include: nonunion, malunion, avascular necrosis of femoral head, secondary degenerative joint disease, and infection.

TAKE-HOME POINTS

- Prevalence of hip fracture increases with age.
- Clinical judgment should guide diagnostic workup; X-ray may not be sufficient.
- Definitive studies comparing conservative medical management and operative treatment of hip fracture in older patients are not available. However, most hip fracture patients do currently receive operative treatment.
- Making the surgical vs. non-surgical management decision requires a conversation between the patient, the family, and physician about prognosis and achievable goals of care.
- Careful attention should be paid to minimizing complications of fracture in both surgical and non-surgical patients.

REFERENCES

1. Manaster BJ, May DA, Disler DG. *Musculoskeletal Imaging*. Third edition. Philadelphia: Mosby Elsevier; 2007.
2. Morrison RS, Siu AL. Survival in end-stage dementia following acute illness. *JAMA*. July 5, 2000;*284*(1):47–52.
3. Handoll HHG, Parker MJ. Non-surgical options. Conservative versus operative treatment for hip fractures in adults (Review). *The Cochrane Collaboration*. 2009;1–20.

87

Osteoarthritis

CASE
Ms. D is an 85-year-old female with a history of coronary artery disease, diverticulosis, macular degeneration, and mild cognitive impairment. She comes to her clinic visit with the complaint of aches in her hands and knees, especially in the morning. She says that it is affecting her daily activities, especially her knitting and gardening. It is also making it difficult to tie her shoes and button her clothes. She says her mother had a lot of pain in her hands and legs later in life as well.

DEFINITION
Osteoarthritis (OA) is not just normal wear and tear, and it is not merely part of aging. It is a complex common pathway of multiple factors, including joint integrity, genetic predisposition, local inflammation, and chemical and biochemical processes. It occurs when the equilibrium between the breakdown and repair of joint tissues is overwhelmed.

OA can be categorized into two categories: idiopathic or secondary.

- Idiopathic OA can be localized or generalized (three or more joints); often affects the hands, hips, and knees, and less commonly the shoulders, elbows, wrists, ankles, and sacroiliac joints.
- Secondary OA often occurs with specific conditions that can predispose to OA, such as trauma, congenital/developmental disorders, diabetes mellitus, acromegaly, Paget's disease, or a history of septic arthritis; presents more atypically and potentially more acutely than idiopathic arthritis.

PREVALENCE
- It's estimated that one in three Americans experience significant symptoms from OA. Prevalence of OA increases with age.[1]
- Radiologic findings often do not correlate with clinical symptoms. Two studies found the prevalence of symptomatic knee OA to be only 29% and radiologically defined disease to be 43%.[2,3]
- OA is the most common cause of disability in the elderly. At a younger age, it is equally common in men or women, but it becomes more prevalent in women after the age of 50.
- The number of people affected with symptomatic OA is likely to increase due to the aging of the population and the obesity epidemic.

LIKELY ETIOLOGIES
- There is no single cause of OA. The interplay of multiple risk factors, mechanical stress, and biochemical processes likely all contribute to the formation of OA, particularly in weight-bearing joints.
- Systemic and local factors that play a significant role include old age, female gender, obesity, knee injury, repetitive use of joints, bone density, muscle weakness, and joint laxity.[4]

Physical Activity as a Risk Factor
Patients may ask, "How much is too much exercise?" They also may wonder what recreational sports put them at higher risk for developing osteoarthritis. Patients may be advised as follows[5]:

- Normal joints are at increased risk of OA without adequate exercise.
- Normal joints are not at risk with low-impact, repetitive recreational exercise (such as cycling). Normal joints are at risk with high-impact, repetitive exercise (such as running).
- Abnormal joints are at risk with low-impact, repetitive recreational exercise.

Ms. D worked in a textile factory for about 12 years. She thinks the repetitive movements led to pain in her hands.

DIAGNOSIS

Diagnosis is based on a combination of history, exam findings, and radiographic evidence.

History

- An achy, somewhat localized pain when the affected joint is being used
- Morning stiffness for less than 30 minutes (moving around helps it feel better)
- Gelling phenomenon: joints can become stiffer after a period of inactivity and improve with movement
- Older patients will likely have more joints involved.
- Increased pain/inflammation with changes in the weather (although there is no strong evidence for this observation)
- Swelling of the joints is often hard and bony, as opposed to soft and warm as seen in rheumatoid arthritis (RA).

Exam

General signs and symptoms:

- Palpation of involved joint reveals tenderness, often without signs of inflammation.
- Crepitus
- Osteophytes may be palpable (bony enlargements at the periphery of the joint).
- Joint effusions may be present.

Upper extremities:

- Most common joints affected (in order of frequency) are proximal interphalangeal (PIP), the first carpometacarpal joint, and, rarely, metacarpophalangeal (MCP) joints.
- Heberden's nodes are usually at the dorsomedial and dorsolateral aspects of the distal interphalangeal joints (DIP). This condition is 10 times more common in elderly women than men; often familial.
- Bouchard's nodes found at the PIPs.
- Carpometacarpal joints, when involved, often hurt and give the hands a squared-off appearance.

Knees:

- Patient may complain that the knee feels like it will "give out." (On exam, the ligaments are often fine; the sense of instability is most likely caused by weakness and pain.)
- Patient may have pain in the opposite, normal knee because it has to compensate.
- Elderly patients with dementia may not complain of pain but may present with gait problems or falls. Sometimes the leg on the unaffected side is swung quickly to avoid more time on the opposite affected knee.
- Findings on physical exam may underestimate the degree of involvement.
- Osteophytes, effusions, crepitus are common.
- Limited range of motion is seen in exacerbations of pain and with advanced disease.
- Malalignment can be seen in advanced cases, with varus (bow-legged) appearance more common than valgus because medial cartilage is more commonly affected.
- Baker's cysts are common (fluctuant swelling in the popliteal fossa) because effusions will follow the path of least resistance, which is posterior in the knee.
- Compartments in order of likely involvement are the medial, the patellofemoral, and the lateral (usually in one compartment).
- Effusions can be appreciated by milking fluid from the medial compartment and feeling it flow back when palpating the lateral compartment, and by balloting the patella. (With the patient lying down, press the patella downward and quickly release it. If the patella visibly rebounds, excess fluid in the knee is present.)

Hips:

- Pain is often vague and harder to locate.
- Pain should be more prominent in the groin, but can radiate to the buttock or along the obturator nerve of the knee (which can be confusing in diagnosis).
- Patients often confuse trochanteric bursitis with hip arthritis (bursitis will have palpable pain on the lateral thigh and will not limit range of motion).
- Consider L2-L3 problems, which can refer pain to the groin, or L5-S1, which can refer pain to the buttocks.
- Early in disease process there is loss of internal rotation and abduction on exam.
- Thomas test: Push the uninvolved knee to the chest of the patient while supine to flatten lumbar lordosis. If the involved leg lifts off the table, there is a flexion

contracture (permanent flexion of hip is a sign of severe hip OA).

- Gait may be characterized by patient leaning over toward the involved weight-bearing hip. This is due to less hip extension of involved hip (attempting to minimize pain) during gait, which leads to earlier heel planting of affected hip with more weight-bearing.

Spinal involvement:

- Most common at levels C5, T8, and L3 (the most flexible areas of the spine).
- Osteophytes from the margins of the vertebral body can narrow the spinal canal. This can lead to spinal stenosis and even cord compression. Spinal stenosis can present like claudication (worse with walking, resolution with rest).
- If stenosis is present, flexion helps, and extension can worsen symptoms.
- Severe stenosis may cause sensory and motor deficits, but usually does not. Can (rarely) lead to bowel and bladder problems.
- Spondylolisthesis (slipping of one vertebral body anteriorly on another) can occur in severe OA, often at L4-L5 or C5.

Tests

- Joint aspiration should be attempted if patient presents with severe, acute joint pain with an effusion. The synovial WBC count should be less than 2000/mm^3. If there are more than 2000 WBC/mm present, other processes, such as a septic arthritis, should be considered.
- There are very few other labs indicated, and they are most helpful only when atypical joints are involved. Be aware of potential for false positives when ordering the following labs:
  - ESR (erythrocyte sedimentation rate): Any inflammatory process can increase the ESR. Remember that the normal value is less than age/2 in men and (age + 10)/2 in women. ESR should be much higher in RA than in OA.
  - The rheumatoid factor (RF) can be helpful in distinguishing OA from RA. In RA the RF titer is usually greater than 1:40. The RF can also be elevated simply from old age.

Imaging

- X-ray is the most important imaging option for evaluation of OA and is most useful for confirming diagnosis, assessing progression, and deciding on when to perform surgical correction. Radiographic evidence of pathology in joints atypical of OA may help point to a different diagnosis. Importantly, X-ray findings often do not correlate with symptoms.
- Classic X-ray findings include:
  - Osteophytes in OA are larger than small age-related marginal osteophytes.
  - Joint space narrowing: Bone on bone often means that severe OA is present.
  - Subchondral cysts from synovial fluid entering small microfractures under pressure
  - Subchondral sclerosis or subchondral bone formation occurs as cartilage loss increases and appears as an area of increased density on the radiograph.

EXPECTED DISEASE COURSE

- OA may initially seem like a minor nuisance to patients and their caregivers, but as the population ages, OA has becomes the leading cause of disability in the United States. A 2005 meta-analysis found that arthritis was the most common cause of disability, followed by back or spine problems.[6]
- OA is also the most common cause of total hip and total knee replacement.[7]
- Factors associated with disability in OA patients include pain, depression, muscle weakness, and poor aerobic capacity.[2]

MANAGEMENT GOALS

- Once OA is diagnosed, educating patient and caregivers about achievable goals of care, stabilization, and treatment options is imperative.
- Management goals include:
  - Minimize pain and swelling
  - Minimize disability
  - Educate the patient about his or her role in minimizing symptoms
  - Maintain, and try to improve, quality of life

Ms. D remembers that her mother had trouble getting out of her apartment due to arthritis. She worries that she have will the same trouble staying active, getting out to visit with her friends and family, and keeping up with the social activities that are such an important part of her life.

Treatment Options

Nonpharmacologic

- Weight reduction decreases stress on joints.
- Physical therapy: Pain results in less joint use, which leads to weakness and increased pain. Strengthening the muscles around the affected joint improves joint mechanics, which reduces pain.
- Low-impact exercise improves proprioception and joint stability, helping with minor adjustments throughout the day needed to prevent injury. Stretching and flexibility exercises (such as yoga) increase range of motion, improve reaction time, and prevent falls and injury.[8]
- Bandaging and neoprene sleeves provide some support, but also improve proprioception by allowing stimulation of superficial nerves.
- Assist devices such as canes, walkers, and wheelchairs should be utilized when indicated. Canes should be held on the opposite side of the most affected leg, at a height holding arm flexion at 30 degrees, and should be moved with the affected leg.
- Elevated toilet seats and chairs can improve functionality and reduce falls at home.
- Insoles/orthotics can improve gait by decreasing the stress on the medial compartment, and should be fitted properly by a podiatrist.
- Occupational therapy can provide tips/strategies for helping with activities of daily life; other treatments include thermal therapy (paraffin wax and water), ultrasound therapy, and transcutaneous nerve stimulation (TENS).
- Psychosocial support and education: A telephone-based study found that monthly phone calls for one year focusing on education about OA, goals related to OA symptoms and management, and action plans to achieve those goals significantly reduced pain from OA compared to levels of pain experienced by patients who did not have monthly discussions about goals and action plans.[9]

Pharmacologic

- The American College of Rheumatology suggests a stepwise pharmacologic approach for OA (Tables 87.1 and 87.2).
- Managing severe pain: If pain becomes intolerable or function is negatively affected, the pharmacological choices in Tables 87.1 and 87.2 continue to be a part of treatment, but evaluation by an orthopedic surgeon is warranted.

Surgical Options

- Indications for surgery depend on the patient's long-term goals, the joint affected, the quality and severity of pain, and the mechanism of the arthritis.
- Surgical techniques include:
  - Total joint replacement
  - Debridement of the joint with arthroscopy
  - Joint fusion
  - Realignment osteotomy: redirection of the load bearing to a less affected part of the joint

SYMPTOM MANAGEMENT TO IMPROVE QUALITY OF LIFE

If surgery is not an option for OA patients with severe pain (either because of patient comorbidities or patient preference), clinicians should focus on symptom management, including modifications in the home and assistive devices to minimize disabilities and improve quality of life (Table 87.3).

TAKE-HOME POINTS

- OA patients and their caregivers should be educated about achievable goals of care, stabilization, and treatment options.
- OA patients should be encouraged to exercise; older adults can still exercise despite comorbidities.
- Nonpharmacological treatment is effective; assistive devices should be utilized to minimize disabilities and improve quality of life.
- NSAIDs should be used with caution in the elderly; opioids (properly managed) are safer than NSAIDs in this age group.
- Indications for surgery depend on the patient's long-term goals, the joint affected, the quality and severity of pain, and the mechanism of the arthritis.

TABLE 87.1: PHARMACOLOGIC TREATMENT OF MILD PAIN: ACETAMINOPHEN IS THE FIRST LINE TREATMENT

Class of Medication	Examples	Properties
Acetaminophen		Lacks anti-inflammatory properties, but not as effective as NSAIDs for hip and knee pain Can increase the half life of warfarin Dosing considerations: No liver conditions—up to 4 grams per day Older adults—up to 3 grams per day Liver failure—no more than 2 grams per day
Oral NSAIDs are potentially acceptable alternative in selected patients[a]	Ibuprofen, Salicylates Diclofenac, Etodolac COX-2 inhibitors[b]	NSAIDs have added anti-inflammatory properties, but overall effect on mild pain is similar to acetaminophen Contraindicated in patients with: Diabetes, renal insufficiency, diuretic therapy because of markedly increased risk of NSAID-associated renal failure due to intrarenal prostaglandin inhibition Anticoagulation therapy (increases bleeding risk) Concomitant steroid therapy or history of GI bleeding (increased risk of GI toxicity) High risk for heart disease, due to increased risk of congestive heart failure Dosing considerations: Low-dose ibuprofen (less than 1600 mg/day) may have fewer GI side effects (bleeding, perforation) Salsalate and Sulindac may have less renal toxicity GI risks increase with age. Kidney function should be monitored within a week of initiation of therapy and regularly thereafter; suspect damage to the kidney if there is a rise in blood pressure
Topical agents	NSAIDs Diclofenac gel (1%) Diclofenac epolamine analgesic patch (1.3%)	FDA approved for use in OA, in a 1% strength formulation Systemic levels may be achieved with risks and toxicities as above
	Capsaicin cream	Helpful in trials, but 40% of patients experience burning and erythema at application site Do not use in patients who cannot follow proper directions, as contact with mucosal membrane after medication application can cause severe burning
	Lidocaine patches	Can be helpful when applied to a painful site Insurance often does not cover use in OA

[a] The multiple possible effects of NSAIDs on renal function, cardiac function, and potential GI side effects make it very difficult to use this class of drugs for pain relief in the geriatric population. NSAIDs should be used with caution and only in carefully selected patients.[10]
[b] COX-2 inhibitors have not been shown to be more effective than NSAIDs with concomitant use of a proton pump inhibitor; therefore, the same precautions apply to COX-2 inhibitors as NSAIDs.[11]

TABLE 87.2: PHARMACOLOGIC TREATMENT OF MODERATE PAIN; CONSIDER OPIOIDS IN ADDITION TO AGENTS USED FOR MILD PAIN

Class of Medication	Examples	Properties
Opioids	Morphine Oxycodone Hydromorphone Fentanyl patch	Use with caution in the elderly—start low, go slow (See guidelines for opioid use in Chapter 29: Managing of Pain in Older Adults) Dosing considerations: Intermittent pain: As needed use with short-acting medications Constant pain: Switch over to long-acting medications once properly titrated See pain management section for renal and hepatic considerations and management/prevention of side effects
Corticosteroid injections		May be helpful but not FDA-approved for hip OA General rule for administration is 1 injection every 3 months, with no more than 3 injections per joint per year
Systemic corticosteroids		Not usually recommended for OA, but low doses of prednisone, about 5 mg daily, can be helpful for severe exacerbations of pain

TABLE 87.3: MANAGEMENT OF OSTEOARTHRITIS SYMPTOMS

Symptom or Disability	Management Recommendations
Hand/wrist pain	Automated utensils, Velcro shoes, attention to ergonomics for repetitive movements
Knee/hip pain	Low-impact exercise, avoid prolonged sitting and low chairs
Low back pain	Proper lifting, avoid sudden movements, limit weight lifted
Neck/upper back pain	Good posture, ergonomics with sitting, regular eye exams
Shoulder pain	Posture, hands-free phone, avoid overloaded luggage, pocketbooks, and bags

REFERENCES

1. Centers for Disease Control and Prevention (CDC). Prevalence of self-reported arthritis or chronic joint symptoms among adults—United States, 2001. *MMWR Morb Mortal Wkly Rep.* 2002;*51*(42):948–950.
2. Felson DT. The epidemiology of knee osteoarthritis: results from the Framingham study. *Semin Arthritis Rheum.* 1990;*20*:42–50.
3. Davis MA, Ettinger WH, Neuhaus JM. Obesity and osteoarthritis of the knee: evidence from the National Health and Nutrition Examination Survey (NHANES I). *Semin Arthritis Rheum.* 1990;*20*:42–50.
4. Zhang Y, Jordan JM. Epidemiology of osteoarthritis. *Clin Geriatr Med.* Aug 2010;*26*(3):355–369.
5. Lane NE. Exercise: a cause of osteoarthritis. *J Rheumatol Suppl.* 1995;*43*:3–6.
6. Centers for Disease Control and Prevention (CDC). Prevalence of disabilities and associated health conditions among adults—United States, 1999. *MMWR Morb Mortal Wkly Rep.* 2001;*50*(7):120–125.
7. Guccione AA, Felson DT, Anderson JJ, et al. The effects of specific medical conditions on the functional limitations of elders in the Framingham study. *Am J Public Health.* 1994;*84*(3):351–358.
8. Grabiner MD, Koh TJ, Lundin TM, et al. Kinematics of recovery from a stumble. *J Gerontol.* 1993;*48*:M97–M102.
9. Allen KD, Oddone EZ, et al. Telephone-based self-management of osteoarthritis (a randomized trial). *Ann Intern Med.* 2010;*153*:570–579.
10. Barkin RL, Beckerman M, et al. Should nonsteroidal anti-inflammatory drugs (NSAIDs) be prescribed to the older adult? *Drugs Aging.* Oct 1, 2010;*27*(10):775–789.
11. Savage R. Cyclo-oxygenase-2 inhibitors: when should they be used in the elderly? *Drugs Aging.* 2005;*22*(3):185–200.

88

Lumbar Spinal Stenosis

CASE

Mr. X is an 81-year-old man with diabetes, hypertension, and osteoarthritis. He reports having a history of intermittent chronic low back pain "for at least 30 years," but has developed subsequent extension of this pain into his buttocks and thighs. He reports the pain is dull and "heavy," and worsens when he is walking or standing for extended periods of time. He finds that the pain resolves fairly rapidly when he rests and sits. He notes that this pain has progressed gradually over several years and now limits the distance he can travel.

DEFINITION

Spinal stenosis is the narrowing of the intraspinal canal.

PREVALENCE

- Lumbar spinal stenosis (LSS) is frequently a cause of low back and thigh pain in the older adults.
- Accounts for 1.2 million yearly office visits in the United States.
- Most common cause for back surgery in the over-65 population; rate of lumbar fusion surgery for degenerative conditions increased 200% from 1990 to 2001.[1]
- About 20% of patients who demonstrate anatomically significant canal narrowing on imaging studies have no symptoms.

LIKELY ETIOLOGIES[2]

Lumbar stenosis can be either congenital or acquired. Congenital stenosis is a well-known feature of achondroplastic dwarfism; usually idiopathic and less likely to be a cause of LSS in older adults. Acquired stenosis is more common and can be caused by several different factors:

1. **Spondylosis or spinal degeneration**: Most frequently the result of deterioration and desiccation of the intervertebral discs leading to reduced disc integrity, bulging and protrusion of disc into the canal, and diminished disc height. This decrease in vertebral interspace distance causes ligamentous buckling and increased stress to the facets. Subsequent synovial changes and bony hypertrophy result in reduction in the caliber of the spinal canal.

2. **Spondylolithesis**: Degenerative process leads to slippage of one vertebral body relative to an adjacent body. Mild spondylolithesis is common and often discovered incidentally on X-rays. Significant spondylolithesis is important to recognize because it is frequently the cause of severe canal stenosis and may necessitate further imaging studies to determine if surgery or epidural corticosteroid injections may be therapeutic options.

3. **Other causes**: Tumors, bone fragments from severe fracture, osteomyelitis, postoperative fibrosis, hardware from prior spinal surgery, Pott's disease, pseudogout, renal osteodystrophy, Paget's disease, rheumatoid arthritis, and intraspinal synovial cysts.
   - The specific mechanism by which canal compression leads to pain and sensorimotor deficits is not entirely apparent. The constellation of pain quality, rapid onset and relief with positional changes, and lack of claudication in many patients with anatomic stenosis leads most researchers to believe that these symptoms stem from neurovascular compromise rather than direct mechanical compression.

DIAGNOSIS

History

- Age is a strongly-associated factor for attribution of a patient's back pain to LSS.

- When symptomatic, patients present with a picture of intermittent neurogenic claudication:
  - Low back pain without radiation
  - Pain that is "dull," "achey," and with perception of "heaviness" in the lateral back, buttocks, and thighs
  - Lower extremity pain, with improvement or resolution of symptoms while seated or leaning forward
- Any maneuver that further shrinks the effective diameter of the spinal canal and foramina (such as lumbar extension) can produce increased compression and therefore elicit increased discomfort.

Mr. X has lumbar spinal stenosis, which generally has a specific territory (low back and legs) and pattern of presentation (worse with lumbar extension, standing erect). There is usually rapid alleviation of these symptoms with forward flexion of the spine, such as rest in a sitting position. On further questioning, you learn that Mr. X can increase his walking ability by using a shopping cart.

Exam

- Active lumbar extension: Will often provoke or increase a patient's pain if done for 30 seconds.
- Stance and gait: Pain from lumbar spinal stenosis will often cause a wide-based gait.
- Sensory and motor exam: Deficits are commonly found but are usually mild and can be subtle.
- Proprioception and vibratory sense: May be altered due to involvement of the dorsal columns.
- Romberg maneuver (patient stands with eyes closed and is observed for imbalance) is a rapid test for source of ataxia; sign of dorsal column dysfunction versus cerebellar disease.
- Differential diagnosis for neurogenic claudication:
  - Vascular claudication in the lower limbs may present like neurogenic claudication but is usually not improved or worsened by positional changes.
  - Peripheral neuropathy superimposed on central low back pain may also mimic pain from lumbar stenosis, but is not usually modified with position; also commonly presents with paraesthesias or a "burning" quality in a more distal distribution to the legs.

- Trochanteric bursitis and hip osteoarthritis: Will demonstrate tenderness or pain with limb movement that is not typical for spinal stenosis.
- Other possibilities: Infection, visceral pain, neoplasm, and systemic inflammatory diseases

Tests

- Van Gelderen's Bicycle Test: A simple method to help differentiate between vascular and neurogenic claudication. In this test, patients who demonstrate pain-limited ability to ride a stationary bike while upright, but who have increased endurance while leaning forward, are more likely to have a neurogenic source of pain.

Imaging

- The majority of patients with lower back pain do not require diagnostic imaging because the history and physical examination should be sufficient to make the diagnosis of symptomatic lumbar stenosis. Imaging studies do have a role, however, when there are clear clinical indications. These include:[3]
  - New symptom of low back pain in an older individual (>50)
  - Recent significant trauma, or milder trauma >50
  - Severe or progressive neurological deficits are present, or serious underlying conditions are suspected based on history and physical exam.
  - When consideration is being given to epidural steroid injection or surgery
- Imaging options include:
  - Radiography in an upright position can often show spondylolisthesis, joint hypertrophy, osteophytes, and disc-height reductions.
  - CT scan can provide a clear, cross-sectional view of the spinal canal, as well as bony pathologies. MRI also gives an axial view, with better soft tissue visualization.
  - Myelography can be performed in conjunction with CT scanning to give a sensitive picture of soft-tissue compression as well as good bony imaging, but is an invasive process involving the use of spinal contrast, with attendant risk of complications. MRI is generally preferred, but CT

myelography is an alternative when MRI is contraindicated.

- Doppler ultrasound of the lower extremities can be used to assist in discriminating vascular from neurogenic claudication.
- Electromyography (EMG) can assist in differentiating between neurogenic claudication and peripheral neuropathy.

EXPECTED DISEASE COURSE[4]

- The natural progression of symptomatic spinal stenosis can fluctuate, but typically is slow or nonprogressive. Untreated patients do not demonstrate significant neurological decline or progressive deficits.
- Symptoms do wax and wane, however, and even though nonprogressive, they can eventually limit a patient's functional ability and significantly affect quality of life.

TREATMENT OPTIONS

Non-Surgical Management

- Except in the event of serious or progressive neurologic deficits, an initial course of conservative non-surgical management is recommended for patients with LSS.[2,5,6]
- The evidence to guide decision-making about non-surgical treatment of LSS is lacking, but clinical practice guidelines on the treatment of low back pain from the American College of Physicians and the American Pain Society recommend trials of selected medications, spinal manipulation, interdisciplinary rehabilitation, exercise therapy, acupuncture, massage therapy, and cognitive behavioral therapy.[3]

Pharmacologic[3]

- Medications in several classes can provide moderate, usually short term, benefit for back pain. Clinicians should evaluate the severity of the pain and functional impairment, and analyze the potential benefits and risks before initiating pharmacologic therapy.
- Acetaminophen and NSAIDs are common first-line drugs for a variety of chronic or recurring pain complaints. Adverse side effects from these drugs are not uncommon, however, and occur more frequently in the geriatric population.
- Topical treatments such as lidoderm and capsaicin and topical NSAIDs can be helpful (e.g., diclofinac).

- Gabapentin is an anticonvulsant that is also frequently used to alleviate neuropathic pain symptoms; there is some evidence that it may help decrease pain and increase functionality in patients with neurogenic claudication, but further studies are needed.
- Opioids have also been prescribed for neurogenic claudication, but conclusive studies are lacking and side effects must be monitored.

Physical Therapy[5,7,8]

- Although physical therapy interventions are not standardized, most programs include an individual regimen of strengthening, stretching, walking, muscle coordination training, and lumbar flexion exercises (cycling).
- Epidural steroid injections are commonly given, but conclusive evidence as to effectiveness is lacking. There may be symptomatic and functional gains, but the duration of effect may be limited.

Surgical Options

- When conservative medical management has failed to relieve pain and restore function, surgical intervention may be offered to patients whose perceived quality of life is significantly diminished by their condition.[2,3,4] The most common surgical intervention is laminectomy, with or without arthrodesis.
- All surgical treatments used currently are based on the concept of decompression of the spinal canal; procedures differ in how that decompression is achieved. Other less invasive surgeries are being developed.
- Operative management has been shown to provide severely afflicted patients with rapid functional and symptomatic improvement. Symptoms can recur, however, and in some trials benefits have diminished over time.[9,10]
- In the geriatric population, the risk of adverse events associated with spinal surgery is small, but not insignificant.
- Delaying surgery in favor of an initial trial of conservative management does not appear to affect the surgical outcome.[10]
- While there is relatively robust evidence for efficacy of surgical intervention for severely afflicted patients, there is lack of consensus about optimal timing for surgery,

the advantages of new techniques, the duration of functional improvement, and the comparative effectiveness of surgical vs. non-surgical treatment.[4]

PALLIATIVE CARE ISSUES

- The use of pain medications for LSS in the geriatric population increases the risk of falls, cognitive deficits, constipation, bladder dysfunction, and other adverse events.
- Because most surgical interventions for LSS are elective in nature, a collaborative decision-making process will allow a patient who is fully informed about the benefits and burdens of surgery to make a decision based on his or her preferences, values, and goals for care.
- The demand for aggressive treatment of LSS appears to be driven by the impact of chronic pain on perceived quality of life, high expectations for functionality, and the value put on the goal of independent living. The consideration of spinal surgery for older adults should be weighed carefully, however, given the fact that comorbidities increase the risk of post-surgical complications and also possibly contribute to less favorable outcomes.

TAKE-HOME POINTS

- Spinal stenosis usually presents insidiously with low back pain, lower extremity heaviness, and gait impairments.
- It is critically important to distinguish spinal stenosis from other disorders with similar presentations, notably vascular claudication.
- The clinical course of symptomatic spinal stenosis can fluctuate but typically is slow or nonprogressive.
- An initial course of conservative non-surgical management is recommended for patients with lumbar spinal stenosis, except in the setting of serious or progressive neurologic deficits.
- After an initial course of conservative non-operative management, surgical intervention may be offered to patients whose perceived quality of life is significantly diminished by pain and functional impairment.
- Surgical intervention can provide relief for severely afflicted patients, but there is lack of consensus about surgical timing, technique for surgery, duration of functional improvement, and the comparative effectiveness of surgical vs. non-surgical treatment.

REFERENCES

1. Deyo RA, Gray DT, Kreuter W, et al. United States trends in lumbar fusion surgery for degenerative conditions. *Spine*. 2005;*30*(12):1441–1445.
2. Katz JN, Harris MB. Lumbar spinal stenosis. *N Engl J Med*. 2008;*358*:818–825.
3. Chou R, Qaseem A, Snow V, et al. Diagnosis and treatment of low back pain: a joint clinical practice guideline from the American College of Physicians and the American Pain Society. *Ann Intern Med*. 2007;*147*:478–491.
4. Markman JD, Gaud KG. Lumbar spinal stenosis in older adults: current understanding and future directions. *Clin Geriatr Med*. 2008;*24*:369–388.
5. Haig AJ, Tompkins CC. Diagnosis and management of lumbar spinal stenosis. *JAMA*. 2010;*303*(1): 71–72.
6. Gunzburg R, Szpalski M. The conservative surgical treatment of lumbar spinal stenosis in the elderly. *Eur Spine J*. 2003;*12*(S2):S176–S180.
7. Whitman JM, Flynn TW, Childs JD, et al. A comparison between two physical therapy treatment programs for patients with lumbar spinal stenosis. *Spine*. 2006;*31*(22):2541–2549.
8. Chou R, Huffman LH. Non-pharmacologic therapies for acute and chronic low back pain: a review of the evidence for an American Society/American College of Physicians clinical practice guideline. *Ann Intern Med*. 2007;*147*:492–504.
9. Chou R, Baisden J, Carragee EJ, et al. Surgery for low back pain. *Spine*. 2009;*34*(1):1094–1109.
10. Amundsen T, Weber H, Nordat HJ, et al. Lumbar spinal stenosis: conservative or surgical management? *Spine*. 2000;*25*:1424–1436.

89

Osteoporotic Fracture

CASE
Mrs. K, a 79-year-old Caucasian woman with moderate dementia, osteoporosis, and kyphosis, was brought in by her daughter for acute onset of excruciating back pain. The pain started when the patient stood up to leave the dining table after breakfast. Initially her daughter thought that her mother had pulled a muscle, and gave her some acetaminophen without relief. The patient cannot get into a comfortable position and is crying in the office.

DEFINITION
Osteoporotic fracture is defined as fracture due to osteoporosis. Osteoporosis is the loss of bone mass and micro architecture that leads to fragility and susceptibility to fracture.

PREVALENCE
- Osteoporosis is most common bone disease in humans, but it typically goes undiagnosed until a fracture occurs.
- The National Osteoporosis Foundation has estimated that more than 10 million Americans have osteoporosis, and an additional 33.6 million have low bone density of the hip.[1]
- Approximately 50% of Caucasian females and 20% of men in the United States will experience an osteoporotic fracture during their lifetimes.[2]
- Fractures associated with osteoporosis are responsible for approximately 500,000 hospitalizations, 800,000 emergency department visits, 2,600,000 physician visits, and 180,000 nursing home placements in the United States each year.[2]

LIKELY ETIOLOGIES
The best predictor of future fracture risk is a spine or hip bone density test plus identification of risk factors (Table 89.1).

Mrs. K is 5 feet tall and weighs 90 pounds. She is currently taking calcium, vitamin D, Aricept, and Fosamax. She has no history of alcohol or cigarette use. She has been a homemaker all her life. She has no other medical illnesses.

DIAGNOSIS

History
Focus should be on risk factors listed in Table 89.1.

Exam
- Height loss
- Abnormal gait
- Kyphosis

Tests
Comprehensive blood panel (CBC, PTH, TSH, protein electrophoresis, vitamin D-25 OH, electrolytes, LFTs, creatinine clearance).

Imaging
Bone Densitometry:
- Central devices, such as Dual X-Ray Absorptiometry (DXA) of hip and spine, are better predictors of fracture risk than peripheral (forearm) measures.
- DXA uses low-dose radiation to measure density of spine, hip, or forearm.
- Serial measurements are helpful to follow progression of bone loss and assess efficacy of therapy.
- For peri-menopausal females, the first site of bone loss is the spine. Bone loss in the hip occurs later. Therefore, DXA of spine is more sensitive in this age group.
- For older females and males, the hip is the most sensitive site; recommend ordering DXA of both spine and hip or better assessment of both trabecular and cortical bone.
- DXA of forearm is sensitive for secondary causes of osteoporosis (hyperthyroidism, hyperparathyroidism,

TABLE 89.1: RISK FACTORS FOR OSTEOPOROTIC FRACTURE

Demographics:	Medications:	Medical Conditions:
Age	Corticosteroids	Renal failure
Female	Antacids containing aluminum	Liver failure
Caucasian, Asian	Methotrexate	Thyroid disease
Hispanic	Cyclosporine	Cushing's syndrome
	Aromatase inhibitors	GI malabsorption
Lifestyle	Anticonvulsants	Diabetes mellitus
Alcohol (> 3 drinks per day)	Heparin	Malignancies
Cigarette smoking	Loop diuretics	COPD
Sedentary	Thyroid hormone	Hypogonadism
	Isoniazid	Hyperparathyroid
		AIDS/HIV
		Rheumatoid arthritis
Nutritional/Diet:		Dementia
Malnutrition/Anorexia		Depression
Low body weight (<127 lbs)		Frailty
Low calcium intake		Vitamin D deficiency
Low Vit D—25 OH (<30 ng/ml)		**Other:**
		Prior fracture as an adult
		Fracture in a first-degree relative
		Exercise-induced amenorrhea
		Early menopause (<45 years)

renal and liver failure, malabsorption syndromes).

- To confirm a vertebral fracture, an X-ray is required.

BMD TESTING[3]

For Screening Purposes

- All postmenopausal women age 65 and older and all men age 70 and older
- Postmenopausal women and men age 50–69 with additional risk factors for osteoporosis.

For Clinical Management

- Men and women with fractures after age 50
- Anyone being treated for osteoporosis, to monitor response to therapy.

Testing Frequency

Although evidence is limited for optimal frequency of testing, results of a recent risk analysis study indicate intervals of approximately 15 years for women with normal bone density or mild osteopenia, five years for women with moderate osteopenia, and one year for women with advanced osteopenia. Intervals for men were not studied.[4]

Determining Risk of Fracture

Use the FRAX tool, a web-based algorithm that uses clinical risk factors and femoral neck BMD (if available) to estimate an individual's 10-year osteoporotic and hip fracture probability[5] (available online at http://www.shef.ac.uk/FRAX/).

TREATMENT OPTIONS

Nonpharmacologic

Universal recommendations for all postmenopausal women and men age 50 and older include the following:[3]

- Calcium: 1,200 mg/day (Encourage dietary sources over supplements; to avoid excess calcium, include calculation of dietary intake in daily dose recommendation.)
- A balanced diet, including adequate protein intake, helps prevent weight loss, muscle wasting, and sarcopenia.
- Vitamin D 1,000 units/day
- Regular weight-bearing exercise
- Falls prevention (See Chapter 63: Falls)
- Avoidance of tobacco use
- Avoid excess alcohol, caffeine, and phosphate-containing drinks (coffee, cola soft drinks)

Pharmacologic

- For postmenopausal women and men age 50 and older, pharmacologic treatment is recommended if:
  - Prior history of prior hip or vertebral fracture
  - T-score of –2.5 or less at femoral neck or spine
  - For patients with mild osteopenia (T-score of –1 to –2.5 at femoral neck, total hip or spine), pharmacologic intervention should be considered if increased risk of fracture is determined.
- Multiple agents have been shown to reduce the risk of osteoporotic fracture. Head-to-head studies have not been conducted, however, to determine which drug is more effective.
- In placebo studies, alendronate, risedronate, and zoledronic acid reduced the risk of vertebral, non-vertebral, and hip fractures. Denosumab reduced vertebral and hip fracture, while raloxifene, ibandronate, calcitonin, and teriparatide reduced vertebral fracture only (Table 89.2).

EXPECTED DISEASE COURSE

- While osteoporosis is a chronic and potentially debilitating disease, it is preventable with timely measures. Early treatment may slow bone loss and prevent fractures.
- Some common initial symptoms include:
  - Back pain
  - Height loss (> 1½ inches)
  - Stooped posture (due to kyphosis)
  - Fractures as a result of low-impact injury
  - Compression fractures
- With disease progression, there is increased risk of hip fracture, increased symptom burden, as well as progressive debility and functional decline.

MANAGEMENT OF ACUTE FRACTURE

- Osteoporosis is often not diagnosed until a fracture occurs. Prevention of further fractures is important, but clinicians should also be aware of the treatment options for spinal compression fractures, since they are the most common form of osteoporotic fracture and often lead to severe pain and debility in older adults.

- Although the paucity of strong evidence limits the ability to make recommendations, treatment options for patients who present with osteoporotic spinal compression fracture, treatment options include:
  1. **Pain management:** Acute spinal compression fractures may not be painful, and patients may not notice them until kyphosis develops. But for patients who do present with pain, aggressive management and support should be provided as necessary. (See Chapter 29: Management of Pain in Older Adults.)
  2. **Bed rest:** Patient should be encouraged to resume activity as soon as possible. If pain is difficult to manage, short-term best rest can be considered. Prolonged bed rest is not recommended, however, as it may lead to further bone loss.
  3. **Braces:** External support may be helpful to some patients for pain relief. Rigid orthoses not recommended, however, due to impaired respiration and low compliance. Soft corset is a better option in this patient population.[9]
  4. **Continue anti-osteoporosis medications:** Although there is some question of whether fracture healing is affected by anti-osteoporosis treatment, there is currently no evidence-based reason to discontinue or withhold anti-resorptive therapy while a fracture heals.[10]

Surgical Options

- Currently, the evidence supporting surgical intervention for osteoporotic compression fracture is limited. The American Academy of Orthopedic Surgeons clinical practice guidelines therefore recommend against vertebroplasty for relief of pain associated with osteoporotic compression fractures of the spine.[11]
- Surgical options are frequently considered, however, when conservative management outlined above is not effective. The two most commonly performed surgical techniques for osteoporotic compression facture are vertebroplasty and kyphoplasty. In both procedures, bone cement is percutaneously injected into a collapsed vertebra under fluoroscopic guidance.

TABLE 89.2: PHARMACOLOGIC TREATMENT OPTIONS[6,7,8]

Class	Drug	Reduction of Fracture Risk
Biphosphonates	Alendronate (Fosamax)	Spine, hip, wrist fracture by 50% in patients with prior spine fracture
	Risedronate (Actonel)	Spine by 48% in patients with no prior spine fracture
	Zoledronic acid (Reclast, Aclasta, Zometa)	Spine fracture by 41%--9%
		Non-spine fractures by 36% with prior spine fracture
		Spine fractures by 70% and hip fractures by 41% in patients with prior spine/hip fracture or osteoporosis of hip
	Ibandronate (Boniva)	Spine fracture by 50% Currently no evidence for reduction of hip fracture
Selective estrogen receptor modulator (SERM)	Raloxifene (Evista)	Spine fracture by 39% in patients with osteoporosis
Other agents	Calcitonin (Miacalcin, Calcimar, Fortical)	New vertebral fractures by 33% in postmenopausal women with osteoporosis, and 36% in pts with one to five prior vertebral fractures
	Denosumab (humanized monoclonal antibody)	New vertebral fractures by 68% in postmenopausal women Hip fracture by 41% in postmenopausal women
	Parathyroid hormone Teriparatide (Forteo)	New vertebral fracture by 65% in postmenopausal women with prior vertebral fracture

- In balloon kyphoplasty, inflatable bone tamps are inserted into the veterbral body, pushing the end plates apart with the objective of restoring vertebral body height and correcting angular deformity. Once the balloon is removed, the void is filled with bone cement. In vertebroplasty, liquid cement is injected into the vertebral body without creating a cavity.[12]
- Of the two procedures, there is limited evidence for the efficacy of kyphoplasty for patients with clinical and imaging signs of osteoporotic fracture and who are neurologically intact. Benefits include pain relief, improved physical function, and quality of life.[12]
- Surgical intervention is not without risk and therefore should not be considered as first-line treatment. The main adverse effects of vertebroplasty and kyphoplasty are related to leakage of cement from the vertebral body and may include increased

pain and, less commonly, pulmonary embolization. There is also an increased long-term risk of fracture in adjacent vertebras.[13]

PALLIATIVE CARE ISSUES

With time and progression of disease, osteoporosis has a serious impact on older adults and their caregivers:

- Reduced health-related quality of life
- Undertreatment of pain associated with hip fracture is a risk factor for delirium;[14] inadequate analgesia can also contribute to immobility, deconditioning, debility, anorexia, constipation, depression, and social isolation. (See Chapter 29: Management of Pain in Older Adults, for assessment of pain in patients with cognitive impairment.)
- Increased morbidity and mortality: Twenty to thirty percent of patients who sustain hip

fracture die in the first year post-fracture, with mortality higher for males. Declines in functional status scores range from 29% on fine motor skills to 56% on mobility index.[15]

- Spinal compression fractures may result in limitation of ambulation, depression, loss of independence, and chronic pain.
- Kyphosis causes many debilitating conditions including:
  - Restricted lung function, leading to shortness of breath
  - Compression of abdominal organs, causing pain, constipation, distention, reduced appetite, and premature satiety
  - Pain and discomfort, contributing to reduced mobility and increased physical dependency and debility
  - Disfigurement, causing depression, anxiety, and loss of self-esteem
- Management of kyphosis-related symptoms to improve quality of life includes:
  - Referral to physical therapy for assistive device and home safety evaluation
  - Psychological screening and, if indicated, referral for evaluation appropriate treatment

Mrs. K. was given 10 mg of oxycodone, and she reported her pain improved from severe to mild. She was discharged with an opioid pain regimen, a bowel regimen, and a prescription for a back brace. A follow-up phone call is scheduled for the day after discharge to reassess her pain and to arrange for an evaluation of home safety and fall risk reduction.

TAKE-HOME POINTS

- Osteoporosis is common is older adults and is increasing dramatically due to increased longevity.
- Osteoporosis often goes undiagnosed until a fracture occurs.
- Both primary and secondary treatment strategies are keys to fracture prevention.
- The best site for screening the elderly for bone loss with bone density testing is the hip; for younger, peri-menopausal females the optimal site is the spine.
- Osteoporotic fractures in older adults can lead to reduced quality of life, high symptom burden, and increased debility.

- Currently, the evidence supporting surgical intervention for osteoporotic compression fracture is limited. Surgical options are frequently considered, however, when conservative management is not effective.
- Quality of life may be improved with lifestyle modifications, physical therapy, and symptom management.

REFERENCES

1. *America's Bone Health: The State of Osteoporosis and Low Bone Mass in Our Nation.* Washington, DC: National Osteoporosis Foundation; 2002.
2. U.S. Department of Health and Human Services. *Bone Health and Osteoporosis: A report of the Surgeon General.* Rockville. MD: U.S Department of Health and Human Services: Office of the Surgeon General; 2004.
3. Clinician's Guide to Prevention and Treatment of Osteoporosis. National Osteoporosis Foundation (NOF).http://www.nof.org/sites/default/files/pdfs/NOF_ClinicianGuide2009_v7 (accessed January 12, 2012).
4. Gourlay ML, Fine JP, Preisser JS, et al. Bone-density testing testing interval and transition to osteoporosis in women. *N Engl J Med.* 2012;*366*(3): 225–233.
5. Kanis JA, Oden A, Johansson H, et al. 2009. FRAX and its applications to clinical practice. *Bone.* 2009;*44*:734–743.
6. MacLean C, Newberry S, Maglione M, et al. Comparative effectiveness of treatments to prevent fractures in men and women with low bone density or osteoporosis. *Ann Intern Med.* 2008;*148*:197–213.
7. Reginster J. Antifracture efficacy of currently available therapies for postmenopausal osteoporosis. *Drugs.* 2011;*71*(1):65–78.
8. Chestnut CH, Silverman S, Andriano K, et al. A randomized trial of nasal spray salmon calcitonin in postmenopausal women with established osteoporosis. *Am J Med.* 2000;*109*(4):267–276.
9. Agabegi SS, Asghar FA, Herkowitz HN. Spinal orthoses. *J Am Acad Othop Surg.* 2010;*18*:657–667.
10. Ip TP, Leung J, Kung AWC. Management of osteoporosis in patients hospitalized for hop fractures. *Osteoporos Int.* 2010;*21*(suppl 4):S605–S614.
11. Esses SI, McGuire R, Jenkins J, et al. The treatment of symptomatic osteoporotic spinal compression fractures. *J Am Acad Orthop Surg.* 2011;*19*: 176–182.
12. Boonen S, Van Meirhaeghe J, Bastian L, et al. Balloon kyphoplasty for the treatment of acute vertebral compression fractures: 2-year results

from a randomized trial. *J Bone Miner Res.* 2011; *26*(7):1627–1637.

13. Cortet B, Chastanet P, Laredo J-D. Osteoporotic vertebral fractures: a role for verteboplasty or kyphoplasty? *Joint Bone Spine.* 2010;*77*:380–381.

14. Morrison RS, Magaziner J, Gilbert M, et al. Relationship between pain and opioid analgesics on the development of delirium following hip fracture. *J Gerontol A Biol Sci Med Sci.* Jan 2003;*58*(1): 76–81.

15. Bentler SE, Liu L, Obrizan M. The aftermath of hip fracture: discharge placement, functional status change, and mortality. *Am J Epidemiol.* 2009;*170*: 1290–1299.

90
Polymyalgia Rheumatica

CASE
Mrs. S is a 78-year-old woman with a history of osteoporosis, hypertension, and osteoarthritis of the hands manifested by Heberden's nodes. She always has functioned quite well and was able to take care of herself. Recently she had a relatively sudden onset of pain in her neck, upper arms, and thigh, accompanied by marked morning stiffness and nocturnal pain that made it difficult to turn in bed. She also has difficulty rising from a chair, climbing stairs, and combing her hair. Mrs. S has no fever or skin rash. Her joints are not swollen.

DEFINITION
Polymyalgia rheumatica (PMR) is an inflammatory disease that occurs predominately in the elderly. Women are affected somewhat more than men. The onset is usually sudden or subacute. It is characterized by pain and stiffness in the shoulder and hip girdles, accompanied by morning stiffness, gelling phenomenon, and fatigue. The joints are not inflamed.[1]

PREVALENCE
The prevalence of the disease is not known, although it is quite common and more frequent in the elderly than rheumatoid arthritis.

LIKELY ETIOLOGIES
PMR is believed to be immunologically mediated.

DIAGNOSIS

Exam
- There are no specific findings. The joints are not swollen with the exception that sometimes patients have small effusions in the knees.
- Patients may have evidence of osteoarthritis particularly in the hands, knees, and feet. There may be limitation of motion due to pain. There is no muscle weakness. Tenderness of the upper arms and thighs is common. On rare occasions, there is a low-grade fever.
- Hypothyroidism, occult malignancy, or infection could present with polymyalgia rheumatica-like symptoms. However, the proper laboratory studies and response to a small dose of corticosteroids would usually distinguish these entities.

Tests
- ESR: elevated sedimentation rate often higher than 80 mm/hour.
- CBC: A mild anemia may be seen.
- CK and aldolase are normal.
- TSH: rule out hypothyroidism.
- Protein electrophoreses often indicates slightly low albumin, elevated alpha-2 globulin and diffuse hypergammaglobulinemia. Patients do not have monoclonal "spikes."

Imaging
X-rays are negative. Evidence of degenerative changes and X-rays of cervical and lumbar spine are not of great value as abnormalities are common in the elderly.

Biopsy
Muscle biopsies show no signs of inflammation, though at times type II fiber atrophy may be found.

DIFFERENTIAL DIAGNOSIS
- In a small percentage of patients, polymyalgia rheumatica may be a manifestation of an underlying cranial arteritis. If the patient has symptoms of temporal arteritis such as severe headaches, vision disturbance, swollen and tender temporal arteries, or jaw claudication, and does not respond to a small dose of prednisone, then temporal arteritis must be considered.

- Temporal artery biopsy should be performed, and a much higher dose of corticosteroids should be given immediately to prevent vision loss. Prednisone or its equivalent is recommended at a dose between 60 mg and 100 mg daily for two weeks. If the patient responds, dose should be tapered slowly to maintain freedom from symptoms, independent of ESR.

On examination, Mrs. S has no active sinusitis. Her BP is 150/90, her lungs are clear, her heart rate is regular, and her abdomen is soft. There is mild tenderness of the upper arms and thighs, though when the joints are in a position where she is not in pain, there is no obvious weakness. Laboratory examination reveals hemoglobin of 11.9, sedimentation rate of 78, negative rheumatoid factor, and antinuclear antibody, and her chemistries are otherwise normal.

EXPECTED DISEASE COURSE

- Polymyalgia rheumatica usually responds rather dramatically to a small dose of corticosteroids (e.g., prednisone 10 mg daily). The duration of treatment generally is between six months and three years, although occasionally small doses of steroids are still required for many years.
- Patients who are not treated with corticosteroids generally will get better over a period of two to three years. In general, about 90% of patients are able to stop treatment within two years.

PROGNOSIS

- Polymyalgia rheumatica is an inflammatory disease of unknown etiology. Unlike rheumatoid arthritis, synovitis is not a major characteristic, and patients do not develop the progressive joints destruction seen in rheumatoid arthritis. Muscle weakness also does not occur.
- Once a diagnosis is made and treatment is initiated, pain and stiffness respond very rapidly, and other types of analgesia are usually not necessary. The illness is usually gone after two years and leaves no residual joint deformities as might occur in rheumatoid arthritis.
- It is important, however, to monitor patients for potential side effects of corticosteroids, particularly osteoporosis

and steroid myopathy which are quite frequent in the elderly.

TREATMENT OPTIONS

Nonpharmacologic

- Early mobilization and encouragement of activity are important to keep the patient functioning as independently as possible.
- Supplementation with calcium and vitamin D and possibly bisphosphonates should be considered, especially if prolonged or high-dose corticosteroids are required.
- Facilitating return to premorbid function is important, and referral to physical therapy should be employed when indicated.

Pharmacologic

- If not absolutely contraindicated, small doses of corticosteroids are the preferred pharmacologic treatment.[2] Either prednisone between 10 mg and 15 mg a day or methylprednisolone between 8 mg and 12 mg a day is usually sufficient for an older adult.
- Once the patient has responded clinically, the corticosteroids should be decreased to the lowest dose that keeps the patient well, independent of sedimentation rate. A slight degree of discomfort and stiffness is an indication that patient is not being overtreated.
- Aspirin or nonsteroidal anti-inflammatory agents can occasionally be of benefit, but the potential for gastrointestinal and renal side effects pose a problem when ASA and NSAIDs are used.
- If the patient does not respond to small dose of corticosteroids, consideration must be given to alternate explanations.

Note on Corticosteroid Use

- Patients must be closely monitored for steroid side effects or complications. These complications may include glucose elevation, fluid retention, delirium, osteoporosis, weakness, particularly of the hip flexors, and steroid myopathy. Should steroid myopathy occur, it responds to a decreased level of corticosteroids.
- Although the pain of PMR is more difficult to treat without steroids, the presence of pre-existing congestive heart failure, diabetes, or severe osteoporosis may

also influence the decision of whether corticosteroids should be used.

After treatment with 12 mg of methylpred-nisolone for a week, Mrs. S is symptom-free. Her ESR has fallen to 26 and hemoglobin is 12.6. After 18 months, she can be tapered off all corticoste-roids. She continues to take 1200 mg of calcium and 1000 units of vitamin D. A subsequent BMD (Bone Mineral Density) test shows a T score of –1.8 at the femoral neck, and she is prescribed 70 mg of alendronate weekly. When the corticosteroids are discontinued, so is the alendronate, but the vitamin D and calcium are maintained indefinitely.

PALLIATIVE CARE ISSUES

- Palliative care can support patients during the treatment period with management of pain, fatigue, and depression, as well as potential side effects of treatment, which may include debility and delirium.
- Should there be delays in treatment and if musculoskeletal deformities do occur, palliative care management can help minimize functional debility and maintain the best possible quality of life.

TAKE-HOME POINTS

- Polymyalgia rheumatica is a common illness of elderly patients who present with pain and stiffness of the shoulder and hip girdle.

- Diagnosis is strongly suggested by the presence of an elevated sedimentation rate, otherwise unexplained.
- The lowest dose of steroids sufficient to control symptoms should be used independently of the sedimentation rate. Patients should be closely monitored for steroid side effects and complications.
- In a small percentage of patients, polymyalgia rheumatica may be a manifestation of cranial arteritis. If symptoms of cranial arteritis are present or patients have not responded to small doses of corticosteroids, a temporal artery biopsy should be performed and a much higher dose of corticosteroids immediately administered to prevent vision loss.
- Palliative care can support patients during the treatment period with management of pain, fatigue, and depression, as well as potential side effects of treatment, which may include debility and delirium.

REFERENCES

1. Spiera R, Spiera H. Inflammatory disease in older adults. *Geriatrics.* 2004;59(11):39–43.
2. Spiera H, Davison S. Long-term follow-up of polymyalgia rheumatica. *Mt Sinai J Med.* 1978;45: 225–229.

91

Rheumatoid Arthritis in Older Adults

CASE 1

Mr. R is an 82-year-old man who presents with a three-month history of gradually increasing pain and swelling affecting his shoulders, wrists, and fingers. These symptoms are accompanied by two hours of diffuse stiffness in the morning. He is incapacitated by the inability to grasp objects and awakens at night due to shoulder pain. Pertinent findings on exam are that he is afebrile. His temporal arteries are nontender. There is evidence of mild synovitis of both shoulders with decreased range of motion, marked soft tissue swelling of the wrists, dorsum of both hands as well as the metacarpophalangeal (MCP) and proximal interphalangeal (PIP) joints. He is unable to fully close his hands. In the lower extremities, there is mild synovitis of the metatarsophalangeal (MTP) joints only. The remainder of his exam is normal. Pertinent labs consist of an ESR of 80 mm/h Westergren, a negative rheumatoid factor, a negative anti-cyclic citrullinated protein (CCP) antibody, and a normal level of thyroid stimulating hormone (TS)H. X-rays of his hands reveal prominent soft tissue swelling around the small joints of his fingers as well as periarticular osteopenia. No joint space narrowing or erosions are seen.

CASE 2

Mrs. T is a 75-year-old woman who presents with a 45-year history of rheumatoid arthritis (RA), as well as complaints of pain in multiple joints. She currently experiences more than an hour of morning stiffness. Treatment in the past included multiple disease-modifying anti-rheumatic drugs (DMARDs) and low-dose steroids, and she is status post-bilateral total knee replacements. Pertinent findings on physical exam consist of marked limitation of cervical spine range of motion, bilateral frozen shoulders, bilateral 5-degree elbow flexion contractures with palpable rheumatoid nodules in the olecranon bursae, mild bilateral soft tissue swelling in both wrists with bilateral swan neck deformities, and decreased grip strength bilaterally.

Range of motion in the hips and bilateral knees is normal with well-healed total knee replacement scars. There is active synovitis of both ankles and bilateral MTP joints with hammertoe deformities. Pertinent laboratories reveal a sedimentation rate of 60 mm/h Westergren, a strongly positive Rheumatoid Factor (RF), and positive anti-CCP antibodies. X-rays demonstrate marked soft tissue swelling and periarticular osteopenia around the small joints of her hands as well as multiple erosions in the wrists, MCPs, PIP joints, as well as in the shoulders and the MTPs.

DEFINITION

These two cases exemplify the clinical spectrum of *rheumatoid arthritis* (RA) affecting persons over the age of 65:[1]

- Presentation later in life: the de novo onset of the disease in later life (Case 1)
- Presentation earlier in life: RA patients whose established disease developed in young middle age (Case 2)

Both cases meet the American College of Rheumatology (ACR) clinical criteria for the diagnosis of RA (Table 91.1):

- Polyarthritis
- Small hand joint involvement
- Symmetrical involvement
- Significant morning stiffness
- Chronicity of their symptoms of greater than six weeks' duration

PREVALENCE

Estimates of the prevalence of RA range from 1% to 2% of the world's population.[2]

LIKELY ETIOLOGIES

- Despite a century of research, the etiology of RA remains unknown. Thus, the diagnosis is based upon the ACR clinical criteria.

TABLE 91.1: AMERICAN RHEUMATISM ASSOCIATION 1987 CRITERIA FOR THE CLASSIFICATION OF RHEUMATOID ARTHRITIS (REVISED)**

Symptom	Definition
1. Morning stiffness	Morning stiffness in and around the joints, lasting at least 1 hour before maximal improvement
2. Arthritis of 3 or more joint areas	At least 3 joint areas simultaneously have had soft tissue swelling or fluid (not bony overgrowth alone) observed by a physician. The 14 possible areas are right or left PIP, MCP, wrist, elbow, knee, ankle, and MTP joints.
3. Arthritis of hand joints	At least 1 area swollen (as defined above) in a wrist, MCP, or PIP joint
4. Symmetric arthritis	Simultaneous involvement of the same joint areas (as defined in 2) on both sides of the body (bilateral involvement of PIPs, MCPs, or MTPs is acceptable without absolute symmetry)
5. Rheumatoid nodules	Subcutaneous nodules, over bony prominences, or extensor surfaces, or in juxtaarticular regions, observed by a physician
6. Serum rheumatoid factor	Demonstration of abnormal amounts of serum rheumatoid factor by any method for which the result has been positive in < 5% of normal control subjects
7. Radiographic changes	Radiographic changes typical of rheumatoid arthritis on posteroanterior hand and wrist radiographs, which must include erosions or unequivocal bony decalcification localized in or most marked adjacent to the involved joints (osteoarthritis changes alone do not qualify)

For classification purposes, a patient shall be said to have rheumatoid arthritis if he/she has satisfied at least 4 of these 7 criteria. Criteria 1 through 4 must have been present for at least 6 weeks. Arnett FC, Edworthy SM, Bloch DA, McShane DJ, Fries JF, Cooper NS, et al. The American Rheumatism Association 1987 revised criteria for the classification of rheumatoid arthritis. *Arthritis Rheum.* 1988;31:315–324.
**ACR 2010 criteria are more expansive, and useful for diagnosing very early RA in order to enable research and clinical trials. The 1987 criteria above remain the most clinically relevant diagnostic guidelines.

- The presence of rheumatoid factor (RF) and/or erosive changes on X-ray are not required for the diagnosis.

DIAGNOSIS[3]

Exam

- The most important finding on physical exam is the presence of objective, symmetric polyarthritis/synovitis, by which the examiner perceives signs of inflammation localized to the joints with or without visible deformities.
- These objective findings consist of increased heat, erythema, soft tissue swelling, effusion, tenderness to palpation, and decreased range of motion around the joints, or any combination of these signs.
- The presence of objective synovitis enables the distinction of RA from polymyalgia rheumatica (PMR), in which objective synovitis on exam is absent.
- The differential diagnosis includes crystal synovitis such as gout and the pseudorheumatoid pattern of pseudogout.

Tests

- ESR/CRP: Expect an elevation.
- RF or Anti-CCP: Positive RF or anti-CCP is helpful, but is rarely positive in the de novo onset (late onset) RA patient group.
- Synovial fluid aspirate (if applicable): Can document inflammatory fluid and rule out crystal synovitis.

Imaging

X-rays: Critical to medical decision-making because in both types of RA, the X-ray would reveal prominent soft tissue swelling and periarticular osteopenia.

COMPLICATIONS

- Joint space narrowing indicative of cartilage destruction as well as marginal erosions are commonly seen in RA patients with longstanding disease, as witnessed by their clinical deformities and prior need for joint replacement.
- Joint space narrowing is only rarely found in the de novo elderly-onset rheumatoid arthritis group.

TREATMENT OPTIONS[2,3]

- Although both clinical cases described above fulfill the ACR criteria for the definition of RA, the diagnostic evaluation and approach to therapy is significantly different in each instance.
- The ability to appropriately treat RA patients is largely predicated upon the presence and extent of radiographic and clinical joint damage and the severity of the synovitis.

Nonpharmacologic

For both early onset RA and onset in later life, the nonpharmacological treatment strategies are the same:

- Assistive devices such as wrist splints, canes, and walkers
- Occupational therapy and physical therapy to help prevent further functional decline and to improve joint function
- Judicious joint repair and/or joint replacement can be considered for patients with severe pain localized to one or two joint areas, and who are suitable surgical and rehab candidates.

Pharmacologic

Pharmacologic treatment options will often differ based on patient age at onset of disease.

1. **Late onset:** For late onset RA patients (Case 1, Mr. R), steroid therapy can be very effective:
   - Low-dose steroids such as prednisone 10 mg per day or less, and most often 5 mg per day or less, are the preferred treatment modality to alleviate symptomatic rheumatoid synovitis.
   - Low-dose steroids have dramatic efficacy, particularly in this type of rheumatoid arthritis patient. Shortly after the initiation of steroid therapy, these patients rapidly regain the use of their hands and an overall sense of well-being.
   - Once symptom control has occurred, the steroids can usually be tapered to a maintenance dose of 5 mg of prednisone per day or less with minimal toxicity.
   - When used for symptom control, nonsteroidal anti-inflammatory drugs (NSAIDs) are quite effective, but high doses must be given daily. In the older rheumatoid arthritis patient, the use of these drugs is especially hazardous, with gastrointestinal toxicity, renal insufficiency, and mental status changes seen frequently.

2. **Established disease:** RA patients with a longer history of disease (Case 2, Mrs. T), present a more difficult management challenge:
   - Low-dose steroids offer some symptomatic, but incomplete, relief of synovitis and may not confer protection from continued joint destruction.
   - The presence of erosions is an important poor prognostic factor, and as such is an indication for the use of disease-modifying antirheumatic drug (DMARD) therapy. Examples include medications in the following classes:

   Immunosuppressive agents:
   - Auranofin
   - Methotrexate
   - Hydroxychloroquine sulfate
   - Sulfasalazine
   - Cyclosporine
   - Azathioprine
   - Leflunomide
   - Mycophenolate mofetil
   - Cyclophosphamide

   Biologic agents (not often used in the older adult):
   - Etanercept
   - Infliximab
   - Anakinra
   - Adalimumab
   - Rituximab

- The choice of a specific therapeutic option should be made based upon the individual patient's comorbidities and prior history of efficacy and/or adverse reaction to specific DMARDs.

PHARMACOLOGIC CONSIDERATIONS FOR OLDER PATIENTS

- Use of the DMARDs hydroxychloroquine (Plaquenil) or sulfasalazine (Azulfidine) have an important role in the treatment of the elderly RA patient. These drugs have relatively little toxicity or need for frequent monitoring as compared with the other DMARDs listed.

- Biologic therapies such as the anti-tumor necrosis factor alpha agents are particularly fraught with hazard in the older age group because many elderly patients have positive PPDs, suffer from chronic infections (such as venous stasis ulcers or recurrent urinary tract infections), or have been treated for malignancy such as skin, breast, or prostate cancers. Although commonly used for severe erosive rheumatoid arthritis in younger patients, these agents are therefore used less frequently in the older age group.

- If the pain is severe and not relieved by clinical management strategies, or if related to chronic, irreversible damage caused by the disease, consideration should be given to using opioids for pain management in older adults.

- For the older RA patient, the benefits and risks of joint repair or replacement should be evaluated in the context of achievable goals for care, comorbidities and their associated prognosis, cognitive and functional status, and the ability to comply with a postoperative rehabilitation program.

TAKE-HOME POINTS

- Rheumatoid arthritis is common in the geriatric population and will be encountered frequently in older patients.

- Recognition and diagnosis depend upon the presence of objective polyarticular synovitis, significant morning stiffness and chronicity; do not depend upon the presence of serologies such as rheumatoid factor or anti-CCP antibodies.

- Treatment with low-dose steroids alone is highly effective and relatively nontoxic in the de novo onset subset of rheumatoid arthritis patients, and as an adjunct to

DMARD therapy in longstanding erosive rheumatoid arthritis patients.

- In view of the many comorbidities commonly encountered in the geriatric population, hydroxychloroquine and sulfasalazine have a more favorable risk-to-benefit ratio as compared with other DMARDs. Anti-TNF alpha agents pose increased risks in this population.

- Nonpharmacologic therapies such as OT, PT, supportive devices, and judicious joint replacement therapy also play an important role in restoring the patient's quality of life and functional status.

- For the older RA patient, the option of joint repair or replacement should be evaluated in the context of achievable goals for care, comorbidities and their associated prognosis, cognitive and functional status, and ability to comply with postoperative rehabilitation program.

- The choice of disease-modifying antirheumatic drug (DMARD) therapy should be made based upon the individual patient's comorbidities and prior history of efficacy and/or adverse reaction to specific DMARD medications.

- If the joint pain is severe and not relieved by specific clinical management strategies, consideration should be given to using opioids for pain management in older adults.

GENERAL REFERENCES

1. Ehrlich GE, Katz WA, Cohen SH. Rheumatoid arthritis in the aged. *Geriatrics.* 1970;25(2): 103–113.
2. Kerr LD. Inflammatory arthritis in the elderly. *Mt Sinai J Med.* 2003;70(1):23–26.
3. Kerr LD. Inflammatory arthropathy—a review of rheumatoid arthritis in older patients. *Geriatrics.* 2004;59(10):32–35.

92

Osteomyelitis in Older Adults

CASE

Mrs. K is a 94-year-old woman from a nursing home with Alzheimer's dementia and diabetes mellitus complicated by neuropathy who is brought to the hospital with a left foot heel ulcer. She has had this ulcer for two months and now presents with fever and purulent drainage from the ulcer. On physical examination, she has a temperature of 38.2, pulse of 90, and blood pressure of 130/80. She has a 2.2 × 1.5 cm ulcer on the plantar surface of the foot near the heel, with purulent drainage that probes to bone. Laboratory examination reveals a white blood cell count of 9.5 with an erythrocyte sedimentation rate of 75. How likely is osteomyelitis?

DEFINITION

Osteomyelitis is an infection of the bone caused by a microorganism and accompanied by inflammatory destruction. The infection can involve one part of the bone or several regions, including the periosteum, cortex, and/or medullary cavity.

PREVALENCE

- Osteomyelitis is a common infection among older adults, who are often predisposed because of other medical disorders such as diabetes mellitus and peripheral vascular disease, as in the case above.
- Foot-related complications in patients with diabetes account for 20% of all hospitalizations among diabetics in North America. The prevalence of osteomyelitis in patients with diabetic foot ulcers can vary widely, and in a recent review of 21 published studies, the prevalence of osteomyelitis ranged from 12% to 100%.[1] This variability is most likely related to the challenges associated with diagnosing osteomyelitis in patients with diabetic foot ulcers.

CLASSIFICATION

- There are different types of osteomyelitis, and two classification systems are often

used to describe them. Waldwogel and coworkers classified bone infections as one of three types:[2]
  - Osteomyelitis secondary to hematogenous spread
  - Osteomyelitis due to local spread from a contiguous source
  - Osteomyelitis secondary to vascular insufficiency
- An alternative classification system by Cierny and Mader takes into account the anatomic location of the infection and the physiologic health of the host.[3] This system is best utilized when considering treatment and prognostic factors, as local and systemic factors that may affect treatment response are considered.

LIKELY ETIOLOGIES

The causative microorganisms associated with the various types of osteomyelitis, as classified by the Waldwogel system, are listed in Table 92.1.

DIAGNOSIS

Exam

Osteomyelitis is frequently difficult to diagnose. On physical examination, the clinician should assess for the following:

- Fever
- Tenderness over the bone
- Presence of foreign body
- In diabetic foot ulcers, Presence and appearance of ulcer/wound—erythema, size and depth, drainage
  - Larger than 2 cm increases likelihood of osteomyelitis (LR 7.2, 95% CI 1.1–49)[2]
  - Probes to bone—strong likelihood of osteomyelitis (LR 6.4, CI 3.6–11)[2]
- The presence of other foot deformities, neuropathy, and signs of arterial insufficiency should also be noted.

TABLE 92.1: CAUSATIVE MICROORGANISMS ASSOCIATED WITH OSTEOMYELITIS

Type of Osteomyelitis	Examples	Causative Microorganisms
Hematogenous osteomyelitis: Seen in young children and older adults Involves seeding of the bone by bacteria present in the blood	Vertebral osteomyelitis (lumbar 45%, thoracic 35%, cervical 20%)[4]	*Staphylococcus aureus* Gram-negative uropathogens (gain access to the vertebra through Batson's plexus in elderly men) *Mycobacterium tuberculosis*
Osteomyelitis secondary to contiguous source: Follows trauma, surgery, or joint replacement	Osteomyelitis after joint replacement (i.e., hip or knee)	*Staphylococcus aureus* Organisms of low pathogenicity can be present such as coagulase-negative staphylococci *or Propionibacterium* spp.
	Sternal osteomyelitis (after open-heart procedure)	*Staphylococcus aureus* Coagulase-negative staphylococci Aerobic gram-negative bacteria
	Mandibular osteomyelitis (dental abscess)	Oral anaerobic flora
	Osteomyelitis secondary to pressure ulcer	*Staphylococcus aureus* Streptococci Gram negative bacteria Anaerobes are also commonly isolated especially when the ulcer involves the sacral or perianal area (i.e., *Bacteroides*)
Osteomyelitis secondary to vascular insufficiency: Soft-tissue infections and non-healing ulcers found on the plantar surface or between the toes that spread to bone	Osteomyelitis secondary to diabetes mellitus or peripheral vascular disease	Often polymicrobial, multiple organisms may be isolated including *Staphylococcus aureus*, coagulase-negative staphylococci, β-hemolytic streptococci, gram negative bacilli including *Pseudomonas* and anaerobic organisms.

In Mrs. K's case, a large ulcer that probes to bone with a high erythrocyte sedimentation rate is consistent with the diagnosis of osteomyelitis.

Tests
- WBC may or may not be elevated
- ESR greater than 70 (LR 11, CI 1.6–79)[2]

Imaging
- **Plain imaging**
  - Plain films show cortical erosion, periosteal reaction, or narrowing/widening of joint spaces.
  - Radiographic changes take at least two weeks to be visible on plain film; therefore the diagnosis of acute osteomyelitis cannot be excluded if plain films are negative.
  - Serial radiographs may be useful in more chronic cases.

- **Nuclear imaging**
  - Technetium, indium, and white blood cell scans are more sensitive than plain films for detecting osteomyelitis, but recent studies have shown that they lack specificity.[2]
- **MRI**
  - MRI is the preferred imaging study, with a sensitivity of 90% and specificity of 83% in all patients.
  - A positive MRI increases the likelihood of osteomyelitis (LR 3.8, 95% CI 2.5–5.8), while a normal MRI makes osteomyelitis much less likely (LR.14, 95% CI 0.08–0.26).[2]

Bone Biopsy
- The gold standard for diagnosing osteomyelitis and isolating the organism; important for guiding antimicrobial therapy.

- A swab taken from an open sinus tract or draining wound often detects only microorganisms colonizing the site and may not correlate with organisms infecting the bone. Therefore, a bone biopsy should be done and sent for aerobic and anaerobic culture, fungal, and mycobacterial cultures and histopathology.

EXPECTED DISEASE COURSE

- Acute osteomyelitis occurs over days to weeks, and patients often present with pain and possibly fever.
- Chronic osteomyelitis is a long-standing infection that persists for months to years as a result of necrotic bone, ongoing inflammation, and presence of microorganisms. Patients usually present with flares involving pain, erythema, swelling, drainage, and possibly fever.
- Most commonly, elderly patients suffer from chronic osteomyelitis secondary to diabetes or peripheral vascular disease, as described in the case of Mrs. K above; these patients may or may not have pain because of diabetic neuropathic changes.[4]

TREATMENT OPTIONS

Osteomyelitis is a difficult infection to treat. Most cases of osteomyelitis in the older adult are a form of chronic osteomyelitis, which is essentially incurable with medical therapy alone. The goal of therapy in many cases is therefore not to cure, but to arrest infection. Relapses and repeated infections are common. Surgical therapy is almost always needed for cure but may not be feasible or optimal due to host factors.

Nonpharmacologic

- In patients with underlying vascular insufficiency, restoring blood supply is a key part of management.
- Optimal nutrition, glucose control, and smoking cessation are particularly important in diabetic patients.
- Hyperbaric oxygen therapy is another forms of nonpharmacologic therapy in which oxygen is supplied to the wound to promote angiogenesis and rapid healing. Although no randomized clinical trials have been done, some retrospective studies and a few prospective studies

have shown encouraging results for this approach.[5]

Pharmacologic

- In acute osteomyelitis, antimicrobial therapy alone may be adequate. Four to six weeks of intravenous antibiotics are recommended based on animal studies that show that bone revascularization after debridement takes four weeks. If quinolones or other antibiotics with good oral bioavailability and bone penetration are used, then the transition to oral antibiotics may be made much earlier, for example after two weeks. Pathogen-specific antibiotic regimens are listed in Table 92.2.[3]
- In chronic osteomyelitis, appropriate therapy requires a combination of surgical management that includes adequate debridement and medical management with appropriate antimicrobial therapy.
- Patients with chronic osteomyelitis who do not undergo surgical debridement may experience relapses and recurrent infections. In certain situations, suppressive antimicrobial therapy may be given in order to prevent the development of complications and to avoid bacteremia and frequent hospitalizations.

PALLIATIVE CARE ISSUES

- Older adults often present with the following special circumstances that should prompt consideration of the non-surgical management option for osteomyelits:
  - The physician and patient agree that the surgical risks outweigh the benefit.
  - Surgery is not desirable because it may cause an unacceptable loss of function/limb.
  - Surgical approach is not concordant with the patient's goals for care.
- In these special circumstances, an alternative approach should be instituted. The treatment plan may include:
  - A discussion with the patient and family about the likely course of disease without surgical intervention (see Expected Disease Course, above)
  - Local wound care with daily inspection and dressing changes
  - Careful attention to pain and symptom management

TABLE 92.2: ANTIBIOTIC TREATMENT OF OSTEOMYELITIS IN ADULTS

Microorganism Isolated	Treatment of Choice[a]	Alternatives
Methicillin-sensitive *Staphylococcus aureus*	Nafcillin 2 gm IV every 6 hours or cefazolin 2 gm IV every 8 hours	Ceftriaxone 2 gm IV daily Ciprofloxacin 750 mg orally every 12 hours or levofloxacin in combination with rifampin 600 mg daily
Methicillin-resistant *S. aureus*	Vancomycin 1 gm IV every 12 hours	Trimethoprim-sulfamethoxazole (if sensitive)
Various streptococci (group A or B β-hemolytic)	Penicillin G (12–20 million units daily)	Ceftriaxone Vancomycin
Enteric gram-negative bacilli	Quinolone (i.e., ciprofloxacin 400–750 mg every 12 hours with early switch to oral)	Ceftriaxone
Serratia sp.; *Pseudomonas aeuroginosa*	Piperacillin-tazobactam 3.375 gm IV q6	Cefepime 2 gm IV every 12 hours Quinolone (if sensitive)
Anaerobes	Ampicillin-sulbactam 3.375 gm IV q6	Metronidazole 500 mg every 8 hours for gram-negative anaerobes
Mixed infection (aerobic and anaerobic microorganisms)	Ampicillin-sulbactam 3 gm IV every 6–8 hours	Imipenem 500 mg IV every 6 hours

Note: Lew DP, Waldvogel FA. Osteomyelitis. *Lancet.* 2004;364:369–379.
[a] All doses are given for normal hepatic/renal function; doses should be calculated using Cockcroft/Gault equation to take into account age and body weight.

- Measures aimed at pressure reduction (see Chapter 59: Pressure Ulcers)

SPECIAL SETTINGS

Vertebral Osteomyelitis

- Vertebral osteomyelitis is commonly seen in the elderly population and increases progressively with each successive decade of life; men are affected about twice as often as women.
- Sources of infection: An arterial route involving the segmental arteries supplying the vertebrae bifurcates; therefore two adjacent vertebrae and the intervertebral disk are commonly involved.
- Diagnosis is often made based on narrowing of the disk space or destruction of the vertebra, as seen by MRI or bone scan. Biopsy under CT guidance should be done and sent for routine aerobic and anaerobic culture, fungal, and mycobacterial culture.
- Treatment is based on the causative organism and usually lasts four to six weeks. Skeletal tuberculosis is treated with anti-tuberculosis

therapy for at least six months. The decision about whether surgical involvement is necessary should be based on the degree of bony destruction and need to manage complications such epidural or paraspinal abscesses requiring drainage, or emergency decompression for cord compression.[3]

- Prognosis: Neurological complications including motor weakness or paralysis or intractable pain related to bone destruction can occur, particularly in patients with cervical spine osteomyelitis. However, with prompt diagnosis and antibiotic treatment, mortality is low.

Prosthetic Joint Infections

- Prosthetic joint infections are often seen in elderly patients following total hip replacement or total knee replacement.
- Source and timing of infection: The first two years after joint replacement[3]
- Presentation: Prosthesis loosening with or without fever
- Diagnosis: ESR is often elevated, and imaging is used to differentiate between osteomyelitis and mechanical loosening.

- Treatment necessitates the removal of the prosthesis and debridement of involved bone. Cultures sent from the joint space are used to guide therapy, which usually involves four to six weeks of intravenous antibiotics, followed by replacement of the joint.[3]
- Prognosis: Surgical removal of the prosthesis can often result in significant morbidity and functional impairment in older patients. If the surgical risk or anticipated loss of function is deemed unacceptable, a conservative approach using suppressive antimicrobial therapy may be considered.

TAKE-HOME POINTS

- Osteomyelitis can be difficult to diagnose. In diabetic patients, the likelihood of osteomyelitis is increased with an ulcer larger than 2 cm, a positive probe-to-bone test, ESR greater than 70, and abnormal plain films. A negative MRI makes the diagnosis less likely.
- The gold standard for diagnosis of osteomyelitis is bone biopsy. Cultures are important for both diagnosis and choosing the correct antimicrobial to help guide therapy.

- Management of osteomyelitis requires a multidisciplinary approach that almost always includes antimicrobial therapy, surgical debridement, meticulous local wound care, and efforts to optimize other host factors.
- If surgery is not an option because risks outweigh the benefit, or if it is not concordant with patient goals and preference, a conservative approach should be instituted including pain and symptom management, local wound care with daily inspection and dressings, pressure reduction measures, and discussion of expected disease course.

REFERENCES

1. Butalia S, Palda VA, Sargeant RJ, Detsky AS, Pourad O. Does this patient with diabetes have osteomyelitis of the lower extremity? *JAMA*. Feb 20, 2008;*299*(7):806–813.
2. Lew DP, Waldvogel FA. Osteomyelitis. *Lancet*. 2004;*364*:369–379.
3. Calhoun JH, Manring MM. Adult osteomyelitis. *Infect Dis Clin North Am*. 2005;*19*:765–786.
4. Cunha BA. Osteomyelitis in elderly patients. *Clin Infect Dis*. 2002;*35*:287–293.
5. Lipsky BA, Berendt AR, Deery HG, et al. IDSA Guidelines. Diagnosis and treatment of diabetic foot infections. *Clin Infect Dis*. 2004;*39*:885–910.

93

Herpes Zoster in Older Adults

CASE

Mr. B, a 72-year-old male with a history of hypertension and osteoarthritis, presents to an outpatient clinic with four days of right-sided burning chest pain. The pain does not seem to be related to activity and is not associated with shortness of breath. The patient had been seen in an emergency room two days ago and had been discharged after an EKG and three serial cardiac enzyme measurements were found to be normal. This morning he noticed a vesicular rash beginning over his right chest and extending onto his right flank below the axilla.

DEFINITION

Herpes zoster (also referred to as "shingles") is a reactivation of varicella-zoster virus (VZV), the etiological agent of primary varicella infection or chicken pox.

PREVALENCE

- Prevalence and incidence increase with age, with an incidence of approximately one case per 1000 person-years in those between 20 and 30 years of age to over 10 cases per 1000 person-years in persons over the age of 85.[1]
- Approximately 50% of persons living to the age of 85 will experience at least one episode of herpes zoster.[1]

LIKELY ETIOLOGIES

VZV infects sensory nerve fibers during primary infection and establishes permanent latency in neuronal bodies located in regional sensory ganglia. It is reactivated in susceptible hosts.

RISK FACTORS

- History of primary varicella: Most adults over the age of over 40 have serological evidence of prior infection despite the fact that many will not remember or will deny a history of primary varicella.[1]
- Age: Risk increases with age

- Immunocompromised hosts:
  - Especially those with deficits in T-cell mediated immunity
  - Also HIV, lymphoproliferative diseases, solid organ or bone marrow transplantation
- Inflammatory diseases:
  - SLE, rheumatoid arthritis, Wegener's granulomatosis, Crohn's disease, and ulcerative colitis
  - Unclear if this is related to the actual disease process or its treatment[1]

DIAGNOSIS

Exam

- Herpes zoster is typically a clinical diagnosis based on the rash's characteristic appearance, distribution, associated prodrome, and time course of disease.
- The case presented above is a classic presentation of herpes zoster, which is typically characterized by a painful, vesicular rash in a unilateral, dermatomal distribution with occasional involvement of two or three adjacent dermatomes.
- The pain is frequently described as burning, throbbing, or stabbing and is often associated with tactile hyperesthesia, although occasionally pruritis is the dominant complaint. Pain generally precedes the appearance of the rash by several days and, depending on the sensory dermatome involved, can be confused with other acute medical conditions such as unstable angina (as in this case), cholecystitis, or renal colic.
- Although virtually any peripheral sensory nerve can be a source of reactivation, the most common sites in immunocompetent hosts are the thoracic sensory nerves, followed by the ophthalmic division of the trigeminal nerve (herpes zoster opthalmicus).

- Herpes zoster can present in atypical or severe forms, especially in patients with deficits in cell-mediated immunity. Examples include disseminated cutaneous disease (vesicles appearing at a distance or contralaterally from the original dermatome), meningoencephalitis, or visceral disease (e.g., pneumonitis, hepatitis, pancreatitis, etc.).[2,3]

Tests

Additional tests are helpful only in patients who present with atypical rash or disseminated disease. Relevant tests may include the following:

- Direct Fluorescent Antigen (DFA)
  - Involves skin scrapings
  - Provides rapid diagnosis
  - Detects both HSV and VZV
- Real-time Polymerase Chain Reaction (PCR)
  - Can be performed on a variety of clinical samples, hence particularly useful in patients with meningoencephalitis or visceral disease
  - Provides a faster turnaround time compared to cultures
- Viral Culture
  - Less useful because of its longer turnaround time

EXPECTED DISEASE COURSE

- Herpes zoster is transmitted via the airborne route and can cause primary varicella in susceptible contacts.
- Patients with zoster are infectious from the onset of the rash until the lesions crust. Transmission can be greatly reduced by covering the affected area.
- Patients should be advised to avoid contact with susceptible or immunocompromised persons until all of their lesions crust.[1]
- Patients should also be instructed on local care to skin lesions.

COMPLICATIONS

Most complications of herpes zoster are related to the specific area of involvement.

- Post-herpetic neuralgia (PHN): Persistence of pain after resolution of skin lesions:
  - Incidence: 18%, 13%, and 10% at 30, 60, and 90 days after resolution of the rash in the pre-vaccine era; increases with age;

approximately 20% of patients over the age of 80 experience PHN three months after resolution of rash.[4]
- PHN can be debilitating, leading to loss of employment, depression, social isolation, and increased medical costs. Bacterial superinfection of the vesicular lesions, typically with normal skin flora, can also occur.
- Herpes zoster opthalmicus:
  - Can affect almost all structures of the ipsilateral eye
  - Requires immediate evaluation by an ophthalmologist
  - Requires prompt antiviral therapy to prevent loss of vision
- Ramsey-Hunt syndrome:
  - May result from involvement of the mucocutaneous division of cranial nerve VII and/or VIII
  - Characterized by facial paralysis, associated hearing and vestibulatory symptoms, and vesicular lesions in the external auditory canal
  - Facial nerve involvement can occur without the presence of vesicular lesions.
- Other serious complications such as encephalitis, meningitis, retinitis, myelitis, or death are uncommon, and usually occur in immunocompromised hosts.

TREATMENT OPTIONS

- Systemic antiviral therapy, specifically with acyclovir, famciclovir, or valacyclovir, is the mainstay of treatment and has been shown to reduce viral shedding, duration of rash, and PHN.[3] (Box 93.1) Duration of treatment is usually seven days. Adjust dosing if renal function is impaired.
- The preferred medication for older adults is valacyclovir (or famciclovir) because of its convenient dosing schedule. Most common side effects include nausea and headache.
- Antiviral therapy is strongly recommended in immunocompetent patients with any of the following criteria:[3]
  - Age > 50
  - Nontruncal involvement
  - Moderate to severe pain and/or rash
  - Presentation within 72 hours of the onset of symptoms
- Given their benign side-effect profile, many experts recommend considering the use of antivirals in all patients with herpes

BOX 93.1   SYSTEMIC ANTIVIRAL THERAPY FOR HERPES ZOSTER

Medication	Dosage
Acyclovir	Oral dose: 800 mg five times/day IV Dose: 10 mg/kg every eight hours
Valacyclovir	Oral dose: 1000 mg three times/day
Famciclovir	Oral dose: 500 mg three times/day

zoster, even those at low risk for severe complications or those who present more than 72 hours after the onset of symptoms.[3]

- Oral therapy is appropriate in most cases of herpes zoster. Intravenous acyclovir is recommended in patients with serious or disseminated disease, depressed cell-mediated immunity, or herpes zoster opthalmicus. Consultation with an infectious diseases specialist is useful in these cases.

Role of Corticosteroids

- In a randomized, placebo-controlled study of immunocompetent adults over the age of 50 (median age: 61.2), adjunctive corticosteroids combined with acyclovir were shown to reduce the pain of acute neuritis, decrease analgesia use, accelerate the healing of vesicular lesions, and reduce the duration of time before resumption of normal activities. There was no effect on the development of PHN, however. It should be noted that patients at risk for complications related to steroids, such as those with diabetes and gastritis, were excluded.[5]
- Corticosteroids should also be considered in patients with facial paralysis or cranial nerve polyneuritis to improve motor outcomes.[3]

Management of Post-Herpetic Neuralgia (PHN)

- Nonsteroidal anti-inflammatory drugs are often used for PHN but with questionable effectiveness.

- Topical medications (lidocaine patches and capsaicin cream) have been used with some success.
- Opioids are useful in patients with severe or debilitating PHN. However, if there is little or no improvement despite appropriate titration, seek the expertise of a pain specialist.
- Tricyclic antidepressants (TCAs) can be tried in patients who do not respond to short courses of opioids. However, side effects may limit their use in older adults.[6,7] If it is an option, use TCAs with less anticholinergic property such as nortryptiline and desipramine.
- Gabapentin is approved by the FDA and frequently used for PHN. However, it often is effective only at high doses that may be associated with side effects, most notably sedation, in the elderly.[3]
- Long-term, intractable pain should be treated in collaboration with an experienced pain-management specialist.

PREVENTION

- A live vaccine for herpes zoster (Zostavax) is now licensed in the United States for use in adults at least 60 years old. In a large phase 3 trial of adults 60 years of age or older, vaccine recipients had a reduced risk from herpes zoster and PHN.
- Although the efficacy of the vaccine decreased with increasing age at vaccination, there was still benefit in all age groups.[8] There was no reduction in other complications associated with severe herpes zoster (e.g., bacterial super-infections, scarring, nerve palsies, or visceral complications). Side effects were mild and included injection site reactions.
- The Centers for Disease Control and Prevention (CDC) recommends routine administration of the herpes zoster vaccine in adults 60 years of age or older. The vaccine should not be administered to previously vaccinated patients, pregnant women, or patients with impaired cell-mediated immunity (e.g., uncontrolled AIDS, leukemia, solid organ transplant, receipt of high dose corticosteroids). However, it can be given to some patients receiving

certain immunosuppressant medications such as low-dose methotrexate, 6-MP, azathioprine, or corticosteroids.[1]

TAKE-HOME POINTS

- Herpes zoster is a common illness in the geriatric population.
- Antiviral medications are the mainstay of treating acute zoster.
- PHN can be treated with topical analgesics, gabapentin, opioids, and TCAs.
- Long-term, intractable pain should be treated in collaboration with an experienced pain-management specialist.
- Vaccination is recommended in all immunocompetent adults over the age of 60.

REFERENCES

1. Harpaz R, Ortega-Sanchez IR, Seward JF. Prevention of herpes zoster: recommendations of the Advisory Committee on Immunization Practices (ACIP). *MMWR Recomm Rep.* 2008;*57*(RR-5): 1–30; quiz CE2-4.

2. Wareham DW, Breuer J. Herpes zoster. *BMJ.* 2007;*334*(7605):1211–1215.

3. Dworkin RH et al. Recommendations for the management of herpes zoster. *Clin Infect Dis.* 2007;*44*(suppl 1):S1–S26.

4. Yawn BP et al. A population-based study of the incidence and complication rates of herpes zoster before zoster vaccine introduction. *Mayo Clin Proc.* 2007;*82*(11):1341–1349.

5. Whitley RJ et al. Acyclovir with and without prednisone for the treatment of herpes zoster. A randomized, placebo-controlled trial. The National Institute of Allergy and Infectious Diseases Collaborative Antiviral Study Group. *Ann Intern Med.* 1996;*125*(5):376–383.

6. McQuay HJ et al. A systematic review of antidepressants in neuropathic pain. *Pain.* 1996;*68*(2–3): 217–227.

7. Kost RG, Straus SE. Postherpetic neuralgia—pathogenesis, treatment, and prevention. *N Engl J Med.* 1996;*335*(1):32–42.

8. Oxman MN et al. A vaccine to prevent herpes zoster and postherpetic neuralgia in older adults. *N Engl J Med.* 2005;*352*(22):2271–2284.

94

HIV/AIDS

CASE

Mr. G is a 75-year-old man with a history of hypertension and atrial fibrillation on anticoagulation. He lives alone in his apartment and until recently has been able to perform all his activities of daily living, including cooking, cleaning, and shopping. He is accompanied his daughter, who has noticed a slow decline in his cognitive function. Because of this decline he undergoes a dementia workup, which includes folate, B12, TSH, RPR, and MRI of the brain. All findings are normal, including the MRI, which reveals only age-related atrophy. The patient is started on Aricept. When his son brings him in for follow-up, the patient reveals that he is bisexual and has remained sexually active. HIV testing is performed and he is found to be HIV-positive with CD4 count of 180.

DEFINITION

The *human immunodeficiency virus* (HIV) is a retrovirus that causes acquired immune deficiency syndrome (AIDS) by depleting T-helper cells. HIV progresses to AIDS usually over a period of 10 years. AIDS is defined as a CD4 < 200 and/or an AIDS-defining infection. Individuals with AIDS are at risk for opportunistic infections and some malignancies.

PREVALENCE

- The CDC estimates that 1.1 million adults and adolescents were living with diagnosed or undiagnosed HIV infection in the United States at the end of 2006.[1]
- Because of improved survival among HIV-infected individuals since the advent of Highly Active Antiretroviral Therapy (HAART), there has been a steady increase in the numbers of older adults living with HIV/AIDS.
- Adults age 50 and older accounted for approximately:
  - 10% of new HIV infections in the United States in 2006
  - 21% of AIDS diagnoses in 2006 and 2007

- 28% of persons living with HIV/AIDS in 2007
- 34% of those living with AIDS in 2007, up from 24% in 2003[2]
- Prevalence is likely underestimated in older adults due to delayed screening and recognition of HIV infection.

LIKELY ETIOLOGIES

- Infection with HIV occurs by transfer of blood, semen, pre-ejaculate, vaginal fluid, or breast milk.
- The major routes of transmission are unprotected sex, contaminated needles, breast milk, and vertical transmission.

RISK FACTORS

While virtually anyone can be infected with HIV, the greatest risk occurs in individuals who:

- Have unprotected sex with multiple partners, including same-sex and heterosexual partners
- Are men who have sex with men
- Have unprotected sex with someone who is known to be HIV-positive
- Have another sexually transmitted infection (e.g., herpes, syphilis, chlamydia, gonorrhea, bacterial vaginosis)
- Share needles during intravenous drug use
- Received a blood transfusion or blood products before 1985

Mr. G's initial evaluation did not reveal that he was still sexually active and that he has sex with both men and women. It is important to recognize that many geriatric patients are sexually active and may have risk factors associated with transmission of HIV. Some members of Mr. G's family were not aware of his HIV risk factors but were supportive when he received his diagnosis. His son was frustrated that it had taken the physicians so long to consider the diagnosis and to test his father.

OLDER ADULTS AND HIV

- Older individuals may be at risk for HIV for several reasons:
  - Aging of the HIV-infected population due to improved survival with HAART
  - Late recognition of HIV due to long incubation period
  - Newly acquired infection at an older age
- There is a misperception that older individuals are not sexually active. However, a 1999 AARP survey revealed that nearly 50% of all Americans age 60 or older engage in sexual activity at least once a month.[3] These older individuals may be at higher risk for sexually transmitted infections due to the following factors:
  - Decreased use of condoms because there is no longer a need for birth control
  - Age-related decrease in vaginal lubrication puts older women at increased risk of transmission
  - Increased sexual activity due to availability of medications to treat erectile dysfunction
  - Lack of knowledge about HIV, leading to increased fear and stigma, which may in turn inhibit honesty about sexual activity and delay treatment

DIAGNOSIS

History and Exam

- A complete history and physical should be performed for all patients, with particular attention given to both current and past sexual history, history of drug use, and history of sexually transmitted infections.
- For patients not known to be HIV-infected, HIV should nonetheless be considered by health care providers as part of the differential diagnosis.
- Many HIV-related conditions are nonspecific and overlap with geriatric conditions; these include memory loss, dementia, weight loss, anemia, diarrhea, loss of appetite, and unexplained fevers.
- Although HIV screening is not a routine part of a dementia workup, older adults with risk factors for HIV should be tested.

Mr. G had an extensive workup for memory loss before he was HIV-tested and was finally diagnosed with HIV dementia.

HIV Testing

- The CDC recommendations for HIV testing in all health care settings are as follows:
  - HIV screening is recommended for patients (age 13–64) in all health care settings, after the patient is notified that testing will be performed, and unless the patient declines.
  - Persons at high risk for HIV infection should be screened for HIV at least annually.
  - Separate written consent for HIV testing should not be required; general consent for medical care should be considered sufficient to encompass consent for HIV testing.
  - Prevention counseling should not be required with HIV diagnostic testing, or as part of HIV screening programs in health-care settings.
- Note that above are *recommendations* regarding HIV testing from the CDC. However, every state does require that a positive HIV test be reported to the relevant state department of health. All states now have confidential name-based reporting, and some states also have anonymous testing; the CDC collects this information from the individual state departments of health.
- Requirements for HIV testing and counseling and consent for HIV testing vary from state to state and can be found at the following site: http://www.nccc.ucsf.edu/consultation_library/state_hiv_testing_laws/.

Tests

- For patients with unknown HIV status: ELISA and western blot confirmatory test
- For patients with known HIV positive status, initial workup includes:
  - CD4 count
  - HIV viral load
  - Complete blood count
  - Complete metabolic panel
  - Hepatitis B and C serologies (risk factors for transmission are the same and there is often coinfection)
  - Toxoplasmosis IgG
  - CMV IgG
  - RPR
  - GC/Chlamydia screening

- Lipid panel
- Cervical pap smear for women
- Anal pap smear
- PPD

EXPECTED DISEASE COURSE

- Untreated HIV infection usually progresses to AIDS. The median incubation period from HIV infection until development of AIDS is approximately 10 years for young adults.
- HIV can progress to AIDS more rapidly in older adults. In addition, older adults are more likely to have AIDS at presentation and have a shorter mean time from diagnosis to death (6.3 months compared to 16.5 months).[4]
- AIDS is defined as a CD 4 <200 and/or an AIDS-defining infection. Individuals with AIDS are at risk for opportunistic infections—bacteria, viruses, fungi, and parasites—which are normally controlled in persons with intact immune systems but that become acute or chronic infections in a person with AIDS. Examples of common opportunistic infections are:
  - Pneumocystis jiroveci pneumonia (PCP)
  - Candidiasis (oral or esophageal)
  - Toxoplasmosis
  - Cryptococcus (usually cryptococcal meningitis)
  - Mycobacterium avium complex (MAC)
  - Cytomegalovirus (CMV)
  - Progressive multifocal leukoencephalopathy
  - Extrapulmonary or disseminated tuberculosis
- In addition to infection, individuals with AIDS are at risk for the following malignancies:
  - Invasive cervical cancer
  - Kaposi's sarcoma
  - Non-Hodgkin's lymphoma

PROGNOSIS

- Since the advent of effective therapy for HIV, people are living longer with HIV infection with relatively intact CD4 counts. People with HIV with a CD4 above 200 are not at risk for opportunistic infections associated with AIDS; however, they are at higher risk for tuberculosis and pneumococcal pneumonia.

- HIV-infected individuals are at higher risk than their noninfected peers for the following conditions:
  - Dyslipidemia
  - Hypogonadism
  - Osteopenia and osteoporosis
  - Diabetes mellitus
  - Coronary artery disease
  - Renal and hepatic dysfunction
  - Non-Hodgkin's lymphoma
  - Psychiatric illness
  - Neurocognitive impairment
- These conditions may be due to HIV itself, antiretroviral therapy, concomitant infection with chronic hepatitis B or C, and/or substance abuse. Many of these conditions occur in the non-HIV-infected population as well, but it is important to note that in HIV-infected adults, these conditions may be hastened or exacerbated by HIV (e.g., dementia) or long-term exposure to antiretrovirals (e.g., insulin resistance, lipids).

Mr. G had a gradual neurocognitive decline and developed other medical conditions that were initially attributed to his comorbid medical conditions. However, the diagnosis of AIDS (CD4 180) suggests that HIV may be playing a role in his dementia and that HIV treatment may be beneficial.

PALLIATIVE CARE ISSUES

Older individuals with HIV benefit from HIV treatment, just as younger patients do. However, there are several complicating issues particular to older adults with HIV.

- Polypharmacy: Older patients in general are more likely to be on a high number of medications. In addition, there is a decline in renal and hepatic function with advancing age, and the provider should be aware of potentially altered drug metabolism. Antiretrovirals for HIV treatment may add to the polypharmacy burden, reducing adherence and increasing side effects.
- Some patients may seek to discontinue medications because of disease progression and/or changing goals of care. In these situations, HAART medications may be discontinued without taper.
- Symptom burden: HIV/AIDS is associated with a significant level of physical and

psychological symptom distress that requires routine screening and expert management. These symptoms include:

- Depression: Depression is prevalent in the older HIV-positive population. One study found that depression in HIV-infected individuals over the age of 50 was related to increased HIV-associated stigma, increased loneliness, decreased cognitive functioning, and reduced level of energy.[5]
- Delirium: Delirium is the most common neuropsychiatric complication in hospitalized patients with AIDS. Occasionally, patients may present with early signs of delirium in the primary care setting. Clinicians should assess for delirium when there is a sudden change in a patient's cognitive functioning, consciousness, or behavior.
- Dementia: HIV itself has an effect on the central nervous system. Advanced age is associated with an increased risk of HIV-associated dementia as the first AIDS-defining illness.[6] It is also important to note that there has been an overall decrease in incidence of HIV dementia with the advent of HAART, so treatment of HIV may benefit neurocognitive functioning.[7]
- Health care disparities: In a resource-rich country such as the United States, HIV can be seen as a chronic illness managed with effective antiretroviral treatment. But it is important to understand that minority and disenfranchised populations (e.g., substance abuse, chronic mental illness) are both disproportionately affected by HIV and more likely to have HIV progress to AIDS. These populations have difficulties accessing and engaging in medical treatment, and adhering to an HIV regimen for many reasons, including lack of social support, depression, stigma, and poverty.

TREATMENT OPTIONS

Once the diagnosis of HIV was made, Mr. G was started on Atripla (a combination of three medications: efavirenz, tenofovir, and lamivudine), which was chosen for its efficacy and ease of use (one pill once a day). He became acutely more confused and dizzy. Workup for CNS infection was negative and his symptoms were attributed to the HIV medication. His mental status returned to baseline when *the Atripla was withdrawn. He was subsequently started on another antiretroviral regimen, which he tolerated well.*

Treatment Guidelines

The U.S. Department of Health and Human Services has published guidelines on initiation of therapy for individuals with an HIV infection.[8]

- *HIV testing and counseling*: Issued by Center for Disease Control and Prevention (CDC). "Revised Guidelines for HIV Counseling, Testing, and Referral" (http://www.cdc.gov/mmwr/pdf/rr/rr5019.pdf).
- *Antiretroviral therapy for adults*: Issued by U.S. Department of Health and Human Services. "Guidelines for the Use of Antiretroviral Agents in HIV-1 Infected Adults and Adolescents" (http://www.aidsinfo.nih.gov/ContentFiles/AdultandAdolescentGL.pdf) and http://aidsinfo.nih.gov/contentfiles/AA_Tables.pdf).
- *Opportunistic Infections:* Issued by U.S. Public Health Service and Infectious Disease Society of America (IDSA). "Guidelines for Preventing Opportunistic Infections Among HIV-Infected Persons" (http://www.cdc.gov/mmwr/PDF/rr/rr5108.PDF).
- *Mental Health*: Issued by New York State Department of Health AIDS Institute, in collaboration with Johns Hopkins University Division of Infectious Diseases. "The Role of the Primary Care Practitioner in Assessing and Treating Mental Health in Persons with HIV" (http://www.hivguidelines.org.php5-1.dfw1-2.websitetestlink.com/?page_id=353).

Pharmacologic Management

- Typically, a patient is started on three active HIV medications from at least two different classes of medications. In addition, depending on CD4 count, a patient may require prophylaxis for opportunistic infections. Treatment guidelines recommend that therapy be managed by a provider with HIV expertise because evidence demonstrates improved patient outcomes. Providers in rural or underserved areas should therefore work in conjunction with experts in the region.

- None of the current HIV medications is absolutely contraindicated in older adults. However, it is important to note that the medication efavirenz—one of the first-line non-nucleoside reverse transcriptase inhibitors (NNRTI)—can cause neuropsychiatric side effects and dizziness. These side effects may exacerbate pre-existing conditions in the older patient (e.g., dementia).

MANAGING SYMPTOMS TO IMPROVE QUALITY OF LIFE

- Patients with HIV may not have any specific symptoms related to their diagnosis, especially if they have a CD4 > 200. However, patients with AIDS (CD4 < 200) may experience some of the symptoms described in Table 94.1,

often due to concurrent opportunistic infections.
- Often the symptoms can be managed through diagnosing and treating the opportunistic infection and treating the HIV itself.
- Some of the symptoms can be related to the side effect profile of the HIV medications.

RESOURCES

Older adults with HIV benefit from resources specifically targeted to their age demographic. The following is a list of resources for individuals over the age of 50 dealing with issues surrounding HIV infection, including a new diagnosis of HIV:

- National Association on HIV Over Fifty (NAHOF)
  Jim Campbell 617-233-7107
  www.hivoverfifty.org

TABLE 94.1: MANAGEMENT OF AIDS SYMPTOMS

Symptoms	Management
Fatigue	Treat HIV infection Screen for depression and refer and treat (*See also Chapter 30: Fatigue*)
Dysphagia Odynophagia	Treat HIV infection Look for oral thrush (candida) and treat empirically for thrush If treatment for candiasis does not alleviate symptoms, obtain EGD to rule out HSV, CMV, or aphthous ulcers (*See also Chapter 49: Dysphagia*)
Diarrhea	Treat HIV infection Workup for infectious diarrhea including clostridium difficile and ova and parasites and treat if appropriate If patient has CD4 < 50, workup additionally for MAI and CMV- related diarrhea and treat if appropriate Evaluate as possible side effect of HIV medications and consider changing regimen (*See also Chapter 46: Diarrhea*)
Hiccups	(*See also Chapter 52: Hiccups*)
Neuropsychiatric disorders	Rule out infection, especially with CD4 < 50 (e.g., PML) Treat HIV infection
Pain	(*See Chapter 29: Management of Pain in Older Adults*)
Pruritis	(*See Chapter 60: Pruritis*)
Sleep disturbances	Evaluate for possible side effect of HIV medications and consider changing regimen (*See also Chapter 36: Sleep Disorders*)
Wasting and anorexia	Treat HIV infection Rule out MAI (common cause of wasting) and treat if appropriate (*See also Chapter 42: Anorexia/Cachexia*)
Xerostomia/dry mouth	(*See Chapter 47: Mucositis*)

- New York Association on HIV Over Fifty
  Katy Nokes, PhD 212-481-7594 or
  kathynokes@aol.com
  www.nyahof.org
- HIV Wisdom for Older Women
  Jane P. Fowler 913-722-3100
  or jane@hivwisdom.org
  www.hivwisdom.org
- Chicago Association on HIV Over Fifty
  William W. Rydwels 773-283-0101
- Senior HIV Intervention Project (SHIP) in
  three Florida counties:
  Broward: 954-467-4779
  Dade: 305-377-5022
  Palm Beach: 561-586-4843
- American Association of Retired
  Persons (AARP)
  Social Outreach and Support (SOS)
  601 E Street, NW, Washington, DC 20049
  202-434-2260
  http://www.aarp.org
- National Institute on Aging
  http://www.nih.gov/nia/

TAKE-HOME POINTS

- Geriatric patients are at risk for HIV/AIDS.
  Physicians should be screening patients
  for sexual activity and reinforcing safe-sex
  behaviors.
- Consider HIV in differential diagnosis
  and remember that nonspecific symptoms
  experienced by older adults may overlap
  with symptomatic HIV.
- Increased survival of HIV-infected
  individuals has led to a growing prevalence
  of older adults with HIV.
- Older adults derive significant benefit from
  HIV treatment.
- Older adults may have less information
  on HIV risks and may be less willing to

disclose high-risk behaviors, and so it is
important for clinicians to provide HIV
education, testing, and prevention.
- Physical, mental health, and social support
  issues should be incorporated into HIV
  primary care.
- HIV AIDS is associated with a high burden
  of physical and psychological symptom
  distress requiring routine screening and
  expert clinical management.

REFERENCES

1. CDC. HIV Prevalence Estimates—United States,
   2006. *MMWR* 2008;*57*(39):1073–1076.
2. Centers for Disease Control and Prevention. HIV/
   AIDS Surveillance Report, 2007. Vol. 19. Atlanta:
   U.S. Department of Health and Human Services,
   Ceneters for Disease Control and Prevention;
   2009:1–63.
3. Jacoby S. Great sex: special report: the 1999 AARP/
   Modern Maturity survey on sexual attitudes and
   behavior. *Modern Maturity.* Sep-Oct 1999.
4. Shah S, Mildvan D. HIV and aging. *Curr Infect Dis
   Rep.* 2006;*8*:241–247.
5. Grov C, Golub SA, et al. Loneliness and
   HIV-related stigma explain depression among
   older HIV-positive adults. *AIDS Care.* 2010;16:
   1–10, i.
6. Janssen RS, Nwanyanwu OC, Selik RM, et al.
   Epidemiology of human immunodeficiency virus
   encephalopathy in the United States. *Neurology.*
   1992;*42*:1472–1476.
7. Saktor N, Lyles RH, Skolasky R, et al. HIV-associated
   neurologic disease incidence changes: Multicenter
   AIDS Cohort Study, 1990-1998. *Neurology.* Jan 23,
   2001;*56*(2):257–260.
8. Appelbaum JS. Chapter 3.1: HIV and Aging.
   In: Hardy D, ed. *AAHIVM Fundamentals of HIV
   Medicine: 2010-2011.* Washiington, DC:American
   Academy of HIV Medicine; 2010:2–8.

95

Skin Cancer

PART A: BASAL CELL CARCINOMA

Case

A 78-year-old Caucasian male with past medical history of coronary artery disease, hypercholesterolemia, and dementia presents with a lesion of the right nose. He is of Northern European extraction. On exam, a pearly papule with rolled borders and central ulceration is present on the right nasal ala and cheek. These findings triggered a total body skin examination, which revealed sun damage of the chest. Biopsy of the papule revealed an infiltrating basal cell carcinoma. The tumor was excised with three stages of Mohs micrographic surgery, as some perineural invasion was present. The defect was repaired with a bilobed transposition flap. The patient will follow up in three months to check for local recurrence. Caretakers were counseled on sun avoidance and sun protection.

DEFINITION

Basal cell carcinoma (BCC) is a slow-growing form of non-melanoma skin cancer that starts from cells that originate in the basal layer of the epidermis. It is painless, may bleed and ulcerate, but rarely metastasizes. The majority of these cancers occur on sun-exposed skin, especially on the face and most frequently on the nose.

PREVALENCE

- BCC accounts for approximately 80% of all skin cancers and 25% of all cancers diagnosed in the United States.[1,2]
- Formerly more common in elderly individuals but is increasingly more frequent in those under 50 years of age[1,2]

RISK FACTORS

- Overexposure to ultraviolet light and other forms of radiation (including therapeutic radiation)[1-3]

- Light-colored skin; blue or green eyes; blond or red hair; inability to tan[1-3]
- Northern European ancestry[2]

DIAGNOSIS

Presentation

- May appear as a skin papule that is pearly or waxy, white or light pink, flesh-colored or brown (rarely)
- A skin bump that is non-healing, friable, has irregular blood vessels in or around it, is ulcerated, swollen, bleeds easily, is crusted, or has a depressed center
- Appearance of a scar-like sore without having injured the area

Exam

Examine the size, shape, color, and texture of any suspicious areas.

Tests

Refer to a dermatologist for a biopsy if there are any lesions of concern.

EXPECTED DISEASE COURSE

BCC rarely metastasizes. However, if left untreated it can cause local invasion and destruction of surrounding areas and nearby tissues and bone. This is most worrisome around the nose, eyes, and ears. Early detection and treatment usually leads to a cure.

TREATMENT OPTIONS

Treatment varies depending on the size, depth, and location of the BCC.

- Biopsy-proven lesions will be removed using one of the procedures shown in Table 95.1.
- Nonsurgical treatment modalities for BCC include topical agents, photodynamic therapy, and radiation therapy. Examples are shown in Table 95.2.

TABLE 95.1: SURGICAL TREATMENTS FOR BCC

Surgical Treatment	Indications	Side Effects/Benefits	Prognosis
Surgical excision	Aggressive tumor on trunk or extremities[2]	Scarring Rapid healing Allows for histological evaluation compared to non-excisional treatments[1-3]	Up to 10% recurrence rate[1-3]
Electrodessication and curettage	Non-aggressive tumor on trunk or extremities[2]	Scarring, slow-healing No tissue removed for histological confirmation of cure Scar tissue may obscure recurrence Maximum tissue conservation[1-3]	Up to 10% recurrence rate[1-3]
Mohs micrographic surgery (MMS)	Aggressive tumor on trunk or extremities[2] Tumor location in high-risk anatomic site (e.g., periorbital, canthus, nasolabial fold, postauricular area, etc)[1,2] Tumor size >2 cm[1-3] Recurrent lesions of any size or location[1-3]	Expensive Highest cure rate, maximum tissue conservation, high cosmetic acceptability[1-3]	Recurrence rate of 1% for primary BCCs[1,3]
Cryosurgery	Nonrecurrent lesions <1 cm[3,4]	No tissue removed for histological confirmation of cure, tissue necrosis, edema, and blister formation; eschar formation (may last up to 4 weeks); pigment loss; hypertrophic scarring Cost-effective, minimal time requirements[1-3]	Up to 10% recurrence rate[1-3]

PREVENTION

- The best way to prevent skin cancer is to reduce exposure to UV light. Ultraviolet light is most intense at midday. Protect the skin by wearing hats, long-sleeved shirts, or pants.
- Always use sunscreen. Apply broad-spectrum sunscreens with SPF (sun protection factor) ratings of at least 15.
- Look for sunscreens that block both UVA and UVB light, and reapply every 1–2 hours.
- Use sunscreens in winter (e.g., facial moisturizer with SPF 15 sunscreen).
- Examine skin regularly for development of suspicious growths, non-healing lesions, or those with changes in color, size, texture, or appearance.
- People with a history of BCC should follow up every three to six months with a dermatologist.

TAKE-HOME POINTS

- Basal cell carcinoma (BCC) is a slow-growing form of non-melanoma skin cancer that typically occurs on sun-exposed skin (primarily on the face and especially on the nose).
- BCC rarely metastasizes, but if left untreated can be locally invasive and destructive of surrounding areas and nearby tissues, including bone.
- Early detection and treatment usually results in cure.

REFERENCES

1. Rubin AI, Chen EH, Ratner D. Basal-cell carcinoma. *N Engl J Med.* 2005;353:2262–2269.
2. Wolff K, Goldsmith LA, Katz SI, Gilchrest BA, Paller AS, Leffell DJ, eds. *Fitzpatrick's Dermatology in General Medicine.* New York: McGraw-Hill Professional; 2007.

TABLE 95.2: NON-SURGICAL TREATMENTS FOR BCC

Treatment	Indications	Side Effects
Topical agent		
Imiquimod (Aldara®)	FDA-approved for superficial BCC[1,4,5]	Local skin reactions including erythema, pruritus, pain, and erosion of the treated area (indicative of efficacy)[4,5]
5-Fluorouracil (Efudex®)	FDA-approved for superficial BCC, also used when multiple lesions preclude surgical options[4,5]	Local skin reactions including erythema, pruritus, pain, and erosion of the treated area (indicative of efficacy)[4,5]
Photodynamic therapy (PDT)		
Photodynamic therapy (e.g., aminolevulinic acid in combination with blue light)	As an adjunct to surgical procedures and/or radiation[3]	Painful burning sensation during treatment; edema post-treatment (may last up to one week), erythema (may last up to two weeks), high recurrence rates[1-3]
Radiation Therapy (XRT)		
Radiation	Large lesions on areas not amenable to closure or graft Positive postsurgical margins Palliation of metastatic BCC Patients who cannot tolerate or prefer non-surgical treatment[2,3,6,7] *Note:* Cannot be used in basal cell nevus syndrome or xeroderma pigmentosum[6]	Deteriorating cosmetic results over long term, inferior cosmesis overall, prolonged treatment course (i.e., requires multiple visits), no tissue removed for histological confirmation of cure, and up to 10% recurrence rate[2,3,6].

3. Bolognia JL, Lorizzo JL, Rapini RP, eds. *Dermatology*. New York: Mosby; 2003.
4. Galiczynski EM, Vidimos AT. Nonsurgical treatment of nonmelanoma skin cancer. *Dermatol Clin.* 2011;29:297–309.
5. Love WE, Bernhard JD, Bordeaux JS. Topical imiquimod or fluorouracil therapy for basal and squamous cell carcinoma: a systematic review. *Arch Dermatol.* 2009;145:1431–1438.
6. Hulyalkar R, Rakkhit T, Garcia-Zuazaga J. The role of radiation therapy in the management of skin cancers. *Dermatol Clin.* 2011;29:287–296.
7. Martinez JC, Otley CC. The management of melanoma and nonmelanoma skin cancer: a review for the primary care physician. *Mayo Clin Proc.* 2001;76(12):1253–1265.

PART B: SQUAMOUS CELL CARCINOMA

Case

A 63-year-old male with no contributory past medical history comes to your office for a routine health maintenance exam. You cannot help but notice various dry, scaly lesions of his dorsal hands and forearms. Your questioning about past sun exposure reveals that he was a recreational sailor since he was a boy. On exam, multiple hyperkeratotic papules of the scalp and helices of the ears, dorsal hands, and forearms are present, along with one particularly red lesion of the left forearm. Biopsy reveals squamous cell carcinoma in situ (Bowen's disease). He declines surgery but agrees to apply imiquimod cream daily to this lesion, as well as to allowing you to perform cryotherapy to the numerous actinic keratoses of his scalp, ears, forearms, and hands. At his one month follow-up, the Bowen's disease has resolved. You negotiate treatment of his scalp, ears, forearms, and hands with 5-fluorouracil cream twice daily in hope of resolving the numerous actinic keratoses as well as any subclinical lesions. Finally, you also choose to perform cryotherapy at one cycle of 10–15 seconds to the worst actinic keratoses. He is scheduled to follow up again in three months.

DEFINITION

Squamous cell carcinoma (SCC) is a form of non-melanoma skin cancer that originates in skin cells above the basal layer of the epidermis. Unlike basal cell carcinoma (BCC), it can grow faster and metastasize to other locations, including other organs. While rarely lethal, SCC can nonetheless cause significant morbidity.

FORMS OF SCC

- Actinic (solar) keratosis ("AK"):
  - Precursor lesion to SCC
  - Rate of transformation to SCC is estimated to be 1% to 20% over 10 years.[1,2]
  - Appears clinically as a rough, scaly, red plaque or papule on sun-exposed areas of the body, including the scalp, face, ears, forearms, and backs of hands (often better felt than seen)
- Keratoacanthoma:
  - Rapidly-growing form of SCC that forms a mound-like lesion with a central crater and frequently grows back to the same shape after incomplete excision
- Actinic cheilitis:
  - Precursor lesion to SCC, involving the lip (usually vermillion border of lower lip). Lesions typically are dry, scaly, and painless, with a mixture of white discoloration and erythema.
- Bowen's disease (SCC in situ):
  - Appears as scaly patches on sun-exposed parts of the trunk and extremities
  - On the penis, human papilloma virus types 16, 18, 31, & 33 can induce SCC in situ, called erythroplasia of Queyrat.[1-4]

PREVALENCE

SCC is the second most common non-melanoma skin cancer after BCC.[1,3]

RISK FACTORS

SCC is most often seen in people over the age of 50. Other risk factors include:

- Light-colored skin; blue or green eyes; blond or red hair[2,3]
- Overexposure to UV light and other forms of radiation (including therapeutic radiation)[1-4]
- Exposure to chemicals including arsenic, tar, paraffin, or coal[1]
- Smoking history[2,3]
- Predisposing conditions include scarring processes such as burns, leg ulcers, discoid lupus, hidradenitis suppurativa, and scars (Marjolin's ulcer)[1-4]

- Human papilloma virus (HPV), especially types 16, 18, 31, and 33[1-4]
- Immunosuppression (especially transplant patients)[1-3]

RISK FACTORS ASSOCIATED WITH METASTASIS[1]

- Location: Lips, ears, areas of inflammation or injury
- Size > 2 cm in diameter
- Histology reveals poor differentiation, perineural involvement, or tumor depth > 4 mm.
- Immunosuppression
- Local recurrence

DIAGNOSIS

Presentation

- Cutaneous SCCs most frequently occur on sun-exposed skin (face, neck, arms, scalp, backs of the hands, and ears). They can also occur on the lips, inside the mouth, on the genitalia, and other locations on the body.
- SCCs usually appear as a) crusted, scaly, or hyperkeratotic papule or plaque on the skin with a red, inflamed base; b) growing tumor, sometimes weeping; c) non-healing ulcer; d) change in an existing wart, mole, or other skin lesion; or e) cutaneous horn.
- Careful attention should also be paid to the regional lymph nodes draining the anatomical region on which the SCC is found.

Exam

Examine the size, shape, color, and texture of any suspicious areas.

Tests

- Refer to a dermatologist for a biopsy if there are any lesions of concern.
- Advanced disease may require imaging:
  - CT to evaluate for lymph node involvement
  - MRI to evaluate for nerve as well as head and neck involvement

PROGNOSIS

- SCC is usually locally destructive. If left untreated, SCC can metastasize.
- The majority of SCC tumors can be cured by prompt removal.

TABLE 95.3: AJCC TNM STAGING OF SCC[5]

TNM Stage	Tumor	Node	Metastasis
0	In situ	N0	M0
I	T1	N0	M0
II	T2	N0	M0
III	T3	N0 or N1	M0
	T1 or T2	N1	M0
IV	T1, T2 or T3	N2	M0
	Any T	N3	M0
	T4	Any N	M0
	Any T	Any N	M1

	Primary Tumor (T) **T0**: No evidence of primary tumor **T1**: Tumor ≤2 cm **T2**: Tumor >2 cm but ≤ 5 cm **T3**: Tumor with invasion of maxilla, mandible, orbit, or temporal bone **T4**: Tumor with invasion of skeleton or perineural invasion of skull base	**Regional Lymph Nodes (N)** **N0**: No regional lymph node metastasis **N1**: Solitary ipsilateral lymph node, <3 cm in greatest dimension **N2**: Metastasis in single ipsilateral lymph node, >3 cm but not >6 cm; or multiple ipsilateral lymph nodes, none >6 cm; arm bilateral or contralateral lymph nodes, none >6 cm	**M0**: No distant metastasis **M1**: Distant metastasis present

[5]Adapted from Edge SE, Byrd DR, Compton CC, et al. *AJCC Cancer Staging Manual.* New York, NY: Springer; 2009.

- Stage I and II SCC of the head and neck have a five-year survival in the range of 95%; Stage III and IV have a five-year survival of < 50%.[6]

TREATMENT OPTIONS

Treatment depends on tumor size, location, and extent of spread. See Table 95.3 for clinical staging guidelines.

Non-Surgical

Non-surgical treatment modalities for SCC include topical agents and radiation therapy. Examples are shown in Table 95.4.

Surgical

Please see surgical treatments for BCC above.

TAKE-HOME POINTS

- Unlike basal cell carcinoma, squamous cell carcinoma can metastasize. Therefore, prevention and early treatment are important.

- Any lesions of concern should be referred to a dermatologist for evaluation.
- After diagnosis and removal of SCC, patients should be closely monitored for new tumors. Suggested frequency of skin surveillance is every three months for two years, and then every six months for life.
- In transplant patients with a large number of actinic keratoses, daily acitretin (10-25 mg orally) can be used to suppress SCC development; however, discontinuation of the medication can cause rebound worsening of existing lesions and/or development of more numerous and more aggressive lesions.

REFERENCES

1. Alam M, Ratner D. Cutaneous squamous-cell carcinoma. *N Engl J Med.* 2001;344:975–983.
2. Bolognia JL, Lorizzo JL, Rapini RP, eds. *Dermatology.* New York: Mosby; 2003.
3. Wolff K, Goldsmith LA, Katz SI, Gilchrest BA, Paller AS, Leffell DJ, eds. *Fitzpatrick's Dermatology*

TABLE 95.4: NON-SURGICAL TREATMENT FOR SCC

Treatment	Indications	Side Effects
Topical agent		
5-fluorouracil (5-FU, Carac®, Efudex®, Fluorplex®)	SCC in situ (off-label use); actinic keratosis/AK (SCC precursor lesion)[7-9]	Erythema and erosion of AK and SCC lesions; may last up to two weeks; identifies subclinical actinic keratoses in the treated area
Imiquimod (Aldara®)	SCC in situ (off-label use); actinic keratosis/AK (SCC precursor lesion)[7-9]	Erythema and erosion of AK and SCC lesions; may last up to two weeks; identifies subclinical actinic keratoses in the treated area
Acitretin (Soriatane®)	Transplant patients with a large number of AKs. Can be used to suppress SCC development[8]	Discontinuation can cause rebound worsening of existing lesions and/or development of more numerous and more aggressive lesions
Radiation Therapy		
Radiation	Large lesions on areas not amenable to closure or graft Positive postsurgical margins Palliation of metastatic SCC Patients who cannot tolerate or prefer non-surgical treatment[10,11]	Deteriorating cosmetic results over long term; inferior cosmesis overall; prolonged treatment course (i.e., requires multiple visits); no tissue removed for histological confirmation of cure; up to 10% recurrence rate

in General Medicine. New York: McGraw-Hill Professional; 2007.

4. James WD, Berger TG, Elston D, eds. *Andrews' Diseases of the Skin Clinical Dermatology*. New York: W.B. Saunders Company; 2005.

5. Edge SB, Compton CC, et al. *AJCC Cancer Staging Manual*. New York: Springer; 2009.

6. Gurudutt VV, Genden EM. Cutaneous squamous cell carcinoma of the head and neck. *J Skin Cancer*. 2011;*2011*:502–723.

7. Galiczynski EM, Vidimos AT. Nonsurgical treatment of nonmelanoma skin cancer. *Dermatol Clin*. 2011;*29*:297–309.

8. Lebwohl MG, Heymann W, Berth-Jones J, Coulson I,, eds. *Treatment of Skin Disease Comprehensive Therapeutic Strategies*. New York: Mosby; 2002.

9. Love WE, Bernhard JD, Bordeaux JS. Topical imiquimod or fluorouracil therapy for basal and squamous cell carcinoma: a systematic review. *Arch Dermatol*. 2009;*145*:1431–1438.

10. Hulyalkar R, Rakkhit T, Garcia-Zuazaga J. The role of radiation therapy in the management of skin cancers. *Dermatol Clin*. 2011;*29*:287–296.

11. Martinez JC, Otley CC. The management of melanoma and nonmelanoma skin cancer: a review for the primary care physician. *Mayo Clin Proc*. 2001;*76*(12):1253–1265.

PART C: MELANOMA

Case

A 71-year-old Caucasian male presents with a cough. Past medical history is significant for chronic obstructive pulmonary disease. Upon auscultation of his chest, you notice a variety of hyperpigmented macules, with one that is particularly dark and irregular. Upon further questioning, he recalls getting several blistering sunburns in his youth. On exam, an oval brown-black macule with irregular borders and asymmetry, about 13 mm in diameter, is noted on his left chest. Lymph nodes, liver, and spleen are normal. The remainder of his total body skin exam is unremarkable. The lesion is too large for you to excise; however, punch biopsy of the darkest area reveals a thin melanoma, 0.25 mm in depth. You refer him to a surgeon for definitive excision with 1 cm margins. He is scheduled to follow up with you in three months and is encouraged to avoid excess sun and to perform self-skin exams monthly.

DEFINITION

Melanoma is a malignant proliferation of melanocytes. It arises mostly from cutaneous melanocytes but can also arise from melanocytes of the mucosal epithelium, retina, and leptomeninges. (Note: Moles (aka "nevi") are benign proliferations of melanocytes. Most are benign, but dysplastic nevi are potential precursors of melanoma.)

PREVALENCE
- In the United States, melanoma is the fifth most common cancer diagnosed among men and the seventh most common cancer diagnosed among women.[1]
- Accounts for < 5% of all skin cancers[1-3]
- Accounts for > 75% of skin cancer deaths[1-3]
- May affect individuals at any age, but incidence increases with age and is highest among individuals in their 70s and 80s.[4]

RISK FACTORS[1-3]
- Numerous dysplastic nevi
- Personal history of melanoma
- Family history of melanoma
- Immunosuppression
- History of excessive exposure to UV light
- Fair complexion, light skin, and blond/red hair
- Xeroderma pigmentosum
- Personal history of pancreatic cancer (CDKN2A gene)
- Most common location: back in men; lower extremities in women
- Palms and soles of darker skin types

DIAGNOSIS

Presentation
Moles or lesions exhibiting the following criteria should be considered warning signs of early melanoma:

- Asymmetry (one-half of lesion appears different from other half)
- Border irregularity (blurry or ragged edges)
- Color change (more than two colors or non-uniform pigmentation)
- Diameter > 6 mm (equal to or greater than the size of a pencil eraser)
- Evolving (changes in lesion over time)

History and Exam
- Initial interview of a patient suspected of having melanoma should include:

- Thorough medical history of the risk factors
- Focus on size, shape, color, and texture of the lesion(s) of concern
- A survey of the entire body looking for other potential lesions and for lymphadenopathy
- A helpful clue is the "Ugly Duckling Sign"—a mole that does not look like a group of similar-looking moles.
- If melanoma is suspected, refer to a dermatologist.

Biopsy
- The dermatologist is likely to diagnose a suspected melanoma with the use of dermoscopy (surface microscopy) followed by a biopsy.
- Punch biopsy allows for depth, a prognostic indicator, to be measured properly. Shave biopsies of pigmented lesions should be avoided. *Note*: Misdiagnosis is more likely when non-dermatologists perform biopsies, or when non-dermatopathologists read the histopathology from a suspect lesion.

Staging Work-Up
Once a patient is diagnosed with a melanoma that is > 1mm in depth, staging workup should include:

- Presence or absence of ulceration
- Mitotic rate
- LDH (two readings, 24 hours apart)
- Chest X-ray and CT scan with contrast (chest, abdomen, pelvis)
- MRI (brain)
- Sentinel lymph node biopsy (SLNB), which helps with staging and prognosis but not with therapy

Staging and Survival
Table 95.5 outlines clinical staging and five-year survival rates for patients with melanoma.

TREATMENT OPTIONS
- A treatment plan should be developed after a comprehensive assessment and in discussion with patient and family.
- Considerations influencing treatment decisions include performance status, stage of disease, safety of surgical intervention,

TABLE 95.5: AJCC MELANOMA CLINICAL STAGING SYSTEM[5] AND SURVIVAL[†]

TNM Stage	Tumor	Node	Metastasis	5-year Survival[†]
0	Tis	N0	M0	99.9%
IA	T1a	N0	M0	97%
IB	T1b	N0	M0	92%
	T2a	N0	M0	
IIA	T2b	N0	M0	81%
	T3a	N0	M0	
IIB	T3b	N0	M0	70%
	T4a	N0	M0	
IIC	T4b	N0	M0	53%
III	Any T	N > N0	M0	
IIIA	Note: Stages IIIA-IIIC are staged pathologically after partial or complete lymphadenectomy and include information about the nodal metastatic burden: micrometastasis,* macrometastasis,[†] and in-transit metastases/satellites without metastatic nodes.			78%
IIIB				59%
IIIC				40%
IV	Any T	Any N	M1	15% to 20%

Primary Tumor (T)	No. of metastatic nodes and metastatic burden:
T1: Thickness ≤1.0 mm	**N0:** No metastatic node, no metastatic burden
a: without ulceration and mitosis <1/mm^2	**N1:** 1 metastatic node
b: with ulceration and mitosis ≥1/mm^2	**N2:** 2–3 metastatic nodes
T2: Thickness between 1.01 and 2.00 mm	**N3:** 4+ metastatic nodes, or matted nodes, or in transit
a: without ulceration	metastases/satellites with metastatic nodes
b: with ulceration	*Micrometastases are diagnosed after sentinel lymph
T3: Thickness between 2.01 and 4.00 mm	node biopsy.
a: without ulceration	[†]Macrometastates are nodal metastases that
b: with ulceration	can be detected clinically but are confirmed
T4: Thickness > 4.00mm	histopathologically.
a: without ulceration	
b: with ulceration	

[5]Adapted from Balch CM, Gershenwald JE, et al. Final version of 2009 AJCC melanoma staging and classification. *J Clin Oncol.* 2009;27:6199–206. [†]Survival rates for melanoma. American Cancer Society. www.cancer.org. Retrieved April 25, 2011.

risks and benefits of adjuvant therapy, and patient's informed preferences.

Surgical

- Surgical excision with a wide margin (aka "wide local excision") followed by histologic confirmation of tumor-free margins is standard therapy for primary cutaneous melanoma[3,6] (Table 95.6).
- Sentinel lymph node biopsy (SLNB) (and/or lymph node dissection, if necessary)[1,3,6]
- Once melanoma is metastatic, surgery is used to decrease tumor burden and relieve symptoms, but is rarely curative.[6]

Chemotherapy

- There are chemotherapy regimens available to treat advanced melanoma (e.g. brain metastases) (Table 95.7). These agents can relieve burdensome symptoms and may also extend survival in some patients.
- Because the effectiveness of these treatments is limited, careful consideration should be given to an analysis of the risks vs. benefits of treatment. Factors include prognosis, goals for care, comorbidities, and the patient's preference for aggressive therapy or desire to avoid the toxicities associated with chemotherapy.

TABLE 95.6: SURGICAL MARGINS FOR
MELANOMA[1]

Primary Tumor Thickness	Recommended Excision Margins
Melanoma *in situ*	5 mm
≤ 1.00 mm	1 cm
> 1.00 mm–2.00 mm	1 cm–2 cm
> 2.00 mm	2 cm

- The following treatment approaches are also available, but they have not been proven to extend overall survival in randomized trials:
  - Biochemotherapy or chemoimmunotherapy: Combines chemotherapy with immunotherapy in Stage IV patients. Commonly used drugs include interleukin-2 and ipilimumab.
  - Isolated Limb Perfusion (ILP): Regional chemotherapy (typically with melphalan). Used to treat multiple, advanced, in-transit melanoma lesions when surgical resection is not possible.

- Clinical trials are also being conducted to test effectiveness of new chemotherapeutic agents and melanoma vaccines.

PALLIATIVE CARE ISSUES

- The common sites of metastatic melanoma are lymph nodes, lung, liver, brain, bone, and GI tract. Brain metastasis usually occurs late in Stage IV disease and is associated with the worst prognosis.
- Treatment goals for metastatic melanoma include controlling spread of disease, prolonging survival, and aggressive management of symptoms associated with the disease process and treatment regimens.
- Symptoms associated with advanced melanoma include pain, fatigue, shortness of breath, anorexia, cachexia, and constipation or diarrhea. Management of disease or treatment related symptoms should be a key focus of the comprehensive care plan. (See Chapter 29: Management of Pain in Older Adults, Chapter 30: Fatigue, Chapter 40: Cough and Secretions, Chapter 42: Anorexia/Cachexia,

TABLE 95.7: CHEMOTHERAPY/IMMUNOTHERAPY THAT MAY BE
USED IN MELANOMA

Agent	Indications	Toxicity
Dacarbazine (DTIC) (Avg effect 3–6 months)	Metastatic melanoma, Stage IV[1,3,6]	Nausea and vomiting, loss of appetite
Temozolomide (Temador®) (Available in pill form)	Metastatic melanoma, Stage IV[1,3,6]	Nausea and vomiting, fatigue, constipation, headache, seizure
Melphalan (Alkeran®)	Metastatic melanoma of the extremity, Stage III[6]	Nausea and vomiting, diarrhea, aphthous ulcers
Interferon alpha (Adjuvant therapy)	Metastatic melanoma, Stage III and IV[1,3,6]	Fever, chills, muscle or joint aches, depression, fatigue, anorexia, drowsiness, and pancytopenia
Interleukin 2	Metastatic melanoma, Stage III and IV[1,3,6]	Fever, chills, aches, fatigue, drowsiness, edema, and pancytopenia
Peginterferon alfa-2b (Sylatron®)	Metastatic melanoma, Stage III, microscopic or gross nodal involvement, must be given within 84 days of definitive surgical lymph node resection (including complete lymphadenectomy)[7]	Fever, chills, muscle or joint aches, fatigue, anorexia, drowsiness, injection site reaction Mental changes include aggressive behavior, memory changes, confusion, depression[8]
Ipilimumab (Yervoy®)	Unresectable or metastatic melanoma, Stage IV[9]	Fatigue, diarrhea, pruritus, rash, and colitis[10]

Chapter 45: Constipation, and
Chapter 46: Diarrhea.)

TAKE-HOME POINTS

- Melanoma is preventable with annual total-body skin examination.
- Biopsy should be performed by a dermatologist, and histopathology should be read by a dermatopathologist.
- Cutaneous melanoma is curable in more than 95% of the cases, especially when caught early.
- Treatment decisions should be made after a comprehensive assessment and in discussion with patient and family. Considerations include performance status, stage of disease, safety of surgical intervention, risks and benefits of adjuvant therapy, and patient's informed preferences.
- Systemic chemotherapy is used primarily for Stage III and IV disease, but overall response rates are very low and neither single agent nor combination chemotherapy has been shown to consistently improve overall survival. Careful consideration should therefore be given to an analysis of the risks vs. benefits of chemotherapy, especially in view of severe toxicity associated with many agents.

REFERENCES

1. Tsao H, Atkins MB, Sober AJ. Management of cutaneous melanoma. *N Engl J Med.* 2004;*351*: 998–1012.
2. Cummins DL, Cummins JM, Pantle H, Silverman MA, Leonard AL, Chanmugam A. Cutaneous malignant melanoma. *Mayo Clin Proc.* 2006;*81*:500–507.
3. Bolognia JL, Lorizzo JL, Rapini RP, eds. *Dermatology.* New York: Mosby; 2003.
4. Howlader N, Noone AM, Krapcho M, et al., eds. *SEER Cancer Statistics Review, 1975-2008*, National Cancer Institute. Bethesda, MD. http://seer.cancer.gov/csr/1975_2008/, based on November 2010 SEER data submission, posted to the SEER web site, 2011.
5. Balch CM, Gershenwald JE, Soong SJ, et al. Final version of 2009 AJCC melanoma staging and classification. *J Clin Oncol.* 2009;*27*:6199–6206.
6. Wolff K, Goldsmith LA, Katz SI, Gilchrest BA, Paller AS, Leffell DJ, eds. *Fitzpatrick's Dermatology in General Medicine.* New York: McGraw-Hill Professional; 2007.
7. U.S. Food and Drug Administration, Center for Drug Evaluation and Research. Peginterferon alfa-2b (Sylatron®), March 29, 2011. Retrieved April 25, 2011, from http://www.fda.gov/AboutFDA/CentersOffices/CDER/ucm249263.htm.
8. U.S. Food and Drug Administration, Center for Drug Evaluation and Research. Medication Guide, Sylatron® (peginterferon alfa-2b). Retrieved April 25, 2011, from http://www.fda.gov/downloads/Drugs/DrugSafety/UCM249397.pdf.
9. U.S. Food and Drug Administration, Center for Drug Evaluation and Research. Ipilimumab (Yervoy®), March 25, 2011. Retrieved April 25, 2011, from http://www.fda.gov/AboutFDA/CentersOffices/CDER/ucm248478.htm.
10. U.S. Food and Drug Administration, Center for Drug Evaluation and Research. Highlights of Prescribing Information Yervoy® (Ipilimumab). Retrieved April 25, 2011, from http://www.accessdata.fda.gov/drugsatfda_docs/label/2011/125377s0000lbl.pdf.

96

Colorectal Cancer

CASE

Mr. K is a 76-year-old man with diabetes mellitus, hypertension, and peripheral vascular disease with limited exercise tolerance. He presents with complaints of progressively worsening constipation over the last three to four months. He noted some bright red blood per rectum this morning, which caused him to seek medical attention. On presentation he is noted to have skin pallor. Colonoscopy reveals a large, partially obstructing mass in the right colon. Pathological review demonstrates an adenocarcinoma.

DEFINITION

Colon cancer can occur at any point in the large intestine from the ascending colon through the sigmoid colon. *Rectal cancer* is any cancer that occurs in the intestines 12 cm or less from the anal verge.[1] The majority of colorectal cancers are adenocarcinomas. This chapter will address colorectal adenocarcinoma.

PREVALENCE

- Colorectal cancer is the third most common cancer diagnosed in the United States, and the third most common cause of cancer-associated mortality in the United States.[1]
- It is a disease of older age with median age at diagnosis of 71 years.[2]

RISK FACTORS[1]

Increased Risk

- First-degree relative with colorectal cancer
- Hereditary syndromes (e.g., Familial Adenomatous Polyposis)
- Personal history of colorectal polyp
- Inflammatory bowel disease
- Physical inactivity
- Diabetes mellitus
- Obesity
- Smoking
- Alcohol intake
- Diet high in red and processed meat

Decreased Risk

- NSAID use
- Diet high in fiber
- Multivitamins

DIAGNOSIS

Presentation

The most common presenting signs and symptoms of colorectal cancer are:

- Fatigue due to iron deficiency anemia
- New onset of constipation
- Change in caliber of stool
- Abdominal pain/cramping
- Observation of blood in the stool

Exam

- Initial physical examination of a patient suspected of having colorectal cancer should include a rectal exam with fecal occult blood testing, followed by colonoscopy and biopsy of any lesions.
- All geriatric patients should also have an assessment of medical comorbidities, performance status, cognitive ability, and social support structure.

Tests

After a patient is diagnosed with colorectal carcinoma, staging workup should include:

- Chest X-ray
- CT scan of the abdomen and pelvis
- Lab work:
  - Complete blood count
  - Liver and kidney function tests
  - Carcinoembryonic antigen (CEA) level

Mr. K's staging workup is significant for an Hgb of 10.3 and a CEA of 22 ng/mL. CT scan and chest X-ray are unremarkable. He undergoes a partial colectomy with en bloc removal of lymph nodes.

STAGING AND SURVIVAL

- Complete staging of colorectal cancer requires surgical resection of the primary tumor and removal and pathological evaluation of a minimum of 12 regional lymph nodes.[4]
- Survival is dependent on extent or depth of invasion of the primary tumor, involvement of regional lymph nodes, and presence of distant metastases (Table 96.1).

TREATMENT OPTIONS

- After assessment of patient by a medical oncologist, treatment decisions should be made in discussion with patients and families. Factors to be weighed include performance status, stage of disease, safety of surgical intervention, risks and benefits of adjuvant therapy, and patient preference.
- The treatment options for colorectal cancer vary with stage of disease and location of primary tumor (colon versus rectum).

Colon Cancer Treatment

Surgical

- Surgical resection is the intervention of choice for both staging and treatment of colon cancer. The exceptions are patients who are at increased surgical risk due to significant medical comorbidities and patients with asymptomatic primary lesions but bulky, unresectable metastatic disease.
- In general, the surgical approach for colon cancer is colectomy and resection of regional lymph nodes with placement of diverting ostomy in any patient with an obstruction and un-prepped intestine.
- Patient age alone should not play a primary role in determining whether or not a patient is a surgical candidate.

Mr. K's post-op course is complicated by a urinary tract infection and debility requiring a stay in subacute rehab prior to returning home. Pathologic evaluation reveals a T3 lesion with 0/12 lymph node involvement (Stage IIA). Postoperative CEA level is 0.4 ng/mL.

Chemotherapy

- All patients with Stage II or higher colon cancer should be evaluated for adjuvant chemotherapy (Table 96.2).
- Decisions about adjuvant chemotherapy for patients with Stage II colon cancer should take into consideration factors that may increase risk of recurrence, including histological findings of lymphovascular invasion, poorly differentiated cells, and suboptimal lymph node sampling.[4]
- Adjuvant chemotherapy is the standard of care for patients with Stage III colon cancer;

TABLE 96.1: COLORECTAL CANCER STAGING AND SURVIVAL[3,4]

TNM Stage	Tumor	Node	Metastasis	5-year Survival
I	T1–T2	N0	0	93.2%
IIA	T3	N0	0	84.7%
IIB	T4	N0	0	72.2%
IIIA	T1–T2	N1	0	83.4%
IIIB	T2–T4	N1	0	64.1%
IIIC	Any T	N2	0	44.3%
IV	Any T	Any N	+	8.1%

Primary Tumor (T)
T1: Tumor invades submucosa
T2: Tumor invades muscularis propria
T3: Tumor invades into subserosa or pericolic or perirectal tissues
T4: Tumor invades other organs and or perforates visceral peritoneum

Regional Lymph Nodes (N)
N1: Involves 1–3 regional lymph nodes
N2: Involves ≥ 4 regional lymph nodes

Dukes A corresponds to Stage 1, Dukes B to Stage IIA-B, Dukes C to Stage III A–C

TABLE 96.2: CHEMOTHERAPY REGIMENS FOR COLON CANCER[4,6]

Chemotherapy Regimen	Indications	Toxicity
Fluorouracil (5FU)/Leucovorin	Stage IIA or higher	Stomatitis (infusional 5FU) Bone marrow suppression (bolus 5FU) Alopecia Diarrhea Nausea/vomiting
Capecitabine	Stage IIA or higher	Diarrhea Stomatitis Nausea/vomiting Fatigue Hand-foot syndrome Bone marrow suppression Hyperbilirubinemia
FOLFOX *Fluorouracil (5FU)/Leucovorin/* *Oxaliplatin*	Stage IIA or higher	Diarrhea Nausea/emesis Stomatitis Bone marrow suppression Peripheral neuropathy (especially with cold exposure) Fatigue
CapOx or XelOx *Capecitabine/* *Oxaliplatin*	Stage IIA or higher	Peripheral neuropathy (especially with cold exposure) Nausea/vomiting Diarrhea Stomatitis Fatigue Hand-foot syndrome Bone marrow suppression

older patients receive the same benefit from adjuvant chemotherapy as younger patients.[2]

- There are online decision-making tools available to assess the benefits of adjuvant chemotherapy for colon cancer and to help guide patient decision-making. www.adjuvantonline.org is one such tool that is individualized based on a patient's age, gender, comorbidities, T and N status, and histological grade. The site produces a handout that the physician can use to explain the mortality benefit and decreased risk of relapse that a patient can hope to achieve with the addition of adjuvant chemotherapy.[5]
- With increasing age, there is decreased tolerance of fluorinated pyrimidines such as fluorouracil (5-FU) that are key active agents in the treatment of colorectal cancer. Dose modifications

may therefore be necessary in older patients.

Given his complicated postoperative course, Mr. K decides against adjuvant chemotherapy, especially after learning that a 5-FU-based chemo regimen would offer only an 18% risk reduction.[5]

Rectal Cancer Treatment

- Surgery is the primary curative strategy for Stage I rectal cancer. The rate of local recurrence increases significantly with increasing depth of invasion and with the presence of lymph node involvement.[1]
- Rectal cancer tends to recur locally in at least half of cases. The treatment approach therefore requires more aggressive local treatment.
- The rate of local control in Stage II and III rectal cancer is significantly improved by the addition of adjuvant therapy.

Surgery

- For patients with distal and/or early stage (T1-2) rectal cancer, a trans-anal surgical approach may be used. For all other patients, a trans-abdominal approach is indicated.
- In those patients with known T3-T4 rectal cancer, consideration should be given to neoadjuvant chemoradiation therapy, with the intention of down-staging the primary tumor to increase resectability and decrease risk of recurrence.[4]

Chemotherapy and Radiation Therapy

- Concurrent chemotherapy and radiation therapy result in similar survival rates but achieve a higher rate of local control of disease than radiation therapy alone.
- Patients are treated with 5-FU and concurrent radiation. Infusional 5-FU is used as an antineoplastic therapy as well as a radiosensitizer.[4]

- Side effects of concurrent 5-FU and radiation therapy include acute GI symptoms, including severe diarrhea and long-term risk of more frequent bowel movements and occasional bowel incontinence.

Advanced Colorectal Cancer Treatment

- There are several treatment options for patients who have advanced colorectal cancer at time of presentation, and for patients who experience recurrent colorectal cancer but who also have good performance status, minimal comorbidities, and interest in receiving disease-modifying therapies.
- The mainstay of disease-modifying therapy for advanced colorectal cancer is chemotherapy (Table 96.3).
- Particularly in the setting of advanced disease, the physician should assist patients with medical decision-making, taking into consideration patient preferences and

TABLE 96.3: CHEMOTHERAPY REGIMENS FOR ADVANCED COLORECTAL CANCER[4,6]

Chemotherapy Regimen	Indications	Toxicity
FOLFIRI *Fluorouracil (5FU)/* *Leucovorin/Irinotecan*	Stage IV	Nausea/vomiting Stomatitis Diarrhea (may be severe) Bone marrow suppression Anorexia Fatigue
Irinotecan	Stage IV *Used as a single agent for* *second-line treatment*	Diarrhea (may be severe) Bone marrow suppression Nausea/emesis Anorexia Abdominal pain Lethargy
Bevacizumab	Stage IV *Used in combination with* *5FU-based therapy*	Diarrhea Hypertension Fatigue Intestinal perforation Intra-abdominal thrombosis Loss of appetite
Cetuximab	Stage IV *Used in combination with 5FU or* *irinotecan-based therapy*	Acneform rash Diarrhea Nausea/vomiting Infusion reaction Fever Fatigue

Note: All regimens in Table 96.3 are also indicated for the treatment of advanced colorectal cancer.

goals of care as well as ability to tolerate chemotherapy.

- Patients who are expected to tolerate therapy are offered combination chemotherapy. Patients generally continue to receive up to three lines of chemotherapy regimens that are rotated at time of disease progression, or when therapy is not tolerated.
- Patients who are interested in receiving disease-modifying therapy but who are unlikely to tolerate intensive chemotherapy can be considered for treatment with single agent chemotherapy.[4]
- Patients with solitary metastatic disease to the liver or lung may also be candidates for surgical resection or metastatectomy.[4]

EXPECTED DISEASE COURSE

- More than 20% of patients present with metastatic (Stage IV) colorectal cancer at the time of diagnosis.[1]

- Approximately half of patients with colorectal cancer will develop metastatic disease.[4] The most common site of metastatic disease for colorectal carcinoma is the liver. Colorectal adenocarcinoma also commonly metastasizes to peritoneum and lung.
- Rectal cancers are more likely to metastasize to the lung than are colon cancers and are also more likely to present with locoregional recurrence.[4]
- Complications of advanced colorectal cancer include intestinal obstruction, bleeding, anemia, liver failure, pulmonary embolism, abdominal pain, fatigue, and cachexia (Table 96.4).

PALLIATIVE CARE ISSUES

- The addition of palliative care to standard oncology care for colorectal cancer ensures that a broad range of patient and family care needs will be addressed, including pain

TABLE 96.4: COMMON COMPLICATIONS OF ADVANCED COLORECTAL CANCER

Complication	Associated Symptoms	Treatment Options
Obstruction	Constipation Abdominal pain Nausea Vomiting Loss of appetite	Surgical intervention Resection, decompression, diverting ostomy Octreotide can be used to decrease GI secretions
GI bleeding	Melena Bright red blood per rectum	Surgical resection if bleeding is excessive and patient is surgical candidate Radiation therapy
Anemia (May be due to acute GI bleeding, iron deficiency anemia, anemia of chronic disease, or chemotherapy)	Fatigue Dyspnea Palpitations Decreased exercise tolerance	Transfusion RBC growth factor Iron therapy
Liver metastases	Jaundice Edema Ascites Encephalopathy	Surgical resection (if isolated recurrence) Diuretics
Pulmonary metastases	Dyspnea Chest pain	Opioids Anxiolytics Oxygen
Pulmonary embolus	Dyspnea	Opioids Anxiolytics Oxygen Anticoagulation, if appropriate
Local recurrence in rectum/pelvis	Pain Bleeding	Opioids Radiation

and symptom management, advance care planning, psychosocial support, coordination of resources, and establishing achievable goals of care based on performance status, prognosis, and patient preferences.

- Physicians should assist patients and their families with informed medical decision-making about available treatment options. Factors to be weighed include performance status, stage of disease, safety of surgical intervention, risks and benefits of adjuvant therapy, and patient goals and preferences for care.
- Management of common treatment-related symptoms associated with chemotherapy, radiation, and surgical procedures should be a key focus of the care plan.
- Treatments that increase the survival rate for colorectal cancer patients may also result in physical, social, and psychological issues that negatively impact health-related quality of life in the post-treatment period. These detriments may persist, especially for older patients, over time. Areas of impairment include role and identity issues, emotional and cognitive functioning, social relationships, and financial difficulty.[7]

TAKE-HOME POINTS

- Treatment decisions for patients with colon cancer should not be made on the basis of age alone. Elderly patients receive the same benefit from adjuvant chemotherapy.
- Surgical intervention should be considered for all patients, as surgery is necessary for complete staging of colorectal cancer; surgery also minimizes risk of symptomatic obstruction by the cancer and of local recurrence in rectal cancer.

- Surgical risk should be carefully weighed for patients with significant medical comorbidities and for those patients with asymptomatic primary lesions but bulky, un-resectable metastatic disease.
- The addition of palliative care to standard oncology care will provide patients and their families with a range of care options, including pain and symptom management and psychosocial support, and will also help patients successfully complete life-sustaining treatments while achieving the best possible quality of life.
- Online tools such as www.adjuvantonline. com can be helpful in assessing benefits of adjuvant chemotherapy for patients with colon cancer, and also provide guidance for patient decision-making.

REFERENCES

1. www.cancer.org. Accessed December 15, 2013.
2. Ades S. Adjuvant chemotherapy for colon cancer in the elderly: Moving from evidence to practice. *Oncology.* 2009;*23*(2):162–167.
3. Greene FL, Page DL, Fleming ID, et al, eds. *AJCC Cancer Staging Manual*, 6th Ed. New York: Springer-Verlag; 2002.
4. National Comprehensive Cancer Network. www.nccn.org. Accessed December 15, 2013.
5. www.adjuvantonline.org. Accessed July 23, 2012.
6. Beveridge RA, Reitan JF eds. *Guide to selected cancer chemotherapy regimens and associated adverse events*, 5th Ed. Guilford, CT: RJM Marketing and Research Assoc.; 2004.
7. Jansen L, Herrmann A, Stegmaier C, et al. Health-related quality of life during the 10 years after diagnosis of colorectal cancer: a population-based study. *J Clin Oncol.* 2011;*29*: 3263–3269.

97

Head and Neck Cancer

CASE

Ms. J is a 68-year-old woman with a 50-pack/ year smoking history who has been drinking two bottles of beer five or six times per week for more than 40 years. She presents to your office with complaints of chronic cough. While taking her history, you note that her voice is hoarse. Her physical exam is remarkable for a small, firm, mildly tender, nonmobile lymph node inferior to the left omohyoid. Laryngoscopic exam reveals a left-sided laryngeal mass, and fine needle aspiration of the lymph node demonstrates squamous cell carcinoma.

DEFINITION

The term *head and neck cancer* is used to refer to any malignancy that arises in the nasal cavity, sinuses, lips, mouth, salivary glands, pharynx, or larynx.

Head and neck cancer includes a heterogeneous group of diseases. The vast majority of these cancers are squamous cell carcinomas.

The staging, natural history, and treatment options vary by site of disease. This chapter will provide a general overview of issues pertinent for geriatric patients diagnosed with squamous cell cancers of the head and neck.

PREVALENCE

- Head and neck cancers account for less than 5% of all cancers diagnosed in the United States.
- The majority of patients present with advanced disease; 43% have lymph node involvement, and 10% have metastatic disease.[1]
- Most patients are between 50 and 70 years old at the time of diagnosis.[1]

RISK FACTORS[1]

- Tobacco*
- Alcohol*

- Occupational exposures:
  - Wood dust
  - Nickel
- UV light exposure
- Radiation exposure
- Marijuana
- Viruses:
  - HIV
  - HPV

*Synergistic

DIAGNOSIS

Presentation

The presenting signs and symptoms of head and neck cancer vary with the site of disease.

Common presenting symptoms include:[1]
- Nose bleeds
- Dysphagia
- Painful swallowing
- Sensation of "lump" in throat
- Hoarseness
- Dysphonia
- Earache
- Coughing up blood
- Stuffiness of ears
- Inability to open mouth normally

History and Exam

- A whole patient assessment should be conducted to assess the patient's symptoms, performance status, medical comorbidities, and social support.
- A detailed physical exam for head and neck cancer should include assessment of the skin/scalp, cranial nerves, eyes, ears, nose, oral cavity, and neck.

Ms. J is referred for bronchoscopy, upper GI endoscopy, and PET/CT, which demonstrate the left laryngeal mass and a 2.5 cm left-sided lymph node with no evidence of metastatic disease or synchronous malignancy.

Tests

Endoscopy

The factors that increase the risk of developing head and neck cancer (particularly tobacco and alcohol) increase the risk for all aerodigestive tumors. All patients diagnosed with head and neck cancer should therefore undergo "triple endoscopy": laryngoscopy, bronchoscopy, and esophagascopy.[1]

Biopsy

In a patient presenting with a palpable lymph node in the neck, a fine needle aspiration is diagnostic in the majority of cases.

Imaging

Imaging to assess extent of local disease can be accomplished by CT scan or MRI with contrast, or PET/CT scanning. Assessment for distant metastases can be achieved by CT scan of chest/abdomen/pelvis or PET/CT scanning.

STAGING AND SURVIVAL

- The staging of head and neck cancers varies by site of disease and will not be reviewed in this chapter.
- The majority of patients diagnosed with squamous cell carcinoma of the head and neck present with advanced disease.
- Stage of disease has a very strong correlation with prognosis.[1] In general, survival for Stage I disease is greater than 80%, and survival for Stage III-IV disease is less than 40%[1] (Table 97.1).

TREATMENT OPTIONS

- Treatment options vary with site of disease. In general, interventions for the treatment of squamous cell cancer include surgery, chemotherapy, and radiation therapy.
- The treatment regimens can be intensive with significant symptom burden. It is therefore of utmost importance that patients are cared for by an interdisciplinary team.
- Clincians on the team should include the following disciplines:[2]
  - Head and neck surgery
  - Radiation oncology
  - Medical oncology
  - Plastic surgery
  - Specialized nursing care
  - Palliative medicine
  - Physical medicine and rehabilitation
  - Speech language pathologist
  - Social work
  - Dietician
  - Psychiatry
  - Dental
- Treatment options include surgical resection, chemotherapy, radiation, and concurrent chemoradiation (Table 97.2). Selection of treatment options depends on location of tumor, stage of disease, and patient performance status. Particularly in the case of laryngeal cancer, treatment choice should take into account side effects and organ preservation. Full discussion of specific treatments is beyond the scope of this chapter.

Ms. J is evaluated by the interdisciplinary team, undergoes a full geriatric assessment, and is referred for support for smoking cessation and Alcoholics Anonymous. Given her Stage III disease and her wish to preserve her vocal cords, she opts to receive concurrent chemoradiation.

TABLE 97.1: FIVE-YEAR SURVIVAL RATES[1]

Site	Stage I	Stage II	Stage III	Stage IV
Oral cavity*	70–100%	50–90%	25–90%	25–60%
Oropharynx*	60–100%	50–100%	20–75%	14–50%
Nasopharynx*	65–95%	50–65%	30–60%	5–50%
Hypopharynx*	50–90%	50–80%	30–70%	15–40%
Larynx*	75–95%	30–80%	45–75%	10–35%
Paranasal sinuses*	60–70%	60–70%	25–35%	10–25%
Salivary glands	90%	55%	45%	10%

* Ranges are provided as each site has multiple sub-sites with varying prognosis.

TABLE 97.2: THERAPY FOR HEAD AND NECK CANCER[3,4]

For Localized Disease

Treatment Options	Associated Toxicities/Symptoms	Specific Issues for Older Adults
Surgical resection	Site-specific side effects include cosmetic deformities, impairment of speech or swallowing, temporomandibular joint dysfunction, airway compromise requiring tracheostomy	Similar efficacy outcomes, but older patients have higher complication rates that increase with increasing comorbidities
Chemoradiation (may be primary therapy or adjuvant) Radiation plus: Cisplatin alone (preferred) Cisplatin-based doublet 5-FU- based doublet	Mucositis, dysphagia, nausea, vomiting, thrombocytopenia Cisplatin-based: nephrotoxicity, peripheral neuropathy	Limited evidence for or against use in patients >65 Increased toxicity in older patients
Induction/Adjuvant chemotherapy Docetaxel/cisplatin/5-FU + surgery	5-FU-based: diarrhea, hand-foot syndrome Neutropenia, neutropenic infection, anemia, mucositis, nausea, anorexia, diarrhea Many patients require delays in treatment as a result of toxicities	Limited evidence, as too few patients over the age of 70 are enrolled in clinical trials Increased toxicity in older patients
	Site-specific side effects include mucositis, dysphagia, pain, hoarseness, dermatitis, loss of taste, xerostomia, thick sputum, and secretions	Similar overall survival Increased incidence of acute mucositis

For Advanced Disease (Metastatic or Recurrent)

Combination chemotherapy:
Cisplatin or Carboplatin + 5-FU ± cetuximab
Cisplatin or Carboplatin + Docetaxel or Paclitaxel, or
Cisplatin/Cetuximab

Single agent chemotherapy:

Cisplatin	Methotrexate
Carboplatin	Ifosfamide
Paclitaxel	Bleomycin
Docetaxel	Cetuximab
5-FU	

Radiation/Re-irradiation

- Many of the treatment options have the potential to significantly impact a patient's ability to reliably eat or take oral medications, either temporarily or permanently. For many patients, it is therefore appropriate to consider enteral feeding tube placement early in the course of treatment to maintain adequate nutritional status. For some patients, the feeding tube may be removed after the completion of therapy. (See Chapter 77: Feeding Tube Management.)
- The final choice of treatment plan should be made in discussion with the patient and family, taking into account patient performance status, medical comorbidities, benefits and burdens of treatment, and individual patient preference.

EXPECTED DISEASE COURSE

- The majority of patients present with Stage III-IV disease.
- Approximately 80% of recurrent head and neck cancers present with loco-regional disease.[1] Relatively few patients develop distant metastasis.
- The ultimate cause of death for patients with head and neck cancer is generally related to poor nutritional status and local complications.

PALLIATIVE CARE ISSUES[5]

- Patients with head and neck cancer struggle with physical symptoms and psychological stressors that are caused by the disease and treatment interventions (Table 97.3).
- The addition of palliative care to standard oncology care provides patients and their families with a range of care options, including pain and symptom management, advance care planning, psychosocial support, coordination of resources, and establishing achievable goals of care based on performance status, prognosis, and patient preferences. These comprehensive supportive services can help patients successfully complete life-sustaining treatments and obtain the best possible quality of life.
- Optimal care for patients with head and neck cancer is based on the interdisciplinary team approach that is a key principle of palliative care. In addition to the expertise of the oncology treatment team, these patients benefit from the coordinated care offered by nursing, chaplaincy, dentists, clinical social workers, physical and occupational therapists, and nutritionists.
- Patients with advanced head and neck cancer may experience serious complications as their disease progresses (Table 97.4). Referral to an inpatient

TABLE 97.3: COMMON SYMPTOMS ASSOCIATED WITH HEAD AND NECK CANCER AND ITS TREATMENT[5]

Symptom	Management Strategies
Pain	Opioids: Consider non-oral route of administration (e.g., fentanyl) Consider which medications may be administered via feeding tubes Methadone can be very effective for patients with neuropathic component to pain due to either direct tumor involvement of nerves, postoperative complication, or chemotherapy-induced peripheral neuropathy. (See Chapter 29: Management of Pain in Older Adults)
Mucositis	Bland rinses: Grade 0 mouthwash (saline/sodium bicarbonate solution) Analgesics: Opioids Topical anesthetics: e.g., Lidocaine-containing mouth rinse Mucosal coating agents: Gelclair, Kaopectate (See Chapter 47: Mucositis)
Dermatitis	Unscented, lanolin-free hydrophilic cream
Dysphagia	Referral to speech language pathologist and dietician Enteral tube placement: May be temporary for nutritional support while patient is undergoing therapy, or may be permanent (See Chapter 49: Dysphagia)
Xerostomia	Frequent water, ice chips Sugarless candy or gum Saliva substitutes Pilocarpine, Evoxac (See Chapter 47: Mucositis)

(continued)

TABLE 97.3: (CONTINUED)

Symptom	Management Strategies
Dental	Referral to dentist Pretreatment for tooth extractions and preventive dental hygiene, as treatment will also predispose to poor wound healing
Change in speech and communications	Referral to speech and language therapist Adaptive devices
Decreased quality of life	Supportive counseling and psychotherapy
Alteration in body image	Supportive counseling and psychotherapy
Depression	Supportive counseling and psychotherapy Antidepressant medications (See Chapter 64: Depression)
Anxiety	Supportive counseling and psychotherapy Anxiolytics (See Chapter 65: Anxiety)

TABLE 97.4: COMMON COMPLICATIONS OF ADVANCED HEAD AND NECK CANCER

Complication	Presentation	Approach to Treatment
Burdens of artificial nutrition and hydration	At the end of life, artificial nutrition and hydration may become burdensome, causing symptoms such as nausea, vomiting, and fluid overload with peripheral edema, and pulmonary edema.	Clinician should meet with patients and families to discuss prognosis and goals of care and assess the benefit/burden ratio of continued artificial nutrition and hydration. (See Chapter 27: Artificial Nutrition and Hydration)
Airway obstruction	Shortness of breath Stridor Coughing	Radiation therapy may be helpful if patient is able to receive further treatment to that area. Placement of tracheotomy if obstruction is proximal Steroids may be of minimal benefit. (See Chapter 41: Dyspnea)
"Carotid blowout"	Tumor invasion into carotid artery leads to exsanguinations.	Strong consideration should be given to inpatient management. Keep dark (red or black) towels at bedside. Available medication for sedation Caregiver preparedness (See Chapter 14: Palliative Care Emergencies)
"SVC syndrome"	Tumor obstruction of the superior vena cava results in shortness of breath, swelling of the arms and face, dilation of veins on the skin surface, cough, and chest pain.	Radiation therapy may be helpful if patient is able to receive further treatment to that area. Steroids may be of benefit. (See Chapter 14: Palliative Care Emergencies)
Aspiration pneumonia	Coughing Fever Elevated white blood cell count	Antibiotics Enteral feeding will not decrease the risk for aspiration in a patient unable to protect his/her airway. (See Chapter 73: Aspiration Pneumonia)

palliative care unit or home hospice care should be considered to ensure expert medical management as well as the necessary emotional and psychological support.

TAKE-HOME POINTS

- Head and neck cancer refers to a diverse group of tumors that often present with late-stage disease.
- There is significant morbidity and mortality associated with head and neck cancer and with its treatment. Patients with head and neck cancer also struggle with physical symptoms and psychological stressors that are caused not only by the disease, but also by treatment interventions.
- Patients and families need the support of a full interdisciplinary team to help guide treatment decisions, coordinate the management of disease and treatment-related symptoms and complications, and cope with the psychosocial impact/disfigurement associated with head and neck cancers.
- The addition of palliative care to standard oncology care provides patients and their families with a range of care options including pain and symptom management, advance care planning, psychosocial support, coordination of resources, and establishing achievable goals of care based on performance status, prognosis, and patient preferences.

REFERENCES

1. Pazdur R, Coia LR, Hoskins WJ, et al., eds. *Cancer Management a Multidisciplinary Approach*, 8th ed. New York, NY: CMP Healthcare Media; 2004.
2. http://training.seer.cancer.gov/head-neck/intro/survival.html. Accessed April 10, 2012.
3. National Comprehensive Network. NCCN Clinical Practice Guidelines in Oncology: Head and Neck Cancers. v 2.2011. www.nccn.org. Accessed April 10, 2012.
4. Beveridge RA, Reitan JF, eds. *Guide to Selected Cancer Chemotherapy Regimens and Associated Adverse Events*, 5th ed. Guilford, CT: RJM Marketing and Research Assoc.; 2004.
5. Goldstein NE, Genden E, Morrison RS. Palliative care for patients with head and neck cancer: "I would like a quick return to a normal lifestyle." *JAMA*. 2008;299(15):1818–1826.

98

Breast Cancer

CASE

Mrs. G is a 78-year-old female with a history of diabetes, hypertension, and osteopenia who presents with a left breast mass that she noticed while showering. She does not have any other concerns and has an excellent performance status. She has never had an abnormal mammogram but notes that it has been many years since her last one. Her examination is remarkable for a 2 cm mass in the upper-outer quadrant of her left breast. No lymphadenopathy is appreciated. A diagnostic mammogram and an ultrasound-guided core biopsy of the lesion are performed. The pathology demonstrates an estrogen receptor-positive, HER2-negative invasive ductal carcinoma.

DEFINITION

Cancer that forms in tissues of the breast. *Breast cancer* occurs in both men and women, although male breast cancer is rare.

CLASSIFICATION

Histopathology

- Noninvasive breast cancers include ductal carcinoma *in situ* (DCIS) and lobular carcinoma *in situ* (LCIS).
- Invasive breast cancers include adenocarcinomas, invasive ductal carcinomas (~80%), and invasive lobular carcinomas (~10%).
- Inflammatory carcinomas: Uncommon (~1%); often have a more aggressive clinical course; involve the lymphatic structures of the dermis, producing breast erythema and edema (the "peau d'orange" appearance).

Molecular Markers

- Molecular markers are used to identify estrogen receptor/progesterone receptor (ER/PR)-positive and negative cancers, and HER2-positive and negative cancers.
- The ER/PR and HER2 status of a breast cancer has important implications for prognosis and treatment. Absence of all three markers ("triple negative" breast cancers) portends a worse prognosis. ER/PR-positive tumors may be treated with endocrine therapies, and HER2-positive tumors may be treated with HER2-targeted treatments.

PREVALENCE

- Most common cancer in women in the United States: 1 in 8 women will develop breast cancer during their lifetime.
- Second most common cause of cancer death in women in the United States.
- Approximately 40% of cases of breast cancer are diagnosed in women older than 65 years. Median age at diagnosis is 61 years.[1]

RISK FACTORS[2]

- With the exception of gender and age, the relative risk associated with each of these risk factors is fairly modest, and most women do not have any other identifiable risk factors.
  - Gender: Women are 100 times more likely than men to have breast cancer.
  - Age
  - Family history of breast cancer in a first-degree relative
  - Early menarche, late menopause
  - Older age at first live childbirth
  - Hormone replacement therapy
  - Obesity, primarily in post-menopausal women
  - Alcohol intake: Risk increases with the amount consumed.
  - History of therapeutic chest wall irradiation
  - History of benign proliferative breast disease: Lesions with atypia (atypical ductal hyperplasia, atypical lobular hyperplasia) have a stronger effect on breast cancer risk than lesions without

atypia (usual ductal hyperplasia, fibroadenoma, sclerosing adenosis, papillomatosis, radial scar).
- History of breast cancer
- Although many women may inquire about genetic mutations in the BRCA gene (BRCA 1 and 2), these mutations are found in only 5% to 7% of all breast cancer cases (usually diagnosed at younger ages) and are unlikely to be a risk factor in an older woman diagnosed with breast cancer.

DIAGNOSIS

Presentation

- Many women will present with a painless breast mass. Some patients may experience pain, nipple discharge, or skin changes.
- A more extensive breast mass may be associated with ulceration and drainage, lymphadenopathy, or symptoms due to metastatic disease.
- Many women present after screening mammography identifies a suspicious lesion for which a biopsy is recommended.

History

- A careful history should include a review of systems to discern whether the patient is experiencing any symptoms from metastatic disease. Questions addressing abdominal symptoms, pulmonary symptoms, bone pain, and localized neurologic symptoms may be helpful. A family history and questions addressing other risk factors are usually included in the history of a patient with a new breast mass.
- In the geriatric population, a thorough assessment of a patient's performance status, medical comorbidities, cognitive ability, and social support structure is essential.
- Clinicians should also assess a patient and family's goals of care if cancer is suspected. These goals may range from symptom management to attempts at cure despite the burdens of treatment. An understanding of the goals of care is critical to determining the extent of workup, as well as selecting the appropriate treatment options.

Exam

- The physical examination should include careful inspection and palpation of the breast, skin, and the nipple-areolar complex.

- A complete lymph node examination, including particular attention to the axillary and supraclavicular lymph nodes, should also be completed.

Tests

In selecting tests to recommend for a patient, the clinician should have an ongoing, open discussion with a patient regarding her goals of care. A physician should carefully consider the patient in the context of her comorbidities, performance status, social support, and goals of care.[2]

Imaging

- Diagnostic mammogram with additional views to further evaluate a lesion
- Ultrasound to further evaluate a lesion

Tissue Biopsy

- Tissue biopsy may be obtained by fine-needle aspiration, ultrasound or stereotactic-guided core biopsy, or an excisional biopsy.
- A core biopsy is usually preferred since the sample provides adequate tissue for confirmation of invasive disease and hormone receptor and HER2 testing.
- Pathology review including determination of the hormone receptor (ER/PR) and HER2 status of the tumor.

Labs

- Labs include complete blood count, chemistries, liver and kidney function tests.

Other

- Additional tests may be considered, depending on the stage of the breast cancer and at the oncologist's discretion. These include breast MRI, bone scan, chest radiograph, chest/abdomen/pelvis CT, PET CT scan, and tumor markers (CA 15-3, CA 27-29, CEA).

PROGNOSIS

- Many women with early-stage breast cancer may be cured of their disease with the appropriate therapy.
- Patients with metastatic disease, especially those with non-visceral metastases, may live for years with breast cancer as a chronic disease.
- In older adults, breast cancer is considered a more indolent disease. Tumors of women older than 65 years are more often ER/

PR-positive (~85%) than in younger women, and HER2 overexpression is less common in older patients. In addition, older women with metastatic disease are more likely to have metastases to the skin and bone, with lower rates of lung and liver metastases, which are associated with a worse prognosis.

- Despite less aggressive tumor characteristics, older women tend to have lower breast cancer-specific survival rates. This has been attributed to undertreatment as well as a more advanced disease stage at diagnosis.[3,4]

BREAST CANCER STAGING AND SURVIVAL

Disease staging is used to determine prognosis and guide treatment decisions (Table 98.1). For stage distribution and five-year relative survival rates, please see Table 98.2.

TREATMENT OPTIONS

- Older women with breast cancer have poorer outcomes when compared to younger women. This is thought to be due in part to undertreatment. Patients of advanced age are less likely to receive standard therapies such as breast-conserving therapy (as compared to mastectomy), axillary lymph node dissection, radiation therapy after breast-conserving therapy, and chemotherapy. In addition, older women are underrepresented in randomized trials, limiting the ability to optimally guide treatments in this patient population.
- There are many treatments for patients who have decided to pursue breast cancer-related therapies. Clinicians should be aware, however, that symptom management is also a treatment option that should always be pursued, with or without cancer disease management interventions. Common symptoms associated with advanced cancer are addressed later in this chapter (Table 98.8).

TREATMENT OF NONINVASIVE BREAST CANCER

Ductal Carcinoma In Situ (DCIS)

- DCIS is a precursor of invasive breast cancer and is managed surgically. The options for treatment include lumpectomy followed by radiation, total mastectomy, or lumpectomy alone. There is no survival difference between these three treatment options, although there are lower rates of in-breast recurrence when radiotherapy is added to lumpectomy.[2] Since DCIS is a noninvasive breast cancer, chemotherapy is not indicated.
- In women with ER-positive DCIS treated with lumpectomy and radiation, tamoxifen for five years can decrease the risk of both noninvasive and invasive breast cancer. In older women, however, the burdens of therapy may outweigh the potential benefit because the absolute benefit of tamoxifen is small (e.g., the cumulative incidence of invasive breast cancer at five years in the ipsilateral breast was 4.2% and 2.1% in women receiving placebo and tamoxifen, respectively[6]), and there is no survival benefit.

Lobular Carcinoma In Situ (LCIS)

- Women who have LCIS are at an increased risk of developing invasive carcinoma in bilateral breasts (~20% over 15 years). Unlike DCIS, it is not a precursor of invasive breast cancer. Therefore, no additional local management (i.e., surgery or radiation) is necessary. It is generally recommended to follow these women with regular history and physical examinations as well as annual diagnostic mammograms.
- Given the increased risk of developing invasive breast cancer, women who have a life expectancy of ≥ 10 years may consider risk reduction strategies like bilateral prophylactic mastectomies or five years of tamoxifen or raloxifene.[2] However, especially in women of advanced age, the burdens of these interventions must be weighed against the potential benefits.

TREATMENT OF INVASIVE BREAST CANCER (EARLY-STAGE)

Surgery

- Surgery remains the cornerstone of curative therapy for breast cancer. Healthy older patients often tolerate breast-conserving surgery and mastectomy as well as younger patients.[7] Comorbidities are the main risk factors that influence surgical morbidity and mortality.

TABLE 98.1: TNM STAGING SYSTEM FOR BREAST CANCER[5]

Primary Tumor (T)

Tis	Ductal carcinoma in situ (DCIS)
	Lobular carcinoma in situ (LCIS)
	Paget's disease of the nipple not associated with invasive carcinoma or carcinoma in situ in the underlying breast parenchyma
T1	Tumor ≤ 2 cm in greatest dimension
T2	Tumor > 2 cm but ≤ 5 cm in greatest dimension
T3	Tumor > 5 cm in greatest dimension
T4	Tumor of any size with direction extension to the chest wall and/or skin (ulceration or skin nodules)

Regional Lymph Nodes (N)

N0	No regional lymph node metastases
N1	Metastases in movable ipsilateral axillary lymph node(s)
N2	Metastases in ipsilateral axillary lymph nodes that are clinically fixed or matted **OR** in clinically apparent ipsilateral internal mammary nodes in the *absence* of clinically evident axillary lymph node metastasis
N3	Metastases in ipsilateral infraclavicular lymph node(s) with or without axillary lymph node involvement **OR** in clinically apparent ipsilateral internal mammary lymph node(s) with clinically evident axillary lymph node metastases **OR** metastases in ipsilateral supraclavicular lymph node(s) with or without axillary or internal mammary lymph node involvement

Distant Metastasis (M)

M0	No distant metastasis
M1	Distant metastasis

Stage Groupings

Stage 0	Tis	N0	M0
Stage I	T1	N0	M0
Stage IIA	T0	N1	M0
Stage IIB	T1	N1	M0
	T2	N0	M0
	T2	N1	M0
	T3	N0	M0
Stage IIIA	T0	N2	M0
Stage IIIB	T1	N2	M0
Stage IIIC	T2	N2	M0
	T3	N1	M0
	T3	N2	M0
	T4	N0	M0
	T4	N1	M0
	T4	N2	M0
	Any T	N3	M0
Stage IV	Any T	Any N	M1

- Older women should be offered the option of breast-conserving therapy (lumpectomy followed by radiation) if they are fit for surgery and if their tumor size less than 4–5 cm.

- In some women with larger tumors, neoadjuvant therapy with endocrine therapy or chemotherapy may be used to shrink the tumor with the hope of making breast-conserving surgery possible.

TABLE 98.2: STAGE DISTRIBUTION AND FIVE-YEAR RELATIVE SURVIVAL RATES[1]

Stage at Diagnosis	Stage Distribution (%)	5-year Relative Survival (%)
Localized (confined to the primary site)	60%	98%
Regional (spread to the regional lymph nodes)	33%	83.6%
Distant (metastatic disease)	5%	23.4%
Unknown	2%	57.9%

- Mastectomy may be recommended for older patients who have larger tumors, those with persistently positive resection margins after attempts at re-excision, or those who cannot or will not undergo radiation therapy.
- Patients who will be undergoing a mastectomy should also be offered a consultation with a reconstructive surgeon, since the loss of a breast may influence the quality of life for patients of all ages.

Procedures to Address the Axillary Lymph Nodes

- An important prognostic factor in early-stage breast cancer is whether or not the ipsilateral axillary lymph nodes are involved with cancer. The status of the axillary nodes also guides decisions about adjuvant chemotherapy and radiation therapy.
- A sentinel lymph node (SLN) biopsy is recommended in women with early-stage breast cancer (clinical stage I and II) and a clinically negative axilla.
- In patients with a positive SLN biopsy, an axillary lymph node dissection (ALND) may be considered to reduce the risk of ipsilateral lymph node recurrence. However, definitive data showing a survival benefit with ALND are lacking, and some experts suggest that this may be considered optional in elderly patients.[2]
- It may not be necessary to perform a lymph node assessment for some older women who have small (<2 cm), ER/PR-positive, clinically node-negative tumors and who will be treated with adjuvant endocrine therapy.
- In women with a palpable lymph node, an axillary ultrasound-guided fine needle or core needle biopsy may be performed. If nodal metastases are found, an ALND is recommended.

Note on potential complications: Both ALND and to a lesser extent SLN biopsy have been associated with lymphedema (Table 98.7). There is some data suggesting that older patients have more arm morbidity associated with ALND.

Radiation Therapy

- After lumpectomy, breast radiation is recommended as part of breast conservation therapy. Radiation decreases the rate of local recurrence, although the risk of local recurrence is lower in older patients. Breast irradiation may be omitted in women older than 70 years of age with small (< 2 cm), ER/PR-positive, clinically node-negative tumors who will be treated with adjuvant endocrine therapy.[2]
- After mastectomy, radiation therapy is recommended for women with high-risk breast cancers: breast cancers with ≥ 4 positive axillary lymph nodes and/or T3/T4 tumors. These recommendations are based on trials that demonstrated a reduction in the risk of local recurrence and death from breast cancer as well as an increase in disease-free survival. Although women over 70 years of age were largely excluded from these trials, there are cohort studies that support the use of post-mastectomy radiation therapy in elderly women with high-risk breast cancers.
- If a patient is going to be treated with adjuvant chemotherapy, radiation therapy usually follows the completion of chemotherapy.
- Complications of breast radiation therapy may include erythema and dryness of the treated area, itching, and in some cases a burning sensation. In the six months after completion of radiation, patients may experience breast edema and thickening of the skin of the breast. The edema usually resolves 12 to 18 months after radiation therapy is completed.[8] Fatigue is also a

common side effect of breast radiotherapy. Potential serious side effects from radiation (< 1%) include radiation pneumonitis, pericarditis, and coronary vessel damage.

Endocrine Therapy

- Patients with ER/PR-positive cancers benefit from adjuvant endocrine therapy, and all patients should be considered for treatment, regardless of age[2] (Table 98.3). Although both aromatase inhibitors and tamoxifen are effective in post-menopausal women, aromatase inhibitors provide a greater survival benefit and are the standard adjuvant endocrine therapy for this population of patients.
- For women who will also be undergoing adjuvant chemotherapy and/or radiation therapy, endocrine therapy is started after these therapies are completed and is continued for five years.
- In patients with favorable, very small (≤ 1 cm), ER/PR-positive, lymph node-negative tumors, observation or endocrine therapy are both appropriate options.
- In older patients with serious comorbidities who are not candidates for surgery or who have a limited life expectancy, endocrine therapy alone may provide local control of ER/PR-positive tumors.

Chemotherapy

- The recommendations for adjuvant chemotherapy are highly individualized and depend upon patient characteristics (e.g., performance status, comorbidities, life expectancy), patient preference, and tumor characteristics (e.g., tumor size, ER/PR and HER2 status, lymph node involvement).
- An oncologist must weigh the benefits of lowering the risk of cancer recurrence with issues that are particularly pertinent to older patients, such as a more limited life expectancy as well as a greater risk of toxicity from treatments. Experts have varying opinions regarding which patients should be recommended for adjuvant chemotherapy.
- There are helpful tools that practitioners may utilize when weighing the benefits and burdens of adjuvant chemotherapy.
  - **Adjuvant! Online** (www.adjuvantonline.com) estimates the benefits of endocrine therapy, chemotherapy, or both according to patient data (including age) as well as tumor information.
  - **Oncotype DX**, is a multigene assay performed on the tumor sample that calculates the risk of distant recurrence in women with early-stage, ER/PR-positive, node-negative breast cancer who will be treated with

---

TABLE 98.3: ENDOCRINE THERAPIES USED IN THE ADJUVANT SETTING AND TOXICITIES[9]

Endocrine Therapy	Toxicities
Aromatase inhibitors (oral, once daily): Anastrozole Letrozole Exemestane	Arthralgias Loss of bone density[a] Fatigue Hot flashes Vaginal dryness
Tamoxifen (oral, once daily)	Hot flashes Vaginal discharge and/or dryness Thromboembolic events Endometrial hyperplasia, polyps, and cancer[b] Hair thinning Fluid retention, peripheral edema Tumor flare in the first two weeks after therapy is initiated may manifest with increase in bone pain, back pain with spinal cord compression, and/or hypercalcemia

[a] Obtain a baseline and serial DEXA scans in patients treated with aromatase inhibitors since they are associated with a loss of bone density and an increased risk of bone fractures.
[b] Vaginal bleeding should be evaluated promptly.

endocrine therapy. This calculated risk of distant recurrence is called the Recurrence Score and suggests whether a patient is likely to benefit from adjuvant chemotherapy. In general, conditions that may benefit from adjuvant chemotherapy include: (1) ER/PR-positive, node-negative tumors with a high Oncotype DX Recurrence Score; (2) ER/PR-positive, node-positive tumors; (3) ER/PR-negative tumors that are either node-positive or > 1 cm in size; and (4) HER2-positive tumors that are either node-positive or > 1 cm in size.

- Healthy older adults may be offered the same chemotherapy regimens as younger patients; four cycles of an anthracycline-containing regimen (usually doxorubicin and cyclophosphamide) are usually considered standard.
- Anthracycline-related cardiac toxicity is more common in patients over the age of 70, but this does not preclude healthy older women from being treated with these agents. Serial monitoring of ejection fraction should be obtained.
- An alternative to an anthracycline-containing regimen is docetaxel with cyclophosphamide. This regimen may also be helpful in patients at risk for the cardiac complications of anthracyclines.
- In fit elderly patients with node-positive disease, four cycles of a taxane (usually paclitaxel) may be added to four cycles of an anthracycline-containing regimen.
- In general, the chemotherapies used in the adjuvant setting have share the common side effects of myelosuppression, nausea/vomiting, mucositis, alopecia, and fatigue. Additional chemotherapy-specific toxicities are listed below (Table 98.4).

Targeted Therapies
- Trastuzumab, a monoclonal antibody that specifically targets HER2, is recommended for the treatment of women with HER2-positive breast cancers.
- When used in conjunction with adjuvant chemotherapy, trastuzumab has been shown to improve survival and decrease the risk of cancer recurrence.
- After chemotherapy has been completed, trastuzumab is given every three weeks to complete one total year of therapy.

TABLE 98.4: CHEMOTHERAPIES USED IN THE ADJUVANT SETTING AND TOXICITIES[9]

Chemotherapy	Toxicities
Anthracyclines: Doxorubicin Epirubicin	Cardiotoxicity—may limit use in older adults with cardiac comorbidities Red-orange discoloration of the urine Sun sensitivity, nail changes
Cyclophosphamide	Taste and smell changes
Paclitaxel	Peripheral neuropathy—dose-dependent Onycholysis
Docetaxel	Arthralgias, myalgias Fluid retention Peripheral neuropathy Maculopapular skin rash, dry/pruritic skin

- Approximately 2% to 3% of patients treated with one year of trastuzumab after an anthracycline-containing adjuvant chemotherapy regimen will develop symptomatic congestive heart failure. Serial monitoring of cardiac function is therefore necessary. This may limit the use of trastuzumab in older adults with comorbidities.

Mrs. G undergoes a left breast lumpectomy and sentinel lymph node biopsy. The pathology demonstrates a 1.5 cm invasive ductal breast cancer with negative margins and no involvement of her sentinel lymph nodes. After a discussion with her oncologist, she decides to forgo breast radiation therapy. The Oncotype DX score for her cancer correlates with a low risk of recurrence, and her oncologist informs her that she does not need chemotherapy. Her oncologist recommends treatment with five years of an aromatase inhibitor. Since Mrs. G. has a history of osteopenia, her oncologist orders a baseline DEXA scan.

TREATMENT OF METASTATIC BREAST CANCER

Prognosis
- The average survival for patients with metastatic breast cancer is often measured in months to years, making quality-of-life

issues critically important. Factors that predict a longer survival in patients with metastatic breast cancer include:

- Lower disease stage: Smaller initial tumor size, fewer positive lymph nodes
- Longer interval without recurrent disease
- ER/PR-positive status
- Non-visceral dominant site of disease recurrence (e.g., bone, soft tissue)
- Breast cancer most commonly metastasizes to the lung, liver, and bones. It is important to biopsy the site of suspected metastasis to confirm the diagnosis of metastatic disease and to check for ER/PR and HER2 status, which can occasionally be different than that of the primary tumor.

Treatment Options

- The treatment options for metastatic breast cancer in elderly patients are dependent on many variables, including both patient characteristics (e.g., performance status, cognition, comorbidities) and tumor characteristics (e.g., ER/PR and HER2 status, site of disease, extent of disease).
- With this information supplementing the prognostic factors listed previously, a physician often has a good understanding of the patient's disease trajectory and how likely she is to benefit from disease-directed therapies. These options may then be presented to a patient in the context of her achievable goals of care.
- It is important to revisit this discussion of goals of care when the disease progresses during therapy and the physician is considering whether to recommend another disease-directed therapeutic option.

Endocrine Therapy

- Regardless of ER/PR status, some experts recommend that all older women with metastatic breast cancer (without life-threatening or rapidly progressive metastatic disease) be treated with a trial of endocrine therapy. Endocrine therapies have fewer toxicities than chemotherapy and may even benefit some ER/PR-negative tumors[10] (Table 98.5).
- An aromatase inhibitor (AI) like anastrozole or letrozole is commonly used in the first-line setting. Depending on the interval from initial diagnosis to

TABLE 98.5: ENDOCRINE THERAPIES USED TO TREAT METASTATIC BREAST CANCER AND TOXICITIES[9]

Endocrine Therapy	Toxicities
Aromatase inhibitors (oral, once daily): Anastrozole Letrozole Exemestane	See Table 98.3
Tamoxifen (oral, once daily)	See Table 98.3
Fulvestrant (intramuscular injection, monthly)	Asthenia Hot flashes Mild nausea/vomiting Flu-like syndrome—fever, malaise, myalgias (10%)
Megace (oral, four times/day)	Weight gain Rare thromboembolic events

progression, women who were treated with an AI in the adjuvant setting may again be treated with an AI in the metastatic setting.

- Single-agent endocrine therapy is continued until disease progression is noted, with different agents tried in succession for the longest period of time.

Chemotherapy

- Chemotherapy may be an option once a tumor progresses on endocrine therapy, or if a patient presents with rapidly progressing or life-threatening visceral disease.
- Overall, chemotherapy usually results in a more rapid but shorter duration of response than endocrine therapy. The response rates tend to be higher in first-line therapy, diminishing with each subsequent regimen.
- Incremental advances in chemotherapy treatments have resulted in statistically significant improvements in overall survival rates for metastatic cancer patients.
- Combination chemotherapy, while associated with significant treatment-related toxicity, is also associated with higher response rates and may be appropriate in treating patients with life-threatening visceral disease or rapidly progressing symptoms.

- Combination therapies have shown only a modest over-all survival benefit compared to single-agent chemotherapy. Utilizing sequential single-agent therapy is therefore a valid approach to minimize toxicities and improve quality of life in older women with metastatic breast cancer.
- See Table 98.6 for various chemotherapies that may be used to treat metastatic breast cancer. As mentioned previously, most chemotherapy regimens cause myelosuppression, nausea/vomiting, mucositis, alopecia, and fatigue.
- In general, elderly patients experience more chemotherapy-related side effects than younger patients. Lower doses of certain therapies (e.g., capecitabine) or alternative dosing schedules (e.g., weekly dosing) may be warranted in patients of advanced age.

HER2-Targeted Therapy

- HER2-targeted therapies have provided new treatment options for women with HER2-positive breast cancer. Trastuzumab may be used in conjunction with chemotherapy to treat HER2-positive cancers. In the metastatic setting, one may consider trastuzumab monotherapy.
- Lapatinib is an orally active dual tyrosine kinase inhibitor of both HER2 and epidermal growth factor receptor (EGFR) and has been approved in combination with capecitabine in women with HER2-positive cancers previously treated with anthracyclines, taxanes, and trastuzumab.

Radiation Therapy

- Radiation therapy may be used to palliate symptoms of pain in patients with bone and chest wall metastases. Radiation may also be utilized to treat patients with brain metastases.
- There are data to support the use of single fraction radiotherapy for the palliation of pain from bony metastases, although the re-treatment and pathological fracture

---

TABLE 98.6: CHEMOTHERAPIES USED TO TREAT METASTATIC BREAST CANCER AND TOXICITIES[9]

Chemotherapy	Toxicities
Anthracyclines: Doxorubicin Epirubicin Pegylated liposomal doxorubicin	See Table 98.4 Pegylated liposomal doxorubicin has less cardiotoxicity than doxorubicin.
Paclitaxel	See Table 98.4
Docetaxel	See Table 98.4
Albumin-bound paclitaxel	Peripheral neuropathy—dose-dependent, less than with paclitaxel Asthenia
Capecitabine (oral, twice daily)	Diarrhea (dose-limiting), mucositis, anorexia Hand-foot syndrome—paresthesias, pain, erythema, rash, dryness, pruritis of the hands and/or feet *Note:* less risk of alopecia
Gemcitabine	Flu-like syndrome—fever, chills, headache, myalgias Pulmonary toxicity—mild dyspnea, drug-induced pneumonitis *Note:* less risk of alopecia
Vinorelbine	Constipation Peripheral neuropathy
Ixabepilone	Peripheral neuropathy Asthenia Diarrhea
Eribulin	Peripheral neuropathy Constipation

BOX 98.1 HER2-TARGETED THERAPIES AND TOXICITIES[9]

Therapy	Toxicities
Trastuzumab (*intravenous, every 3 weeks*)	Cardiotoxicity with reduced LV function Nausea/vomiting, diarrhea Myelosuppression
Lapatinib (*oral, once daily*)	Diarrhea (dose-limiting) Nausea/vomiting Cardiotoxicity with reduced LV function Myelosuppression (mostly anemia) Hand-foot syndrome and skin rash

rates may be higher when compared to patients treated with multiple fraction radiotherapy.[11]

- Because single-fraction radiotherapy is a more efficient, less costly, and better tolerated treatment, it should be recommended for palliative pain management in older or seriously ill patients.

PALLIATIVE CARE ISSUES

- Women treated for breast cancer may have cancer-related as well as comorbid disease issues that impact their quality of life. These challenges may include physical and psychosocial impairments as well as treatment-related complications (Table 98.7). These issues can occur in patients who are considered cured, as well as in those who are living with chronic or advanced disease.
- Complications of advanced cancer and associated symptoms are described in Table 98.8. As patients may live for years with metastatic breast cancer (especially those with non-visceral metastases), effective management of these issues is critically important to maintain and optimize a patient's quality of life.

TAKE-HOME POINTS

- Although breast cancers in older patients have less aggressive tumor characteristics than in younger patients, patients of advanced age may present with more advanced-stage disease and may have poorer outcomes due to undertreatment.

TABLE 98.7: COMPLICATIONS OF BREAST CANCER THERAPIES

Complication	Associated Symptoms	Treatment Options
Lymphedema—most commonly in the upper extremities after lymph node dissection but may occur after sentinel lymph node biopsy[12]	Edema Paresthesias Sensation of heaviness/tightness	Prevention includes elevation, exercise, massage, wraps, and compression garments Advised to avoid venipuncture and blood pressure measurements on the side of the lymph node surgery Treatment includes manual therapies (massage technique performed by certified lymphedema therapists), compression bandaging, exercises Referral to a specialist is recommended (See Chapter 58: Lymphedema)
Shoulder dysfunction after breast cancer surgery[8]	Shoulder immobility Fibrous tissue deposits ("cords") in the axillary and chest wall area	Home exercise program in the early postoperative period Physical therapy
Chronic pain after mastectomy	Breast pain	Home exercises Physical therapy Acetaminophen or NSAIDs for mild-to-moderate pain Opioids for more severe or increasing pain Adjuvant analgesics such as TCA, anticonvulsants, and neuroleptics may also be helpful
Neuropathy due to chemotherapy	Usually decreases or goes away after treatment is stopped Occasionally residual symptoms persist	Gabapentin TCAs (See Chapter 29: Management of Pain in Older Adults)
Hot flashes due to endocrine therapy		Venlafaxine Gabapentin Clonidine Acupuncture therapy

TABLE 98.8: COMPLICATIONS OF ADVANCED BREAST CANCER

Complication	Associated Symptoms	Treatment Options
Progressive disease (local or metastatic lesions)	Pain	Acetaminophen or NSAIDs for mild-to-moderate pain Opioids for more severe or increasing pain (See Chapter 29: Management of Pain in Older Adults) Adjuvant analgesics such as TCA, anticonvulsants, and neuroleptics may also be helpful. (See Chapter 29: Management of Pain in Older Adults)
Lung metastases	Dyspnea	Opioids (See Chapter 41: Dyspnea) Oxygen (See Chapter 41: Dyspnea) Bronchodilators
Liver metastases	Edema Ascites Encephalopathy Pain	Diuretics (See Chapter 76: End-Stage Liver Disease) For pain, opioids and corticosteroids should be used. (See Chapter 76: End-Stage Liver Disease)
Bone metastases	Pain Pathologic fractures	Bisphosphonates—have been shown to prevent skeletal-related events (e.g., bone fractures, bone pain requiring radiation therapy, spinal cord compression, and hypercalcemia)[2] NSAIDS Opioids (See Chapter 29: Management of Pain in Older Adults) Corticosteroids Radiation therapy Surgical stabilization or repair may be indicated For widespread bone disease, systemic radionuclides in patients with life expectancy of > 3 months (e.g., strontium-89 chloride)
Brain metastases	Change in mental status Focal neurologic symptoms Headache Nausea/vomiting	Corticosteroids Radiation Surgical resection may be considered in selected patients
Spinal cord metastases	Back pain	Corticosteroids Radiation Neurosurgical intervention may be indicated. (See Chapter 14: Palliative Care Emergencies)
Leptomeningeal metastases [12]	Headache Nausea/vomiting Seizure Altered mental status Cauda equina syndrome Cranial nerve abnormalities Polyradiculopathy	Corticosteroids Whole brain radiation and intrathecal chemotherapy may be considered. (See Chapter 102: Intracranial Malignancies)

- In early-stage breast cancers, surgery is indicated for those patients who are able to tolerate it. Older women may also benefit from radiotherapy, adjuvant chemotherapy, and/or adjuvant endocrine therapy. The

Adjuvant! Online tool and the Oncotype DX assay can help guide decisions about adjuvant therapy.
- Patients may live for years with metastatic breast cancer and will often benefit from

endocrine or chemotherapy treatments. Continual symptom assessment and treatment of the complications of metastatic disease are key strategies for maintaining a patient's quality of life.

- Palliation of treatment-related side effects, symptom management and psychosocial/ spiritual support are essential from the point of diagnosis throughout the course of the illness.

RESOURCES

Breastcancer.org:
www.breastcancer.org (English)
Living Beyond Breast Cancer:
www.lbbc.org (English)
888-753-5222 (English and Spanish)
SHARE: Self-help for Women with Breast or Ovarian Cancer:
www.sharecancersupport.org (English and Spanish)
212-382-2111 (English)
Susan G. Komen Breast Cancer Foundation:
www.komen.org (English and Spanish)
800-462-9273 (English and Spanish)
Y-ME National Breast Cancer Organization:
www.y-me.org (English)
www.y-me.org/espanol (Spanish)
800-221-2141 (English)
800-986-9505 (Spanish)

REFERENCES

1. Altekruse S et al. *SEER Cancer Statistics Review, 1975–2007*. Available from: http://seer.cancer.gov/csr/1975_2007/.

2. *Breast Cancer*. NCCN Clinical Practice Guidelines in Oncology 2011; Version 2.2011: Available from: www.nccn.org.

3. Bouchardy C et al. Undertreatment strongly decreases prognosis of breast cancer in elderly women. *J Clin Oncol.* 2003;*21*(19):3580–3587.

4. Gennari R et al. Breast carcinoma in elderly women: features of disease presentation, choice of local and systemic treatments compared with younger postmenopasual patients. *Cancer.* 2004;*101*(6): 1302–1310.

5. Edge S et al., eds. *AJCC Cancer Staging Manual.* 7th ed. New York, NY: Springer-Verlag; 2009.

6. Fisher B et al. Tamoxifen in treatment of intraductal breast cancer: National Surgical Adjuvant Breast and Bowel Project B-24 randomised controlled trial. *Lancet.* 1999;*353*(9169):1993–2000.

7. Crivellari D et al. Breast cancer in the elderly. *J Clin Oncol.* 2007;25(14):1882–1890.

8. Hunt KK, Robb GL, Strom EA, et al., eds. *Breast Cancer.* 2nd ed. New York, NY: Springer; 2008.

9. Chu E, Devita VT Jr., eds. *Physicians' Cancer Chemotherapy Drug Manual.* Sudbury, MA: Jones and Bartlett Publishers; 2008.

10. Petrakis IE, Paraskakis S. Breast cancer in the elderly. *Arch Gerontol Geriatr.* 2010;*50*(2):179–184.

11. Sze WM, Shelley M, Held I, Mason M. Palliation of metastatic bone pain: single fraction versus multifraction radiotherapy. *Cochrane Database of Systematic Reviews* 2002;Issue 1. Art. No.: CD004721.

12. Devita VT, Lawrence TS, Rosenberg SA, eds. *Cancer Principles and Practice of Oncology.* 8th ed. Philadelphia: Lippincott, Williams, & Wilkins; 2008.

99

Prostate Cancer

CASE

Mr. W is an 81-year-old man with a history of hypertension and benign prostatic hypertrophy who presents to his primary medical doctor with complaints of progressively worsening back pain over the last six weeks.

DEFINITION

Prostate cancer is the most common cancer diagnosed in men in the United States. The vast majority of prostate cancers are adenocarcinoma.[1]

INCIDENCE

- Prostate cancer is typically a disease of the elderly. The median age at diagnosis is 68 years, and the incidence increases with age, peaking at 80.[1]
- Additional risk factors for prostate cancer include race (the highest incidence of prostate cancer is in African-American men who often present with more advanced disease) and obesity.[1]

DIAGNOSIS

Presentation

- In the past, the most common presenting signs and symptoms of prostate cancer were obstructive urinary symptoms and/or abnormalities found on digital rectal exam (DRE).
- Since the introduction of prostate-specific antigen (PSA) screening, prostate cancer is most commonly diagnosed at earlier stages, when patients are asymptomatic.[1] (See note below on USPSTF screening guidelines.)

Exam

- Initial physical examination of a patient suspected of having prostate cancer should include a DRE to assess the prostate for nodularity or induration.
- All geriatric patients should also have an assessment of medical comorbidities, performance status, cognitive ability, and social support.

Tests

- The U.S. Preventive Services Task Force (USPSTF) recommends that healthy men without symptoms should not be screened for prostate cancer. This advisory is based on evidence that PSA screening does not save lives overall and often leads to treatments that carry the risk of serious complications, including impotence and incontinence.[2]
- An elevated PSA alone is not diagnostic of prostate cancer; PSA may be elevated as a result of benign prostatic hypertrophy as well as prostatitis.
- While PSA testing should be used judiciously and not as a routine screening process, once a patient is suspected of having prostate cancer, initial staging workup should include PSA testing and prostate biopsy with histologic grading.

On physical examination, the doctor notes decreased strength in Mr. W's lower extremities with hyperreflexia and decreased anal sphincter tone. MRI of the spine reveals cord compression at L1-L2 with evidence of metastatic disease in the vertebrae. Blood work reveals a PSA level of 27.

STAGING AND SURVIVAL

- The most widely used cancer staging system for prostate cancer is the TNM system (Table 99.1).
- Survival is dependent on patient age, comorbidities, tumor grade, and stage at time of diagnosis.[1] The standard histologic grading system used for prostate cancer is the Gleason score.[4]

Grade	Degree of Differentiation	Gleason Score
GX	Grade cannot be assessed	
G1	Well differentiated	Gleason 2–4
G2	Moderately differentiated	Gleason 5–6
G3–4	Poorly differentiated or undifferentiated	Gleason 7–10

TABLE 99.1: STAGING OF PROSTATE CANCER[4]

	TNM Staging
Localized disease	T1a—incidental histologic finding involving ≤ 5% of resected tissue
	T1b—incidental histologic finding involving > 5% of resected tissue
	T1c—identified by needle biopsy
	T2a involves ≤ ½ of one lobe
	T2b involves > ½ of one lobe
	T2c involves both lobes
Locally advanced disease	T3a—extracapsular extension
	T3b—tumor invades seminal vesicle
	T4—invades bladder, pelvic side wall, or adjacent structures
Metastatic disease	N1—positive regional lymph nodes
	M1—distant metastasis
Stage 1: T1a, G1	Stage 3: T3
Stage 2: T1a(G2–4)–T2	Stage 4: T4, N0; N1; or M1

- After excluding patients whose cause of death is a diagnosis other than prostate cancer, the relative five-year survival rate for men with prostate cancer is 100%, the relative 10-year survival rate is 91%, and the relative 15-year survival rate is 76%.[1] Therefore, further decision-making about staging workup should take into account the patient's life expectancy, presence of symptoms, PSA level, and Gleason score.
- Patients with a life expectancy greater than five years who have symptoms, a higher PSA level (>20), locally advanced disease (T3–4), or Gleason score ≥ 8 should undergo further workup and treatment.[3]
- Further evaluation should include bone scan and a pelvic CT or MRI for all patients with T3–T4 disease or T1–T2 disease with high suspicion of lymph node involvement.[3]

TREATMENT OPTIONS

Localized Disease

There are several treatment options for clinically localized (T1 or T2) prostate cancer (Table 99.2).

- Selecting the appropriate treatment option should take into account the risks and benefits of each option, patient performance status, ability to tolerate therapy, and individual patient preference.
- PSA levels should be followed after completion of definitive therapy because rising PSA level indicates evidence of recurrent disease.[3]

Locally Advanced Disease

- Treatment options for locally advanced prostate cancer include:
  - Radiation therapy (XRT)
  - Hormonal therapy with XRT
  - Radical prostatectomy +/– hormonal therapy
- Making a decision about treatment options should take into consideration a patient's medical comorbidities, life expectancy, treatment-related side effects, and personal preference.

Mr. W receives high-dose steroids followed by emergent neurosurgical intervention for treatment of his spinal cord compression. After a period of physical rehabilitation, Mr. W regains 90% of his strength and begins treatment with every-three-month leuprolide acetate.

Advanced Systemic (Metastatic) Disease

- Whether patients are presenting with recurrent systemic disease after treatment of more localized prostate cancer, or are presenting with advanced systemic disease at the point of diagnosis, the primary treatment approach is medical or surgical castration (Table 99.3).
- First-line hormonal therapy generally controls symptoms for one and a half to two years.[5]

Hormone-Refractory Disease

- After the development of hormone-refractory disease, the median survival is nine to twelve months.[5]

TABLE 99.2: PRIMARY MANAGEMENT OPTIONS FOR CLINICALLY LOCALIZED PROSTATE CANCER[3]

Treatment Option	Approach	Advantages	Disadvantages
Active surveillance	Staging Assessment of life expectancy Regular follow-up DRE and PSA every 6 months Repeat biopsy as clinically indicated Plan for intervention if cancer progresses	Avoid side effects of aggressive therapy Quality of life maintained Risk of unnecessary treatment of indolent disease reduced	Potential to miss opportunity for cure Potential to need more aggressive interventions Frequent medical follow-up Potential need for repeated biopsies
Radiation	External beam radiotherapy	Avoids complications associated with surgery Low risk of urinary incontinence and stricture Less risk of acute erectile dysfunction	Treatment course of 8–9 weeks Up to 50% of patients have temporary bladder or bowel symptoms Radiation proctitis Risk of erectile dysfunction increases over time
	Brachytherapy (*Placement of permanent or temporary radioactive implants into prostate*)	Treatment is completed in 1 day Quick recovery time Control rate for low-risk tumors comparable to surgery	Requires general anesthesia Risk of acute urinary retention
Surgery	Radical prostatectomy	Average hospital stay is 3 days High control rate for localized tumors	Risk of bleeding Anesthesia risks (e.g., MI, PE) Urinary incontinence is common in first few months; most patients recover Risk of erectile dysfunction
	Nerve sparing radical prostatectomy	Higher erection recovery rate than standard surgery Appropriate for men with small-volume disease	

- Chemotherapy regimens that have been used for the treatment of prostate cancer include mitoxantrone and prednisone and docetaxel-based regimens.
- The preferred first-line chemotherapy is docetaxel + prednisone.[3] A docetaxel-based regimen administered every three weeks results in improved pain relief and a small (<2.5 month) survival benefit.[6]
- There are no age-related differences in docetaxel efficacy. Strong consideration should be given to the use of growth factor support in patients over the age of 65.[3]

- The major chemotherapy-related toxicities are myelosuppression, gastrointestinal toxicity, neuropathy, and alopecia.
- Abiraterone acetate, an inhibitor of androgen biosynthesis, prolongs survival by approximately four months in patients who have progressed through a docetaxel-based regimen.[8]
- Bisphosphonate therapy significantly decreases pain and the incidence of pathologic fractures in patients receiving chemotherapy for prostate cancer.[5]

TABLE 99.3: HORMONAL THERAPY FOR PROSTATE CANCER[4]

Class	Medications	Indications/Advantages	Side Effects
LHRH analogs* (*can cause transient "flare" response with initial treatment)	Leuprolide acetate Goserelin acetate	Produce chemical castration, sparing the psychological trauma of surgery Injectable medication given every 3, 4, 6, or 12 months	Hot flashes (50%) Fatigue Mild gynecomastia Erectile dysfunction Depression
Antiandrogens	Flutamide Bicalutamide Nilutamide Ketoconazole	Block transient "flare" caused by LHRH agonists Added to LHRH when patients stop responding to those agents alone Ketoconazole (+/−hydrocortisone) can be used as a second-line hormonal agent	Abnormal liver function tests Diarrhea (10%) Erectile dysfunction Depression
Combined androgen blockade	LHRH agonist + antiandrogen	Most beneficial for patients presenting with minimal symptoms and minimal systemic disease At time of progression of disease, removal of antiandrogen can cause paradoxical decrease in disease burden	Hot flashes Fatigue Mild gynecomastia Abnormal liver function tests Diarrhea Erectile dysfunction Depression
Estrogens	Diethylstilbestrol (DES)	Can be considered for second-line hormonal therapy	Gynecomastia Cardiovascular risks at high doses Erectile dysfunction Depression
Inhibitor of androgen biosynthesis	Abiraterone acetate	Indicated for second line for hormone-refractory disease after docetaxel failure Consider for patients with hormone-refractory disease who are not candidates for chemotherapy	Hypertension Hypokalemia Peripheral edema Liver injury Fatigue

COMPLICATIONS OF ADVANCED PROSTATE CANCER

The complications experienced by patients with advanced prostate cancer are listed in Table 94.4.

PALLIATIVE CARE ISSUES

- Palliative care should be integrated into the collaborative treatment model for prostate cancer patients (surgeon, oncologist, radiologist). Concurrent care assures that patients and their families will be offered pain and symptom management, advance care planning, psychosocial support, and coordination of resources.
- Palliative care comanagement also ensures enhanced provider-patient-caregiver communication on the topics of

establishing achievable goals of care, what to expect as disease progresses, and fully informed decision-making regarding transitions between care settings, including timely and appropriate referral to hospice.[7]

- Health-related quality of life (HRQOL) issues should be discussed with patients in order to set realistic expectations and facilitate informed treatment decisions. HRQOL domains commonly affected by prostate cancer treatment include urinary, bowel, vitality, and sexual function.[9]

TAKE-HOME POINTS

- Screening for prostate cancer should be offered to patients, but decisions to

TABLE 99.4: COMMON COMPLICATIONS OF ADVANCED PROSTATE CANCER

Complication	Associated Signs and Symptoms	Treatment Options
Bone metastasis	Pain Pathologic fracture	Opioids Bisphosphonates Steroids XRT to specific painful lesions Strontium-89 Samarium-153
Cord compression[a]	Back pain Bowel/bladder incontinence Weakness Inability to ambulate	Steroids Radiation Surgery
Ureteral obstruction	Pain Nausea Acute renal failure	Nephrostomy tube placement
Pulmonary embolus	Dyspnea Pleuritic chest pain	Opioids Anxiolytics Oxygen Anticoagulation, if appropriate

[a] Cord compression is a medical and palliative care emergency. Failure to treat immediately may lead to neurological compromise, including loss of bowel and bladder continence as well as loss of lower extremity sensation and function. (See Chapter 71: Malignant Spinal Cord Compression.)

proceed with testing should include a discussion of the benefits and burdens, taking into account the patient's risk factors, age, life expectancy, and personal preferences.

- Treatment options for localized prostate cancer include watchful waiting, radiation therapy, and surgery. Treatment decisions must take into consideration a patient's medical comorbidities, life expectancy, treatment-related side effects, and personal preference.
- The mainstay of treatment for patients with metastatic prostate cancer is hormonal therapy and bisphosphonates.
- Chemotherapy for hormone refractory disease may offer palliation of symptoms and a small survival advantage, and should therefore be considered for patients with good performance status who will be able to tolerate expected chemotherapy-related toxicities.
- A concurrent care approach, integrating palliative care with the collaborative oncology treatment model (surgeon, oncologist, radiologist), assures that patients and families will be offered pain and symptom management, advance care planning, psychosocial support and coordination of resources.

REFERENCES

1. American Cancer Society. Available online at: http://www.cancer.org/Cancer/ProstateCancer/DetailedGuide/index. Accessed March, 2012.
2. U.S. Preventive Services Task Force. Available online at: http://www.uspreventiveservicestaskforce.org/uspstf/uspsprca.htm. Accessed on March 15, 2012.
3. National Comprehensive Cancer Network (NCCN) guidelines. Available online at: www.nccn.org. Accessed March 15, 2012.
4. Greene FL, Page DL, Fleming ID, et al., eds. *AJCC Cancer Staging Manual*, 6th ed. New York, NY: Springer-Verlag; 2002.
5. Pazdur R, Coia LR, Hoskins WJ, et al., eds. *Cancer Management a Multidisciplinary Approach*, 8th ed. New York, NY: CMP Healthcare Media; 2004.
6. Mike S, Harrison C, Coles B, et al. Chemotherapy for hormone-refractory prostate cancer. *Cochrane Database Syst Rev*. Oct 18, 2006;(4):CD005247.
7. Bruera E, Hui D. Integrating supportive and palliative care in the trajectory of cancer: establishing goals and models of care. *J Clin Oncol*. 2010;28(25):4013–4017.
8. De Bono JS, Logothetis CJ, Molina A, et al. Abiraterone and increased survival in metastatic prostate cancer. *N Engl J Med*. 2011;364:1995–2005.
9. Alemozaffer M, Regan M, Cooperberg MR, Wei J, et al. Prediction of erectile function following treatment for prostate cancer. *JAMA*. 2011;506(11):1205–1214.

100

Lung Cancer

CASE

Mr. R is a 72-year-old male with hypertension and a 20 pack-year history of tobacco use who presents with progressive dyspnea on exertion over the last two months. His examination reveals diminished breath sounds at the left base. A chest radiograph and chest CT scan show a 5 cm left upper lobe mass and a left pleural effusion. A bronchoscopy with biopsy is performed, and the pathology demonstrates a lung adenocarcinoma.

DEFINITION

The term *lung cancer* refers to malignancies that originate in the airways or pulmonary parenchyma.

CLASSIFICATION

Non-small-cell lung cancer (NSCLC):

- Represents 80% to 85% of lung cancers
- Includes adenocarcinoma, squamous carcinoma, and large-cell carcinoma

Small-cell lung cancer (SCLC):

- Represents 15% of lung cancers
- Has a faster doubling time, a higher growth fraction, and an earlier development of metastases than non-small-cell lung cancer

PREVALENCE

- Most common cancer in the world
- Second most common cancer in both men and women in the United States.
- Leading cause of cancer-related deaths in the United States
- Incidence increases with age, with a median age at diagnosis of 71 years old.[1]
- More than 65% of cases of lung cancer are diagnosed in patients > 65 years old.[1]

RISK FACTORS

- Cigarette smoking: More than 85% of all cases of lung cancer are related to smoking.
- Asbestos exposure: Increases risk by 90-fold, particularly in smokers.
- Radioactive dust and radon exposure.

DIAGNOSIS

Presentation

A patient's presentation is dependent on the location and extent of tumor involvement. Symptoms may include the following:

- Cough: Smokers with a chronic cough may experience a change in the frequency or severity of their cough.
- Dyspnea
- Hemoptysis
- Weight loss
- Post-obstructive pneumonia, due to bronchial obstruction
- Chest pain, from tumor invasion of the chest wall
- Shoulder/arm pain and Horner's syndrome, from apical tumors
- Symptoms attributed to distant metastatic disease. Most common sites of metastases are the brain, bone, and liver.
- Endocrine and neurologic paraneoplastic syndromes. Small-cell lung cancer is associated with SIADH (syndrome of inappropriate antidiuretic hormone), Cushing's syndrome, Lambert-Eaton syndrome, encephalomyelitis, and sensory neuropathy.

History and Exam

- A thorough history includes an assessment of performance status, weight loss, comorbidities, cognitive ability, social support structure.
- A complete physical examination should include a lung examination with careful auscultation and percussion as well as a thorough lymph node examination of the neck and supraclavicular fossa.

Tests

- Chest imaging (chest X-ray, chest CT scan) to locate the lesion
- Tissue diagnosis:
  - Sputum cytology and flexible bronchoscopy for centrally located lesions
  - CT-guided needle biopsy for peripheral lesions
  - Peripheral lymph node biopsy for palpable cervical or supraclavicular nodes
  - Thoracentesis for suspected malignant pleural effusion
- Staging evaluation:
  - CT scan of the chest and upper abdomen, including the adrenals (to assess for liver and adrenal metastases)
- Lab work: Complete blood count, chemistries, liver and kidney function tests
- For non-small-cell lung cancer staging, other testing may be necessary if the patient is a potential surgical candidate. This may include a brain MRI, PET CT, and mediastinoscopy.
- For small-cell lung cancer staging, a brain MRI and PET CT are recommended, given its highly metastatic nature.

STAGING

- The revised TNM (Tumor/Node/Met) staging system for lung cancer was released in 2010. These staging criteria pertain

---

TABLE 100.1: TNM STAGING SYSTEM FOR LUNG CANCER[2]

Primary Tumor (T)

T1	Tumor ≤ 3 cm in greatest dimension, surrounded by lung or visceral pleura, without invasion more proximal than the lobar bronchus
T1a	Tumor ≤ 2 cm in greatest dimension
T1b	Tumor > 2 cm but ≤ 3 cm in greatest dimension
T2	Tumor > 3 cm diameter but ≤ 7 cm in greatest dimension **OR** tumor with any of the following features:
	Involves main bronchus, ≥ 2 cm distal to the carina
	Invades the visceral pleura
	Associated atelectasis or obstructive pneumonitis that extends to the hilar region but does not involve the entire lung
T2a	Tumor > 3 cm but ≤ 5 cm
T2b	Tumor > 5 cm but ≤ 7 cm
T3	Tumor > 7 cm **OR** any of the following:
	Invasion of the chest wall (including superior sulcus tumors), diaphragm, mediastinal pleura, parietal pleura, parietal pericardium, phrenic nerve
	Tumor in the main bronchus < 2 cm distal to the carina (not involving the carina)
	Associated atelectasis or obstructive pneumonitis of the entire lung
	Separate tumor nodule(s) in the same lobe
T4	Tumor of any size with any of the following:
	Invasion of the mediastinum, heart, great vessels, trachea, esophagus, vertebral body, carina, recurrent laryngeal nerve
	Separate tumor nodules in a different ipsilateral lobe

Regional Lymph Nodes (N)

N0	No regional lymph node metastasis
N1	Metastasis in ipsilateral peribronchial and/or ipsilateral hilar lymph nodes and intrapulmonary nodes, including involvement by direct extension

(continued)

TABLE 100.1: (CONTINUED)

N2	Metastasis in ipsilateral mediastinal and/or subcarinal lymph node(s)	
N3	Metastasis in contralateral mediastinal, contralateral hilar, ipsilateral or contralateral scalene, or supraclavicular lymph node(s)	

Distant Metastasis (M)

M0	No distant metastasis
M1	Distant metastasis
M1a	Separate tumor nodule(s) in a contralateral lobeTumor with pleural nodules Malignant pleural or pericardial effusion
M1b	Distant metastasis

Stage Groupings

Stage IA	T1a or T1b	N0	M0
Stage IB	T2a	N0	M0
Stage IIA	T2b	N0	M0
Stage IIB	T1a, T1b, or T2a	N1	M0
	T2b	N1	M0
	T3	N0	M0
Stage IIIA	T1a, T1b, T2a, or T2b	N2	M0
Stage IIIB	T3	N1 or N2	M0
	T4	N0 or N1	M0
	T4	N2	M0
	Any T	N3	M0
Stage IV	Any T	Any N	M1a or M1b

mostly to non-small-cell lung cancer (Table 100.1).

- Small-cell lung cancer is usually classified into limited-stage and extensive-stage disease.[3]

  Limited-stage: Disease confined to the ipsilateral hemithorax; can be safely encompassed within a tolerable radiation field

  Extensive-stage: Disease beyond the ipsilateral hemithorax; may include malignant pleural or pericardial effusion or hematogenous metastases

PROGNOSIS

- Lung cancer typically has a poor prognosis because most patients present with advanced or metastatic disease at the time of diagnosis.
- Numerous prognostic factors have been studied, but the most prominent and widely used is disease stage (Table 100.2).

TREATMENT OPTIONS

Non-Small-Cell Lung Cancer
Early Stage NSCLC

- Unfortunately, only a minority of patients present with potentially curable disease.

TABLE 100.2: LUNG CANCER STAGE DISTRIBUTION AND FIVE-YEAR SURVIVAL RATES[1]

Stage Distribution	Stage Distribution at Diagnosis	5-year Survival
Localized stage (confined to the primary site)	15%	52.9%
Regional spread (cancer has spread to regional lymph nodes or directly beyond the primary site)	22%	24%
Distant stage (cancer has metastasized)	56%	3.5%
Unknown	8%	8.7%

- Surgery, chemotherapy, radiation, or combined modalities may be offered to older adults with curative intent.
- Treatment decisions are dependent on a host of patient characteristics, including but not limited to a patient's functional status, comorbidities, organ function, prognosis, and goals of care.
- For those patients who decline surgery or who are not appropriate candidates, definitive radiation may be a possibility. Some patients may be cured with radiation alone.
- The acute side effects of radiation may include odynophagia, dysphagia, cough, and hoarseness as well as pneumonitis and carditis. The late sequelae of radiation include progressive pulmonary fibrosis, dyspnea, and chronic cough. Esophageal strictures have also been observed.

Advanced Stage NSCLC

- Chemotherapy is the cornerstone of management for patients with advanced non-small-cell lung cancer (Table 100.3). However, the medical and physiological complexity of older adults often puts older patients at risk for undertreatment.[4]
- Age alone has not been shown to have an impact on survival in patients with advanced non-small-cell lung cancer. Rather, a patient's performance status, extent of disease, and weight loss in the last six months are the most important prognostic factors for survival.[4]
- It is important to recognize that older adults are underrepresented in clinical trials. As a result, therapeutic guidelines have been largely derived from prospective trials and retrospective subgroup analyses.[4]
- Older adults who have minimal comorbidities and a good performance status may be considered for treatment with combination chemotherapy, usually with carboplatin in addition to another agent (e.g., paclitaxel). Recent data looking at combination therapy in patients older than 70 years indicate that that survival is prolonged and that therapy is generally well tolerated.[5]
- Older adults with advanced non-small-cell lung cancer who are not deemed candidates for combination chemotherapy may be considered for single-agent chemotherapy. Commonly used chemotherapies include vinorelbine, gemcitabine, docetaxel, paclitaxel, and pemetrexed. Factors that need to be considered include chemotherapy toxicities, organ function, and the comorbidities of the patient. There

TABLE 100.3: CHEMOTHERAPIES USED TO TREAT NON-SMALL-CELL LUNG CANCER[8]

Chemotherapy	Toxicities
Vinorelbine	Myelosuppression Nausea/vomiting Constipation, diarrhea, stomatitis, anorexia Peripheral neuropathy Alopecia Fatigue
Gemcitabine	Myelosuppression Nausea/vomiting, diarrhea, mucositis Flu-like syndrome (fever, chills, headache, myalgias)
Paclitaxel	Myelosuppression Peripheral neuropathy Alopecia Mucositis, diarrhea, nausea/vomiting
Docetaxel	Myelosuppression Fluid retention (weight gain, edema, pleural effusion, ascites) Alopecia Mucositis, diarrhea, nausea/vomiting Peripheral neuropathy Fatigue, arthralgias, myalgias
Pemetrexed (for non-squamous histology)	Myelosuppression Skin rash Mouth ulcers Nausea/vomiting, diarrhea
Cisplatin	Nephrotoxicity Nausea/vomiting Myelosuppression Peripheral neuropathy Ototoxicity Metallic taste of food, anorexia Alopecia
Carboplatin	Myelosuppression Nausea/vomiting Nephrotoxicity Peripheral neuropathy

is data to support not only prolonged survival with chemotherapy but also palliation of lung cancer-related symptoms and improved quality of life.

- Tumors that have a non-squamous histology should be tested for a mutation in the epidermal growth factor receptor (EGFR).[6] In those patients whose tumors have this mutation, erlotinib is recommended as first-line therapy.[6]
- Patients who refuse or are unlikely to tolerate chemotherapy may also be considered for erlotinib, even if they do not have an EGFR mutation (although a benefit is less likely to be seen). Erlotinib is a daily oral therapy that is generally well tolerated, although common side effects include an acneiform rash and diarrhea.
- The addition of palliative care in conjunction with anticancer therapies provides patients and their families with a range of care needs including symptom management, advance care planning, psychosocial support, coordination of resources, and establishing achievable goals of care based on performance status, prognosis, and patient preferences.
- Early palliative care in addition to standard oncology care for patients with newly diagnosed non-small-cell lung cancer is associated with improved quality of life, improved mood, and longer survival.[7]

Mr. R undergoes a left thoracentesis, and the cytology shows malignant cells. A brain MRI does not show metastases. Given the malignant pleural effusion, Mr. R has Stage IV lung cancer. His tumor does not contain an EGFR mutation. Since he has an excellent performance status, Mr. R's oncologist discusses palliative combination chemotherapy with Mr. R. The oncologist explains that combination chemotherapy has been shown to prolong survival even in older patients, without compromising quality of life. After Mr. R discusses this information with his family, he agrees to proceed with chemotherapy.

Small-Cell Lung Cancer

- Due to the aggressive nature of small-cell lung cancer, staging and evaluation by an oncologist should be expedited, and treatment should be initiated within one week of diagnosis.[3] Treatment delays may precipitate a rapid clinical decline. The median survival of patients with untreated

small-cell lung cancer is two to four months.[9]
- Unfortunately, most patients, including those initially diagnosed with limited-stage disease, will eventually die from recurrent disease. Factors that portend a poor prognosis include extensive-stage disease, a poor performance status, and weight loss.
- Older patients with a good functional status are treated with standard combination chemotherapy +/− radiotherapy. They have prognoses similar to younger patients.[3]
- In patients who are less fit, reduction in treatment cycles, reduction in chemotherapy/radiotherapy dose, or single-agent chemotherapy may be options.
- As in non-small-cell lung cancer, both survival and quality of life are improved in treated patients.[9] However, the practitioner should be aware that treatment-related myelosuppression, fatigue, and diminished organ reserves are more commonly seen in patients of advanced age.

Limited-Stage SCLC (20–30%)

- Surgery: Only a small minority of patients (2% to 5%) present with disease amenable to surgical resection. Staging of the mediastinum to rule out mediastinal lymph node involvement is important to pursue prior to surgical resection. Patients who undergo resection should then be treated with adjuvant chemotherapy.
- Concurrent chemotherapy and thoracic radiotherapy: Small cell lung cancer is very sensitive to chemotherapy and radiation, and patients with limited-stage disease are treated with curative intent. Etoposide and cisplatin with concurrent thoracic radiotherapy are the standard of care. Carboplatin may be substituted for cisplatin in order to reduce the risk of emesis, nephropathy, and neuropathy, but this is recommended only when cisplatin is contraindicated or poorly tolerated.
- Prophylactic cranial irradiation (PCI): PCI decreases the incidence of cerebral metastases and improves both disease-free and overall survival in patients who experience a complete remission.[3] In those patients who have a complete response to chemotherapy, PCI should be administered after the completion of chemotherapy in order to reduce the neurologic toxicity. PCI is not recommended for patients

with a poor performance status, multiple comorbidities, or cognitive dysfunction.

Extensive-Stage SCLC

- Chemotherapy: Most patients unfortunately present with extensive-stage disease, and for these patients combination platinum-based chemotherapy alone (cisplatin, carboplatin, etoposide) is the standard of care. Chemotherapy may help prolong survival and palliate symptoms.
- Carboplatin is usually substituted for cisplatin in extensive-stage disease, given its diminished toxicities and some data suggesting equivalence of the two drugs. (See Table 100.4 for toxicities associated with cisplatin and carboplatin. Etoposide toxicities include myelosuppression, nausea/vomiting, anorexia, alopecia, mucositis, and diarrhea.)
- Prophylactic cranial irradiation: Patients who respond to chemotherapy may be considered for PCI.
- Whole-brain radiation therapy (WBRT): Patients who have extensive-stage disease and brain metastases may be offered whole-brain radiation therapy before or after chemotherapy. Decisions regarding WBRT should be made based on patient's neurologic status and a benefit/burden assessment to determine whether the

treatment is in line with patient's achievable goals of care.

EXPECTED DISEASE COURSE

- Unfortunately, most lung cancers are metastatic at the time of diagnosis. Only 15% of patients with lung cancer survive five or more years after their diagnosis.
- The most common sites of metastatic disease are bone, brain, liver, adrenal glands, and the lung. Small-cell lung cancer also metastasizes to the bone marrow.
- Complications of advance lung cancer are shown in Table 100.5 below.

PALLIATIVE CARE ISSUES

- At the time of diagnosis, the majority of patients with lung cancer have metastatic disease. Palliative treatments that augment the length and/or quality of life are therefore critically important.
- The goals of treatment for lung cancer are to prolong survival and strive for the best possible quality of life. The addition of palliative care in conjunction with standard oncology care (radiation therapy, chemotherapy, and surgery) assures that patients and their families will be offered symptom management, advance care planning, psychosocial support, coordination of resources, and establishment of achievable goals of care based on performance status, prognosis, and patient preferences.
- Palliative care comanagement also ensures enhanced provider-patient-caregiver communication on the topics of establishing achievable goals of care, what to expect as disease progresses, and fully informed decision-making regarding transitions between care settings, including timely and appropriate referral to hospice.
- Lung cancer patients experience significant symptom distress, including pain, dyspnea, cough, and fatigue (Tables 100.4 and 100.5). Aggressive palliation of symptoms is indicated commencing at the time of diagnosis.
- Significant psychological stress has been identified among advanced cancer patient caregivers, indicating the need for more attention to mental health needs of this group.[11]

TABLE 100.4: CHEMOTHERAPIES USED TO TREAT SMALL-CELL LUNG CANCER[8]

Chemotherapy	Toxicities
Cisplatin	Nephrotoxicity Nausea/vomiting Myelosuppression Peripheral neuropathy Ototoxicity Metallic taste of food, anorexia Alopecia
Carboplatin	Myelosuppression Nausea/vomiting Nephrotoxicity Peripheral neuropathy
Etoposide	Myelosuppression Nausea/vomiting Anorexia Alopecia Mucositis, diarrhea

TABLE 100.5: COMPLICATIONS OF ADVANCED LUNG CANCER[10]

Complication	Associated Symptoms	Treatment Options
Progressive disease, chest wall invasion	Pain	Acetaminophen or NSAIDs for mild pain Opioids for more severe or increasing pain Adjuvant analgesics such as TCAs, anticonvulsants, and neuroleptics may also be helpful. Palliative radiotherapy, palliative chemotherapy (See Chapter 29: Management of Pain in Older Adults)
Progressive disease (first rule out potentially reversible etiologies like effusion, PE, CHF/COPD flare)	Dyspnea Cough	Opioids Oxygen Bronchodilators Corticosteroids Relaxation techniques, fans, psychosocial support (See Chapter 40: Cough and Secretions, and Chapter 41: Dyspnea)
Bone metastases	Pain Pathologic fractures	Analgesics Radiation therapy Bisphosphonates If refractory, consider radiopharmaceuticals Surgical stabilization or repair may be indicated. (See Chapter 29: Management of Pain in Older Adults)
Brain metastases (seen in more than 50% of patients with small-cell lung cancer)	Change in mental status Focal neurologic symptoms Headache Nausea/vomiting	Corticosteroids Resection or radiosurgical ablation may be indicated in patients with resectable non-small-cell lung cancer and a solitary brain metastasis; whole brain radiation should follow Whole brain radiation
Spinal cord metastases	Back pain	Corticosteroids Radiation Neurosurgical intervention may be indicated
Airway obstruction	Dyspnea Hemoptysis	*For endobronchial lesions:* Bronchoscopy with endobronchial management such as stenting, laser, electrocautery *For extrinsic compression by lymph nodes:* Radiation
Malignant pleural effusion	Dyspnea	Thoracentesis If recurrent, consider pleurex catheter placement or pleurodesis
Superior vena cava obstruction	Dyspnea Facial fullness Venous engorgement of the neck/chest wall Cyanosis Upper extremity edema	*If due to small-cell lung cancer:* Chemotherapy (stenting if no response) *If due to non-small cell lung cancer:* Stent and/or radiation therapy
Malignant tracheoesophageal fistula or bronchoesophageal fistula	Aspiration Cough Dyspnea Recurrent pneumonia Increased secretions	Stenting of the esophagus, airway, or both

TAKE-HOME POINTS

- Because the majority of patients with lung cancer present with incurable, advanced disease, palliative treatments should be offered in conjunction with standard oncology therapies.
- Patients should be routinely assessed and treated for complications related to their cancer.
- Decisions about lung cancer treatment are dependent on a host of patient characteristics, including but not limited to a patient's functional status, comorbidities, organ function, prognosis, and goals of care.
- Older patients with lung cancer are commonly undertreated, despite the ability of chemotherapy to prolong survival and improve the quality of life in many patients.
- In addition to pain and symptom management, psychosocial support, and coordination of resources, palliative care comanagement ensures enhanced provider-patient-caregiver communication about goals of care, disease progression, and appropriate settings and levels of care, including timely referral to hospice.

REFERENCES

1. Altekruse S et al. *SEER Cancer Statistics Review, 1975–2007*. Available from: http://seer.cancer.gov/csr/1975_2007/.
2. Edge S. et al., eds. *AJCC Cancer Staging Manual*. 7th ed. New York, NY: Springer-Verlag; 2009.
3. Small Cell Lung Cancer. NCCN Clinical Practice Guidelines in Oncology 2011; Version 1.2011: Available from: www.nccn.org.
4. Gridelli C et al. Treatment of advanced non-small-cell lung cancer in the elderly: results of an international expert panel. *J Clin Oncol*. 2005;23(13): 3125–3137.
5. Quoix E et al. Weekly paclitaxel combined with monthly carboplatin versus single-agent therapy in patients age 70 to 89: IFCT-0501 randomized phase III study in advanced non-small cell lung cancer (NSCLC). *J Clin Oncol*. 2010;28(18S): suppl; abstr 2.
6. Non-Small Cell Lung Cancer. NCCN Clinical Practice Guidelines in Oncology 2011; Version 3.2011. Available from: www.nccn.org.
7. Temel JS, Greer JA, Muzikansky A, Gallagher ER, et al. Early palliative care for patients with metastatic non-small-cell lung cancer. *N Engl J Med*. Aug 19, 2010;363(8):733–742.
8. Chu E, Devita Jr VT, eds. *Physicians' Cancer Chemotherapy Drug Manual*. Sudbury, MA: Jones and Bartlett Publishers; 2008.
9. Weinmann M et al. Treatment of lung cancer in elderly part II: small cell lung cancer. *Lung Cancer*. 2003;40(1):1–16.
10. Kvale PA, Selecky PA, Prakash UB. Palliative care in lung cancer: ACCP evidence-based clinical practice guidelines (2nd edition). *Chest*. 2007;132(suppl 3): 368S–403S.
11. Vanderwerker LC, Laff RE, Kadan-Lottick ND, et al. Psychiatric disorders and mental health service use among caregivers of advanced cancer patients. *J Clin Oncol*. 2005;23(28):6899–6907.

101

Leukemia

CASE

Mr. S is a 75-year-old gentleman with a history of hypertension who presented to his primary care physician with complaints of fatigue, dyspnea on exertion, and easy bruising for the prior two weeks.

DEFINITION

Leukemia is predominantly a disease of older adults. It can present acutely or follow a more chronic course (Table 101.1). Increased white blood cell count is common.

INCIDENCE

- Leukemia is much less common than breast, lung, or colon cancer.
- In 2009 there were an estimated 44,790 newly diagnosed cases of leukemia in the United States.
- Acute myeloid leukemia (AML):
  - Most common acute leukemia in adults; overall incidence of 2.7 cases/100,000 population

- Median age of diagnosis 65 years; incidence dramatically increases in adults over 65 years old
- Incidence in people over 65 years old is 12.2 cases/100,000 population, compared with 1.3 cases/100,000 in people less than 65.
- Acute lymphoid leukemia (ALL):
  - Overall incidence of 1.5 cases/100,000 population
  - Sixty percent of cases diagnosed in childhood; much less common in adults
  - A second ALL peak is seen in adults older than 60 years old.
- Chronic lymphoid leukemia (CLL):
  - Incidence of 3.9 cases/100,000 population
  - Most common chronic leukemia
  - Disease of older adults; median age at diagnosis is 72 years old.
- Chronic myeloid leukemia (CML):

TABLE 101.1: ACUTE VS. CHRONIC LEUKEMIA

Acute

Acute myeloid leukemia (AML)	Proliferation of a clone of malignant myeloblasts (AML) or lymphoblasts (ALL)
Acute lymphoid leukemia (ALL)	Leukemic blasts replace normal bone marrow function, resulting in low blood counts or cytopenias. Cytopenias can result in an increased risk of infection, anemia, and bleeding.

Chronic

Chronic myeloid leukemia (CML)	Myeloproliferative disorder
	Proliferation of all blood cells, including full range of myeloid cells
	Defined by the "Philadelphia chromosome":
	    Translocation between chromosomes 9 and 22 forms a bcr-abl tyrosine kinase
	    which stimulates cell proliferation

Chronic lymphocytic leukemia (CLL)	Malignant cell is the lymphocyte.
	Lymphocytes replace other blood cell precursors.
	Patients present with:
	    Lymphadenopathy
	    Symptoms due to hepatosplenomegaly
	    B-symptoms: fevers, sweats, weight loss

- Overall incidence is 1.7 cases/100,000 population
- Much less common than CLL
- Accounts for 15% of leukemia diagnoses
- Median age at diagnosis is 66 years old

LIKELY ETIOLOGIES

The development of leukemia has been associated with prior chemical exposure as well as with chemotherapy and radiation treatment.

- Prolonged exposure to benzene and petroleum products can increase risk of AML 10 to 30 years following exposure.
- Prior chemotherapy or radiation therapy for cancer (breast and ovarian cancer, lymphoma, myeloma); AML is often preceded by myelodysplastic syndrome (MDS) in these cases.
- Leukemic cells often have characteristic chromosomal abnormalities.
- There is no clearly established association with chemical exposure and disease development in ALL, CML, and CLL.

MYELODYSPLASTIC SYNDROME (MDS)

- MDS is a clonal bone marrow disorder commonly seen in older adults that often precedes acute myeloid leukemia (AML):
  - Incidence increases with age.
  - Median age at diagnosis is 70 years old.
  - Maturation of bone marrow elements is impaired, resulting in a decreased number of functioning blood cells.
  - Presents with anemia alone or with leukopenia +/− thrombocytopenia
- Risk of transformation to AML is related to:
  - Number of cytopenias
  - Cytogenetic abnormalities
  - Number of bone marrow blast cells
- Treatment/Supportive care:
  - Erythropoeitic stimulating factors to boost red cells (erythropoietin)
  - Transfusion support with red cells and platelets
  - Hypomethylating agents (azacytidine and decitabine)
- Transformation to AML:
  - Disease can be very resistant to treatment in context of advanced patient age and comorbidities.
  - Outcomes are poor with or without treatment.

DIAGNOSIS

History and Exam

Patients present with symptoms related to their abnormal blood counts, coagulopathy, enlargement of liver and spleen, lymphadenopathy, or systemic B-symptoms. These symptoms may include:

- Fatigue
- Weight loss
- Shortness of breath
- Easy bruising or bleeding (especially from the gums or mouth)
- Gingival hyperplasia
- Upper respiratory infections, sinusitis
- Bloating, early satiety, abdominal discomfort and distension (due to hepatosplenomegaly and more common in CLL and CML)
- Lymphadenopathy (CLL)
- Fevers, drenching night sweats, and weight loss of more than 10% of body weight (systemic B-symptoms)

Tests

- Complete blood count (CBC); If abnormal, a referral to a hematologist/oncologist should be made.
- AML and ALL commonly present with an elevated white blood cell count; may also present with leukopenia; hemoglobin and platelets are typically decreased.
- Chronic leukemias (CML and CLL) may be asymptomatic; incidental finding of elevated white blood cell count is often found on routine testing.

Biopsy

Bone marrow aspirate and biopsy:

- Outpatient procedure performed with local anesthesia
- Samples are sent for pathologic review, flow cytometry, and cytogenetic analysis to characterize the type of leukemia, and to stratify patients according to risk for treatment selection and outcome.

Imaging

CT scan: Consider for initial staging and evaluation of patients with CLL and lymphadenopathy.

On exam, Mr. S was found to be pale, and pete-chiae and ecchymoses were observed over his arms and legs. A blood count demonstrated a decreased white blood cell count of 2x10(3)/uL, a reduced hemoglobin of 8 g/dL and platelets of 30x10(3)/uL.

Mr. S was referred to a hematologist, and a bone marrow examination was diagnostic for myelodys-plastic syndrome (MDS). Mr. S initially received treatment with erythropoietin but then became blood and platelet transfusion dependent and started treatment with azacytidine.

EXPECTED DISEASE COURSE
Patients who achieve remission have improved quality of life and improved survival, but the disease course of acute and chronic leukemias can be highly variable.

Acute Myeloid Leukemia (AML) and Acute Lymphoid Leukemia (ALL)[1,2]
- These are aggressive diseases in the older adult population that carry a poor prognosis due to:
  - Advanced patient age
  - Comorbid conditions
  - Patient performance status
  - Increased drug resistance and poor risk tumor cytogenetics
  - History of antecedent MDS or prior chemotherapy/radiation (for AML)
- Median survival of patients 66 to 75 years old treated with induction chemotherapy is 14 months.
- Median survival of patients 76 to 89 years old treated with induction chemotherapy is six months.[3]
- Overall survival is poor and decreases with increasing age. Patients are at high risk from both the underlying disease and complications of treatment. These include:
  - Infections (viral, bacterial, and fungal) due to neutropenia and impaired immunity
  - Bleeding due to low platelets and coagulation defects
  - Complications can be life-threatening and often a cause of death.

Chronic Lymphoid Leukemia (CLL)
- The disease course for CLL is highly variable. Early stage CLL (elevated WBC +/- enlarged lymph nodes) is often diagnosed on routine blood work. If asymptomatic, observation with periodic follow-up is recommended.
- For advanced stage CLL (hepatosplenomegaly, anemia, thrombocytopenia or systemic B-symptoms), overall survival is based on risk according to disease stage:
  - Low risk (early stage): more than 10 years
  - Intermediate risk: six 6 years
  - High risk (advanced stage): two years

Chronic Myeloid Leukemia (CML)
- CML is characterized by chronic phase, accelerated phase, and blast phase disease. The majority of patients are diagnosed in chronic phase.
- At diagnosis, 25% to 50% of patients are asymptomatic. Median survival is 3.5 to 5 years if untreated.
- Patients treated with tyrosine kinase inhibitors can expect 5-year overall survival rate of greater than 80%.
- Greatest risk is disease transformation to accelerated or blast phase, in which survival is poor.

Six months later, Mr. S continued to require regular transfusions. However, his white blood cell count was now noted to be increased to 30 x10(3)/ul, and a repeat bone marrow examination was diagnostic for acute myeloid leukemia.

TREATMENT OPTIONS
Multiple treatment options are available for each type of leukemia. Selecting the appropriate treatment strategy treatment should include careful consultation with the patient and family about goals and preferences for care, and consideration of the following factors:

- Patient age
- Performance status: Eastern Cooperative Oncology Group Score (ECOG) (Table 101.2), or Karnofsky Performance Score (KPS), or Palliative Performance Scale (PPSV2)
- Comorbid conditions (including cardiac, renal or hepatic insufficiency, frailty, debility, dementia)
- Side effect profile
- Duration and location of treatment (inpatient or outpatient)[5]

TABLE 101.2: EASTERN COOPERATIVE ONCOLOGY GROUP (ECOG) PERFORMANCE SCALE

Performance Status	Definition
0	Fully active, no performance restrictions
1	Strenuous physical activity restricted; fully ambulatory and able to carry out light work
2	Capable of all self-care but unable to carry out any work activities; up and about > 50% of waking hours
3	Capable of only limited self-care; confined to bed or chair > 50% of waking hours
4	Completely disabled; cannot carry out any self-care; totally confined to bed or chair

Oken MM, Creech RH, Tormey DC, et al. Toxicity and response criteria of the Eastern Cooperative Oncology Group. *Am J Clin Oncol.* 1982;5:649–655.

Acute Myeloid Leukemia (Newly Diagnosed)

- Treatment options vary from standard, conventional induction chemotherapy to palliative therapies (Table 101.3).
- There is no single preferred therapy for AML in the older adult. Chronologic age does not predict response to therapy or treatment-related morbidity. Strong consideration should be given to induction chemotherapy in older, healthy adults after individualized treatment decision based on favorable tumor biology, good functional status (ECOG performance status of 0–2), and minimal comorbidities.[2]
- Any treatment decisions should incorporate the factors above and include collaborative consultation with the patient and family.
- Bone Marrow or stem cell transplantation:
  - Less intensive pre-transplant chemotherapy regimens (reduced-intensity and "mini" transplants) have broadened upper age limit for bone marrow or stem cell transplantation.

- May be a therapeutic option following initial therapy for patients up to 70 years old.
- Careful patient selection essential; based on disease status; performance status; comorbid conditions; psychosocial assessment of home condition and patient support.

Acute Lymphoid Leukemia (Newly Diagnosed)

- A range of therapeutic options available for newly diagnosed ALL patients are presented in Table 101.4.
- Older patients can be treated with traditional combination chemotherapy with age-adjusted dose modifications if they are suitable candidates.
- A less intensive and more palliative approach is also an optioon, including oral corticosteroids or chemotherapy, hydroxyurea to decrease elevated white blood cell counts, and transfusion or antibiotic support.
- For patients diagnosed with Philadelphia chromosome-positive ALL, treatment with an oral tyrosine kinase inhibitor (imatinib, dasatinib, and nilotinib) may be an option as well.

Chronic Myeloid Leukemia (CML)

- Imatinib, a "designer" drug targeting the bcr-abl kinase, has revolutionized the treatment of CML.
- Prior to the development of the tyrosine kinase inhibitors, CML was treated with hydroxyurea, busulfan, interferon, and stem cell transplantation.
- Today, CML has become a chronic disease with excellent disease-free survival with oral therapy. The tyrosine kinase inhibitors and alternate therapeutic options are outlined below in Table 101.5.

Chronic Lymphocytic Leukemia (CLL)

- CLL may be asymptomatic and indolent for many years, and some patients may never require therapy.
- If treatment is indicated, there are many options to choose from, including chemotherapy or immunotherapy (Table 101.6). Patient age, comorbidities, performance status, and goals for care should be considered when making decisions about treatment.

TABLE 101.3: THERAPEUTIC OPTIONS: ACUTE MYELOID LEUKEMIA (AML)[1,2]

Therapy	Route	Side Effects	Indications
Chemotherapy			
Conventional Induction Chemotherapy (7 + 3) (cytarabine + idarubicin)	IV	N, V, A, C	Strongly consider in patients > 65 if: Excellent performance status No comorbid conditions Inpatient therapy
Clofarabine	IV	N, V, D	Inpatient therapy
Hypomethylating agents			Consider if prior history of MDS Can be given on an outpatient basis
Azacytidine	IV/SQ	N, V, D, Fa, Fe	
Decitabine	IV	F, Co, D	
Investigational agent (clinical trials)	?	?	Strongly consider if patient is eligible Research may lead to more therapeutic choices in future for older patients with AML
Palliative chemotherapy			For patients who are not candidates for more intensive therapy
Low-dose cytarabine	IV, SQ	N, V	To treat elevated WBC
Hydroxyurea	PO	N, V, D, Co, S	To treat elevated WBC
Supportive care			
Antibiotics	IV, PO		To treat infection
Transfusion support	IV	Transfusion reactions	To treat symptoms associated with anemia and bleeding due to low platelets
Hospice care			Hospice care in the setting that best meets existing care needs and psychosocial considerations— home, inpatient, or nursing home hospice (See Chapter 12: The Hospice Model of Palliative Care)

Key for common side effects: alopecia (A), cardiotoxicity (C), constipation (Co), diarrhea (D), fatigue (Fa), fever (Fe), nausea (N), pancytopenia (P), stomatitis (S), vomiting (V).

PALLIATIVE CARE ISSUES

- Palliative care should be an integral component of a leukemia patient's care from the point of diagnosis and throughout the disease trajectory. Careful consideration should be given to the following factors before diagnostic procedures and treatment interventions are implemented, especially in older adults:
  - Performance status and comorbidities, especially end organ failure and cognitive decline
  - Prognosis associated with comorbidities
  - Organ function (kidney, liver, cardiac, and bone marrow function)
  - Common treatment-related toxicities and ability to tolerate full-dose treatment

- In patients with a good performance status, advanced age should not limit treatment.
- A patient-centered approach to treatment should include establishing goals of care and identifying quality of life priorities. Financial implications of diagnostic and treatment recommendations should be taken into account.
- Prevention and/or management of common symptoms should be a key focus of care plan. These include:
  - Anxiety/depression
  - Anorexia
  - Fatigue, weakness, malaise
  - Mucositis/stomatitis
  - Nausea/vomiting
  - Pain
  - Weight loss

TABLE 101.4: THERAPEUTIC OPTIONS: ACUTE LYMPHOID LEUKEMIA (ALL)[4]

Therapy	Route	Side Effects	Indications
Chemotherapy			
Standard combination chemotherapy (daunorubicin, cytoxan, steroids, vincristine)	IV	Depending on specific agents	Curative intent Chemotherapy with age-appropriate dose adjustment
Tyrosine kinase inhibitors (TKIs)	PO	See below	For patients with Philadelphia (Ph) + ALL Options include imatinib, dasatinib, nilotinib
Supportive care			
Antibiotics	IV, PO		To treat infection
Transfusion support	IV	Transfusion reactions	To treat symptoms associated with anemia and bleeding due to low platelets
Palliative measures			For patients who are not candidates for more intensive therapy
Chemotherapy +/– corticosteroids	IV, PO, SQ	N, V	To treat elevated WBC
Hydroxyurea	PO	N, V, D, Co, S	To treat elevated WBC
Hospice care			Hospice care in the setting that best meets existing care needs and psychosocial considerations—home, inpatient, or nursing home hospice (See Chapter 12: The Hospice Model of Palliative Care)

Key for common side effects: alopecia (A), cardiotoxicity (C), constipation (Co), diarrhea (D), fatigue (Fa), fever (Fe), nausea (N), pancytopenia (P), stomatitis (S), vomiting (V)

TABLE 101.5: THERAPEUTIC OPTIONS: CHRONIC MYELOID LEUKEMIA (CML)[4]

Therapy	Route	Side Effects	Indications
Tyrosine kinase inhibitors			Targets the bcr-abl kinase binding site and prevents cell proliferation
Imatinib	PO	N, V, D, E, R, M	
Dasatinib	PO	N, D, E, R, M, Fa, H	
Nilotinib	PO	N, Co, E, H, R, Fe, Fa, M, Q, P	
Alternative therapies			For patients intolerant of/or have progressed on TKIs
Hydroxyurea	PO	N, V, D, Co, S	To treat elevated WBC
Interferon	SQ	Fe, Fa, CD, Fl	Can have significant flu-like side effects
Stem cell transplantation			For select patients with progressive, TKI-resistant disease
Supportive care			
Antibiotics	IV, PO		To treat infection
Transfusion support	IV	Transfusion reactions	To treat symptoms associated with anemia and bleeding due to low platelets
Palliative measures			For patients who are not candidates for more intensive therapy
Hospice care			Hospice care in the setting that best meets existing care needs and psychosocial considerations—home, inpatient, or nursing home hospice (See Chapter 12: The Hospice Model of Palliative Care)

Key for common side effects: alopecia (A), cardiotoxicity (C), cognitive disturbances (CD), constipation (Co), diarrhea (D), edema/fluid retention (E), fatigue (Fa), fever (Fe), flu-like symptoms (Fl), headache (H), musculoskeletal pain (M), nausea (N), pancytopenia (P), pruritus (P), Q/T interval prolongation (Q), rash (R), stomatitis (S), vomiting (V)

TABLE 101.6: THERAPEUTIC OPTIONS: CHRONIC LYMPHOCYTIC LEUKEMIA (CLL)[4]

Therapy	Route	Side Effects	
Chemotherapy			
Fludarabine	IV	Fa, Fe, N, V	Commonly given in combination with rituximab +/– cyclophosphamide
Cyclophosphamide	IV	N, V, An, S	
Rituximab	IV	Al, T	Monoclonal antibody to CD20, a protein expressed on the surface of CLL cells
Bendamustine	IV	Fe, N, V, Fa, An	
Alemtuzumab	IV/SQ	Al, Fe, Fa, R, N, V, I	Monoclonal antibody to CD52, a protein expressed on the surface of CLL cells
Supportive care			
Antibiotics	IV, PO		To treat infection
Transfusion support	IV	Transfusion reactions	To treat symptoms associated with anemia and bleeding due to low platelets
Palliative measures			For patients who are not candidates for more intensive therapy
Oral chemotherapy +/– corticosteroids	PO	N, V	To treat elevated WBC
Hydroxyurea	PO	N, V, D, Co, S	To treat elevated WBC
Hospice care			Hospice care in the setting that best meets existing care needs and psychosocial considerations— home, inpatient, or nursing home hospice (See Chapter 12: The Hospice Model of Palliative Care)

Key for common side effects: allergic reaction (Al), alopecia (A), anorexia (An), cardiotoxicity (C), cognitive disturbances (CD), constipation (Co), diarrhea (D), edema/fluid retention (E), fatigue (Fa), fever (Fe), flu-like symptoms (Fl), headache (H), infection (I), musculoskeletal pain (M), nausea (N), pancytopenia (P), pruritus (P), Q/T interval prolongation (Q), rash (R), stomatitis (S), tumor lysis syndrome (T), vomiting (V).

- Family and patient should be supported throughout the disease course, with attention to symptom management and help with practical, spiritual, and social issues.

TAKE-HOME POINTS
- Leukemias in older adults can be acute or chronic.
- Acute myeloid leukemia commonly presents following an antecedent myelodysplastic syndrome.
- Older patients are less likely to achieve remission due to increased drug resistance and adverse tumor cytogenetics.
- Patient-centered approach to treatment should includes establishing achievable goals of care and identifying quality of life priorities.

- Treatment selection must be made very carefully, including thorough consideration of clinical issues such as comorbidities, frailty, dementia, performance status, and organ impairment.
- Treatment of CML has been revolutionized with the introduction and use of tyrosine kinase inhibitors.
- CLL is often an indolent disease and especially in an older adult may not require treatment.
- Prevention and/or management of common symptoms should be a key focus of care plan.

REFERENCES
1. Dohner H, Estey EH, Amadori S, et al. Diagnosis and management of acute myeloid leukemia in adults: recommendations from an international expert

panel, on behalf of the European LeukemiaNet. *Blood.* 2010;*115*:453–474.

2. Kantarjian H, O'Brien S, Cortes J, et al. Therapeutic advances in leukemia and myelodysplastic syndrome over the past 40 years. *Cancer.* 2008;*113*(7):1933–1952.

3. Juliusson G, Antunovic P, Derolf A, et al. Age and acute myeloid leukemia. *Blood.* 2009;*113*(8): 4179–4187.

4. Klepin HD, Balducci L. Acute myelogenous leukemia in older adults. *Oncologist.* 2009;*14*: 222–232.

5. Oken MM, Creech RH, Tormey DC, et al. Toxicity and response criteria of the Eastern Cooperative Oncology Group. *Am J Clin Oncol.* 1982;*5*: 649–655.

102

Non-Hodgkin's Lymphoma

CASE

Mr. P is a 71-year-old gentleman with a history of hypertension, hypercholesterolemia, and mild COPD who presented to his primary care physician with complaints of fevers, night sweats, and loss of appetite, with a growing right neck lump for three months.

DEFINITION

- *Lymphoma* includes a broad spectrum of diseases with many categories and subtypes (Table 102.1). Ninety percent of lymphomas are derived from B-cells.
- Non-Hodgkin's lymphoma (NHL) can be intermediate/high-grade (aggressive) disease, or low-grade (indolent) disease.

PREVALENCE

- NHL accounts for 4.6% of all cancer diagnoses; fifth most common cancer diagnosis in women, sixth in men.
- Estimated 65,908 new cases diagnosed in 2009 with 19,500 deaths (American Cancer Society). Although older and elderly adults are disproportionately affected, the overall incidence is increasing in adults of all ages.
- Disease incidence increases dramatically with age.
  - In 20- to 24-year-olds, incidence is 2.4 cases per 100,000 population.
  - In adults more than 65 years old, incidence is 87.2 per 100,000 population.
  - In older adults aged 80–84, incidence is 119.4 per 100,000 population.
- More than 50% of new NHL diagnoses in North America and Europe occur in people older than 65.

LIKELY ETIOLOGIES

NHL is associated with:

- Viral infections: Epstein-Barr virus, human T-cell lymphotropic virus (HTLV-1), hepatitis C infection, human herpes virus 8 or Kaposi's sarcoma-associated herpes virus

- Bacterial infections: Helicobacter pylori (Gastric MALT lymphoma)
- Chemical exposure: Pesticides and herbicides (2,4-D-organophosphates, chlorophenols), solvents and organic chemicals (benzene, carbon tetrachloride), and wood preservatives
- Treatment with prior chemotherapy or radiation
- Immunosuppression (acquired and congenital)
  Acquired:
  - HIV infection
  - Patients who have undergone organ or stem cell transplants who are on long-term immunosuppressive therapy
  - Celiac and Crohn's disease (GI lymphoma)
  - Autoimmune diseases (systemic lupus erythematosus, rheumatoid arthritis, Sjögren's syndrome)
  Congenital:
  - Ataxia-telangiectasia
  - Wiskott-Aldrich syndrome
  - Common variable hypogammaglobulinemia
  - X-linked lymphoproliferative syndrome
- Severe combined immunodeficiency

DIAGNOSIS

Presentation

- Patients often present with complaints of an enlarging lymph node in the neck, axilla, or groin with or without fever, sweats, and weight loss.
- Symptoms will vary based on the location of lymphadenopathy. Common presenting symptoms include:
  - Enlarged non-tender lymph nodes of the neck, axilla, and inguinal areas:

TABLE 102.1: LYMPHOMA SUBTYPES

Aggressive Lymphoma	Indolent Lymphoma
B-cell	
Diffuse large B-cell*	Follicular*
Burkitt lymphoma/leukemia	Nodal marginal zone
B-lymphoblastic lymphoma	Mucosa-associated lymphoid tissue (MALT) (extranodal)
Mantle cell lymphoma	Splenic marginal zone lymphoma
Mediastinal B-cell lymphoma	Small lymphocytic lymphoma
T-cell	
Peripheral T-cell	Mycosis fungoides/Sezary syndrome
Anaplastic large T-cell (ALCL)	Primary cutaneous anaplastic large cell
T-lymphoblastic lymphoma	
Adult T-cell leukemia/lymphoma (ATLL)	

*Most common histologic subtypes in each category

- Chest pain or pressure, shortness of breath, superior vena cava syndrome
- Abdominal distension, bloating, pain, or early satiety
- Abnormal blood counts with bone marrow involvement
- Fever, drenching night sweats, and weight loss (B-symptoms)

Exam
- Lymphadenopathy—firm, rubbery, and non-tender lymph nodes are most common.
- Hepatosplenomegaly.
- Pallor or petechiae (in advanced disease with bone marrow involvement)

Tests
Refer patients with lymphadenopathy for imaging and biopsy:

- Core biopsy or excisional lymph node biopsy provide adequate tissue for diagnosis. (Fine needle-aspirate is inadequate).
- CT-guided biopsy, mediastinoscopy, or laparoscopy may be necessary.
- Bone marrow biopsy is used to make a diagnosis in patients with bone marrow disease.

Staging
Staging evaluates extent of disease; also used for risk assessment and treatment choice.

- Contributions to staging are obtained from:
  - PET/CT or CT scans (including neck, chest, abdomen, and pelvis)
  - Bone marrow biopsy
  - CBC, chemistries, including lactate dehydrogenase (LDH)
  - Testing for hepatitis B, C, HIV, and HTLV-1
- The most commonly used staging schema is the Ann Arbor Staging.[1]

Stage I	Single lymph node region is involved (I) or Single extralymphatic organ or site (IE)
Stage II	Two or more lymph node regions/lymphatic structures on the same side of the diaphragm (II)
	Two or more lymph nodes/lymphatic structures on the same side of the diaphragm with contiguous extralymphatic organ/tissue (IIE)
Stage III	Involved lymph nodes are found above and below the diaphragm, including the spleen (IIIS) or with contiguous extralymphatic organ or site (IIIE)
Stage IV	Disease within one or more extralymphatic organs/tissues, with or without associated lymphatic involvement

All patients are also classified by the presence (**B**) or absence (**A**) of systemic B symptoms (fevers, nights sweats, and weight loss).

On exam, Mr. P has enlarged, rubbery, and mobile lymph nodes in the bilateral neck as well as in the left axilla. A complete blood count is normal. Mr. P undergoes an excisional lymph node biopsy of the right neck with a diagnosis of diffuse large B-cell lymphoma.

Further staging with a PET/CT scan shows active lymphoma in the neck, axilla, and mediastinum. No disease is present below the diaphragm, and a bone marrow biopsy is negative.

EXPECTED DISEASE COURSE

The disease course is highly variable, depending on the NHL subtype.

1. Indolent lymphoma:
   - Diagnosed at older ages and at a more advanced stage
   - Generally incurable with standard therapies
   - Chronic course with multiple relapses
   - Some patients survive many years with stable disease even without therapy.
   - Early treatment of asymptomatic disease does not increase survival.
   - Median survival is 5 to 10 years, but survival may be more than 15 to 20 years.
2. Aggressive lymphoma:
   - May be responsive to combination chemotherapy
   - Acute presentation
   - Rapid progression
   - Can require emergent, inpatient treatment
   - Disease relapses most commonly seen within the first two years after completion of initial therapy
3. For patients with primary refractory or relapsed disease:
   - Poor outcome
   - May be responsive to high dose chemotherapy and stem cell transplant for patients under 70 years old

PROGNOSIS

- International Prognostic Index (IPI) is used for risk stratification, prediction of overall survival, and complete response rates. Incorporates the following factors:
  - Patient age
  - Performance status
  - Serum lactate dehydrogenase (LDH)
  - Ann Arbor stage
  - Number of extranodal disease sites

- Overall five-year survival rate for patients with NHL between 1990 and 2003 was 63%. Survival is highly variable based on subtype of NHL, risk factors, and age. For high-risk diffuse large B-cell NHL, overall survival at four years is 55%. For high risk follicular NHL, overall survival at five years is 52%.
- Patients who do not achieve remission with first-line therapy can go on to receive salvage chemotherapy, immunotherapy, or radiation depending on disease extent and histology. Response rate will decrease with each subsequent therapy.
- Patients with refractory aggressive lymphoma will have a life expectancy of months. Death is most commonly due to disease progression, organ dysfunction, or infection.

TREATMENT OPTIONS

- There are many treatment options available (Table 102.2). Treatment varies based on NHL subtype. Combination chemotherapy +/– biologic agents is the most common approach.
- For the older adult, treatment decisions should be determined using an integrated approach based on discussions between the physician, patient, and family members.
- In patients with good performance status, advanced age alone should not limit treatment. For a healthy older adult, for example, the plan may be to administer chemotherapy adequate to achieve a long-lasting remission, while minimizing the toxic side effects of treatment.
- For a seriously ill older patient with poor cognitive function and several comorbidities, however, aggressive chemotherapy regimen may not be aligned with patient and family goals for care.

POST-TREATMENT FOLLOW-UP

- Repeat PET/CT after completion of therapy to document remission.
- Physical examination and lab testing every three to six months or as clinically indicated after the completion of therapy.
- Follow-up CT scans every six months for the first two years after treatment completion.

The patient has an excellent performance status and normal cardiac, renal, and liver function.

TABLE 102.2: TREATMENT OPTIONS[2,3]

Therapy	Route	Side Effects	Indications
Observation			Appropriate in asymptomatic patients with indolent NHL
Combination chemotherapy +/– biologic agents			Given as first line or salvage treatment Many options to choose from
R-CHOP or R-CVP (rituximab—cyclophosphamide, doxorubicin, vincristine, prednisone)	IV, PO	A, C, Fe, H, He, Hy, I, N, Ne, P, V	Most common first-line therapy Generally very well tolerated Doxorubicin may be omitted in elderly patients or in those with indolent lymphoma
Rituximab	IV	Fe, H, I, P	Anti-CD20 monoclonal antibody Can be used alone or in combination with chemotherapy Used for initial treatment or for maintenance therapy
Investigational agent (clinical trial)	IV/SQ/PO	?	Strongly consider if patient is eligible May lead to more therapeutic choices in future for older patients with NHL
Radioimmunotherapy			Delivers ionizing radiation to target cells and neighbors Anti-CD20 antibodies Can cause profound myelosuppression
Y-90 ibritumomab	IV	Fa, Fe, I, N, P	
I-131 tositumumab	IV	Fa, Fe, I, N, P	
Vaccine therapy (anti-idiotype)	SQ/IV	?	Active area of investigation
Radiation therapy		Fa, P	Most commonly used for early-stage indolent lymphoma (follicular) Palliation of symptomatic disease sites
Surgery			Reserved for bowel obstruction/emergencies
Stem cell transplantation (autologous and allogeneic)			For select patients with relapsed, chemosensistive disease younger than 70 Careful patient selection essential Disease status Performance status Comorbid conditions Psychosocial assessment of home condition and patient support
Supportive care			
Antibiotics	IV, PO		To treat infection
Transfusion support	IV	Transfusion reactions	To treat symptoms associated with anemia and bleeding due to low platelets
Palliative measures			For patients who are not candidates for more intensive therapy
Palliative radiotherapy			For palliation of symptomatic disease sites
Hospice care			Hospice care in the setting that best meets existing care needs and psychosocial considerations. Hospice settings include home, inpatient, or nursing home hospice.

Key for common side effects: alopecia (A), cardiotoxicity (C), constipation (Co), diarrhea (D), fatigue (Fa), fever (Fe), headache (H), hemorrhagic cystisis (He), hyperglycemia (Hy), infusion reaction (I), nausea (N), peripheral neuropathy (Ne), pancytopenia (P), vomiting (V)

Mr. P's stage II lymphoma is treated with six cycles of R-CHOP chemotherapy. A repeat PET scan after completing therapy is negative.

PALLIATIVE CARE ISSUES

- Palliative care should be an integral component of a NHL patient's care from diagnosis to the end of life.[4] A patient-centered approach to treatment includes establishing goals of care, assigning a health care proxy, and identifying quality-of-life priorities. Financial implications of diagnostic and treatment recommendations should also be taken into account.
- Careful consideration should be given to the benefits/burdens of diagnostic procedures and treatment intervention, especially in older adults. Factors to be weighed include:
  - Performance status and comorbidities, especially end organ failure and cognitive decline
  - Prognosis associated with comorbidities
  - Organ function (kidney, liver, cardiac, and bone marrow function)
  - Common treatment-related toxicities and ability to tolerate full-dose treatment
  - In patients with a good performance status, advanced age should not limit treatment.
- Prevention and/or management of burdensome symptoms are key components of the care plan. Common symptoms include nausea/vomiting, pain, anxiety/depression, and mucositis/stomatitis.
- Patient and family should receive psycho-social and spiritual support throughout disease course. Care near the end of life should be managed to maximize quality of life and minimize burdensome and distressing symptoms. (See Chapter 15: Dying at Home, and Chapter 19: Last Hours of Living.)

TAKE-HOME POINTS

- Lymphomas include a very heterogeneous group of diseases that may be aggressive or indolent.

- Lymphoma is much more common in older adults than in younger adults.
- Disease stage, prognostic factors, and careful consideration of cognitive function,, comorbidities, performance status, and underlying organ impairment are used to determine the best treatment approach for each individual patient.
- Based on the NHL subtype and histology, it may be appropriate to choose from more than one treatment approach.
- Elderly patients generally have an inferior outcome compared to younger patients (including decreased response to initial treatment, disease-free survival, and overall survival) due to therapeutic implications posed by increased comorbidities, altered pharmacokinetics, and reduced performance status.
- Treatment, however, should not be withheld from a patient based solely on age.
- Prevention and/or management of burdensome symptoms are key components of the care plan. Patient and family should also receive psycho-social and spiritual support throughout disease course.

REFERENCES

1. Carbone PP, Kaplan HS, Musshoff K, et al. Report of the Committee on Hodgkin's Disease Staging Classification. *Cancer Res.* Nov 1971;*31*(11): 1860–1861.
2. Keating GM. Rituximab: a review of its use in chronic lymphocytic leukaemia, low-grade or follicular lymphoma and diffuse large B-cell lymphoma. *Drugs.* 2010;*70*:1445–1476.
3. Morrison VA. Evolution of R-CHOP therapy for older patients with diffuse large B-cell lymphoma. *Expert Rev. Anticancer Ther.* 2008;*8*:1651–1658.
4. Thieblemont C, Grossoeuvre A, Houot R, et al. Non-Hodgkin's lymphoma in very elderly patients over 80 years. A descriptive analysis of clinical presentation and outcome. *Ann Oncol.* 2008;*19*: 774–779.

103

Intracranial Malignancies

CASE

JCC is an 82-year-old right-handed man with a two-year history of chronic atrial fibrillation managed with warfarin anticoagulation. He was recently evaluated because of a two-month history of increasing confusion. His family reported that his business judgment had declined and he was losing considerable sums of money in the business he still owned and managed.

DEFINITION

There are two types of intracranial malignancies: Primary intracranial malignancies originate from cells within the nervous system. Secondary (metastatic) intracranial malignancies are metastatic to the brain from another primary site.

PREVALENCE

- Most common primary tumors are astrocytoma and meningioma. High-grade astrocytoma (glioblastoma) is the most common malignant brain tumor in adults. Meningioma prevalence increases with age and most are benign.
- Metastatic tumors are the more common cause of intracranial tumors in older adults; ten times more frequent than primary brain tumors, and occur in 20% to 40% of adults with systemic cancer.
- Twenty percent of intracranial malignancy diagnoses represent new cancer diagnosis, 80% occur in patients who already have history of systemic cancer; 70% have multiple sites of metastases.

RISK FACTORS

Primary tumors:

- Best established risk factor is ionizing radiation, especially for meningiomas and glial tumors, often with a latency period of 10 to more than 20 years between RT and ocurrence.

- Much rarer causes include genetic mutations and deletions that are seen in hereditary syndromes, and chronic immunosuppression due to drugs or disease process.

Metastatic tumors:

- Lung (small-cell and non-small-cell), breast, and melanoma are the most common primary sites of metastatic brain tumors. Others include leukemia, lymphoma, GU, GI, etc. Prostate cancer usually metastasizes to the dura, not to brain parenchyma.
- Usually result from hematogenous spread and are most commonly seen at the junction of gray and white matter where the diameter of blood vessels narrows.

DIAGNOSIS

Presentation

- Since most patients with brain tumor present after onset of symptoms, it is important for clinicians to be sensitive to general and localizing symptoms and signs of intracranial tumors (Tables 103.1 and 103.2).
- Not all brain masses are cancers. Infectious abscesses, "tumifactive" demyelinating lesions, some cerebrovascular accidents, and intracerebral hemorrhages can masquerade as tumors. Conversely, some brain tumors may present as ischemic or hemorrhagic strokes.

Exam

- In addition to the neurological examination, the exam for suspected metastatic cancer without a known primary should also focus on chest, breasts, abdomen, skin (for melanoma), and prostate/testicles (for men).

TABLE 103.1: GENERAL SIGNS AND SYMPTOMS OF INTRACRANIAL TUMORS

General Signs and Symptoms of Intracranial Tumors:

Headache	Common—present in 20% at diagnosis and rises to 60% over the course of the disease Often due to increased intracranial pressure ($\uparrow$ICP) or irritation of cranial nerves V or IX innervated structures Usual headache is a "tension-type" pain—dull ache or bifrontal pressure, worse in morning in 1/3 of patients and day-long in a similar number Characteristic headache syndromes in orbital metastasis, parasellar tumors, jugular foramen tumors, occipital condyle metastasis, and gasserian ganglion metastasis
Nausea, vomiting	More commonly seen in brainstem and posterior fossa tumors Vomiting may occur without nausea May also be a sign of papillary edema associated with $\uparrow$ICP
Seizures	Seen in 30%–50% of brain tumors More commonly seen with slower growing primary tumors May be generalized, focal motor, or focal sensory with or without secondary generalization Focal seizures may be difficult to control
Altered mentation (lethargy to stupor and coma)	Seen in patients with frontal and temporal lobe tumors and in patients with $\uparrow$ICP Forgetfulness, change in personality, decline in concentration, and/or judgment
Visual changes	A sign or symptom of advanced papilledema, present in ~70% of patients Early papilledema does not cause symptomatic loss of visual acuity Advanced papilledema enlarges the physiological blind spot and may restrict vision
Syngultis (hiccups)	Usually caused by tumors in the medulla or those causing medullary compression
Skull pain	Often seen in skull-based metastases, and especially common in cancers of breast, lung, and prostate

Imaging

- MRI brain +/– contrast:
  - Test of choice
  - Contrast dyes contain gadolinium; use with caution in patients with GFR < 60 mL/min.
- CT brain +/– contrast:
  - Use for patients who cannot have MRI (i.e., patients with indwelling pacemakers, certain prosthetic cardiac valves, deep brain and spinal cord stimulators, extreme claustrophobia).
  - Use CT contrast dye with caution in diabetes mellitus, dehydration, myeloma, and renal insufficiency.
- Tissue diagnosis:
  - Usually desirable if there is a single tumor, or if tumors are clustered in small region and in an accessible area.
  - Tissue diagnosis is necessary if no other site of systemic tumor is known or can be safely biopsied.

JCC's evaluation disclosed an irritable elderly man with poor insight and judgment, and a right visual field defect. MRI of his brain without and with contrast revealed an infiltrating left parietotemporal neoplasm. Stereotactic biopsy of the neoplasm disclosed a glioblastoma that probably arose in a pre-existing area of low grade gliomatosis cerebri.

EXPECTED DISEASE COURSE

- Glioblastoma (GBM):[1]
  - Median survival in elderly (> 65 years): 3.9 to 8 months
  - Diminished survival compounded by poor functional status casts doubt on decisions to treat aggressively.
- Brain metastases:
  - Median overall survival: 3 to 6 months
  - Six-month (35%), 1-year (15%), and 2-year survivals (5%)
  - Most patients die of their systemic disease.

TABLE 103.2: FOCAL NEUROLOGICAL DEFECTS: LOCALIZING SIGNS AND SYMPTOMS
OF INTRACRANIAL TUMORS

Localizing Signs and Symptoms of Intracranial Tumors:

Frontal lobe tumors	Signs and symptoms may be vague or nonspecific
	Psychiatric: altered concentration, flattened affect, personality change, forgetfulness
	Disturbance of higher cortical function
	Large tumors may be associated with apathy, bradykinesia, and motor or psychomotor slowing, problems with inhibition of movement, withdrawn, indifferent behavior
	Rarely: hyperactivity, euphoria, disinhibition, instability, hypersexuality, catatonia, changes in posture or gait
	Dysphasia: involvement of Broca's area → nonfluent aphasia
Temporal lobe tumors	Disorders of speech and language—"nonfluent" or "fluent" aphasias (arcuate fasciculus, Wernike's area)
	Visual defects—contralateral hemianopic visual field defects
	Cognitive dysfunction—decline in intellectual function, flattened affect, psychomotor slowing, decline in concentration/attention, progressing to stupor and coma in advanced cases
Parietal lobe tumors	Complex sensory dysfunction—agnosias and apraxias
	Complex visual dysfunction—alexia, visual hallucinations, palinopsia
Occipital lobe tumors	Visual field defects—usually contralateral homonymous hemianopic field defects, often with "macular sparing"
Diencephalic tumors	Hydrocephalus
	Positional headache
	Forgetfulness, confusion, psychomotor slowing
	Endocrine dysfunction—diabetes insipidus, bulimia, obesity, sexual dysfunction, impotence, abnormal sleep patterns, thermoregulatory disturbances, amenorrhea
Brainstem tumors	Cranial nerve palsies
	Nystagmus
	Imbalance
	Dysarthria and aspiration
Cerebellar tumors	Vomiting—often early AM
	Occipital/cervical pain
	Neck stiffness
	Head tilt
	Lateral hemispheral tumors—appendicular ataxia, intention tremor, dysarthria, "loss of check"
	Medial hemispheral tumors—truncal ataxia
Cerebello-pontine angle tumors	Tinnitus
	Progressive hearing loss
	Vertigo is unusual early symptom
	Large tumors also compress brainstem and cause symptoms due to brainstem/corticospinal dysfunction
Pineal region tumors	In the elderly—hydrocephalus due to obstruction of the ventricular system
	Parinaud's syndrome: paresis of upward gaze, convergence retraction nystagmus, pupillary light-near dissociation—due to compression of midbrain tectum

TREATMENT OPTIONS

- Once a brain tumor is diagnosed, it is highly recommended that a neuro-oncologist or medical oncologist be involved in the remainder of the workup, evaluation, and treatment process. Neurosurgeons and radiation oncologists are also commonly part of the treatment team.
- As with all treatment considerations, patient and family goals are taken into consideration after presentation of realistic, achievable options to determine an appropriate treatment plan.
- Establishing the care plan entails one or more meetings between health care professionals and the patient-family unit to discuss what quality of life means to the patient, which treatment options (both disease-fucused and palliative) are available to maintain that quality of life, the benefit and risks of the treatment, and what to expect if the treatment does not achieve the desired outcome.

Palliative Treatment

Palliative treatment options and considerations are presented in Table 103.3.

Disease-Focused Treatment

When neuro-oncologists evaluate patients for disease-focused treatments such as surgery, radiation, and chemotherapy, the following considerations are taken into account:

- Type of brain tumor
- Life expectancy of the patient
- The patient's performance status
- Quality-of-life indicators specific to the patient

Surgery

- Goals of surgery are to safely remove as much tumor as possible (in the case of surgically accessible tumors) in order to establish the correct diagnosis and to debulk the tumor mass without jeopardizing neurologic function.
- Primary brain tumors are highly infiltrative, and complete removal is never possible,

---

TABLE 103.3: PALLIATIVE TREATMENTS AND CONSIDERATIONS

Symptoms	Management Considerations
Headaches	Often respond to dexamethasone, but doses of up to 96 mg/day may be needed Ventriculo-peritoneal fluid diversion in severe obstructive hydrocephalus, but risk of potential spread of tumor to peritoneum
Seizures	Prophylactic anticonvulsant use recommended only in patients who have had seizures Peri-operative antiepileptic prophylaxis is common and poorly researched No established benefit of prophylactic anticonvulsants for patients who have never had a seizure One possible exception—brain metastasis from melanoma, seizure frequency exceeds 50%, so antiepileptic treatment are sensible
Syngultis (hiccups)	Pharmacological measures: chlorpromazine, metoclopramide, carbamazepine, phenytoin, valproic acid, baclofen Folk remedies: numerous, including breath holding, induced vomiting by stimulating posterior pharynx with finger Surgical therapies: phrenic nerve destruction by transection, crushing, or anesthetic blockade is rare and usually done as last resort since it may aggravate respiratory impairment by causing diaphragmatic paralysis
Hydrocephalus	May respond to corticosteroids and palliative radiation Intractable hydrocephalus may require spinal fluid diversion—worthwhile considering if anticipated survival exceeds six-months and good quality of life is achievable
Skull pain	Often seen in skull-based metastasis Radiation therapy—palliative Non-narcotic and opioid drugs often necessary

so patients often receive other therapies, including radiation (Table 103.4) and chemotherapy (Table 103.5).
- Potential side effects of surgery include bleeding, infections, cerebral edema, and loss of brain function.

Radiation

- Stereotactic radiosurgery is a method of delivering high doses of focal radiation to a tumor while minimizing irradiation of the adjacent normal tissue. For the most part, there are very few side effects associated with stereotactic radiation. Transient effects include fatigue and headache.[2]
- Whole brain radiation, on the other hand, can cause alopecia, dermatitis, cerebral edema, memory loss, depression, other cognitive deficits, and symptoms of nausea and vomiting in addition to the transient effects noted in stereotactic radiation.[3]

PROGNOSIS

- Independent variables that predict poor outcome include malignant gliomas in elderly patients (> 65), those with KPS ≤ 60, those with significant comorbid health problems, and biopsy rather than gross total surgical resection of tumor.
- In brain metastasis, 50% of patients with one or two metastases are not surgical candidates because of inaccessibility of tumors, extensiveness of systemic cancer, or other complicating medical factors.
- While up to 50% of patients treated with whole-brain radiation therapy have an objective improvement, and many are sustained for more than six months, relapse is common.[4]
- Because of the poor prognosis associated with any malignant brain tumor, symptom

TABLE 103.4: RADIATION ONCOLOGY

Type of Brain Tumor	Treatment Regimen	Evidence
Low-grade gliomas	3D or conformal radiation	Evolving evidence: prolongs progression-free survival (PFS) but not overall survival (OS)
Malignant gliomas	Standard therapy is 60 Gy/2-Gy fractions/30 days to 6 weeks (for those with KPS ≥ 70)	
	In-field radiation (50 Gy/28-fractions/5 weeks)	Improvement in survival (from 16.9 → 29.1 weeks) without reducing QoL or cognition in the elderly
	Abbreviated radiation (40 Gy/15-fractions/3 weeks) in elderly with GBM	Equivalent median survival time and comparable 1-year survival without sacrificing QoL
Brain metastasis: overall median survival 3–6 months	Surgery + WBRT	Produces better overall survival and QoL than surgery alone in patients with good KPS, stable or limited systemic disease, and surgically accessible single brain metastasis
Brain metastasis: patients with ≤ 3 brain metastases	Stereotactic radiation + WBRT	Very modest OS benefit when compared to WBRT alone.
Brain metastasis: patients with 1–4 brain metastases	SRS + WBRT vs. SRS alone	No demonstrated survival benefit

Abbreviations:
PFS = progression free survival; OS = overall survival; QoL = quality of life; KPS = Karnovsky Performance Scale; WBRT = whole brain radiation therapy; SRS = stereotactic radiation

TABLE 103.5: CHEMOTHERAPY

Type of Brain Tumor	Chemotherapy Role
Low-grade primary gliomas	No defined role presently
Malignant gliomas (anaplastic astrocytomas and oligodendrogliomas, glioblastomas)	Temozolomide, an oral and IV alkylating agent, is generally given as chemotherapy and is then given in monthly cycles for 6–12 months after radiation completed Median OS: 15 months, generally shorter in patients >65 Well tolerated by most but may need dose adjustment in older adults Common side effects include fatigue, headache, nausea/vomiting
Metastatic brain tumors	No well-defined chemotherapy role in treatment Reports of brain metastasis from breast cancer that responds to hormonal or systemic chemotherapy and of NSCLC that responds to EGFR inhibitors (erlotinib, gefitinib)—generally have non-mutated Kras receptor

management should be a primary focus of any treatment regimen.

After discussion of his preferences and goals of care with the patient and his family, a program of palliative care was initiated for symptoms management and psychosocial support. JCC died comfortably four months later.

TAKE-HOME POINTS

- Brain tumors are common (20,000 new cases of primary brain tumors/year, 200,000 new cases of brain metastasis/year).
- Brain tumors (primary and metastatic) pose unique management challenges.
- Primary brain tumors are highly infiltrative, and complete surgical removal is never possible, so appropriately selected patients often receive other therapies, including radiation and chemotherapy.
- Prognosis is measured in months for both primary and secondary brain tumors. Focus should therefore be primarily on preserving

function and quality of life. Burdens of treatment (in terms of treatment side effects and quality of life considerations) should be weighed against benefit.

REFERENCES

1. Brandes A et al. Glioblastoma in the elderly: Current and future trends. Crit Rev Oncol Hematol. 2006;60:256–266.
2. Aoyama H et al. Stereotactic radiosurgery plus whole-brain radiation therapy vs stereotactic radiosurgery alone for treatment of brain metastases: a randomized controlled trial. *JAMA.* 2006;*295:* 2483–2491.
3. Chang EL et al. Neurocognition in patients with brain metastases treated with radiosurgery or radiosurgery plus whole-brain irradiation: a randomized clinical trial. *Lancet Oncol.* 2009;*10:* 1037–1044.
4. Broadbent AM et al. Survival following whole brain radiation treatment for cerebral metastases: an audit of 474 patients. *Radiother Oncol.* 2004;*71:* 259–265.

SECTION VI

The Interdisciplinary Team

104

Clinical/Counseling Psychologist

DEFINITION[1]

Psychologists are doctorally trained professionals with expertise in human behavior. Clinical and counseling psychologists apply this knowledge to the assessment and treatment of psychological problems.

- The clinical activities of clinical and counseling psychologists are very similar, although clinical psychologists tend to deal with more abnormal psychopathology such as schizophrenia, bipolar disorder, autism, severe ADHD, and other types of chronic mental illness or personality disorders. Counseling psychologists traditionally treat mental health issues in a more normally functioning population, dealing with problems such as depression, anxiety, and stress.
- Some psychologists are generalists in diagnosis and treatment, and others specialize in the areas of neuropsychology or specific mental health disorders.
- Psychologists may also administer and interpret standardized psychological tests as needed.

QUALIFICATIONS

- Graduates of doctoral-level clinical and counseling psychology programs are eligible for the same professional benefits, such as psychology licensure, independent practice, and insurance reimbursement.
- Both counseling and clinical psychologists are licensed in all 50 states as "licensed psychologists," and as such are able to practice independently as health care providers.[2]

ROLE ON THE PALLIATIVE CARE TEAM

- Assessment of psychological and cognitive problems

- Supportive counseling to facilitate adjustment to illness, grief, and loss
- Treatment of mental health conditions
- Consultation with interdisciplinary team members on patient and family-related issues and team support/debriefing opportunities

WHEN TO REFER

Referral to psychologist is appropriate for assessment or treatment of the following patient and family issues:[3,4,5]

- Mental health or cognitive problems that impact decision-making or care
- Patient assessment indicates overlapping medical and psychological issues, such as clinical depression, withdrawal, and sadness when coping with serious illness or debility.
- Short-term patient/family-focused counseling related to illness, bereavement
- Anxiety disorder
- Expression of a wish to die

POTENTIAL BENEFITS OF REFERRAL

- Assists team members in understanding patient and family mental health challenges that may complicate care, treatment, and decision-making.
- Helps to differentiate between emotional states that are normal vs. abnormal, and to determine treatment needs and appropriate interventions, including referral to other mental health providers and programs.

ACCESSIBILITY/FINANCING

- Many psychologists have independent practices or work on staff in hospitals or community mental health centers. Accessing services of a psychologist with expertise in palliative care may be challenging, since they are only beginning to be involved in the field.

- Many psychologists are experienced, however, in geriatric psychology, trauma, and bereavement. These areas of specialty offer a bridge to the developing field of palliative psychology.
- Most clinical services offered by psychologists are covered by insurance when there is a diagnosable condition that is the focus of treatment. Testing, psychotherapy, and health and behavior interventions all are billable services.

REFERENCES

1. Roger PR and Stone G. What is the difference between a clinical psychologist and a counseling psychologist? APA Division 17; Society of Counseling Psychology. (http://www.div17.org/about/what-is-counseling-psychology/counseling-vs-clinical)
2. APA Practice Organization. Continuing education and professional development: State licensure (http://www.apapracticecentral.org/ce/state/index.aspx)
3. Block SD. Assessing and managing depression in the terminally ill patient. *Ann Intern Med.* 2000;*132*:209–218.
4. Breitbart W, Rosenfeld B, Pessin H, Kaim M, et al. Depression, hopelessness, and desire for hastened death in terminally ill patients with cancer. *JAMA.* 2000;*284*(22):2907–2911.
5. Goelitz A. Suicidal ideation at end of life: the palliative care team's role. *Palliat Support Care.* 2003;*1*:275–278.

105

Complementary and Alternative Practitioners

DEFINITION

The field of complementary and alternative medicine (CAM), more recently termed "integrative health," describes the integration of complementary therapies with traditional Western medicine to provide the "whole person approach" that is one of the core principles of palliative care.

ROLE ON THE PALLIATIVE CARE TEAM

Complementary and alternative members of palliative care teams may include acupuncturists, yoga instructors, licensed massage therapists, and practitioners of mind-body therapies.

CLINICAL PRACTICE

A number of integrative health modalities are supported by research or empirical evidence and may offer theoretical or demonstrated benefits to palliative care patients.[1,2,3,4] CAM practitioners use these different approaches to help patients who are suffering from physical, emotional, and spiritual distress. (See Chapter 17: Complementary and Alternative Medicine).

WHEN TO REFER

- Patients often seek complementary and alternative therapies when they feel that traditional Western medicine is not providing them with desired results. Practitioners should routinely inquire about the patient and family's use of alternative therapies.
- If the patient reports CAM use, clinician should discuss selected modalities that have been shown to be helpful. Symptoms that can benefit from CAM include anxiety, fatigue, insomnia, nausea and vomiting, pain, shortness of breath, and stress.

POTENTIAL BENEFITS OF REFERRAL

Complementary and alternative medicine modalities may:

- Reduce the need for pharmacological treatment in chronic cancer pain
- Assist in pain alleviation
- Improve mood, fatigue, sleep quality, and general well-being
- Reduce dyspnea in severe COPD
- Reduce fear, anxiety, and stress
- Be energizing and relaxing

(See Chapter 17: Complementary and Alternative Medicine)

ACCESSIBILITY/FINANCE

- Most mind-body therapies are not covered by insurance unless delivered by an MD, PhD, or MSW.
- Some insurance companies will pay for medical massage and manual lymph drainage with a prescription from a doctor.
- For other CAM modalities, patients should ask their insurance company whether treatments are covered in their plan.

REFERENCES

1. Deng G, Cassileth BR. Integrative oncology: Complementary therapies for pain, anxiety and mood disturbance. *CA Cancer J Clin.* 2005;55: 109–116.
2. National Center for Complementary and Alternative Medicine. http://nccam.nih.gov/health/whatiscam. Accessed February 1, 2012.
3. Pan CX, Morrison RS, Ness J, et al. Complementary and alternative medicine in the management of pain, dyspnea, and nausea and vomiting near the end of life: A systematic review. *J Pain Symptom Manage.* 2000;20:374–387.
4. Smith J, Richardson J, Hoffman C, et al. Mindfulness-based stress reduction as supportive therapy in cancer care: systematic review. *J Adv Nurs.* 2005;52:315–327.

106

Registered Dietitian

DEFINITION

A registered dietitian is a food and nutrition professional who has met the minimum academic and professional requirements to qualify for the credential "RD." The majority of RDs work in the treatment and prevention of disease (administering medical nutrition therapy, often part of medical teams), in health-care facilities or private practice. In addition, a large number of RDs work in community and public health settings and academia and research.[1]

QUALIFICATIONS

A registered dietitian (RD) has met the ADA educational and professional criteria for dietetics:[1]

- Completed a minimum of a bachelor's degree at a U.S. accredited university
- Completed a supervised practice program at a health care facility, community agency, or a food service corporation, or combined with undergraduate or graduate studies
- Passed a national examination administered by the Commission on Dietetic Registration (CDR)
- Completed continuing professional educational requirements to maintain registration

ROLE ON THE PALLIATIVE CARE TEAM

The functions of the RD on the palliative care team include:

- Providing dietary consultation and services to the patient and/or the patient's caregiver in accordance with the diagnosis and plan of care (POC)
- Developing nutritional interventions appropriate to the patient's nutritional access, needs, and tolerance
- Revising the nutritional plan of care during interdisciplinary team meetings to meet the patient's evolving needs
- Providing recommendations for diet orders, nutritional supplements, and nutrition support regimens
- Documenting nutritional assessment and plan of care
- Educating staff and associated professionals on nutritional practices in palliative care
- Identifying the patient and family's need for food as a comfort measure

WHEN TO REFER

- Referrals made to the RD are often part of the nursing assessment but may also come from any discipline at any stage of an inpatient admission.
- In the community, referrals are made through a home health agency or hospice program.

POTENTIAL BENEFITS OF REFERRAL

- RD consultation benefits the patient by providing nutritional expertise and recommendations to the clinical team for dietary modifications regarding:
  - Patient safety, particularly around chewing and swallowing
  - Appetite changes and weight loss
  - Symptom control for dry mouth, nausea, and vomiting
  - Adjustments in dietary management that may be indicated by changes in goals for care
  - Enteral feeding decisions, planning, and management
- The RD may also offer supportive counseling to patients and caregivers who may struggle with such issues as decreased intake by mouth in terminal disease progression.

ACCESSIBILITY/FINANCE

The RD on the palliative care team may be employed on per diem, part-time, or full-time basis. The RD is paid from the organizational or institutional budget.

REFERENCE

1. Academy of Nutrition and Dietetics. What is a Registered Dietician? http://www.eatright.org/BecomeanRDorDTR/content.aspx?id=8142. Accessed July 26, 2013.

107

Licensed Massage Therapist

DEFINITION

The licensed massage therapist (LMT) manipulates soft tissue, muscles, and fascia of the body in systematic ways to loosen muscle tension, increase range of motion, reduce stress, and facilitate general circulation.

Massage therapy can complement standard medical care for patients of all ages and stages of illness. Massage therapy techniques (i.e., pressure, speed, and intent) can be modified according to a patient's specific needs and goals.

ROLE ON THE PALLIATIVE CARE TEAM

In geriatric palliative care practice, the LMT:

- Provides direct care to patients, caregivers, and staff
- Educates patient, family, and clinicians about the therapeutic benefits of massage and its application in clinical practice
- Provides training and mentorship to other massage therapists in the utilization of modified massage techniques.

QUALIFICATIONS

Most states and the District of Columbia have laws regulating the practice of massage therapy. Requirements include successful completion of an accredited educational program and passing a national certification examination or a state licensing exam. Individuals may seek advanced training and certification in selected specialty areas.

WHEN TO REFER

- Patient exhibits symptoms amenable to massage therapy intervention, particularly pain, agitation, dyspnea, mood, and sleep disorder.

- Caregiver exhibits signs of fatigue, stress.

POTENTIAL BENEFITS OF REFERRAL

There is growing evidence that massage therapy has therapeutic benefit for health, stress, and symptom management.[1,2] Potential benefits to patients includes:

- Symptom relief of pain, agitation, anxiety, mood, and sleep disturbance
- Comfort and relaxation
- Tactile and sensory stimulation
- Decreased isolation through one-on-one attention

ACCESSIBILITY/ FINANCE

- Comprehensive geriatric palliative care and hospice programs may offer massage therapy under special funding or grants, and also may use a volunteer network of massage therapists to provide services.
- Insurance: Many insurance companies will reimburse for "medical massage," which requires a doctor's prescription. Sessions and billing are done in 15-minute increments. Patients should check with their insurance carrier for reimbursement eligibility.
- Private practice: Massage therapists may offer sessions on a sliding scale basis or at a discount. Prices for massage therapy vary depending upon the massage therapist's level of training, locale, and whether office visit or house call.[3,4]

REFERENCES

1. Massage as CAM: National Center for Complementary and Alternative Medicine, National Institutes of Health. http://nccam.nih.gov/health/massage/
2. Corbin L. Safety and efficacy of massage therapy for patients with cancer. *Cancer Control*. 2005 Jul;*12*(3):158–164.
3. Find a Nationally Certified Massage Practitioner: http://www.ncbtmb.org/consumers_find_practitioner.php
4. NYS Office of Professions, New York State Education Department: Online License Verifications. http://www.op.nysed.gov/opsearches.htm#nme

108

Music Therapist

DEFINITION

Music therapy is defined by the American Music Therapy Association as the clinical and evidence-based use of music interventions by a credentialed professional within a therapeutic relationship.[1]

In geriatrics and palliative care, music promotes a sense of hope in the patient and values him or her as a creative individual. The patient is encouraged to find the realm of the creative self through music rather than living in the realm of the pathology alone.[2]

ROLE ON THE PALLIATIVE CARE TEAM[1]

- The music therapist engages the patient using modalities of music such as listening, singing, and playing along in rhythm to enhance patient comfort and well-being. The therapist assesses the patient's history, favorite genres, ethnic preferences, and spiritual or religious expression through music. Whenever possible, family and friends are encouraged to participate.
- Songwriting, song lyric analysis, singing, guided imagery with breathing techniques, and bedside instrument playing are some of methods utilized by music therapists. The session may be conducted with the patient alone, or in group settings with family members, friends, or other patients.

QUALIFICATIONS

- Completion of an American Music Therapy Association (AMTA) approved college music therapy curriculum and internship, followed by a national examination administered by the Certification Board. Music therapists are required to be a credentialed MT-BC (Board Certified Music Therapist).[1]

- A graduate degree in music therapy (M.A. or M.S.) allows the music therapist to expand and broaden clinical skills and integrate theories and treatment methods into his or her work with specific clinical populations.

WHEN TO REFER

Patients who may be appropriate for referral to music therapy include:

- Patients who have difficulty expressing emotion verbally, including patients with Alzheimer's disease and other brain injuries
- Patients with symptoms such as pain, anxiety, depression, sleeplessness
- Patients who are socially withdrawn

POTENTIAL BENEFITS OF REFERRAL

- Improves quality of life through enjoyment of music
- Can provide a personal record of patient through songwriting
- Helps to lessen anxiety and elevate mood
- Overcomes isolation and increases social relations
- Provides a diversion from discomfort and pain

ACCESSIBILITY/FINANCE

- A music therapist who is regularly employed in a hospital, nursing home, or hospice is not entitled to reimbursements by insurance companies.
- A music therapist in private practice may receive reimbursement from some insurance companies. These companies reimburse for prescribed music therapy services if the CPT codes have been approved by either the insurance adjuster or case manager.

- The American Association for Music Therapy provides a list of CPT codes and can provide a list of board-certified music therapists who are trained to work with geriatric palliative care patients.[1]

RESOURCES

www.musictherapy.org

Aldridge, David. *Music Therapy in Palliative Care: New Voices.* Philadelphia, PA: Jessica Kingsley Publishers; 1999.

Wigram, Tony. *Songwriting Methods: Developing a Working Model.* Philadelphia, PA: Jessica Kingsley Publishers; 2005.

REFERENCES

1. Musictherapy.org
2. Aldridge D, ed. *Music Therapy in Palliative Care.* New Voices. Philadelphia, PA: Jessica Kingsley Publishers 1999.

109
Nursing

DEFINITION
A nurse is a health care professional who is trained to protect, promote, and optimize health and function, prevent illness and injury, alleviate suffering through the diagnosis and treatment of human response, and advocate for the care of individuals, families, and communities.[1]

Although there are many different categories of nursing, each with a different set of responsibilities, all nurses share a consistent approach to patient care known as "the nursing process." The nursing process structures each patient encounter in a series of five steps: assessment, diagnosis, planning, implementation, and evaluation.

QUALIFICATIONS AND ROLE ON THE PALLIATIVE CARE TEAM
- Levels of nursing practice include the registered nurse (RN), the advanced practice nurse (APN), the clinical nurse specialist (CNS), and the licensed practical (vocational) nurse (LP/VN) (Table 109.1).
- Personal care workers with various titles (certified nursing assistant, home health aide, personal care assistant, and home attendant) also assist frail elders and chronically or seriously ill patients with personal care and activities of daily living. The scope of practice and responsibilities of each of these nursing categories on the palliative care team are determined by the nurse's level of education and clinical training, as well as satisfaction of professional licensure and/or certification requirements (Table 109.2).

WHEN TO REFER
- Palliative care nursing promotes quality of life for patients and families facing serious illness by combining the science of expert assessment, symptom management, and critical thinking with the art of compassion, openness, mindfulness, and skillful communication.
- To ensure that all aspects of patient-centered care are addressed, nursing is a core component of every interdisciplinary palliative care and hospice team.
- The level and intensity of nursing care provided is determined by the individual patient and family needs and disease acuity.

POTENTIAL BENEFITS OF REFERRAL[7,8,9]
- RNs trained in palliative care offer expert pain assessment, an ability to listen, skilled communication, comfort when talking about spirituality, expertise in wound care and repositioning strategies, and compassionate and knowledgeable management of distressing physical and existential symptoms. The nurse is also well positioned to be the primary liaison who brings the interdisciplinary team's care plan to the bedside for explanation and implementation.
- In collaboration with attending physicians, advanced practice nurses certified in palliative medicine and hospice care provide a more advanced level of holistic patient/family-centered care. The skills and expertise of APNs include comprehensive history and physical examinations, ordering lab tests and diagnostic tests, prescribing pharmacological and nonpharmacological therapies for the management of symptoms or diseases, and assuring that comprehensive and

coordinated care is consistent with patient and family preferences.

ACCESSIBILITY/FINANCE

- The only nurses who can bill for palliative care services are advanced practice nurses (APNs) who are licensed and certified by an approved credentialing organization to perform independent patient care services within the scope of their certification.
- Centers for Medicare/Medicaid Services (CMS) rules for APN billing are more complex than guidelines for physician billing. Selected rules for independent Medicare billing by a hospital-based APN include:[10,11]
  - APNs must be certified by one of the seven CMS-recognized certifying boards, must be authorized by the state in which they practice, and must possess a master's degree.
- When APN billing is permitted, certified APNs can bill for care at 85% of attending physician billing rates.
- To provide attending physician services, APNs must be directly involved in the patient's care, providing care that is medically necessary, and working in collaboration with one or more physicians. (The collaborating MD does not need to evaluate each patient nor be present with APN when services are furnished.)
- If the care could be offered by another member of the team (e.g., RN, social worker, or physical therapist) then the service cannot be billed separately by an APN.
- For additional information on APN billing for palliative care services, visit the Tool

TABLE 109.1: NURSING LEVELS, QUALIFICATIONS AND ROLE ON THE PALLIATIVE CARE TEAM[2,3,4,5]

Nursing Level	Qualifications/Credentials	Role on the Palliative Care Team
Registered Nurse (RN) A registered nurse protects, promotes, and optimizes the health and abilities of patients; prevents illness and injury; alleviates suffering; diagnoses and treats the human response to suffering; and advocates for patients, families, communities, and populations.	Educational requirements for an RN include completion of a diploma in nursing, a bachelor's degree in nursing (BSN), or an associate degree in nursing (ADN), and satisfactory completion of the nursing certification exam for registered nurses. RNs are licensed in the state where they practice, and their role is governed by the Nurse Practice Act within each individual state. Certification in hospice and palliative care is available for RNs from the National Board for Certification of Hospice and Palliative Nurses (NBCHPN).	*Clinical:* Provides holistic patient-centered care based on the physical, psychological, religious, and cultural needs of the patient and family Coordinates bedside care of patient/family through delegation of tasks to licensed practical nurse (LPN) or nursing assistant (NA) Communicates findings to the medical team responsible for patient's care Conducts/participates in family meetings (depending on skill level and experience) Educates patients/family about disease process, pain and symptom management, and what to expect in the event of disease progression Counsels patients and families on end-of-life issues and decision-making, and provides guidance throughout the trajectory of illness *Administrative:* Depending on team structure and size, may be the administrative coordinator for the palliative care team May assume a leadership/administrative role for a hospital unit or for selected patients

(continued)

TABLE 109.1: (CONTINUED)

Nursing Level	Qualifications/Credentials	Role on the Palliative Care Team
Advanced Practice Nurse (APN) Advanced practice nurse (APN) is an umbrella term for registered nurses who are prepared at the graduate level to provide direct patient care and who have obtained licensure and credentialing reflecting this advanced preparation.	APNs complete a master's or doctoral degree in nursing from an accredited training program, usually with a concentration in a specific specialty. To practice, APNs define their scope of practice to the state based on their educational preparation and the certification they have obtained. The four areas of practice for APNs include the clinical nurse specialist (CNS), the nurse practitioner (NP), the certified nurse midwife (CNM), and the certified registered nurse anesthetist (CRNA). The National Board for Certification of Hospice and Palliative Nurses is the certifying body for APNs in palliative and hospice care. In the field of palliative care, the APN is most often certified as a nurse practitioner (NP) or clinical nurse specialist (CNS). Although APNs have an autonomous role, they are required to work in collaborative practice with an attending medical doctor; this collaboration is governed by each state's Nurse Practice Act.	*Scope of practice for hospice and palliative care APNs includes:* Providing holistic patient-/family-centered care that involves independent judgment, synthesis of assessment data, initiation and evaluation of care plan and treatment regimens Comprehensive history and physical examinations Ordering lab tests and diagnostic tests Prescribing pharmacological and nonpharmacological therapies Making referrals to assure comprehensive and coordinated care Conducting/participating in family meetings Psychosocial counseling Participating in discharge planning Offering patient and family education, as well as education on end-of-life issues in the community Participating in research and public policy initiatives
Licensed Practical (Vocational) Nurse (LP/VN) Licensed practical/vocational nurses provide basic and routine nursing care that is consistent with their education, under the direction of a supervising heath professional in a variety of health care settings.	Becoming an LP/VN requires a 12- to 14-month training program after high school, as well as supervised clinical instruction on the fundamental aspects of nursing care. Once this training is complete, the graduate is required to pass a licensing examination. LP/VNs are licensed in the state of their practice; they must pass state or national boards to renew their license LP/VNs are required to work under the supervision of a registered nurse (RN), nurse practitioner (NP), physician, dentist, or psychologist. LP/VNs can be certified by the National Board of Certification for Hospice and Palliative Nurses.	Scope of practice varies depending on the state and the institution in which the LP/VN practices Duties and tasks are assigned by the supervising health care professional to ensure comprehensive care at the bedside Duties may include: Providing basic nursing care, administering medications, measuring vital signs and other indications of patient health status, keeping records, performing emergency life-saving techniques such as CPR Participating in the development of the plan of care Educating patient and family; attending family meetings Keeping the supervising professional informed of changes in patient's condition Documenting patient/family care events and concerns during the nursing shift With additional training, an LP/VN may perform more specialized tasks, such as catheterization and suctioning, and administering blood products

TABLE 109.2: PERSONAL CARE WORKERS[6]

Home Health Aide (HHA)
Personal Care
Assistant (PCA)
Home Attendant (HA)
Home health aides, personal care assistants, and home attendants belong to a category known as personal care workers in health services. They assist with care for people who are elderly, disabled, chronically ill, or cognitively impaired in a variety of settings (home, hospital, long-term care facility, and hospice).

Home health care aides are not required to have a college degree or high school diploma, and they are often trained on the job by nurses or other medical professionals. Personal care workers who are employed by Medicare/Medicaid-certified hospices or home health agencies must obtain formal training as certified nursing assistants and pass a standardized test.
(*See certified nursing assistant below*)

HHAs assist individuals who have health care needs with personal care activities such as bathing and dressing, and provide bedside care including basic nursing procedures under the supervision of an RN or LP/VN.
In some states, HHAs may also be able to administer certain medications or to check the client's vital signs under the direction of a nurse or other health care practitioner
HHAs and PCAs assist only with personal care and basic activities of daily living, including bathing, dressing, grooming, making patients more comfortable at home, shopping, paying bills, doing laundry, and accompanying patients to medical appointments.

Certified Nursing Assistant (CNA)
CNAs are trained to perform basic patient care under the supervision of an RN or LPN.

Home health aides (HHAs) who are employed by agencies that are funded by Medicare or Medicaid must meet minimum standards of training. Federal training regulations for these nursing aides are mandated in the Omnibus Budget Reconciliation Act of 1987.
Standards include 75 hours of training, 16 hours of supervised practical work, and passing a competency evaluation or state certification program. Some states also require additional training. NAs can become certified nursing assistants by registering completion of their academic achievement and supervised workplace experience with a central certifying body. Certification is available through the National Board of Certification for Hospice and Palliative Care Nurses (NBCHPN).
A national certification is also offered by the National Association of Home Care and Hospice (NAHC).

CNAs assist patients with activities of daily living, measure vital signs, keep the patient's environment clean and safe, and approach and support the patient and family in accordance with their cultural and religious needs. CNAs report findings to supervising LPN or RN. These updates help the nurse to assess the progress of the patient as well as determine any needs the patient might have for medical intervention.
Timely and precise communication is a key element in avoiding errors in patient treatment. The nursing assistant is trained in documentation, observation, and reporting, both to the nurse and to one's replacement at shift change or during the end-of-shift report.

Section of the Center to Advance Palliative Care website (www.capc.org).

REFERENCES

1. Code of Ethics for Nurses. American Nurses Association. http://nursingworld.org/MainMenu Categories/EthicsStandards/CodeofEthics forNurses/. Accessed September 2012.

2. American Nurses Association (ANA). What nurses do. http://www.nursingworld.org. Accessed September 2012.

3. Value of the professional nurse in palliative care. Hospice and Palliative Nurses Association (HPNA) Position Statement. 2011. http://www. hpna.org/DisplayPage.aspx?Title=Position%20 Statements. Accessed September 2012.

4. Value of Advanced Practice Nurse in Palliative Care. Hospice and Palliative Nurses Association (HPNA) Position Statement. 2010. http://www. hpna.org/DisplayPage.aspx?Title=Position%20 Statements. Accessed September 2012.

5. Value of the Licensed Practical/Vocational Nurse in Palliative Care. Hospice and Palliative Nurses Association Position Statement (HPNA). 2012. http://www.hpna.org/DisplayPage.aspx?Title= Position%20Statements. Accessed September 2012.

6. U.S. Department of Labor. Bureau of Labor Statistics Occupational Outlook Handbook. http:// www.bls.gov/ooh/healthcare/home-health-and-personal-care-aides.htm. Accessed Sept 11, 2012.

7. Kramer LM, Martinez J, Jacobs MJ, Williams MB. The nurse's role in interdisciplinary and palliative care. In: Matzo ML, Sherman DW, eds. *Palliative Care Nursing: Quality Care to the End of Life.* New York: Springer; 2001:118–139.

8. Coyle N. Introduction to palliative nursing care. In: Ferrell BR, Coyle N, eds. *Textbook of Palliative Nursing.* New York: Oxford University Press; 2001: 3–6.

9. Horton JR, Indelicato RA. The advanced practice nurse. In Ferrell BR, Coyle N, eds. *Oxford Textbook of Palliative Nursing.* New York: Oxford University Press; 2010:1121–1129.

10. Dahlin C. APN billing for palliative care services: essentials for billing and reimbursement. *Hospice and Palliative Nurses Association Audio Conference,* 7/31/2008. Available at www.capc.org. Accessed September, 2012.

11. Meier DE, Beresford L. Advanced practice nurses in palliative care: a pivotal role and perspective. *J Palliat Med.* 2006;9(3):624–627.

110

Rehabilitation Therapist

DEFINITION

The specialty of physical medicine and rehabilitation deals with the prevention, diagnosis, and treatment of functionally limiting disease or injury. Rehabilitation specialists use physical and pharmacologic regimens to help patients restore function lost due to impairments, disabilities, and illness.

In palliative rehabilitation, the traditional restorative approach of physical medicine is reversed. When chronic or life-limiting illness precludes the return to the pre-morbid level of function, palliative rehabilitation therapists strive to support patients and their families as they face the prospect of inevitable disease progression accompanied by functional decline over time. (See Chapter 25: Rehabilitation).

ROLES ON THE PALLIATIVE CARE TEAM

There are three categories of palliative rehabilitation therapists, each addressing a separate but frequently overlapping range of functional activities:

- Speech therapists specialize in tasks involving the oral-pharyngeal-laryngeal function, as well as cognitive components involved in the process of communication. (For a discussion of palliative speech therapy, see Chapter 113: Speech Language Pathologist.)
- Physical therapists (PT) are concerned with gross functional mobility, sometimes referred to as "transitional movements." Physical therapists traditionally seek to improve strength, flexibility, coordination, and other aspects of general function. Early in the course of a serious illness, palliative physical therapy may concentrate on ambulation training, including teaching the appropriate selection and safe use of walkers, canes, crutches, braces, etc. In the event of disease progression, clinical

PT goals would shift first to supportive interventions, and eventually to palliative strategies to maximize the patient's quality of life and reduce the caregiver burden.

- Occupational therapists (OT) focus on activities of daily living (ADLs), and help patients who have been injured or who are recovering from illness participate in the activities that they want and need to do. Common occupational therapy interventions in the early stages of serious illness would target self-care activities such as grooming and feeding, home management, and the patient or family use of assistive devices and assistive technologies to provide supports for older adults experiencing physical and cognitive changes.[2] As in PT, clinical OT goals would shift toward supportive measures in the event of disease progression.

QUALIFICATIONS

There are specific educational, certification, and licensing requirements that must be satisfied in order to become a physical or an occupational therapist (Table 110.1).

WHEN TO REFER

Palliative patients who are referred for rehabilitation therapy will receive the following services:

- Individualized evaluation, during which the patient, family, and therapist collaboratively determine the goals of care
- Customized intervention to maintain or possibly enhance the patient's ability to perform daily activities and achieve the identified goals
- An outcomes evaluation to assess whether goals are being met and/or to make adjustments to the intervention plan when necessary because of advancing illness

TABLE 110.1: OCCUPATIONAL AND PHYSICAL THERAPISTS: QUALIFICATIONS, EDUCATION, AND CERTIFICATION[3,4]

Rehabilitation Discipline	Education	Certification/License
Occupational therapist	Most occupational therapists enter the occupation with a master's degree in occupational therapy. A small number of programs offer doctoral degrees in occupational therapy. Admission to occupational therapy programs generally requires a bachelor's degree; applicants may also have to demonstrate previous work or volunteer experience in an occupational therapy setting. Both master's and doctoral programs require several months of supervised fieldwork.	Occupational therapists become certified by passing the National Board for Certification of Occupational Therapists (NBCOT) exam. Certification allows therapists to use the title of Occupational Therapist Registered (OTR). To maintain certification, continuing education credits are required. All states require occupational therapists to be licensed. Licensure requires a degree from an accredited educational program and passing the NBCOT certification exam.
Physical therapist	Physical therapists are required to have a postgraduate professional degree, usually a Doctor of Physical Therapy (DPT) degree or a Master of Physical Therapy (MPT) degree. Most programs, either DPT or MPT, require a bachelor's degree for admission. Physical therapists may apply to and complete residency programs after graduation. Residencies last nine months to three years and provide additional training and experience in advanced or specialty areas of care.	All states require physical therapists to be licensed. Licensing requirements vary by state but typically include passing the National Physical Therapy Examination or a similar state-administered exam. A number of states require continuing education for physical therapists to keep their license. After gaining work experience, some physical therapists choose to become board certified in a particular clinical specialty, such as pediatrics or sports physical therapy. Board certification requires passing the relevant examination.

- The appropriate timing for referring to these OT or PT services will be determined by the stage of the illness and by the patient's motivation, prognosis, and cognitive and functional status. The priorities and goals of the patient and family in the face of advancing illness will also guide the appropriate timing for referral (See Chapter 25: Rehabilitation):
  - Early in the disease, referral may be for preserving function and reducing dependency.
  - As illness progresses, priorities will include safety, environment assessment, assisted mobility, falls-prevention measures, and transfer techniques.
  - When the end of life is near, emphasis will shift to quality of life and maximal comfort measures, including bed positioning to preserve skin integrity, pain relief techniques, gentle massage, and support for family caregivers.

POTENTIAL BENEFITS OF REFERRAL

- Palliative rehabilitation emphasizes realistic and achievable goals of care, strategies to control pain and distressing symptoms, and helping patients and caregivers adjust to the discouraging loss of independence and function while maximizing quality of life for both patient and family.
- Rehabilitation therapy alleviates patient fears of being a burden on caregivers, reduces patients' feelings of helplessness, increases their sense of competence and control, and contributes to improved mood and sense of well-being. It also is associated

with enhanced quality of life and improved functional status that can help patients tolerate burdensome treatments such as radiation and chemotherapy.[5]

- For caregivers, maintaining patient capacity and function may provide physical relief and can minimize or delay the need for expensive patient care such as increased home health aide hours, equipment, home modification, crisis intervention, respite care, etc.

ACCESSIBILITY/FINANCING[6]

- For hospice patients, physical therapy and occupational therapy are generally treated as part of the Medicare Part A benefit. Assistive devices such as wheelchairs, walkers, etc., are also part of the hospice benefit.
- For palliative care patients, the following rehabilitation therapy services and equipment are covered by Medicare Part B:
  - Durable medical equipment for use in the home, such as oxygen equipment and supplies, wheelchairs, walkers, and hospital beds ordered by a health care provider enrolled in Medicare.
  - Evaluation and treatment by an occupational or physical therapist to help the patient perform activities of daily living or to help maintain or improve general physical function. Therapy services must be certified as

medically necessary by a health care provider. There may be a cap on the amount Medicare will pay for services in a single year. The patient pays 20% of the Medicare-approved amount, and the Part B deductible applies.

- Coverage for rehabilitation services by private insurance plans is variable.

REFERENCES

1. Wu J, Quill T. Geriatric rehabilitation and palliative care: opportunity for collaboration or oxymoron? *Top Geriatr Rehabil.* 2011;27(1):29–35.
2. American Association of Occupational Therapy (AOTA). Living Life to the Fullest. http://www.aota.org. Accessed on September 12, 2012.
3. Bureau of Labor Statistics, U.S. Department of Labor, Occupational Outlook Handbook, 2012–13 Edition. Physical Therapists. Available at: http://www.bls.gov/ooh/healthcare/physical-therapists.htm. Accessed September 13, 2012.
4. Bureau of Labor Statistics, U.S. Department of Labor, Occupational Outlook Handbook, 2012–13 Edition. Occupational Therapists. Available at: http://www.bls.gov/ooh/healthcare/occupational-therapists.htm. Accessed September 13, 2012.
5. Huang ME, Sliwa JA. Inpatient rehabilitation of patients with cancer: efficacy and treatment considerations. *PM &R.* 2011;3:746–757.
6. Medicare & You. U.S. Department of Health and Human Services: Centers for Medicare and Medicaid Services. *CMS Product #10050-38.* August 2011.

111

Pharmacist

DEFINITION

The American Association of Hospital Pharmacists defines pharmacists as health care professionals responsible for provision of medication-related care for the purpose of achieving definite outcomes that improve a patient's quality of life.[1]

ROLE ON THE PALLIATIVE CARE TEAM

The functions of the pharmacist on the palliative care team are:[2]

- Assessing the appropriateness of medication orders
- Ensuring the timely provision of effective medications for symptom control
- Counseling and educating clinical staff about medication therapy, especially screening for drug-drug interactions when adding a new drug to patient's regimen
- Advising clinicians of potentially inappropriate medications (PIM) that pose more risk than benefit to the patient either because they are ineffective, they pose unnecessary risks, or there are safer alternatives available
- Ensuring that patients and caregivers understand and follow the directions provided with medications
- Providing efficient mechanisms for extemporaneous compounding of nonstandard dosage forms
- Addressing financial concerns/pharmacy costs, alternatives, or resources
- Ensuring safe and legal disposal of all medication after institutional deaths
- Establishing and maintaining effective communication with regulatory and licensing agencies

QUALIFICATIONS

- A registered pharmacist (RPh) is a licensed professional who has met the specific educational requirements established by the Accreditation Council for Pharmacy Education and successfully completed both a national and a state-specific licensing examination.
- Currently, all pharmacy programs require a minimum of six years post-secondary education, and the entry-level degree is a Doctor of Pharmacy (Pharm.D.) degree. Some pharmacists pursue advanced training such as residencies or fellowships, and some may elect to become board certified in a specialty area of practice.

WHEN TO REFER

Pharmacists are consulted by palliative care teams for:

- Development of pain management protocols
- Providing patient-specific pain management recommendations
- Providing patient-specific recommendations for patients with limited options for administration
- Researching alternative forms or routes of medication for patients with limited options for administration

POTENTIAL BENEFITS OF REFERRAL

- The pharmacist is an integral team member whose contributions can potentially improve patients' medication management, thereby reducing their risk of adverse medication events and subsequent hospital re-admissions.
- Pharmacist counseling of patients about drug dosage, administration, and anticipated side effects can aid medication compliance.

ACCESSIBILITY/FINANCING

- Medicare regulations state that a hospice must employ a licensed pharmacist or have a formal agreement with a licensed pharmacist to advise the hospice on ordering, storage, administration, disposal, and record-keeping of medications.

- Some pharmacists serve hospice programs as volunteer consultants and some are employed by the facility, but most provide contract services through a home health care pharmacy or hospital.
- A licensed pharmacist may be required or requested to be part of the hospital-based interdisciplinary palliative care team and would typically be employed by the institution.

REFERENCES

1. American Society of Hospital Pharmacists. ASHP statement on pharmaceutical care. *Am J Hosp Pharm*. 1993;50:1720–3.
2. American Society of Health-system Pharmacists. ASHP statement on the pharmacist's role in hospice and palliative care. http://www.ashp.org/DocLibrary/BestPractices/SpecificStHospice.aspx. Accessed September 1, 2012.

112

Physician

DEFINITION

The palliative care physician usually has MD or DO training, followed by specialty training in one of several fields, most commonly internal medicine, family medicine, or neurology. Common subspecialties include geriatrics and hematology/oncology.

Ideally, the physician will also have subspecialty training and certification in hospice and palliative medicine.

ROLE ON THE PALLIATIVE CARE TEAM[1,2]

The physician has three key roles on the palliative care team:

1. Provider of direct patient care
2. Liaison to the primary care physician or, as a consulting physician, to the health care institution or system
3. Organizational leader within the interdisciplinary team, particularly in traditional settings and as specified by legal-regulatory authorities.
   - These primary roles each have clinical, administrative, and educational aspects that are interrelated, and there is a considerable amount of overlap in the descriptions of physician roles summarized in Tables 112.1, 112.2, and 112.3.

WHEN TO REFER

Palliative care is provided by a team of doctors and nurses and other specialists who work with a patient's other doctors to provide an extra layer of support. It is appropriate at any age and at any stage of a chronic or serious illness, and can be provided together with curative treatment. The provision of palliative care should not be restricted to the end-of-life phase of the disease process.[3]

POTENTIAL BENEFITS OF REFERRAL

- Patients receiving treatment for serious illnesses can experience unrelieved pain and a range of burdensome symptoms related to the disease process or as side effects of the treatment. A palliative care physician has the knowledge and expertise to evaluate the patient and assess and manage distressing symptoms, thus improving the patient's quality of life.
- When treating a serious illness, health care providers are often required to have "difficult" conversations with the patient and family members about advance care planning and decision-making, a difficult diagnosis or prognosis, or transitioning from an approach focused on potential cure to a care plan focused on comfort and/or hospice referral. The palliative care physician has special training in how to communicate with patients and families in these stressful and sometimes very emotionally charged situations[4] (See Chapter 9: Communication Skills).
- Palliative care comanagement (the addition of palliative care in conjunction with specialized medical care) assures that seriously or chronically ill patients and their families will be offered symptom management, advance care planning, psychosocial support, coordination of resources, and establishment of achievable goals of care based on performance status, prognosis, and patient preferences.
- Palliative care involvement also ensures enhanced provider-patient-caregiver communication on the topics of establishing achievable goals of care, what to expect as the disease progresses, and fully informed decision-making regarding transitions between care settings, including timely and appropriate referral to hospice.[5,6]

TABLE 112.1: PHYSICIAN ROLE: PROVIDING PATIENT CARE

Aspect of Role	Responsibilities
Clinical	Provide medical oversight and direction consistent with patient's goals of care Contribute medical assessment, prognosis, symptom management, and treatment recommendations to help establish achievable goals of care; help coordinate and implement care plan Translate hospice and palliative medicine research data into evidence-based treatment options Collaborate and communicate with other physicians who also care for the patient, including patient's primary care physician and other consultants and specialists Assume primary care role if requested When feasible and appropriate, provide physician home visits for patients who are seriously ill and home-bound
Administrative	Determine hospice appropriateness and eligibility Help patient and family caregivers navigate complex health care system, advocating for patient's needs but keeping in mind the real constraints of the system (e.g., knowing what patient's health insurance will and will not cover; obtaining prior authorization for necessary medications that may be costly; not prescribing therapies that may conflict with patient's other needs—such as extensive radiation therapy for patient on hospice)
Educational	Educate patient and family caregivers about importance of good pain and symptom management across settings and programs, including inpatient, outpatient, hospital, home, and hospice Educate patient and family about how to successfully navigate the health care system (e.g., refer patients to their health insurance case manager to discuss what treatments will and will not be covered; explain prior authorization procedures for necessary medications that may be costly) Educate patient and caregivers about the important roles of other interdisciplinary team members and encourage acceptance of their care and support

TABLE 112.2: PHYSICIAN ROLE: LIAISON WITH PRIMARY CARE PHYSICIAN OR HEALTH CARE SYSTEM

Aspect of Role	Responsibilities
Clinical	Help patient and family navigate complex health care system, advocating for patient's needs but keeping in mind the real constraints of the system Collaborate and communicate with other physicians who also care for the patient, including patient's primary care physician and other consultants and specialists Back up the primary care physician as needed, providing 24/7 availability for medical management
Administrative	Determine hospice appropriateness and eligibility Formulate "marketing" strategies to help make palliative care and hospice a visible and well-regarded component of the routine continuum of care
Educational	Provide latest hospice and palliative care research data and evidence-based practice for community physicians to help enhance the care of their patients, especially in the areas of pain and symptom management Educate members of the medical community about the principles, practices, and benefits of palliative care and hospice; audience should also include non-palliative care professionals, CEOs and Boards of Directors of health care facilities as well as community organizations and agencies Assist practicing physicians and trainees with strategies to make palliative care and hospice a visible and relevant part of the medical continuum Work with hospital leadership or CEO of hospice to promote discussion of palliative care and hospice care education in the community, including community-based agencies and skilled nursing facilities Participate in formal teaching settings, including medical, nursing, and other professional grand rounds, workshops, conferences, with special attention to utilization of evidence-based practice and hospice-palliative medicine research data

TABLE 112.3: PHYSICIAN ROLE: ORGANIZATIONAL LEADER ON THE INTERDISCIPLINARY TEAM

Aspect of Role	Responsibilities
Clinical	Contribute medical information relating to patient's care Authorize patient therapies, medications, and services; serve as backup to nurses, social workers, and other team members in support of patient's plan of care Participate in and or facilitate meetings with patient/family Collaborate and communicate with other physicians who also care for the patient, including patient's primary care physician and other consultants and specialists Be available for medical management to back up nurses during home visits
Administrative	Determine hospice appropriateness and eligibility Participate in, facilitate, or direct team meetings
Educational	Educate other physicians about the roles and strengths of other disciplines and the ability of the interdisciplinary team to offer optimal care for patient and family caregivers Mentor nurses to increase their expertise in pain and symptom management Provide latest hospice and palliative medicine research data and evidence-based practice for interdisciplinary members related to the care of their patients (e.g., regular in-service sessions or grand rounds)

ACCESSIBILITY/FINANCE

- Palliative care physician services are paid for as a fee-for-service item under Medicare, Medicaid, or private insurance plans, using CPT (Current Procedural Terminology) codes and hospital DRG (Diagnosis Related Group) codes. Physician care services can also be supported by the core hospital facility and charitable contributions.[1]
- For hospice medical directors, Medicare allows a one-time palliative care consult to evaluate whether a patient is appropriate for hospice. (Hospice medical directors cannot certify patients for hospice, however. This would be considered a conflict of interest.) (See Chapter 5: Financing Hospice and Palliative Care, and Chapter 13: Health Insurance.)
- In addition to per diem payment for overall hospice services, Medicare will reimburse hospice medical directors to provide clinical visits. Most other third-party payers do not reimburse for hospice physician visits.

REFERENCES

1. Teno JM, Connor SR. Referring a patient and family to high-quality palliative care at the close of life. *JAMA.* 2009;*301*(6):651–659.
2. Melvin TA. The primary care physician and palliative care. *Prim Care.* 2001;*28*(2):239–247.
3. National Quality Forum. National framework and preferred practices palliative and hospice care. http://www.qualityforum.org. Accessed September 18, 2012.
4. Back A, Arnold R, Tulsky J. *Mastering Communication with Seriously Ill Patients: Balancing Honesty with Empathy and Hope.* New York: Cambridge University Press; 2009: 26–27.
5. Bruera E, Hui D. Integrating supportive and palliative care in the trajectory of cancer: establishing goals and models of care. *J Clin Oncol.* 2010;*28*(25):4013–4017.
6. Temel JS, Greer JA, Muzikansky A, Gallagher ER, et al. Early palliative care for patients with metastatic non-small-cell lung cancer. *N Engl J Med.* Aug 19, 2010;*363*(8):733–742.

113
Social Work

DEFINITION

Social work is the professional activity of helping individuals, groups, or communities to enhance or restore their capacity for social functioning and to create conditions in society that support this goal.

Social work practice consists of the professional application of social work values, principles, and techniques to achieve one or more of the following ends: helping people obtain tangible services; counseling and psychotherapy with individuals, families, and groups; helping communities or groups provide or improve social and health services; and participating in legislative processes.[1]

QUALIFICATIONS[2]

- A bachelor's degree is the minimum educational requirement for entry into the field, but many positions require an advanced degree. For example, a master's degree in social work (MSW) is typically required for positions in health care settings and is required for clinical work as well. College and university teaching positions and most research appointments normally require a doctorate in social work (DSW or PhD).
- All states and the District of Columbia have licensure, certification, or registration requirements, but these regulations vary by state. In many states, certification also requires sitting for an examination given by the Association of Social Work Boards (ASWB).
- Advanced specialty practice accreditation is available from the National Association of Social Workers (NASW) and the National Hospice and Palliative Care Organization (NHPCO).

ROLE ON THE PALLIATIVE CARE TEAM[3,4]

- Social workers are integral members of the interdisciplinary palliative care team, with a key role in assessing and identifying the social needs of seriously ill patients and their families. Included in the assessment is the exploration of family structure, relationships, lines of communication, existing social and cultural networks, perceived social support, work and school settings, finances, living arrangements, caregiver availability, access to transportation, legal issues, access to community resources, and documentation of patient and family values, goals, and preferences for care.
- After the social needs assessment is complete, the social worker develops a care plan that responds to the identified social and practical needs as effectively as possible, with an added focus on minimizing adverse impact of caregiver burden and promoting caregiver and family goals and well-being.
- A core element of creating a care plan is the discharge planning process, i.e., facilitating the patient's transition out of the hospital and into an appropriate care setting, based on feasibility, safety, available resources, and level of care required.
- The social worker also makes referrals to appropriate services for patients and families when indicated, including help in the home, transportation, rehabilitation, medications, counseling, community resources, and equipment.
- In addition to comprehensive patient and family social assessment and discharge planning, the social worker's role on the team includes:
  - Facilitation of communication within families and between patients/families and health care or interdisciplinary teams through routine organization of and participation in family meetings
  - Direct counseling of patients and family members facing life-limiting illness, the dying process, death, grief, and bereavement

- General family counseling, crisis counseling, information and education counseling, community resource counseling
- Grief and bereavement support
- Advocacy for team self-care and support practices, including guidance on self-reflection and offering debriefing opportunities.

Note: If the interdisciplinary palliative care team does not include a social worker, many of these services can be accessed through collaboration with social workers assigned to specific care units within the hospital or health care facility.

WHEN TO REFER

In addition to the range of clinical care services outlined above, there are special clinical situations when a social work referral is indicated:

- Death is imminent
- Patient has been given a prognosis of less than two weeks
- The patient/family has made a decision to withdraw ventilator support
- Patient and family need help with end-of-life issues, including understanding manifestations of grief/distress/conflict, explaining what is happening to young children in the family, helping to gather information about arrangements for funeral/burial/death certificates, etc.
- Complex or disputed discharge issues:
  - Lack of safe and reasonable plan for discharge
  - Concern that proposed plan is not feasible or appropriate
  - Family conflict over discharge options.

POTENTIAL BENEFITS OF REFERRAL[5]

- Social workers advocate within the palliative care team for the views and

needs of individuals and families and can encourage and assist clients to communicate effectively with team members.
- Patients, families, and team members often rely on the expertise of the social worker in situations requiring problem solving and conflict resolution.
- The psychosocial expertise of the social worker helps the interdisciplinary team to understand the complexity of the clinical situation, analyze appropriate interventions, review decisions, and formulate treatment plans.
- The social worker identifies resources, provides counseling, offers support services, and can research practical interventions.

ACCESSIBILITY/FINANCING

Social workers do not bill for clinical services in the hospital setting; services are usually part of bundled care through Medicare, Medicaid, or other insurance coverage.

REFERENCES

1. National Association of Social Workers (NASW). http://www.socialworkers.org/practice/default. asp. Accessed September 4, 2012.
2. National Association of Social Workers (NASW). http://www.socialworkers.org/pressroom/2011/ HSH-FactSheet2011.pdf.
3. National Consensus Project for Quality Palliative Care. 2009. *Clinical Practice Guidelines for Quality Palliative Care*, Second Edition. http://www. nationalconsensusproject.org.
4. Altilio T, Otis-Green S, eds. *Oxford Textbook of Palliative Social Work*. New York: Oxford University Press; 2011.
5. *NASW Standards for Social Work Practice in Palliative and End of Life Care*. 2009. National Association of Social Workers. http://www.naswdc.org/practice/bereavement/standards/default. asp. Accessed September 4, 2012.

114

Speech-Language Pathologist

DEFINITION

Speech-language pathology is the assessment and treatment of disorders that affect a person's speech, language, cognition, voice, and/or swallowing.

Speech-language pathology focuses on the rehabilitative or corrective treatment of physical and/or cognitive deficits resulting in difficulty with communication and/or swallowing. Communication is defined as including speech, both receptive and expressive language (including reading and writing), and nonverbal communication such as facial expression and gesture.

ROLE ON THE PALLIATIVE CARE TEAM

- The speech-language pathologist's role is to evaluate, diagnose, and treat speech, language, voice, cognitive-communication, and swallowing disorders in individuals of all ages.
- Speech-language pathologists work in a variety of different settings, including hospitals, rehabilitation and nursing facilities, and private practice.

QUALIFICATIONS

- The standard level of education for speech-language pathologists is a master's degree. Graduate programs often include courses in age-specific speech disorders, alternative communication methods, and swallowing disorders. These programs also include supervised clinical practice in addition to course work.
- The Council on Academic Accreditation (CAA), part of the American Speech-Language-Hearing Association (ASHA), accredits education programs in speech-language pathology.
- Speech-language pathologists must be licensed in almost all states. A license requires at least a master's degree and

supervised clinical experience. Additional requirements vary by state.
- Speech-language pathologists can earn a Certificate of Clinical Competence in Speech-Language Pathology (CCC-SLP) offered by the ASHA. Certification satisfies some or all of the requirements for licensure and may be required by some employers.

WHEN TO REFER FOR AN INSTRUMENTAL SWALLOW EVALUATION

- Patients with evidence of or complaints about the following conditions should be referred for an instrumental swallow evaluation:
  - Coughing or choking with swallowing
  - Difficulty initiating a swallow
  - Difficulty with oral containment
  - Residue in oral cavity after swallow
  - Oral, pharyngeal regurgitation
  - Sensation of food sticking in the chest or throat
  - Recurrent aspiration pneumonia
- Instrumental swallow evaluation is not indicated for diagnosis of GERD, esophageal dysmotility, or as routine evaluation in patients with advanced dementia.
- The gold standard for identification of aspiration is the Modified Barium Swallow (MBS), also called a videofluoroscopic evaluation of swallow.
- Benefits of an instrumental swallow evaluation include:
  - Identifying aspiration or penetration and quantifying the amount of aspirate
  - Identifying at what point during swallow patient aspirated
  - Identifying physiological swallow dysfunction and/or anatomical abnormalities

- Testing multiple consistencies of food to determine appropriate diet
- Evaluating strategies and positions to facilitate safer swallows

WHEN TO REFER FOR A SPEECH, LANGUAGE, COGNITIVE EVALUATION

- Refer patients with evidence of, or difficulty with the following:
  - Aphasia
  - Dysarthria
  - Apraxia
  - Anomia
  - Memory
  - Automatic speech/repetition/fluency
  - Reading/writing
  - Comprehension of verbal, visual, written information
- Patients who benefit the most when they are referred in early stages of disease, and thus are able to participate in evaluation, include those who are status post cerebral vascular accident (CVA), who are within two years of traumatic brain injury (TBI), or who may have a diagnosis of neurodegenerative disease.
- Benefits of a speech, language, or cognitive evaluation include:
  - Improved communication
  - Improved patient and caregiver quality of life
  - Introducing alternate means of communication when indicated

ACCESSIBILITY/FINANCE

- All services through hospitals and rehabilitation facilities require a doctor's prescription, including a diagnosis code and the notation "speech therapy evaluation and treat."
- If requesting a swallowing evaluation, clinicians must indicate that an instrumental swallow evaluation is needed. Voice, speech and language, or cognitive therapy may also be specified.

MEDICARE INFORMATION

- The Centers for Medicare and Medicaid Services (CMS) publishes an *Outpatient*

TABLE 114.1: MEDICARE DIAGNOSIS CODES FOR SPEECH/ LANGUAGE EVALUATION

ICD-9 Code	Diagnosis
315.32	Mixed Receptive-Expressive Language Disorder
787.2	Dysphagia
438	Cognitive Deficits, Late Effects Of Cerebrovascular Disease
438.1	Speech And Language Deficit Unspecified
438.11	Aphasia
438.12	Dysphasia
V72.83	Other Specified Pre-Operative Examination

Medicare Physician Fee Schedule (MPFS) for Part B Speech-Language Pathology services (http://www.asha.org/uploadedFiles/2 012-Medicare-Fee-Schedule-SLP.pdf).
- Examples of Medicare diagnoses that support medical necessity are shown in Table 114.1 below.

OTHER INSURANCE INFORMATION

- Coverage by other insurance plans varies. Patients should check with their carrier prior to receiving services to get information on coverage for the specific treatment they will receive.
- In private practice, speech-language pathology fees are based on individual practitioners' billing rates and the types and number of services provided. Patients should check with their insurance carrier for reimbursement eligibility.

INTERNET WEB SITES

Complete resources, including information on support groups for a full range of communication disorders: http://asha.org

To locate a SLP specialist in local area: http://asha.org/ findpro/

115

Chaplain

DEFINITION
A health care chaplain is a clinically trained health care professional, certified by a national pastoral care organization, who is officially engaged by a health care institution to provide spiritual, pastoral, and emotional care to all patients, their families, as well as staff employed by the organization.[1]

ROLE ON THE PALLIATIVE CARE TEAM
The chaplain's role is to provide emotional as well as spiritual support for patients, their families, clinical team members, and support staff. Specific tasks and functions of the chaplain include:

- Provide a pastoral presence for palliative care patients and their families
- Provide a pastoral presence for interdisciplinary team members, support staff, and other clinicians caring for palliative care patients
- Conduct spiritual screening and assessment to identify individuals whose religious/spiritual conflict or distress may compromise their recovery or ability to tolerate treatment interventions
- Conduct memorial services for patients or staff members
- Educate staff, medical students, residents, fellows, and seminarians about the impact of illness on the spiritual life of patient and family
- Mentor seminarians interested in the field of chaplaincy
- Be available as moral and ethical consultant for the clinical team

QUALIFICATIONS[2]
In the United States and Canada, acquiring and maintaining certification as a professional chaplain requires:

- Graduate theological education or its equivalent

- Endorsement by a faith group, or a demonstrated connection to a recognized religious community
- Clinical pastoral education equivalent to one year of post-graduate training in an accredited program recognized by the constituent organizations
- Demonstrated clinical competency
- Completion of annual continuing education requirements
- Adherence to a code of professional ethics for health care chaplains
- Professional growth in competencies as demonstrated in peer review

WHEN TO REFER TO A CHAPLAIN
- Patient or family is spiritually and/or emotionally suffering.
- Patient is actively dying
- Patient or family is struggling to make medical decisions
- Family is bereaved
- Patient or family has received difficult news
- Team member(s) or hospital staff are spiritually and/or emotionally distressed

BENEFITS OF REFERRAL
- When patients or families are in spiritual/emotional crisis, the chaplain facilitates exploration and understanding of the meaning of the distress. Once the source of suffering is identified, referrals or interventions that promote spiritual healing can be made.
- When staff members are at risk for spiritual/emotional crisis, the chaplain is someone to whom they can speak during times of high stress or crisis (professional or personal).
- When a patient is dying, the chaplain provides support, ministering to the patient when alert, providing support for family if

present, and offering staff an outlet for grief or frustration.

- When a patient or family is struggling to make medical choices, the chaplain is trained to be both a sounding board and a facilitator for patients and families working through difficult religious and ethical decisions demanded by treatment recommendations. The chaplain, perceived as a neutral and supportive party, can help reduce patients' and families' anxiety and guide them to an understanding of the options being discussed.
- When the family is bereaved, the chaplain is able to offer a blend of emotional, spiritual, and practical support for the family. The chaplain is also able to answer the "what happens next?" questions on both the logistical and existential levels.
- When a patient/family has received difficult news, the chaplain's presence provides a "safe place" for strong emotions to be expressed. (See also Chapter 21: Spirituality.)

ACCESSIBILITY/FINANCING

- Many hospitals provide round-the-clock pastoral care coverage. In hospitals that do not provide 24-hour pastoral presence, palliative care leaders who are concerned for a patient or family frequently contact the hospital's pastoral care department to identify an appropriate faith resource for support.
- Chaplains are usually employed by the hospital or heath care facility. If they are hired as part of a separate department (other than pastoral care), the position may be grant-funded.

REFERENCES

1. Association of Professional Chaplains. http://www.professionalchaplains.org/uploadedFiles/pdf/hipaa-definition-of-chaplain-template.pdf. Accessed September 2, 2012.
2. Vandercreek L, Burton L, eds. Professional chaplaincy: its role and importance in health care. http://www.healthcarechaplaincy.org/userimages/professional-chaplaincy-its-role-and-importance-in-healthcare.pdf. Accessed September 2, 2012.

INDEX